Hit and Lead Profiling

Edited by
Bernard Faller and Laszlo Urban

Methods and Principles in Medicinal Chemistry

Edited by R. Mannhold, H. Kubinyi, G. Folkers
Editorial Board
H. Timmerman, J. Vacca, H. van de Waterbeemd, T. Wieland

Previous Volumes of this Series:

Wolfgang Jahnke, Daniel A. Erlanson
Fragment-based Approaches in Drug Discovery
Vol. 34
2006, ISBN: 978-3-527-31291-7

Jörg Hüser (Ed.)
High-Throughput Screening in Drug Discovery
Vol. 35
2006, ISBN: 978-3-527-31283-2

Klaus Wanner, Georg Höfner (Eds.)
Mass Spectrometry in Medicinal Chemistry
Applications in Drug Discovery
Vol. 36
2007, ISBN: 978-3-527-31456-0

Raimund Mannhold (Ed.)
Molecular Drug Properties
Measurement and Prediction
Vol. 37
2007, ISBN: 978-3-527-31755-4

Roy J. Vaz, Thomas Klabunde (Eds.)
Antitargets
Prediction and Prevention of Drug Side Effects
Vol. 38
2008, ISBN: 978-3-527-31821-6

Eckhard Ottow, Hilmar Weinmann (Eds.)
Nuclear Receptors as Drug Targets
Vol. 39
2008, ISBN: 978-3-527-31872-8

Han van de Waterbeemd, Bernard Testa (Eds.)
Drug Bioavailability
Estimation of Solubility, Permeability, Absorption and Bioavailability
2., Completely Revised Edition
Vol. 40
2008, ISBN: 978-3-527-32051-6

Roberto Todeschini, Viviana Consonni
Molecular Descriptors for Chemoinformatics
Volume I: Alphabetical Listing
Volume II: Appendices, References
Vol. 41
2009, ISBN: 978-3-527-31852-0

Wolfgang Sippl, Manfred Jung (Eds.)
Epigenetic Targets in Drug Discovery
Vol. 42
2009, ISBN: 978-3-527-32355-5

Hit and Lead Profiling

Identification and Optimization
of Drug-like Molecules

Edited by
Bernard Faller and Laszlo Urban

WILEY-VCH Verlag GmbH & Co. KGaA

Series Editors

Prof. Dr. Raimund Mannhold
Molecular Drug Research Group
Heinrich-Heine-Universität
Universitätsstrasse 1
40225 Düsseldorf
Germany
mannhold@uni-duesseldorf.de

Prof. Dr. Hugo Kubinyi
Donnersbergstrasse 9
67256 Weisenheim am Sand
Germany
kubinyi@t-online.de

Prof. Dr. Gerd Folkers
Collegium Helveticum
STW/ETH Zurich
8092 Zurich
Switzerland
folkers@collegium.ethz.ch

Volume Editors

Dr. Bernard Faller
Novartis Institutes for BioMedical Research
Forum 1
4002 Basel
Switzerland
bernard.faller@novartis.com

Dr. Laszlo Urban
Novartis Institutes for BioMedical Research Inc.
250 Massachusetts Ave.
Cambridge, MA 02139
USA
laszlo.urban@novartis.com

All books published by Wiley-VCH are carefully produced. Nevertheless, authors, editors, and publisher do not warrant the information contained in these books, including this book, to be free of errors. Readers are advised to keep in mind that statements, data, illustrations, procedural details or other items may inadvertently be inaccurate.

Library of Congress Card No.: applied for

British Library Cataloguing-in-Publication Data
A catalogue record for this book is available from the British Library.

Bibliographic information published by the Deutsche Nationalbibliothek
The Deutsche Nationalbibliothek lists this publication in the Deutsche Nationalbibliografie; detailed bibliographic data are available on the Internet at http://dnb.d-nb.de

© 2009 WILEY-VCH Verlag GmbH & Co. KGaA, Weinheim

All rights reserved (including those of translation into other languages). No part of this book may be reproduced in any form – by photoprinting, microfilm, or any other means – nor transmitted or translated into a machine language without written permission from the publishers. Registered names, trademarks, etc. used in this book, even when not specifically marked as such, are not to be considered unprotected by law.

Printed in the Federal Republic of Germany
Printed on acid-free paper

Cover Design Schulz Grafik-Design, Fußgönheim
Composition Thomson Digital, Noida, India
Printing Strauss GmbH, Mörlenbach
Bookbinding Litges & Dopf Buchbinderei GmbH, Heppenheim

ISBN: 978-3-527-32331-9

Contents

List of Contributors   XIX
Preface   XXV
A Personal Foreword   XXVII

Part I

1   Process Logistics, Testing Strategies and Automation Aspects   3
Hansjoerg Haas, Robert S. DeWitte, Robert Dunn-Dufault, and Andreas Stelzer
1.1   Introduction   3
1.2   The Process from Raw Ingredients to Data   3
1.2.1   Compound Management   5
1.2.2   Cell Biology   6
1.2.3   Lead Profiling   7
1.2.4   Liquid Chromatography/Mass Spectrometry   7
1.3   DMPK Testing Strategies: the Process from Data to Decisions   8
1.4   New Questions, New Assays and New Technologies Challenge the Process   10
1.5   Organizational Models to Scale Up the Process   11
1.5.1   Food Court   11
1.5.1.1   The Fast Food Restaurant   12
1.5.1.2   The Family Restaurant Chain   12
1.6   Critical Factors to Improve the Process   13
1.7   Materials in ADME/Tox Screening   14
1.8   Machines and Equipment in ADME/Tox Screening   17
1.8.1   Liquid Handlers   17
1.8.2   Detection and Analysis   17
1.9   Software, Data Retrieval, Analysis, Manipulation and Interpretation   18
1.10   Environment and Management = Organizational Structure in ADME/Tox Screening   19

Hit and Lead Profiling. Edited by Bernard Faller and Laszlo Urban
Copyright © 2009 WILEY-VCH Verlag GmbH & Co. KGaA, Weinheim
ISBN: 978-3-527-32331-9

1.11	Methods in ADME/Tox Screening 20	
1.11.1	Examples of Whole-Process Approaches 20	
1.11.1.1	Automation Islands with Manual Data Upload to a LIMS System 21	
1.11.1.2	Complete Physical Integration and Automation 21	
1.11.1.3	Federated Physical Automation with Software Integration 22	
1.12	Conclusions 22	
	References 23	
2	**Prediction of Drug-Likeness and its Integration into the Drug Discovery Process** 25	
	Ansgar Schuffenhauer and Meir Glick	
2.1	Introduction 25	
2.2	Computational Prediction of Drug-Likeness 26	
2.2.1	Machine Learning 26	
2.2.2	Empirical Rules and Their Basis 30	
2.2.3	Drug-Likeness of Natural Products 32	
2.2.4	Do Ligands of Different Target Classes Differ in Their Drug-Like Properties? 34	
2.2.5	Unwanted Structural Elements 34	
2.3	What is the Best Practice in Utilizing Drug-Likeness in Drug Discovery? 35	
2.4	Concluding Discussions 37	
	References 38	
3	**Integrative Risk Assessment** 41	
	Bernard Faller and Laszlo Urban	
3.1	The Target Compound Profile 41	
3.1.1	Introduction 41	
3.1.2	The Importance of the Projected Clinical Compound Profile in Early Drug Discovery 42	
3.1.3	The Impact of Delivery On the Design of the Drug Discovery Process 43	
3.2	The Concept of Hierarchical Testing in Primary and Follow-Up Assays 45	
3.2.1	Impact of Turn-Around Time 47	
3.2.2	Assay Validation and Reference Compounds 47	
3.2.3	Requirements of Profiling Assay Quality 48	
3.2.4	The Importance of Follow-Up Assays 48	
3.3	Exposure Assays 49	
3.3.1	Basic Absorption Assays 49	
3.3.1.1	Solubility Assays 50	
3.3.1.2	Permeability Assays 50	
3.3.2	Active Transports and Efflux 51	
3.3.3	Metabolism 51	
3.3.4	Distribution and Elimination 51	
3.3.5	Drug–Drug Interactions 53	

3.3.6	iviv Correlations	53
3.4	Iterative Assays: Link Between Assays	54
3.5	Specific Safety Profiling Assays	56
3.5.1	Sensitivity and Specificity of Safety Assays should be Adjusted to the Phase of Drug Discovery	58
3.5.2	Addressing Species Specificity in Early *In Vitro* Assays	58
3.6	Data Reporting and Data Mining	59
3.6.1	Decision Making: Trend Analysis, Go/No Go Decisions	60
3.7	Integrative Risk Assessment	61
	References	64

Part II

4 Solubility and Aggregation 71
William H. Streng

4.1	Importance of Solubility	71
4.2	Factors Influencing Solubility	72
4.3	Methods Used to Determine Solubility	74
4.4	Approaches to Solubility	76
4.5	Solubility in Non-Aqueous Solvents and Co-Solvents	78
4.6	Solubility as a Function of pH	79
4.7	Effect of Aggregation Upon Solubility	83
4.8	Dependence of Dissolution upon Solubility	86
4.9	Partitioning and the Effect of Aggregation	87
4.10	Solubility in Simulated Biological Fluids	89
	References	90

5 *In Silico* Tools and *In Vitro* HTS Approaches to Determine Lipophilicity During the Drug Discovery Process 91
Sophie Martel, Vincent Gasparik, and Pierre-Alain Carrupt

5.1	Introduction	91
5.2	Virtual Filtering: *In Silico* Prediction of log P and log D	92
5.2.1	Lipophilicity of Neutral Substances: *In Silico* Methods to Predict log P_{oct}^{N}	92
5.2.1.1	2D Fragmental Approaches	92
5.2.1.2	Prediction Methods Based on 3-D Molecular Structure	95
5.2.1.3	General Comments on the Prediction of log P_{oct}	96
5.2.2	Prediction Models for log P in Other Solvent/Water Systems of Neutral Compounds	97
5.2.3	Prediction Models for log P of Ionic Species (log P^I)	97
5.3	Experimental Filtering: the ADMET Characterization of a Hit Collection	98
5.3.1	HTS log P/log D Determination Based on Microtiterplate Format	98
5.3.2	Chromatographic Methods	100

5.3.2.1	Reverse-Phase Liquid Chromatography	100
5.3.2.2	Immobilized Artificial Membranes	102
5.3.2.3	Hydrophilic Interaction Chromatography	103
5.3.2.4	Capillary Electrophoresis	104
5.3.3	A Global View On *In Vitro* HTS Methods to Measure log P/log D	104
5.4	Concluding Remarks: Efficacy or Accuracy Dilemma	105
	References	107

6 Membrane Permeability – Measurement and Prediction in Drug Discovery 117

Kiyohiko Sugano, Lourdes Cucurull-Sanchez, and Joanne Bennett

6.1	Overview of Membrane Permeation	117
6.1.1	Structure, Physiology and Chemistry of the Membrane	117
6.1.2	Passive Transcellular Pathway: pH Partition Theory as the Basis of Understanding Membrane Permeability	118
6.1.3	Paracellular Pathway	119
6.1.4	Active Transporters	119
6.1.5	*In Vitro–In Vivo* Extrapolation	119
6.2	*In Vitro* Cell Models	121
6.2.1	Intestinal Cell Culture Models	121
6.2.2	BBB Cell Culture Models	122
6.2.3	Cell Models to Study Active Transporters	123
6.2.4	Correlation of *in Vitro* Models to Human P_{eff} and Fraction Absorbed Data	124
6.2.5	Correlation of Cell Culture Models with *In Vivo* Brain Penetration	124
6.3	Artificial Membranes	125
6.3.1	Partition and Permeation	125
6.3.2	Parallel Artificial Membrane Permeation Assay: Recent Progress	126
6.3.2.1	Understanding PAMPA	126
6.3.2.2	Variation of PAMPA: Recent Progress	127
6.3.2.3	Phospholipid Vesicle PAMPA	127
6.3.2.4	Phospholipid–Octanol PAMPA	127
6.3.2.5	Tri-Layer PAMPA	127
6.3.2.6	Mucus Layer Adhered PAMPA	127
6.3.3	Application of PAMPA for Drug Discovery	128
6.4	Limitation of *In Vitro* Assays	128
6.4.1	Impact of UWL on Permeability	128
6.4.2	Membrane Binding	129
6.4.3	Low Solubility	129
6.4.4	Difference of the Paracellular Pathway	129
6.4.5	Interlaboratory Variability	129
6.5	Computational Approaches/*In Silico* Modeling	130

6.5.1	*In Vivo* Systems 130
6.5.2	*In Vitro* Cellular Membrane Systems 132
6.5.3	Artificial Membranes 134
6.5.4	Perspectives 135
6.6	Outlook 135
	References 136

7	**Drug Metabolism and Reactive Metabolites** 145
	Alan P. Watt
7.1	Introduction to Drug Metabolism 145
7.1.1	Historical Perspective 145
7.1.2	*In Vitro* Metabolism 146
7.1.3	Cytochrome P450 148
7.1.4	Prediction of Drug Metabolism 149
7.2	Adverse Drug Reactions 149
7.2.1	ADR Classification 150
7.2.2	Idiosyncratic Drug Reactions 150
7.3	Bioactivation 151
7.3.1	Definition 151
7.3.2	Reactions of Electrophilic Metabolites 151
7.3.3	Glutathione 151
7.3.4	Detection of GSH Conjugates 151
7.3.5	Acyl Glucuronides 152
7.3.6	Free Radicals and Oxidative Stress 152
7.4	Reactive Metabolites and Idiosyncratic Toxicity 153
7.4.1	The Hapten Hypothesis 153
7.4.1.1	Immune-Mediated Cutaneous Reactions 153
7.4.2	The Danger Hypothesis 153
7.4.3	Alternate Perspectives to Covalent Binding 154
7.4.3.1	Non-Toxicological Covalent Binding 154
7.4.3.2	Covalent Binding as Detoxification 154
7.5	Measurement of Reactive Metabolites 155
7.5.1	Trapping Assays 155
7.5.1.1	Soft Nucleophiles 155
7.5.1.2	Hard Nucleophiles 155
7.5.2	Mass Spectrometric Detection of GSH Conjugates and Mercapturic Acids 155
7.5.3	Radiometric Assays 156
7.5.3.1	Covalent Binding to Liver Microsomes 157
7.5.3.2	*Ex Vivo* Covalent Binding 157
7.5.3.3	^{14}C Cyanide Trapping 157
7.5.3.4	Radiolabeled Soft Nucleophile Trapping 158
7.5.4	Alternate Approaches 158
7.6	Strategies for Minimizing Reactive Metabolite Risk 159
7.6.1	Dose and Exposure 159

7.6.2	Structural Alerts	159
7.6.3	Cascade for Radiolabeled Covalent Binding Experiments	160
7.6.4	Criteria for Progression	160
7.7	Conclusions	160
	References	161

8 Drug–Drug Interactions: Screening for Liability and Assessment of Risk 165

Ruth Hyland, R. Scott Obach, Chad Stoner, Michael West, Michael R. Wester, Kuresh Youdim, and Michael Zientek

8.1	Introduction	165
8.2	*In Silico* Approaches	167
8.3	Perpetrators of Drug–Drug Interactions: Enzyme Inhibition	169
8.3.1	Competitive Inhibition	169
8.3.2	Conventional CYP Inhibition Screen	170
8.3.3	Fluorescent Inhibition Screen	172
8.3.4	DDI Single Point versus IC_{50} Determinations	172
8.3.5	DDI Cocktail Assay	173
8.3.6	Mechanism-Based Inhibition	174
8.4	Perpetrators of Drug–Drug Interactions: Enzyme Induction	176
8.4.1	Ligand Binding Assay	177
8.4.2	Reporter Gene (Transactivation) Assays	178
8.4.3	Overall Evaluation of High-Throughput Induction Assays	179
8.5	Drug–Drug Interactions; Victims of Interaction; Reaction Phenotyping	179
8.5.1	Chemical Inhibition	180
8.5.2	Recombinant Human CYP Enzymes	181
8.6	Predictions of Drug–Drug Interactions	182
8.6.1	New Compounds as Potential DDI Perpetrators	183
8.6.2	New Compounds as Potential DDI Victims	184
8.7	Summary	187
	References	188

9 Plasma Protein Binding and Volume of Distribution: Determination, Prediction and Use in Early Drug Discovery 197

Franco Lombardo, R. Scott Obach, and Nigel J. Waters

9.1	Introduction: Importance of Plasma Protein Binding	197
9.2	Impact of Plasma Protein Binding on PK, Exposure, Safety Margins, Potency Screens and Drug–Drug Interaction	197
9.3	Methodologies for Measuring Plasma Protein Binding	201
9.4	Physicochemical Determinants and *In Silico* Prediction of Plasma Protein Binding	206
9.5	Volume of Distribution: General Considerations and Applications to Experimental Pharmacokinetics and Drug Design	208
9.5.1	Prediction of Human Volume of Distribution	210

9.5.1.1	Prediction of Human Volume of Distribution from Animal Pharmacokinetic Data *210*	
9.5.1.2	Prediction of Human Volume of Distribution from *In Vitro* Data *212*	
9.5.1.3	Prediction of Human Volume of Distribution from *In Silico* Methods *213*	
9.6	Relationship Between Clearance, VDss and Plasma Protein Binding *213*	
9.7	Summary and Conclusions *214*	
	References *215*	
10	**Putting It All Together** *221*	
	Pamela Berry, Neil Parrott, Micaela Reddy, Pascale David-Pierson, and Thierry Lavé	
10.1	Challenges in Drug Discovery *221*	
10.2	Methodological Aspects *222*	
10.2.1	PBPK *222*	
10.2.2	PK/PD *225*	
10.3	Strategic Use of PBPK During Drug Discovery *226*	
10.4	Strategic Use of PK/PD During Drug Discovery *227*	
10.5	Application During Lead Identification *227*	
10.6	Application During Lead Optimization *232*	
10.7	Application During Clinical Lead Selection *235*	
10.8	Limitations with Current Methodology and Approaches *236*	
10.9	Conclusions *238*	
	References *238*	

Part III

11	**Genetic Toxicity: *In Vitro* Approaches for Hit and Lead Profiling** *243*	
	Richard M Walmsley and Nicholas Billinton	
11.1	Introduction *243*	
11.2	Definitions *245*	
11.3	Major Challenges for Early, Predictive Genotoxicity Testing *246*	
11.4	Practical Issues for Genotoxicity Profiling: Vehicle, Dose, Dilution Range and Impurity *248*	
11.4.1	Vehicle and Dose *248*	
11.4.2	Dilution Range *249*	
11.4.3	Purity *249*	
11.5	Computational Approaches to Genotoxicity Assessment: "*In Silico*" Assessment *250*	
11.5.1	How Should *In Silico* Methods be Applied in Hit and Lead Profiling? *252*	
11.6	Genotoxicity Assays for Screening *253*	
11.6.1	Gene Mutation Assays *254*	

11.6.2	The Ames Test and Variants	255
11.6.3	Mammalian Cell Mutation Assays	256
11.6.4	*Saccharomyces cerevisiae* ("Yeast") Mutation Assays	256
11.7	Chromosome Damage and Aberration Assays	256
11.7.1	Aberrations	256
11.7.2	Micronuclei	257
11.7.3	"Comet" Assay	258
11.7.4	DNA Adduct Assessment	258
11.7.5	Gene Expression Assays	259
11.7.5.1	Prokaryotic	259
11.7.5.2	Eukaryotic	259
11.8	Using Data from *In Vitro* Profiling: Confirmatory Tests, Follow-Up Tests, and the Link to Safety Assessment and *In Vivo* Models	260
11.8.1	Annotations from Screening Data	261
11.8.2	Annotations from Positive Screening Data	262
11.8.2.1	Gene Mutation Assays	262
11.8.2.2	Chromosome Damage Assays	262
11.8.2.3	Reporter Assays	263
11.9	Can a Genetic Toxicity Profile Inform *In Vivo* Testing Strategies?	263
11.9.1	Prospects for *In Vivo* Profiling of Hits and Leads for Genotoxicity	264
11.10	What to Test, When and How?	265
11.10.1	Profiling Entire Libraries: >100 000 Compounds/Year	265
11.10.2	Profiling Hits: 10 000–100 000 Compounds/Year	265
11.10.3	Profiling in Lead Optimization: 2000–10 000 Compounds/Year	266
11.11	Summary	267
	References	267
12	***In Vitro* Safety Pharmacology Profiling: an Important Tool to Decrease Attrition**	**273**
	Jacques Hamon and Steven Whitebread	
12.1	What is "*In Vitro* Safety Pharmacology Profiling?"	273
12.2	Examples of Drug Failures Due to Secondary Pharmacology	274
12.2.1	Components	275
12.2.1.1	Target Selection	275
12.2.1.2	Target Annotation	276
12.2.1.3	Examples of *In Vitro* Safety Pharmacology Profiling Panels	277
12.3	Processes	280
12.3.1	Assay Requirements and Technologies	280
12.3.2	Binding and/or Functional Assays	284
12.3.3	Processes and Logistics	286
12.4	Application to Drug Discovery	287
12.4.1	How and When to Use *In Vitro* Safety Pharmacology Profiling	287
12.4.2	Pharmacological Promiscuity and Its Clinical Interpretation	288
12.4.3	Relevance of Potency and Therapeutic Index (TI)	290

12.4.4	Possible Benefits of Off-Target Effects	*291*
12.5	Conclusions and Outlook	*291*
	References	*292*

13 **Knowledge-Based and Computational Approaches to *In Vitro* Safety Pharmacology** *297*
Josef Scheiber, Andreas Bender, Kamal Azzaoui, and Jeremy Jenkins

13.1	Introduction	*297*
13.1.1	The Value of Safety Pharmacology Data: the Value and Relevance of Complete, Standardized Data Matrices for *In Silico* Prediction of Adverse Events	*298*
13.2	"Meta Analysis" of Safety Pharmacology Data: Predicting Compound Promiscuity	*304*
13.2.1	Introduction	*304*
13.2.2	Data Analysis	*305*
13.2.2.1	Hit Rate Parameter and Chemical Profiling	*305*
13.2.2.2	Computational Efforts: Generation of Hypotheses	*307*
13.2.2.3	Promiscuity and Attrition Rate	*308*
13.2.2.4	Conclusion on Promiscuity Prediction	*310*
13.3	Prediction of Off-Target Effects of Molecules Based on Chemical Structure	*310*
13.3.1	Introduction	*310*
13.3.2	Available Databases and Desired Format	*311*
13.3.3	The Best Established Technologies for *In Silico* Target Fishing	*313*
13.3.3.1	Similarity Searching in Databases	*313*
13.3.3.2	Data Mining in Annotated Chemical Databases	*314*
13.3.3.3	Data Mining on Bioactivity Spectra	*314*
13.4	Future Directions	*316*
	References	*317*

Part IV

14 **Discovery Toxicology Screening: Predictive, *In Vitro* Cytotoxicity** *325*
Peter J. O'Brien

14.1	Introduction	*325*
14.2	Basis of Need for Discovery Toxicology Screening	*326*
14.2.1	High Attrition at High Cost	*326*
14.2.2	High Proportion of Attrition Due to Adverse Safety	*326*
14.2.3	Discovery Screening Reduces Attrition by An Order of Magnitude	*326*
14.3	Obstacles to Discovery Toxicology Screening	*327*
14.4	Need to Coordinate Cytotoxicity Screening with Other Discovery Safety Assessments	*327*
14.5	Discovery Cytotoxicology	*329*
14.5.1	Biomarkers for Safety versus Efficacy for Screening	*329*

14.5.2	Past Failure of Cytotoxicity Assessments 329
14.5.2.1	Insufficient Exposure 329
14.5.2.2	Measurement of Cell Death 330
14.5.3	Effective Cell-Based Assays for Marked and Acute Cytotoxicity 331
14.5.4	Characteristics of an Optimally Effective Cell Model of Toxicity 331
14.5.4.1	Need for Morphological and Functional Parameters 333
14.5.4.2	Need for Multiple and Mechanistic Parameters 333
14.5.4.3	Need for Single-Cell Monitoring 333
14.5.4.4	Need for Effective Parameters 334
14.5.4.5	Need for Validation with Human Toxicity Data 336
14.6	High Effectiveness of an HCA Cell Model in Predictive Toxicology 337
14.6.1	Background on HCA 337
14.6.2	Idiosyncratic Hepatotoxicity 337
14.6.3	Characteristic Pattern and Sequence of Cytotoxic Changes 338
14.6.4	Safety Margin 338
14.6.5	Hormesis 338
14.6.6	Implementation of HCA Cytotoxicity Testing in Drug Discovery 339
14.6.7	Limitations of HCA Cytotoxicity Testing in Drug Discovery 340
14.7	Future Impact of Cytotoxicity Testing 340
	References 341
15	**Predicting Drug-Induced Hepatotoxicity: *In Vitro*, *In Silico* and *In Vivo* Approaches 345**
	Jinghai J. Xu, Amit S. Kalgutkar, Yvonne Will, James Dykens, Elizabeth Tengstrand, and Frank Hsieh
15.1	Introduction 345
15.2	Reactive Metabolites 346
15.2.1	Assays and *In Silico* Knowledge to Assess Bioactivation Potential 347
15.2.1.1	*In Vitro* Reactive Metabolite Trapping Studies 347
15.2.1.2	Covalent Binding Determinations 348
15.2.2	Utility of Reactive Metabolite Trapping and Covalent Binding Studies in Drug Discovery 348
15.2.3	Are Reactive Metabolite Trapping and Covalent Binding Studies Reliable Predictors of Hepatotoxic Potential of Drug Candidates? 348
15.2.4	Mitigating Factors Against Hepatotoxicity Risks Due to Bioactivation – a Balanced Approach Towards Candidate Selection in Drug Discovery 351
15.2.5	Future Directions 355
15.3	Mitochondrial Toxicity 356
15.3.1	Uncouplers of Mitochondrial Respiration 358
15.3.2	Drugs that Inhibit OXPHOS Complexes 358
15.3.3	Drugs that Induce the Mitochondrial Permeability Transition Pore (MPT) 359
15.3.4	Drugs Inhibiting mtDNA Synthesis and Mitochondrial Protein Synthesis 359
15.3.5	Inhibition of Fatty Acid β-Oxidation or Depletion of CoA 360

15.3.6	*In Vitro* and *In Vivo* Assessment of Drug-Induced Mitochondrial Dysfunction *360*	
15.4	Oxidative Stress *363*	
15.4.1	Sources of Oxidative Stress *363*	
15.4.2	Measurements of Oxidative Stress *363*	
15.4.3	Critical Review: Is There Sufficient Clinical, Pre-Clinical and *In Vitro* Data to Substantiate the Link Between Oxidative Stress and Idiosyncratic Liver Injury? *364*	
15.5	Inhibition of Bile Salt Efflux Protein and Drug-Induced Cholestasis *365*	
15.5.1	*In Vitro* and *In Vivo* Assays to Measure BSEP Inhibition *365*	
15.5.2	Critical Review: Is There a Link between BSEP Inhibition, Drug-Induced Cholestasis and Idiosyncratic Liver Injury? *368*	
15.6	Biomarkers *369*	
15.6.1	Hepatocellular Injury *370*	
15.6.2	Cholestatic Injury *370*	
15.6.3	Application of Serum Chemistry Markers *370*	
15.6.4	Need for New Biomarkers *371*	
15.6.5	Biomarker Discovery Efforts *372*	
15.6.6	Approaches for Biomarker Discovery *372*	
15.6.6.1	Development of *In Vivo* Biomarkers *373*	
15.6.6.2	Development of *In Vitro* Biomarkers *373*	
15.6.6.3	Biomarker Validation *374*	
15.6.7	Future Biomarker Directions *374*	
15.7	Conclusions *375*	
	References *376*	
16	**Should Cardiosafety be Ruled by hERG Inhibition? Early Testing Scenarios and Integrated Risk Assessment** *387* *Dimitri Mikhailov, Martin Traebert, Qiang Lu, Steven Whitebread, and William Egan*	
16.1	Introduction *387*	
16.2	Role of Ion Channels in Heart Electrophysiology *389*	
16.3	hERG Profiling Assays *391*	
16.3.1	Cell-Free Competition Binding Assays *392*	
16.3.1.1	Radioligand Binding *393*	
16.3.1.2	Fluorescence Polarization *393*	
16.3.2	Non-Electrophysiological Functional Cellular Assays *393*	
16.3.2.1	Rubidium Efflux and Thallium Influx *393*	
16.3.2.2	Membrane Potential-Sensitive Fluorescent Dyes *394*	
16.3.3	Higher-Throughput Planar Patch Technologies *394*	
16.3.4	Non-hERG Ion Channel Assays Related to Cardiotoxicity *395*	
16.3.5	Nonclinical Cardiosafety Assays in Early Drug Development *396*	
16.4	Computational Models for hERG *398*	
16.4.1	Pharmacophore Models *398*	
16.4.2	Docking to Homology Models *399*	

16.4.3	QSAR Models *400*	
16.5	Integrated Risk Assessment *401*	
16.5.1	Cardiosafety Assessment of Early Discovery Projects *401*	
16.5.2	Cardiosafety Assessment of Preclinical Positive Signals *403*	
16.6	Summary *405*	
	References *406*	

17	**Hematotoxicity: *In Vitro* and *Ex Vivo* Compound Profiling** *415*	
	David Brott and Francois Pognan	
17.1	Introduction *415*	
17.2	Known Compounds with Hematotoxic Potential *417*	
17.3	Tiered Cascade of Testing *419*	
17.3.1	Tier 1 Tests *420*	
17.3.2	Tier 2 Tests *426*	
17.3.3	Tier 3 Tests *428*	
17.4	Triggers for Hematotoxicity Testing *430*	
17.5	Conclusions *433*	
	References *433*	

18	**Profiling Adverse Immune Effects** *439*	
	Wim H. De Jong, Raymond Pieters, Kirsten A Baken, Rob J. Vandebriel, Jan-Willem Van Der Laan, and Henk Van Loveren	
18.1	Immunotoxicology *439*	
18.1.1	The Immune System and Immunotoxicology *439*	
18.1.2	Detection of Immunotoxicity *442*	
18.1.3	Evaluation of the Immune System in Toxicity Studies *443*	
18.1.4	Testing for Induction of Allergy *445*	
18.1.5	Testing for Induction of Autoimmunity *446*	
18.1.5.1	Introduction *446*	
18.1.5.2	Assays for Testing the Induction of Autoimmunity *446*	
18.1.5.3	Alternative Approach for Evaluation of Autoimmunity Potential of Chemicals *447*	
18.1.6	Structures Associated with Immunotoxicity *449*	
18.1.7	Immunostimulation by Components of the Immune Systems Used as Therapeutics *450*	
18.2	Non-Animal Approaches for the Determination of Immunotoxicity *451*	
18.2.1	*In Silico* Approaches *451*	
18.2.2	*In Vitro* Approaches to Test Various Aspects of Immunotoxicity *451*	
18.2.2.1	Introduction *451*	
18.2.2.2	Immunosuppression *453*	
18.2.2.3	Chemical Sensitization *454*	
18.2.2.4	Conclusions *456*	
18.2.3	Toxicogenomics *456*	
18.2.3.1	Introduction *456*	
18.2.3.2	Immunotoxicogenomics *456*	

18.2.3.3	Interpretation of Results	*457*
18.2.3.4	Toxicogenomics for Prediction of Effects	*457*
18.2.3.5	Target Organs and Cells for Immunotoxicity	*458*
18.2.3.6	Conclusions	*458*
18.3	Summary	*459*
	References	*459*

19 *In Vitro* Phototoxicity Testing: a Procedure Involving Multiple Endpoints *471*

Laurent Marrot and Jean-Roch Meunier

19.1	Introduction	*471*
19.2	Optical Considerations: Relevant UV Sources and Sunlight Absorption	*472*
19.2.1	Working with the Appropriate Artificial Sunlight Source Determines the Relevance of Phototoxicity Screening	*472*
19.2.2	When to Study the Phototoxicity of a Substance?	*474*
19.3	*In Silico* Methods for Prediction of Phototoxicity – (Q)SAR Models	*474*
19.3.1	Global Models	*475*
19.3.2	Local Models	*475*
19.4	Photoreactivity *In Tubo*: Prescreening of Compounds Producing ROS Upon Sunlight Exposure	*478*
19.4.1.	Biochemical Detection of Photoinduced ROS	*478*
19.4.2	Photo-Cleavage of Isolated Plasmid DNA	*479*
19.4.3	Photo Red Blood Cells Test	*479*
19.5	Microbiological Models for Photomutagenesis Assessment	*480*
19.5.1	Photo-Ames Test	*480*
19.5.2	The Yeast Model	*480*
19.6	Photocytotoxicity and Photogenotoxicity in Mammalian Cells: Regulatory Tests and Beyond	*482*
19.6.1	The 3T3 NRU Assay: a Validated Test for the Assessment of a Photoirritation Potential	*482*
19.6.2	Photogenotoxicity: an Endpoint Without Corresponding *In Vivo* Equivalents	*483*
19.7	Reconstructed Skin: a Model for Mimicking Phototoxicity in the Target Organ	*486*
19.8	Conclusions	*488*
	References	*489*

Index *495*

List of Contributors

Kamal Azzaoui
Novartis Pharma AG
Center for Proteomic Chemistry
Molecular Libraries Informatics
Forum 1
4002 Basel
Switzerland

Kirsten A. Baken
Maastricht University
Department of Health Risk Analysis
and Toxicology
P.O. Box 616
6200 MD Maastricht
The Netherlands

Andreas Bender
Leiden/Amsterdam Center for
Drug Research
Division of Medicinal Chemistry
Einsteinweg 55
2333 CC Leiden
The Netherlands

Joanne Bennett
Pfizer Global Research & Development
Research Formulation
Sandwich, Kent CT13 9NJ
UK

Pamela Berry
Roche Palo Alto LLC
Drug Metabolism and
Pharmacokinetics Department
Modeling and Simulation Group
3431 Hillview Ave.
Palo Alto, CA 94304
USA

Nicholas Billinton
Gentronix Ltd
CTF Building
46 Grafton Street
Manchester M13 9NT
UK

David Brott
AstraZeneca
Global Safety Assessment
Wilmington, DE 19850
USA

Pierre-Alain Carrupt
University of Geneva/University of
Lausanne
School of Pharmaceutical Sciences
30 Quai Ernest-Ansermet
1211 Geneva 4
Switzerland

Hit and Lead Profiling. Edited by Bernard Faller and Laszlo Urban
Copyright © 2009 WILEY-VCH Verlag GmbH & Co. KGaA, Weinheim
ISBN: 978-3-527-32331-9

Lourdes Cucurull-Sanchez
Pfizer Global Research & Development
Pharmacokinetics, Dynamics and
Metabolism
Sandwich, Kent CT13 9NJ
UK

Pascale David-Pierson
F. Hoffmann–La Roche Ltd
Drug Metabolism and
Pharmacokinetics Department
Modeling and Simulation Group
Grenzacher Strasse 124
4070 Basel
Switzerland

Wim H. De Jong
National Institute for Public Health
and the Environment (RIVM)
Laboratory for Health Protection
Research
Antoni van Leeuwenhoeklaan 9
3721 MA Bilthoven
The Netherlands

Robert S. DeWitte
Thermo Fisher Scientific
5344 John Lucas Drive
Burlington, Ontario L7L 6A6
Canada

Robert Dunn-Dufault
Thermo Fisher Scientific
5344 John Lucas Drive
Burlington, Ontario L7L 6A6
Canada

James Dykens
Pfizer Global Research and
Development
Sandwich, Kent CT13 9NJ
UK

William Egan
Novartis Institutes for Biomedical
Research
250 Massachusetts Ave.
Cambridge, MA 02139
USA

Bernard Faller
Novartis Institutes for BioMedical
Research
Novartis Campus
WSJ-350.3.04
4002 Basel
Switzerland

Vincent Gasparik
University of Geneva/University of
Lausanne
School of Pharmaceutical Sciences
30 Quai Ernest-Ansermet
1211 Geneva 4
Switzerland

Meir Glick
Novartis Institutes for Biomedical
Research Inc.
Center for Proteomic Chemistry
250 Massachusetts Ave.
Cambridge, MA 02139
USA

Hansjoerg Haas
Thermo Fisher Scientific
5344 John Lucas Drive
Burlington, Ontario L7L 6A6
Canada

Jacques Hamon
Novartis Institutes for Biomedical
Research
WSJ–360.4.08
4002 Basel
Switzerland

List of Contributors

Frank Hsieh
Nextcea Inc.
600 West Cummings Park #6375
Woburn, MA 01801
USA

Ruth Hyland
Pfizer Global Research & Development
Pharmacokinetics, Dynamics and
Metabolism
Sandwich, Kent CT13 9NJ
UK

Jeremy Jenkins
Novartis Institutes for Biomedical
Research
Center for Proteomic Chemistry
250 Massachusetts Ave.
Cambridge, MA 02139
USA

Amit S. Kalgutkar
Pfizer Global Research and
Development
Eastern Point Road
Groton, CT 06340
USA

Thierry Lavé
F. Hoffmann–La Roche Ltd
Drug Metabolism and
Pharmacokinetics Department
Modeling and Simulation Group
Grenzacher Strasse 124
4070 Basel
Switzerland

Franco Lombardo
Novartis Institutes for BioMedical
Research
Metabolism and Pharmacokinetics
Groups
Cambridge, MA 02139
USA

Qiang Lu
WuXi Pharma Tech Inc.
288 Fute Zhong Rd
Shanghai 200131
PR China

Laurent Marrot
L'OREAL Recherche
International Department of Safety
Research
Phototoxicity Unit
1 Avenue E. Schueller
93600 Aulnay-Sous-Bois
France

Sophie Martel
University of Geneva/University of
Lausanne
School of Pharmaceutical Sciences
30 Quai Ernest-Ansermet
1211 Geneva 4
Switzerland

Jean-Roch Meunier
L'OREAL Recherche
International Department of Safety
Research
Phototoxicity Unit
1 Avenue E. Schueller
93600 Aulnay-Sous-Bois
France

Dimitri Mikhailov
Novartis Institutes for Biomedical
Research
250 Massachusetts Ave.
Cambridge, MA 02139
USA

R. Scott Obach
Pfizer Global Research & Development
Pharmacokinetics, Dynamics and
Metabolism
Groton, CT 06340
USA

Peter J. O'Brien
University College Dublin
School of Agriculture, Food Science
and Veterinary Medicine
Room 013, Veterinary Sciences Centre
Belfield, Dublin 4
Ireland

Neil Parrott
F. Hoffmann–La Roche Ltd
Drug Metabolism and
Pharmacokinetics Department
Modeling and Simulation Group
Grenzacher Strasse 124
4070 Basel
Switzerland

Raymond Pieters
Utrecht University
Institute for Risk Assessment
Sciences (IRAS)
P.O. Box 80178
3508 TD Utrecht
The Netherlands

Francois Pognan
Novartis
Preclinical Safety
Muttenz
4133 Schweitzerhalle
Switzerland

Micaela Reddy
Roche Palo Alto LLC
Drug Metabolism and
Pharmacokinetics Department
Modeling and Simulation Group
3431 Hillview Ave.
Palo Alto, CA 94304
USA

Josef Scheiber
Novartis Pharma AG
Novartis Campus
Forum 1
4056 Basel
Switzerland

Ansgar Schuffenhauer
Novartis Pharma AG
Center for Proteomic Chemistry
Postfach
4002 Basel
Switzerland

Andreas Stelzer
Thermo Fisher Scientific
5344 John Lucas Drive
Burlington, Ontario L7L 6A6
Canada

Chad Stoner
Pfizer Global Research & Development
Pharmacokinetics, Dynamics and
Metabolism
La Jolla, CA 92037
USA

William H. Streng
3021 Pine Island Lake Road
Eagle River, WI 54521
USA

Kiyohiko Sugano
Pfizer Global Research & Development
Research Formulation
Sandwich, Kent CT13 9NJ
UK

Elizabeth Tengstrand
Nextcea Inc.
600 West Cummings Park #6375
Woburn, MA 01801
USA

Martin Traebert
Novartis Pharma AG
4002 Basel
Switzerland

Laszlo Urban
Novartis Institutes for BioMedical
Research
250 Massachusetts Ave.
Cambridge, MA 02139
USA

Rob J. Vandebriel
National Institute for Public Health
and the Environment (RIVM)
Laboratory for Health Protection
Research
Antoni van Leeuwenhoeklaan 9
3721 MA Bilthoven
The Netherlands

Jan-Willem Van Der Laan
National Institute for Public Health
and the Environment (RIVM)
Center for Biological Medicines and
Medical Technology
Antoni van Leeuwenhoeklaan 9
3721 MA Bilthoven
The Netherlands

Henk Van Loveren
National Institute for Public Health
and the Environment (RIVM)
Laboratory for Health Protection
Research
Antoni van Leeuwenhoeklaan 9
3721 MA Bilthoven
The Netherlands
and
Maastricht University
Department of Health Risk Analysis
and Toxicology
P.O. Box 616
6200 MD Maastricht
The Netherlands

Richard M. Walmsley
University of Manchester
Faculty of Life Sciences
Manchester M13 9PL
UK
and
Gentronix Ltd
CTF Building
46 Grafton Street
Manchester M13 9NT
UK

Alan P. Watt
GlaxoSmithKline
Immuno-Inflammation Centre
of Excellence for Drug Discovery
1250 South Collegeville Road
Collegeville, PA 19426
USA

Nigel J. Waters
Pfizer Global Research & Development
Pharmacokinetics Dynamics and
Metabolism
Groton Laboratories
Groton, CT 06340
USA

Michael West
Pfizer Global Research & Development
Pharmacokinetics, Dynamics and
Metabolism
Groton, CT 06340
USA

Michael R. Wester
Pfizer Global Research & Development
Pharmacokinetics, Dynamics and
Metabolism
La Jolla, CA
USA

Steven Whitebread
Novartis Institutes for Biomedical
Research
250 Massachusetts Ave.
Cambridge, MA 02139
USA

Yvonne Will
Pfizer Global Research and
Development
Eastern Point Road
Groton, CT 06340
USA

Jinghai J. Xu
Merck & Co.
Knowledge Discovery & Knowledge
Mining
WP42A–4015
Sumneytown Pike
P.O. Box 4
West Point, PA 19486
USA

Kuresh Youdim
Pfizer Global Research & Development
Pharmacokinetics, Dynamics and
Metabolism
Sandwich, Kent CT13 9NJ
UK

Michael Zientek
Pfizer Global Research & Development
Pharmacokinetics, Dynamics and
Metabolism
La Jolla, CA 92037
USA

Preface

One of the most important tasks in drug discovery is to design a target compound profile for a particular clinical indication. In addition to target validation, drug discovery teams consider drug-like properties which ensure efficacious exposure at the expected site of action without any major safety issues for the patients. Thus, the definition of the target compound profile is essential for the design of a meaningful flowchart for a drug discovery project. The target compound profile is impacted by factors linked to the target itself (i.e., peripheral versus central), the type/class of chemical structure, the projected therapeutic dose, the route of administration, the likelihood of co-medications and the potential off-target side effects which can be anticipated even at early stages of the project. Most of these factors also need to be balanced with respect to the medical value of the treatment or severity of the disease. Optimization of pharmacokinetics, addressing metabolism and drug-drug interactions are now integrated into very early phases of drug discovery. This requires teams of scientists with diverse skills, ranging from theoretical chemistry to medical expertise.

The focus of the present volume by Bernard Faller and Laszlo Urban is on methods and processes designed to predict drug-like properties, exposure and safety during hit and lead discovery. Distinguished authors from industry and academia discuss the current methods to generate pharmacokinetic and safety profiles of drug candidates, as well as how they must be balanced against one other for the best selection of candidates for further development.

Following an introduction to the necessities of filtering and risk assessment of potential new drug molecules before entering lead optimization, the equally important aspects of pharmacokinetic (ADME) and safety (toxicity) profiling are covered in separate parts.

The ADME section covers the profiling of basic physicochemical parameters, such as solubility and permeability, as well as more complex traits, such as the likelihood of drug-drug interactions, metabolic clearance and protein binding properties. The toxicology part addresses, among others, recent advances in early genetic toxicity testing, bioactivation screening, organ-specific toxicity assays for liver, heart, kidney and blood, as well as profiling for autoimmune reactions. By addressing both drug efficiency and drug safety, this volume shows readers how each individual

Hit and Lead Profiling. Edited by Bernard Faller and Laszlo Urban
Copyright © 2009 WILEY-VCH Verlag GmbH & Co. KGaA, Weinheim
ISBN: 978-3-527-32331-9

aspect figures in shaping the key decisions on which the entire drug development process hinges.

The series editors would like to thank Bernard Faller and Laszlo Urban for their enthusiasm to organize this volume and to work with such a fine selection of authors. We also express our thanks to Nicola Oberbeckmann-Winter, Waltraud Wüst and Frank Weinreich from Wiley-VCH for their valuable contributions to this project and to the entire series.

August 2009

Raimund Mannhold, Düsseldorf
Hugo Kubinyi, Weisenheim am Sand
Gerd Folkers, Zürich

A Personal Foreword

The one airplane that flies: selection of the right one molecule for clinical use.

Many years ago, when we started to set up the Preclinical Profiling group at Novartis, an article came to our attention. Authors discussed the unique way pharmaceutical industry achieved success, largely by trial and error. They compared drug development to an imaginary aeronautics engineering company which designs and makes airplanes by the best available knowledge and then tries them all: the one which keeps flying and does not drop out of the skies is the right one and will succeed. While this is bizarre to imagine, it carried some relevance to how drug discovery worked. Early memories about projects in the pharmaceutical industry confirm that basic drug-like properties were fairly neglected during lead optimization and we lost compounds for such reasons as simple, predictable toxic effects or inappropriate pharmacokinetics right before clinical trials. Since then, the industry has moved on and so-called "affinity-driven" drug discovery has changed for a more complex risk-aware process. Nevertheless, with the arsenal of reasonably predictive and refined profiling assays and *in silico* tools, the pharmaceutivcal industry continues to lose a large volume of compounds at later phases of drug discovery or in clinical trials.

This high attrition rate, particularly during late preclinical and clinical development, carries a large price tag for the pharmaceutical and biotechnology industry, which is carried over to health care providers. In addition, compounds which qualify for clinical use but fail due to safety matters raise serious ethical issues and questions concerning the responsibility and competence of the industry and registration authorities.

While all drug candidates go through rigorous testing for their efficacy and safety, this process largely remains the duty of scientists and clinicians during the later phases of drug discovery, resulting in a significant loss of clinical candidates. Furthermore, in some cases, the process cannot detect "idiosynchratic" liabilities which only come to light when a large and diverse patient population is exposed to the new medicine. It is also true that some old drugs in the clinic have to be reevaluated in terms of safety, particularly when safer medications have become available, if they are the perpetrators of drug–drug interactions or in case significant side effects were overlooked. Such a recent example is the discovery that the 5HT-2 antagonist, ketanserin, an antihypertensive drug which turned out to be a potent hERG blocker, although this was not known, while it caused sporadic cases of arrhythmias in the clinic [1].

Recognizing these shortcomings and to produce safe and efficacious medicines, the pharmaceutical industry, in coordination with regulatory authorities, continuously seeks new ways to shift attrition upstream during drug discovery. Development of novel technologies provides less expensive and reliable tests, processes to avoid chemical structures or individual compounds which carry too high a risk to progress towards clinical use. This new approach created a broad-scale, largely automated drug discovery environment, which involves *in silico* and *in vitro* technologies and extensive data analysis during lead selection and the lead optimization phase. It has been a formidable challenge to translate large-scale, expensive *in vivo* assays into tests which use tiny amount of compounds and turn around data at the speed that can match chemistry's synthetic cycle to aid structure–activity relationship (SAR) analysis. Thus, a new drug discovery profiling culture has been created. First came the revolution in ADME with the front runner "rule of five" coined by Lipinski [2], which draws attention to the importance of physicochemical characteristics of molecules highly relevant for drug-like performance. This approach opened the door from the culture of affinity-driven drug discovery towards a more complex, risk-aware approach. More advances followed in the area of metabolism, drug–drug interaction (DDI), and slowly, toxicology–safety started to follow. All of these advances bear fruit, however caution is required not to slow down lead selection and lead optimization by extensive and also expensive tests, sometimes with low or irrelevant predictive value. It is also easy to create a box-checking culture which, if combined with over-sensitive assays, could paralyze projects. Also, one has to be aware that recent investments into early phase drug discovery significantly contribute to the increase of already colossal cost of drug development. Thus, more rigor on the linkage of early data to expected clinical performance and return on investment studies are necessary for the design of a good preclinical profiling portfolio.

The meaning of the word profiling originates from drawing, or rather outlining the contour of something, for example, *profilare* to draw in outline. Today, its meaning has been considerably extended and in the context of the present book we use it to describe "a set of data often in graphic form portraying the significant features of something" (Merriam-Webster's New Collegiate Dictionary, 2008). We came across two distinctive types of criminal profiling, namely inductive and deductive, and realized how easily we can apply this to hit and lead profiling. After all, we try to predict, estimate or (in the worth case) guess the behavior of drug candidates in their future clinical environment. The usual or unusual suspects (in these case molecules) can be characterized either by thorough experimental examination (deductive profiling), or by information obtained from similar medicines in the clinic (inductive profiling). Eventually, both will be applied at the same time and in most cases.

While we do not use directly the above approach in this book, many chapters remind you that hit and lead profiling is close to detective work. It is equally exciting: it carries a large volume of unknown elements which can only be dealt with using refined tools and protocols.. But what is most rewarding in this job is that correction, or to be precise, optimization is built into it.

In this spirit, we outline the many important contribution of compound profiling to the drug discovery process. Drug discovery starts with identification of a target which has a causative link with a disease or symptoms of a disease. While genetic engineering can provide animal or cellular models which can link targets to diseases, it cannot define the therapeutic impact of modulating the function of the target molecule. For this, you need the "magic bullet" which selectively inhibits or excites the target molecule. The bullet has to be potent at the target molecule and be clean of any off-target effects. If it has effects at other targets there could be three possible problems:

1. Its effect on the phenotype (therapeutic effect) can be unrelated to the presumed primary target. An example for this is the "discovery" of the association of the NPY Y5 receptor with feeding behavior [3].

2. Effect is a combination of actions of the drug at the primary target and at various off-targets. Many of the antipsychotic drugs come under this consideration. While those work well which have a certain combination of effects at various receptors, ion channels and transporters, others with a cleaner profile do not have the same therapeutic effect.

3. The third possibility is probably the trickiest: off-target effects balance or antagonize the main effect. This can be of benefit, as in the case of verapamil, which has a potent inhibitory effect at the hERG channel, but this is balanced by an inhibitory effect at the Ca channel and allows safe clinical use of the molecule [4].

While the above examples focus on safety matters associated with pharmacological off-targets, it has to be emphasized that the knowledge of physicochemical properties of compounds is equally important at any phase of drug discovery. For example, poor solubility and permeability can prevent decent exposure and extensive hepatic metabolism might create inactive or toxic metabolites.

As projects progress, the profiling approach at hit expansion phase changes and the focus is now on the identification of liabilities associated with different chemotypes, and if so, whether there is any divergence between the pharmacophores of the primary and off-target. Some therapeutic targets notoriously attract off-target liabilities by having close similarities between their pharmacophores (e.g., antihistamines often inhibit the hERG channel [5]).

We do not wish to go through the many iterations of profiling in this introduction: let the chapters tell you about various aspects of the profiling process. The most important message is that the modern drug discovery process has to be driven by risk awareness but not by being risk aversive. After all, all medicines can cause harm depending on the dose. What is imperative that we can design them with safe therapeutic index. Hit and lead profiling should provide an early tool to do so.

In this book, we would like to take you on this exciting journey towards a better, more predictive drug discovery process, share the achievements, but also warn about bumps and potholes. It was a considerable dilemma for the editors, what should be included in this book. For example, the many facets of organ specific toxicities is difficult to address in one volume. We opted for a restricted approach and addressed generic issues, such as *in vitro* safety pharmacology for the prediction of target-specific adverse drug reactions (ADRs), genetics and cytotoxicity (linked with phototoxicity matters) and we selected three major elements of both late preclinical and clinical attrition, namely hepatotoxicity, cardiac toxicity and bone marrow toxicity.

Finally, the editors would like to thank all contributors for sharing their experience in drug discovery and to the series editors of Wiley VCH for providing the opportunity and support to address this important topic. We are grateful to our associates who provided important data for this book and to all of the family members, friends who always make the difference.

Basel, Switzerland and
Cambridge, USA

Bernard Faller
Laszlo Urban

References

1 Lipinski, C.A. (2000) Drug-like properties and the causes of poor solubility and poor permeability. *Journal of Pharmacological and Toxicological Methods*, **44**, 235–249.

2 Tang, Q., Li, Z.-Q., Li, W., Guo, J., Sun, H.-Y., Zhang, X.-H., Lau, C.-P., Tse, H.-F., Zhang, S. and Li, G.-R. (2008) The 5-HT2 antagonist ketanserin is an open channel blocker of human cardiac ether-a-go-go-related gene (hERG) potassium channels. *British Journal of Pharmacology*, **81**, 1–9.

3 Whitebread, S., Hamon, J., Bojanic, D. and Urban, L. (2005) *In vitro* safety pharmacology profiling: an essential tool for drug development. *Drug Discovery Today*, **10**, 1421–1433.

4 Zhang, S., Zhou, Z., Gong, Q., Makielski, J.C. and January, C.T. (1999) Mechanism of block and identification of the verapamil binding domain to hERG potassium channels. *Circulation Research*, **14**, 989–998.

5 Yap, Y.G. and Camm, A.J. (1999) Arrhythmogenic mechanisms of non-sedating antihistamines. *Clinical and Experimental Allergy*, **29** (Suppl 3), 174–181.

Part I

1
Process Logistics, Testing Strategies and Automation Aspects

Hansjoerg Haas, Robert S. DeWitte, Robert Dunn-Dufault, and Andreas Stelzer

1.1
Introduction

This introductory chapter tries to step outside the details of any particular measurement type, in order to review the organizational landscape in which ADME/Tox experiments are conducted and the different approaches to delivering high-quality, decision-ready data to drug discovery teams. In particular, attention is paid to: (i) the many different groups of scientists involved in the overall process from request to data; (ii) different models for converting data to decisions; and (iii) themes that challenge the process, particularly increasing demand for more and more data; and then (iv) a framework is described for improving the process that should be applicable in any organizational context, following the well trod path of root cause analysis; and (v) finally examples are given of three types of effort to organize the overall process through automation and software.

The authors hope that the overview provided here will help many laboratories organize their talent, technology and people in such a way as to maximize the availability and impact of ADME/Tox data throughout the drug discovery enterprise. With respect to the specific choices of technology, we hope that the discussion of root cause analysis and different organizational models enables groups to develop long-term plans that build toward efficient use of talent and laboratory space through both hardware and software.

1.2
The Process from Raw Ingredients to Data

The overall workflow of ADME/Tox characterization of lead compounds is typically distributed across multiple departments or functional groups within pharmaceutical companies, often with specialized groups for different assays, analysis and interpretation. A representation of the overall workflow is provided in Figure 1.1.

Hit and Lead Profiling. Edited by Bernard Faller and Laszlo Urban
Copyright © 2009 WILEY-VCH Verlag GmbH & Co. KGaA, Weinheim
ISBN: 978-3-527-32331-9

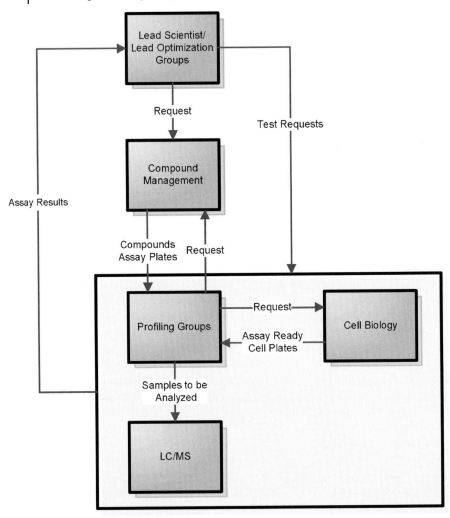

Figure 1.1 A typical DMPK workflow. Requests typically come from the lead optimization group for a set of compounds to be tested in a number of ADME/Tox assays. These could be according to predefined campaign strategy or selected a la carte. Quite often the profiling group initiates the activities of compound management and coordinate the preparation of biological material from cell biology. This may require one to three weeks lead time to get materials to the profiling laboratory. Once materials arrive the testing can commence. Aliquots of the compounds may be sent to the LC/MS for purity and ID confirmation. After completion of the ADME assays by the lead profiling group the results are collected, quality controlled and sent back to the lead optimization group for detailed review as input for subsequent synthesis/optimization cycles.

While the departmental structure varies from company to company and often from site to site, the workload of getting compounds through this process typically breaks down into a few defined areas of functional specialization. Each of these groups have challenges unique to their responsibilities, that impact the overall effectiveness of moving raw materials through to data. Some aspects of these challenges are briefly framed below.

1.2.1
Compound Management

This group manages large chemical libraries containing up to millions of samples (often in different formats) and maintains a complex database of sample inventory. This group typically fills orders received from various screening groups and scientists for thousands to millions of samples. Because rapid order turn around is critical to fuelling materials for the drug discovery process, major investments have been made to enable the compound management group to cope with their essential and demanding role. They are often the most automated group with large storage and sample retrieval systems where samples are typically stored frozen at $-20\,°C$ in large rooms or expandable compartments and retrieved with industrial robotics tolerant of the harsh atmosphere. Once samples are retrieved these groups also have dedicated systems for cherry picking, re-arraying, thawing/freezing and repackaging. When dealing with massive numbers of samples, efficient software is key for inventory management and order fulfillment.

In addition to having tools to aid in the tracking of sample location for retrieval, it is important to monitor sample volumes and to trigger notification when they are critically low. For example, some departments implement consumption-triggered logistics to switch to a "rationing mode" to limit their consumption. Feedback is required to request more samples to replenish their stock when larger supplies exist or can be re-synthesized.

Critical to the effective management of compounds is ensuring the quality or integrity of the samples submitted for testing. For example, compounds that have precipitated or degraded due to water absorption or too many freeze/thaw cycles will confound the results of assays. Often the long-term stability of compounds is not known and samples may be submitted to profiling groups without an integrity check. In these cases, it is up to the profiling group to do a purity and ID confirmation.

Another challenge the compound management group faces is the migration from legacy compound management systems in the face of changing strategies/technologies in screening. Older systems inherently pose limitations in the range of sample volumes and formats in which compounds can be delivered for testing. With the latest in assay technologies trending toward more cell-based assays [1] and miniaturization, additional reformatting is left to occur further down the line. Typically, there is no efficient means of dealing with the valuable excess samples which often end up being wasted. The latest in compound management equipment has greater flexibility in this respect and can even offer samples in dilution series, however turnaround time from order to delivery may start being affected. Ideally the goal is to provide samples with zero waste, in a variety of formatted outputs to be directly consumed by screening facilities, all within a suitable turnaround time. In practice a balance must be struck in each organization between flexible formatting, material conservation and the response time from request to delivery.

1.2.2
Cell Biology

The cell biology group must maintain a continuous culture of various cells, each with unique growth rates and culture conditions to supply cell suspensions or seeded cell plates for the upcoming ADME/Tox assays. It is critical that this group is able to balance all activities to produce cells and deliver "just in time" in order to maintain the optimal window of cell health and density required for the variety of assays performed by the profiling groups. To cope, cell biology groups have had to become adept at predicting demand and managing highly responsive materials supply logistics.

In addition to meeting a sometimes complex delivery schedule, the maintenance of living cells also poses some challenges for this group. Cells that have overgrown or that have had inconsistent feeding cycles can begin to die or differentiate resulting in assay variability and misleading results. Consistent sample processing is paramount. For example, a simple failure to maintain aseptic transfer techniques can result in cross-contamination of samples and a significant loss of time, materials and productivity. These problems require stringent quality control measures, strict sample tracking and sufficient frozen sample supply to ensure a quick recovery.

The vast majority of facilities maintain their cells manually, with several technicians working diligently in front of biological safety cabinets. Even with the best planning, this becomes difficult to scale when some cell-handling steps must occur over the weekend. Some facilities have turned to automation to maintain their standard cell lines; taking some of the routine burden off skilled technicians and effectively achieving 24/7 operation when fully functional.

An alternative approach for alleviating these logistical issues, that may be amendable to some assay, is to use assay-ready frozen stocks. Cells frozen at high concentration would be seeded into assay plates and used later that day or the next. The build-up of frozen stock reserves is then independent of current demand and can even be purchased directly from suppliers. At least one such supplier has taken a step further by also providing ready-to-use assay plates with cells frozen within. By simply adding media it is possible to revitalize the cells and run your assay within hours [2].

It is uncommon that the cell biology department is dedicated solely to providing standard cell lines for consumption by screening groups. With increased focus on cell-based screening there is pressure to constantly develop and modify cell lines to address the current business strategy. With a manual or semi-manual approach it may take several months to develop a suitable cell line that is ready for standard production. More complex and flexible research-scale automation is on the horizon, that may prove to be the key to optimizing cell culture conditions at small scales that are representative of large scale production [3]. This automation, once proven, will allow a dramatic reduction of human resources for the development of culturing conditions with more systematic sampling of environmental parameters and shorter development cycles.

Because of their unique talents and skill sets, profiling groups may also become responsible for broader cell biology functions. One such example would be high content screening (HCS). HCS has proven to be a valuable tool in assays such as toxicology, allowing for more complex mechanistic cell or system responses to be measured, rather than the simple "yes/no" or "how much" type of answers typically afforded by conventional screening assays. With the development of standardized bioassays and consumables used in an automated fashion to enable throughput enhancements and labor reduction, these specialized assays may move out into the mainstream screening battery.

1.2.3
Lead Profiling

We typically find that there is no single laboratory known as the ADME/Tox or DMPK laboratory. In most cases several laboratories are involved in performing one portion or another of the absorption, distribution, metabolism, excretion and toxicology studies, each with their own specialty. Some assays require advanced instrumentation, others must be performed manually, and some require sterile environments for cell-based screens. In general we see manned workstations dedicated to one or perhaps two different assays depending on the overlap of instrumentation required to perform them. Assays such as metabolic stability and cytochrome P450 can usually be performed on the same workstation, whereas CACO-2 and permeability assays may have their own dedicated equipment. To improve consistency and throughput, assays are semi-automated with simple instruments such as bulk dispensers and plate washers, or full liquid handling workstations surrounded by instruments and storage devices.

Considering the success of the intensified focus on ADME testing (i.e., a substantial decrease in drug failure due to poor ADME properties) a continued increase in demand on the profiling groups is to be expected [4]. Where groups are already running at capacity, it is difficult to squeeze through any additional requests without moving to processes and technologies that scale well.

1.2.4
Liquid Chromatography/Mass Spectrometry

Of particular note is liquid chromatography/mass spectrometry (LC/MS) detection. LC/MS technology is a critical technique for DMPK studies due to its ability to analyze samples with very high sensitivity and specificity particularly within complex mixtures. It is not uncommon to find LC/MS based sample analysis residing within its own functional department due to the specialized facility requirements and technical skills of the operators. Additionally with LC/MS instrumentation becoming lower cost and simpler to operate, they are also becoming a workhorse of the profiling groups for certain assays traditionally analyzed with plate readers, such as cytochrome p450 inhibition, PAMPA and solubility.

While sensitive, this technology typically poses some throughput challenges. Even with the relatively large number of instruments seen within the laboratories, LC/MS analysis often remains a bottleneck.

A typical injection and analysis time for LC/MS may be somewhere between several seconds to a few minutes, depending on the complexity of the sample and the LC/MS technology used. More often than not the LC/MS is connected to an auto-sampler capable of handling several 96 or 384 well plates, allowing a high degree of walk-away time once the system is up and running. Only a handful of technicians may be required to manage several units. Technology is now in hand to make the cycle time shorter, further reducing the cost per sample, making the shift to LC/MS analysis more attractive [5].

1.3
DMPK Testing Strategies: the Process from Data to Decisions

Critical to the success of a DMPK testing strategy is the ability to efficiently make decisions that affect the overall drug discovery process. These decisions are made by stakeholders in multiple core disciplines in multiple departments and affect which compounds are carried on to combinatorial library expansion, medicinal chemistry optimization and further biological testing. Within the profiling department itself the ability to deliver critical data to the organization is largely gated by the ability to process and make informed decisions on the quality of data in a timely manner. It is at this stage of the process where significant opportunity exists for efficiency improvements to be made by many organizations.

A common problem experienced under the current automation paradigm, with the demand for greater results in shorter iteration cycles (1–2 weeks), is that screeners are required to collect data from several single assay workstations, often run on different software platforms. With the demand for results on more compounds per week, the screeners must process more samples through the assays, each with fewer data points and replicates. This trade off in quality for quantity can result in lower overall data fidelity.

The management of this screening workload distributed across multiple workstations can be rather labor-intensive and error prone without appropriate sample and data management tools. This places a large resource burden on screeners who could otherwise spend their time on higher-value activities such as more rigorous data evaluation.

As organizations have historically navigated the changing requirements for ADME/Tox testing different decision-making philosophies have evolved that can impact the effectiveness of screening approaches and their underlying logistics.

One common approach is the use of scoring criteria. Typical practice is to run all the compounds under investigation under a battery of assays in parallel without consideration for their interdependence. For example, 500 compounds will be run through several assays within a week or two. When the campaign is complete the data is passed on to the researchers for a score card type of evaluation based on a summary of all the results. The selection of the best compounds is then based on a consultative evaluation of all the available data. This approach can have a few drawbacks depending on how it is implemented. Since all data on all compounds is required prior to decision making, the turn-around time for data evaluation and QC can sometimes be longer than desired for the next iteration of compound synthesis. Additionally, the volume of multivariate data that must be analyzed in order to make the decisions is also very high and can confound the selection process.

Another common approach is the use of cut-off criteria to define which compounds should be carried forward. Each assay in a campaign has a predefined limit for acceptable values and compounds that fail these criteria are abandoned. For example, compounds that fail the cut-off for solubility may be dropped from further consideration. This approach has strengths in promoting the discipline of only advancing the very best compounds and simplifying the decision making process by enforcing a "live with the outcome" culture. In practice some flexibility or relaxation in the strict criteria may be required in order to ensure that sufficient compounds can progress through the pipeline.

It is interesting to note that this approach can be implemented as either a parallel or hierarchical screening approach depending on whether or not the data on failed compounds is required Figure 1.2. For example, when screening a focused library for

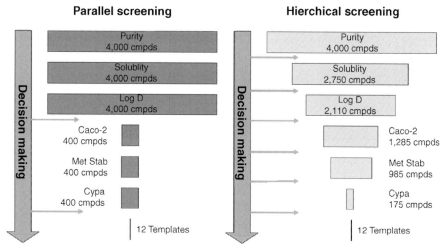

Figure 1.2 Comparison of parallel and hierarchical screening strategies. In the parallel screen the first three assays are run in parallel followed by a manual decision to reduce the candidate compounds down for the subsequent set of three assays. The use of real-time data QC steps and feedback in the hierarchical approach supports the filtering out of failed compounds prior to submission to the next assay. Both strategies depicted defer the lower throughput assays until the end of the campaign. The gradual filtering model in the hierarchical approach is a more informed process when compared to the large single elimination of 3600 compounds seen in the parallel approach. The resulting 12 templates from the hierarchical approach can be viewed as having a greater potential for a marketable drug.

structure–activity relationship (SAR) modeling, all data on failing compounds is of use. In this case running the assays in parallel would make the most sense if the screening capacity is available. However, where a larger number of compounds are to be evaluated, the decision to test the compounds hierarchically can produce a significant resource saving and throughput enhancement. In a hierarchical screen the assays would be conducted in a logical order that enabled the elimination of failing compounds from further testing. This approach defers the time consuming assays until a large number of compounds have been ruled out.

Ideally the ADME/Tox screening laboratory service would be set up to flexibly offer choice in the screening strategy that best fits the current campaign circumstances. It would also provide real-time data feedback both to enable researchers to use the critical information to make decisions on further testing and to reduce cycle times by eliminating compounds midcampaign [6].

1.4
New Questions, New Assays and New Technologies Challenge the Process

In the wake of the impact of LC/MS on rapid bioanalytical method development, no compounds are advancing into first in man studies without explicit assessment of exposure levels in preclinical animal models. As a result, the clinical attrition rate due to poor DMPK has dropped dramatically [7]. Drug hunters are unsatisfied, however, by the arrival of bad news late in their programs: rather than killing compounds and killing programs, scientists would prefer to unravel cause and effect and design their series around the liabilities that increase risk of clinical failure. What has followed, therefore is an ever-expanding sequence of mechanistic assays probing passive and active phenomena for drug uptake, metabolism and elimination.

The main scientific drivers of clinical attrition remain toxicity (30% of failure) and efficacy (additional 30%) [8]. The latter is the domain of the burgeoning field of biomarkers, leading to promising notions of personalized medicines. Whereas the practical application of biomarkers in drug discovery and clinical development is challenged by many logistical and technological concerns, these are generally very closely related to the target under study within the research program, and tend to be handled outside of the ADME/Tox laboratory. Biomarkers that warn for the likelihood of mechanistic toxicities, however, have broad applicability. More and more these assays are invoked during lead selection and lead optimization programs. So, in addition to the biochemical and physicochemical assays exploring ADME phenomena, a new range of predictive Tox assays are growing in popularity [4].

These trends do more to challenge the preclinical profiling process with a growing menu of tests: they introduce new technological paradigms, which must be somehow knit into the scope of the laboratory workflow. Cell-based assays with readouts ranging from simple fluorescence to cell-based imaging to RNA extraction and quantitation by RT-PCR have come alongside solubility assays, PAMPA measurements and cytochrome P450 inhibition studies.

The range of cell types that must be prepared, cultured and manufactured on a just in time basis, the number of detection systems that must be accommodated, the complex scheduling of incubation periods, sample preparation and analysis procedures, the form and fashion of data and post-analytical processing all contribute to a very complex laboratory, balancing a complicated set of demands.

Another dimension of complexity must be layered on top of this description: the demand for these forms of data is growing as drug hunter teams become increasingly reliant on ADME/Tox feedback during the course of their lead optimization programs. Naturally, this growing demand for data is a welcome trend, as it indicates broader opportunity for impact, but of course increased demand exacerbates the complexity of the process.

An apt analogy may be the small intimate bistro restaurant, with a highly complex menu of offerings. With only ten tables the chef and sous chef can preside over each dish, artistically delivering perfect dishes in synchronicity for the customers at each table. The chef continues to invent new dishes, increasing the appeal of his menu, but also increasing the complexity of the process in the kitchen. Everything is fine with only ten tables. But word has gotten out, the bistro is good, and the manager has expanded the dining room. There are now 40 tables and somehow the chef has to figure out how to feed everyone to the same level of satisfaction at the same time. And the menu keeps getting bigger.

1.5
Organizational Models to Scale Up the Process

Like the chef, the laboratory manager has many constraints in moving forward: he cannot merely add staff and cost to the kitchen, he cannot begin to deliver inconsistent product, his responsiveness may not decrease, he cannot achieve quality without well qualified, well trained staff. Instead, he must identify real efficiencies that can be derived from scale.

Laboratories, just like restaurants, have adopted several different models for responding to increased demand: (i) the food court, (ii) the fast food restaurant and (iii) the family restaurant chain.

1.5.1
Food Court

In the food court, there are limited options – combos – to choose from, and each compound is subjected to a predefined battery of tests. This is akin to treating ADME/Tox experimentation as a form of secondary screening, eliminating or severely restricting à la carte testing options. Clear efficiencies can be gained per unit of data, and there are intellectual benefits for collecting wide arrays of information about many compounds, but there will also be a lot of data generated that will not be used. Economically, therefore, the best assays to include as a secondary screening panel are those that are broadly referenced and relatively inexpensive to produce, such as basic physicochemical and biochemical endpoints (e.g., solubility, cytochrome P450 inhibition). Due to its predefined combo menu, the laboratory generally achieves medium to high throughputs at good efficiencies. More expensive or rare tests are disruptive to the workflow and are better handled outside of the generic test regime. Adaptation to changes and implementation of new assays are not easily accommodated by this set up.

1.5.1.1 The Fast Food Restaurant

The kitchen of a fast food restaurant is characterized by islands of automation, with well defined subprocesses focused on producing a certain kind of output, coordinated by a crew chief. The principal advantage of a fast food restaurant is consistency and fast delivery. The dedicated subunits are designed to perform a certain type of process (assay) at a high rate with very little room for change. Economically, this model is difficult to sustain unless each assay type has sufficient demand to justify the existence of dedicated space, equipment and personnel. It is also not as efficient as a secondary screening model. For assays that are routinely, but not always, requested then this model is very appropriate (e.g., CACO-2 permeability, microsomal stability). However, for the more costly and complex assays that are requested less often, the cost of dedicated people and equipment is hard to justify and as a result the assay has to come off the menu. This is why most fast food restaurants have a relatively limited menu, including mostly foods that are simple to prepare.

1.5.1.2 The Family Restaurant Chain

Dotting the landscape of suburban North America, the family restaurant chain lies somewhere between the bistro and the fast food restaurant. Menus are longer, the food preparation is more complex, the kitchen has multi-purpose stations dedicated to types of food and sophisticated systems for communication and tracking. By streamlining the logistics of managing the overall process and improving the duty cycle of kitchen equipment, kitchen staff and kitchen space, these restaurants are able to efficiently offer the restaurant's most popular items and more rarely ordered novelties. The food quality is consistent, the response time is fair and the price is relatively low.

It should be noted that among these three restaurant models, only the third offers the chef broad latitude in creating new recipes, extending and revising the menu, preserving a customer favorite and improving a staple item.

It is also very telling to consider where the investment is made in each scenario. In the secondary screening model (food court), investment is made to completely automate the experimental process, so that scale can be achieved at marginal incremental cost. Many specific engineering challenges are engaged to minimize the manual steps performed by laboratory staff. In the fast food model, investment is made in people, dedicated equipment and additional laboratory space, so that every type of assay can be supported in a timely fashion. In the family restaurant model, investment is made in managing the logistics of the laboratory workflow, so that tasks are not dropped as equipment and people switch from one assay to another.

Preclinical profiling laboratories generally begin as fast food restaurants, employing dedicated people, space and equipment for specific assays. As they grow in throughput and in the scope of assays offered, this proves to be the default model of laboratory growth, with incremental investment in more people, space and equipment to meet the growing demands of the organization. As these resources become more and more difficult to secure, laboratory managers would be well advised to invest in process management technology and to make the jump from fast food to family restaurant.

1.6
Critical Factors to Improve the Process

Notwithstanding the organizational model being pursued (or of course a hybrid of the above approaches), evolving the capabilities within the ADME/Tox laboratory is a complex process engineering exercise that involves detailed considerations of the roles, capabilities and limitations of all of the participating groups. Because each company has its own particular goals, organizational structure, size, scale and style, there are as many potential solutions as there are organizations. Nonetheless, there are common considerations that all groups must bear in mind when identifying opportunities to increase scope, scale, quality or efficiency. Stated in this fashion and viewed at the abstract level, we can see that the laboratory operation has a lot in common with a manufacturing operation and it may therefore be worthwhile to examine a well established methodology for manufacturing process improvement. Here we explore and adapt a typical and widely accepted approach to analyze processes and pinpoint process improvements: the fishbone model for root cause analysis.

Root cause analysis (RCA) is a class of problem solving methods aimed at identifying the root causes of problems or events. The practice of RCA is predicated on the belief that problems are best solved by attempting to correct or eliminate root causes, as opposed to merely addressing the immediately obvious symptoms. By directing corrective measures at root causes, it is hoped that the likelihood of problem recurrence will be minimized. However it is recognized that complete prevention of recurrence by a single intervention is not always possible. Thus RCA is often considered to be an iterative process and is frequently viewed as a tool of continuous improvement.

The following are basic elements the RCA would target in a generic production process.

- Materials
- Machine/Equipment
- Environment
- Management
- Methods

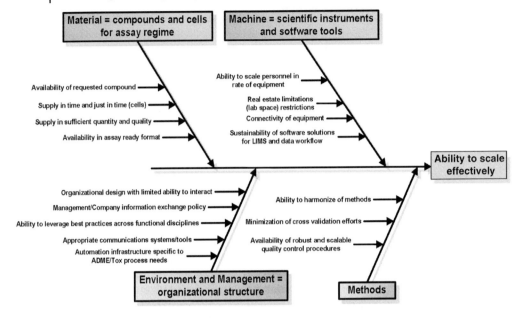

Figure 1.3 Fishbone diagram of ADME/Tox process elements. The scale up of the ADME/Tox screening laboratory requires careful consideration of all crucial elements involved in its process. The commonly accepted approach of route cause analysis has been applied to identify potential hurdles that should be reviewed when planning a significant increase in sample throughput. The importance of individual factors may vary due to the particular goals, organizational structure, size, scale and style of different organizations. The fishbone diagram tries to identify common areas of consideration when identifying opportunities to increase scope, scale, quality and efficiency of the testing process.

Many, though not all, of the factors in a generic production process have an analog within the ADME/Tox process (see Figure 1.3). The following section identifies process elements specific to ADME/Tox screening and potential hurdles an organization might face in scaling their operations.

1.7
Materials in ADME/Tox Screening

Materials in the ADME/Tox screening process relate mainly to consumables (plastic ware, tips, plates, reagents, etc.) and the raw materials the tests will be performed on, which are plates with compounds and cells. To simplify the analysis, it is assumed that access to consumables is not a major issue, since these supplies can easily be ordered through the supply chain and are generally available to the personnel performing the test assays (Figures 1.4 to 1.7).

The just in time supply of plates from the compound management and cell biology groups seems to be a more critical operational hurdle. The ADME/Tox screening

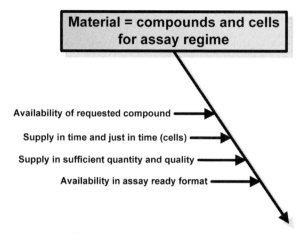

Figure 1.4 Fishbone element "Materials" in the ADME/Tox process.

laboratories receive the compound and cell plates either in a standardized concentration (which usually requires subsequent manipulations to prepare them for the test assay), or in an "assay-ready" format for immediate consumption. Regardless of the delivery format, having the proper compounds and assay-ready plates available at the desired time and in sufficient quantity requires upfront planning and coordination with the compound management and cell biology groups. In our studies, we could identify two generic methods for the supply of compound plates: (i) as stock solutions in DMSO (usually 10 mM) or (ii) as test plates in ready to use form with compounds in appropriate dilution series and buffers, with wells reserved for standards and controls. In the case of compound plates supplied in DMSO, the local laboratory usually performs a reformatting step to prepare test

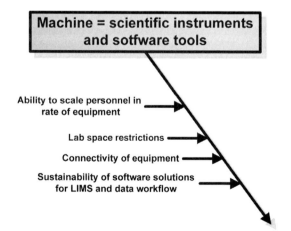

Figure 1.5 Fishbone element "Machine" in the ADME/Tox process.

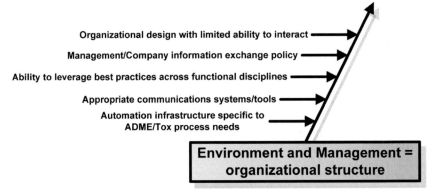

Figure 1.6 Fishbone element "Environment and Management".

plates in the proper pipetting format for subsequent testing. These reformatting steps are often rate limiting unless the local laboratory is equipped to quickly transform them into the desired test format. The reformatting procedures are usually done in a batch mode process that becomes the rate limiting step in the subsequent assay regime. Both the ordering scenarios and the standard format or assay-ready plates require tight linkages of demand and supply between ADME laboratories, compound management and biology groups. In many cases the research organizations put electronic ordering systems in place that allow synchronization between groups similar to supply management systems in production facilities. In most cases these systems prove to be effective, even though the time between request and delivery of compound may sometimes be as long as three weeks, even longer if a compound is in limited supply; in such situations, the library management group has to re-supply this compound from stock or powder solutions or place limitations on its use in ADME/Tox testing. These "long lead time items" determine the pace of research in the laboratory. A similar scenario

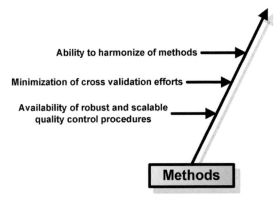

Figure 1.7 Fishbone element "Methods".

is seen with the receipt of assay-ready cell plates with the added complexity of dealing with living material.

1.8 Machines and Equipment in ADME/Tox Screening

The basic equipment in the ADME/Tox laboratory revolves around three major core technologies: (i) liquid handling; (ii) detection and analysis instrumentation; and (iii) software for data retrieval, analysis, interpretation and quality control.

1.8.1 Liquid Handlers

Liquid handling is a basic core function of all physiochemical, biochemical or cell-based assays performed in the ADME/Tox laboratory. Generic tools for these tasks are bench-top liquid handling workstations. The basic interaction with the equipment requires the loading of plates (test plates, assay plates, consumables, etc.), the programming/selection of test assay procedure and the transfer (unloading) of the prepared plates to the next instrument (typically a reader or MS analyzer). These workstations are initially ideal to increase throughput and capacity while gaining walk-away time for the scientist. However, when additional throughput is demanded from this infrastructure of isolated workstations, the laboratories are generally left with two options: (i) increase the number of workstations or (ii) alter the assay to run more compounds during the day.

The strategy of increasing the number of workstations is widely applied since a relatively minor incremental investment is required for each addition, which in theory results in a twofold increase in throughput for that particular assay. Perhaps four or five workstations are required for each overall twofold increase for all assays. Although not a 1:1 ratio, additional personnel is required to man the extra workstations. For a time this approach to scaling up works, however with the anticipated increases for ADME/Tox screening one can expect to see a limit reached relatively soon with the number of additional workstations and personnel that the facility can handle.

A complementary approach is to conduct the assays under high-throughput automated conditions. This can be either through the miniaturization of assays, that is, 96–384 plates and if possible 1536, or through the use of alternative assay technologies (e.g., microfluidics). Both scenarios require studies of equivalency testing and backwards compatibility with previous methods and results.

1.8.2 Detection and Analysis

Most detection and analysis is performed on either optical plate readers or mass spectrometers. While multimode plate readers are relatively compact, inexpensive devices with parallel measurement capabilities (typically providing a fast read of a multiple samples in a 96 or 384 plate format in just a few minutes), LC/MS instruments analyze samples serially and are rate-limited by the chromatographic separation step, such that analysis of each well of a microplate can take several minutes, even with modern multiplexing approaches. In order to cope with the sample throughput demand, companies invest in multiple high-throughput LC/MS units to run analyses in parallel. Similar to the challenge in scaling liquid handling workstations, adding LC/MS analysis units also requires concomitant increase in laboratory space and personnel.

1.9
Software, Data Retrieval, Analysis, Manipulation and Interpretation

While the sample processing bottleneck is well on the way to being solved, the results analysis component still remains a challenge. A variety of software analysis tools exist to automatically analyze and reduce chromatographs to useful interpretive data. However even with automated analysis software, manual review of the data is often required, not only for situations where the chromatograph cannot be analyzed (poor resolution, inappropriate conditions, carryover, etc.), but for all results, where the human eye and experience can spot anomalies that the software simply misses. Much of a LC/MS technician's time is still spent hovering over a computer monitor with the mundane task of clicking chromatograph after chromatograph and rescreening the runs that have failed. With the shift towards the integration of LC/MS detection into automated systems will likely come the inherent benefits of deeper data integration and hopefully intelligent automated data QC algorithms in the sample processing workflow.

One of the major challenges in scaling up operations is the connectivity of instrumentation and the data/results they produce. Any increase in the number of instruments or instrument types also increases the number of necessary software bridges to enable tracking of samples and association of results with samples. Further, data analysis and QC operations often must be conducted using instrumental firmware, introducing further complexity into the overall workflow organization within the laboratory. Many pitfalls arise in this scenario: often instruments cannot be accessed remotely, or data file transfer is not in the inherent design of the instrument's firmware. This leaves scientists to perform tedious, relatively unproductive and error-prone tasks of copying and transferring data. It has been suggested [9] that about 70% of an ADME/Tox scientist's time is spent in data manipulation, interpretation and QC. Since limited commercial solutions for instrument and data interfacing are on the market, companies either produce their own systems (homebrew LIMS infrastructure) or add commercial solutions to their specific need (stitched together). Not only is such an undertaking a "tour de force" for IT groups, the resulting system is typically very difficult and costly to support, maintain and adapt. It is also quite common that a very small number of key individuals have a detailed understanding of the system, leading to potential risks for the organization, in the case of turnover of key personnel.

1.10 Environment and Management = Organizational Structure in ADME/Tox Screening

While most of the environmental elements of the generic RCA model might not be directly applicable to the ADME/Tox screening laboratories, the job designs, layout of the work environment and the organizational design might present significant obstacles to a scale up.

Limitations to gaining efficiencies may include the inability to leverage existing talent and best practices across laboratories, departments and sites. Barriers to exchange are often the use of divergent tools or infrastructure and insufficient communication across departments.

In our experience with organizational designs, we have found instances of decentralized departments with little capacity nor desire to communicate to the department whose subsequent analysis is dependent on their results. This element links closely to the management philosophy and organizational environment they create. Organizing related functions and processes physically close to each other to encourage interaction between departments that depend on one another is an important step to improve interdisciplinary exchange and collaboration. It is understood that spatial closeness of related functions cannot always be achieved, especially when rapid scale up occurs. Advanced communication tools that facilitate intercompany exchange and relationship building can partially compensate for a limited ability of physical personnel interaction. Communication tools that allow scientists to post and discuss methods, best practices and results enable the scientists to better align their specific roles with their counterparts and create alignment. Fostering an environment that enables scale up without breaking crucial information links is largely dependent on the foundation that management has laid in its policies and encouragement for information exchange.

Many pharma organizations have chosen the path of laboratory automation with robotics and software to increase sample throughput. The industry realizes that those tools are most effective when combined with the appropriate in house support structure for implementation, operation and continuous improvement [10]. When in early 2000s the ADME/Tox testing laboratories were asked to provide a higher sample throughput, other areas in research process such as the primary HTS laboratories were already well equipped with robotics devices, automation and the appropriate personnel support structure. In contrast, automation tools and proven implementation strategies were relatively new to the ADME/Tox screening laboratories. Therefore management often looked to the HTS facilities to lend their expertise and potentially unused capacity to run automated ADME/Tox screening assays [11]. HTS systems are designed to process a high number of samples on a relatively limited set of assays. But, ADME/Tox testing deals with relatively small number of compounds that are to be tested on a larger set of assays. Nevertheless, some ADME/Tox screens, mainly fluorescence or cell-based assays (e.g., cytochrome P450, PAMPA) did fit the HTS system designs and could easily be implemented into the testing regime of the primary screening groups.

While utilizing the HTS expertise and capacity might deliver the initial desired results, we recommend that serious considerations are given to the transfer of expertise and build up of a local automation and support infrastructure that is specific to the needs of ADME/Tox testing in order to understand crucial process steps, when a rapid scale up is required.

1.11
Methods in ADME/Tox Screening

Limited standardization of methods, procedures and equipment within a laboratory make it difficult to compare data generated at different points of time, and – within larger organizations – between departments and sites. Companies try to compensate for such incompatibilities through cross-validation efforts. Variability in the results is generally originated by different personnel conducting the experiment, due to different skill sets or deliberate seemingly "minor" changes to improve their own efficiency, variability of different types of equipment used to perform the same assay functions (different manufacturers) or differences in performing the assay manually as compared to an automated procedure. From a process efficiency point of view, cross-validations are wasted effort, since they represent re-work and do not enhance the resulting product (the result). In addition they are a burden in the sense that they have to be documented and maintained separately. Besides those efforts in re-work, cross-validations present a real obstacle to scale, since it isn't clear which process among the many alternatives will routinely deliver the most accurate and precise result. It seems obvious that in order to efficiently leverage scientific resources, equipment and processes a certain level of method standardization is required.

Even once a method is standardized, erroneous results can still be generated. As a result, it is critical to have robust quality control procedures in place. Here, careful attention should be paid to identify opportunity for in-process control measures such as internal standards, calibration, control plates, replicates and so on as opposed to post-processing data review steps. Inline QC approaches allow sources of error to be identified and remedied much more rapidly and help limit costly re-tests, or the possibility of erroneous data leaving the laboratory.

1.11.1
Examples of Whole-Process Approaches

As can be seen through the lens of the root cause analysis discussion above, optimizing the laboratory process is a highly complex undertaking. In as many laboratories as the authors have visited, no specific solution has been seen twice. Here we showcase three general patterns that have arisen, each of which offers distinct characteristics. While all three are drawn from the laboratories of large pharmaceutical companies, the learnings from each should be applicable at any scale.

1.11.1.1 Automation Islands with Manual Data Upload to a LIMS System

This is a common approach. A central LIMS system keeps track of the compounds, layout of plates supplied from compound management and the assays requested for each sample. Scientists track the mapping of samples though the preparation of test plates, sample preparation and analysis with the help of macros (usually programmed in Excel). At the conclusion of the experiment, data is uploaded back into the LIMS system for review and delivery to the requesting scientist.

Depending on the degree of automation, scientists may be preparing test plates and running the experiments manually, or operating preprogrammed liquid handler workstations. Depending on the degree of software integration, scientists may be manually entering data into Excel sheets (though this is rare nowadays), cutting and pasting results from one software package to another (this is very common, even from one Excel workbook to another), or using fully automated data upload macros (this is very rare).

The pros and cons of this approach depend on the degree of automation of the experimental and data analysis processes. When a great deal of manual pipetting and manual data manipulation is required, human error and fatigue can significantly compromise data quality. More automation of these steps can reduce these sources of random error, but may also hide systematic errors, unless the systems also include sophisticated capabilities to highlight deviation from expected performance. This is particularly true with LCMS analyses. Regardless, skilled scientists are spending a disproportionate amount of time performing manual steps.

This approach does have its merits, however, groups can evolve to this sort of system incrementally, automating experimental steps and data manipulations as they become burdensome, often using inhouse programming resources. Also, as no particular experiment format is "hard wired", changing methods is relatively straightforward. However, groups pursuing this approach should bear in mind that such flexibility comes at a cost: maintenance of a growing set of software "scripts" and macros can become unruly; it is not always possible to keep track of which macro version was applied to a specific piece of data, which makes trouble-shooting and retrospective comparison difficult; further it can become difficult to enforce standard operating procedures.

These cautions and the relatively high investment in laboratory staff, space and dedicated equipment make it difficult to scale this approach economically.

1.11.1.2 Complete Physical Integration and Automation

In our experience, very few ADME/Tox groups pursue a complete physical integration and automation strategy. Whereas this approach is very effective in accelerating high-throughput screening, it has proven rather difficult to adapt this to the ADME/Tox workload. Some elements of HTS technologies have been integrated into relevant stages of ADME screens, such as plate replication, sample preparation and analysis running traditional *in vitro* ADME tests in a "HTS like fashion". HTS operates on the basis of campaigns, running a very large, fixed, compound collection through one specific assay as rapidly as possible, followed by re-configuration and another campaign and so on. ADME/Tox laboratories, in contrast, must provide real-time service for a different set of compounds each week, running each of them through a different panel of assays.

The closest example we have seen to a complete physical integration is the ALIAS system at Pfizer, Sandwich [4].

ALIAS is described as a robotic platform with integrated sample submission and LC/MS analytical systems. It consists of systems with centralized robotic arms that combine a series of modular assay workstations. As this example indicates, it is certainly possible to develop a highly integrated system for ADME/Tox application. However, due to their complexity, it is typically rather difficult to adapt such systems to changes in assay types/strategies and detection technologies, unless a fundamental integration infrastructure is designed with such flexibility in mind.

1.11.1.3 Federated Physical Automation with Software Integration

One attempt to build an automated ADME/Tox platform on top of such a flexibility-friendly integration infrastructure is our own work on the LeadStream system. The system is well documented elsewhere in the literature [12], so only a brief description is given here. LeadStream is a system of automated WorkCells, each with specific automation capabilities, tied together through a software system that manages all the data and sample flow through, from request to result (Orchestrator). One module, the Reformatter, receives sample plates from compound management and prepares assay-ready plates, including just those compounds that have been requested for each assay. The laboratory can include any number of ADME WorkCells that can be programmed to carry out any number of complex sample preparation experiments as well as optical readout. Additional LCMS WorkCells provide automated quantitation by LCMS. Both types of WorkCells automate the analysis of data and report results back to the Orchestrator software.

This approach provides certain operational advantages within the ADME/Tox laboratory, such as minimizing manual data and sample handing and improving overall throughput. The method also promises to avoid the main pitfall of more complete physical integration: difficulty in adapting to new assays or changes in experimental method. This platform is best suited for "greenfield" sites that establish a new laboratory infrastructure utilizing the benefits of an integrated approach to automation, sample and data workflow.

1.12
Conclusions

The demand for more ADME data has cascading effects that impact on several key groups within the pharmaceutical industry. It is likely in today's push for more and more productivity that these groups are reaching or are already at capacity, with considerable limitations to cope with future needs. Due to the circular (re-circulating) workflow within ADME testing each group is dependent on the other in one way or another. The benefits in throughput gained through the typical approach of increasing personnel and instrumentation (with or without automation) will quickly reach a plateau without serious consideration for efficient workflow. This is achieved through clear understanding of the barriers that can prevent coordination of all activities and data results, and developing implementation plans that fit into one's current businesses mold.

Abbreviations

ADME/Tox	Absorption, distribution, metabolism, excretion/toxicology
CACO-2	Colonic adenocarcinoma 2 (human cell line)
DMPK	Drug metabolism and pharmacokineticss
DMSO	Dimethylsulfoxide
ID	Compound identification
IT	Information technology
HCS	High content screening
LC/MS	Liquid chromatography/mass spectrometry
LIMS	Laboratory information management system
PAMPA	Parallel artificial membrane permeability assay
QC	Quality control
RT-PCR	Reverse transcriptase–polymerase chain reaction
RNA	Ribonucleic acid
RCA	Root cause analysis
SAR	Structure–activity relationship

References

1 High throughput screening 2007 report: new strategies, success rates, and use of enabling technologies. HighTech Business Decisions, December 2007.
2 CCS Cell Culture Service GmbH. http://www.cellcultureservice.com.
3 Schreyer, H.B., Miller, S.E. and Rodgers, S. (2007) High-throughput process development: MicroBioreactor system simulates large bioreactor process at submilliliter volumes. *Genetic Engineering & Biotechnology News*, **27** (17), 44.
4 Saunders, K.C. (2004) Automation and robotics in ADME Screening. *Drug Discovery Today: Technologies*, **1**, 373–380.
5 Carlson, T.J. and Fisher, M.B. (2008) Recent advances in high throughput screening for ADME properties. *Combinatorial Chemistry High Throughput Screen*, **11**, 258–264.
6 DeWitte, R.S. and Haas, H. (2005) Adding agility to your ADME/Tox screening process. *Next Generation Pharmaceutical*, **2005**, 47–49.
7 Kola, I. and Landis, J. (2004) Can the pharma industry reduce attrition rates. *Nature Reviews. Drug Discovery*, **3**.

8 Booth, B., Glassman, R. and Ma, P. (2003) Oncology's trials. *Nature Reviews. Drug Discovery*, **2**, 609–610.
9 Burdette, D. (2005) Rational robotics for ADMET screening. LabAutomation 2005, San Jose, Calif., USA.
10 Association for Laboratory Automation 2006: Industrial laboratory automation survey, January 2007.
11 High throughput screening 2005: New users, more cell-based assays, and a host of new tools. Hightech Business Decisions, October 2005.
12 DeWitte, R.S. and Robins, R.H. (2006) ADME/Tox screening process. *Expert Opinion on Drug Metabolism and Toxicology*, **2** (5), 805–817.

2
Prediction of Drug-Likeness and its Integration into the Drug Discovery Process
Ansgar Schuffenhauer and Meir Glick

2.1
Introduction

High-throughput screening (HTS) plays an important role in drug discovery. In this process a large collection of accessible compounds is either directly submitted to a high-throughput biological experiment, or assessed by virtual screening techniques followed by medium-throughput biological experiment on the resulting virtual hits [1]. For an HTS campaign to be considered successful – namely a hit to lead chemistry program is initiated – the compounds in the screening collection must meet a number of requirements. Of these, three are deemed important. First, the compounds must be compatible with compound handling and long-term storage conditions in solution and comply with the screening technology at hand. Second, the screening deck must contain compounds with biological relevance and that can modulate the target of interest. Third, the compounds must be amenable to lead optimization. There are considerable synergies between the requirements of technology compatibility and lead optimization. Water solubility is required not only for optimization but also to achieve the desired concentration in the assay system. If the compounds are too lipophilic and have poor solubility, they might precipitate or form aggregates in the screening solution, which can sequester the protein in biochemical assays in a non-specific way and lead to a false positive readout [2]. If a cellular assay format is used to screen intracellular targets, cell membrane penetration is required. Compounds that are chemically reactive may have the potential to react nonspecifically with cellular targets such as DNA, causing mutagenicity. They might equally be chemically unstable for long-term storage in solution or disturb the assay system by covalent binding to assay components. These synergies between technology compatibility and the potential of a compound for lead optimization are no coincidence, but are to some degree an attempt by the assay to model a subset of human biology. Apart from the freedom to operate in the intellectual property space, amenability of a potential hit to lead optimization can be defined as the ability to achieve an efficacious blood–plasma concentration within a reasonable dosing regime. The blood–plasma concentration depends upon the compound's absorption, distribution, metabolism and excretion (ADME). At the same time undesirable side effects for this dosing regime should be minimal. The oral bioavailability of a compound is largely related to its solubility and permeability, the two components of the biopharmaceutical classification system (BCS). In order to maintain the efficacious blood plasma concentration the drug must not be metabolized too rapidly. Unwanted toxic side effects of the drug compound and its metabolites have to be avoided. This requires predicting both metabolism rate and the nature of the metabolites themselves. Ideally a broad range of toxic effects should be predicted from chemical structures. It is noteworthy here that the optimization requirement is to a large extent independent from the individual target and applies for many drugs; therefore, compounds fulfilling these properties are often called drug-like. Typically drug-likeness criteria are targeted towards oral administration of compounds. Drug-likeness is used as a guideline throughout the modern drug discovery pipeline. In this chapter we review the definition of drug-likeness and its impact on screening collections, prioritization of HTS hits and lead optimization where drug-likeness rules are used to guide the synthetic efforts into a desirable physicochemical property space and to avoid unwanted liabilities.

2.2
Computational Prediction of Drug-Likeness

2.2.1
Machine Learning

The evolution of drug-likeness is depicted in Figure 2.1. Below we discuss each of the approaches to predict drug-likeness, starting with machine learning. Before studying predictive models for the individual properties relevant for drug-likeness, it is helpful to understand some common underlying principles of molecular property prediction by machine learning. Most methods use a fixed length descriptor vector to represent the chemical structure. Frequently, binary vectors denoting the presence or absence of structural features are used, which are often called molecular fingerprints. Other frequently used descriptors are occurrence count vectors of structural fragments ("molecular holograms"). Once the structures are encoded as fixed-length descriptor vectors, molecular property prediction is treated as a machine learning problem, for which multivariate statistics offers a wide range of solutions [4]. The machine learning algorithm itself in such a setup does not need to have any built-in chemical knowledge. This separation of the molecular descriptor encoding step and the machine learning step into distinct, sequentially executed processes makes the application of new machine learning algorithms for structural property prediction quite straightforward. This separation is however not, in principle, necessary, and there have been examples reported where the machine learning algorithm operates directly on the structure graphs [5]. Regardless of the algorithm used, the general

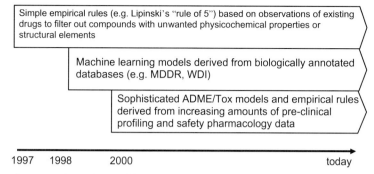

Figure 2.1 The evolution of the drug-likeness concept. Drug-likeness evolved from empirical rules such as Lipinski's rule of 5 through more sophisticated data mining algorithms into utilization of preclinical profiling and safety pharmacology data [3]. Sophisticated drug-likeness models are normally used across a congeneric series of compounds to solve a specific problem in lead optimization. On the other hand, empirical rules are frequently used in lead finding.

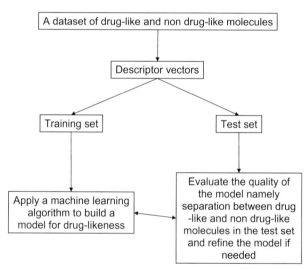

Figure 2.2 The generation of a drug-likeness model includes the following steps. Assemble a set of molecules for which the property to be learned is already known. Calculate descriptors for structures. Divide the dataset into training and test sets. Put the test set aside. Present the training set to the machine learning algorithm to build a model. Sometimes at this stage a validation set is put aside from the molecules in the training set, which is not used in the model building itself, but to detect when to stop refining and adding complexity to the model. Use the test set to evaluate the quality of the model. If the evaluation of the model yielded satisfactory results then the model can now be used to predict if a new molecule is drug-like.

process of drug-likeness prediction based on machine learning is always the same as depicted in Figure 2.2.

Mathematically, the model is a function that predicts the learned property from the descriptor vector. Building the model means finding the optimal prediction function in the solution space defined by the range of possible types of functions and the parameters. The larger the solution space sampled during the machine learning process, the more training data is needed to find the optimal prediction function. The machine learning algorithm determines the range of possible prediction functions. Algorithms which restrict the prediction functions (e.g., to linear functions only) have a smaller solution space and can often be trained with less data. Non-linear models require more training data, but have the benefit of being able to deal with cases where the relationship between the descriptors and the property to be trained is not linear or the property to be predicted can be influenced by several disconnected mechanisms (e.g., active and passive transport in cell permeability). Also one model for toxic side effects can potentially cover multiple causes for a particular effect if they are covered by the training data. The number of parameters to fit also depends on the dimensionality of the input descriptor vector. Higher dimensional descriptor vectors will lead to an increase in the number of parameters and therefore require more training data. This causes problems when fingerprints encoding the absence or presence of structural features are used, which typically have high dimensionality (often ≥ 1000).

Building a model with a machine learning algorithm does not, in principle, require any basic understanding of the property to be modeled. However such knowledge could reduce the solution space by selecting the appropriate descriptors as input variables. This can be done by the machine learning process itself in a feature selection step, for example, with genetic algorithms [6–8]. However, feature selection requires additional training data. There are numerous applications of machine learning algorithms for the prediction of ADME properties described in the literature, of which a selection is given in Table 2.1.

An ideal global model is expected to be predictive across the complete chemistry space, but in reality predictivity across a reasonable wide range of chemotypes or chemical series is already a challenging goal. Often there is insufficient training data available on the property of interest to build a global model, making robust predictions across all compound classes difficult. The physicochemical characterization of a compound is labor-intensive and usually done after the compound has shown some biological activity of interest. Therefore, training data is missing for many chemical classes that have not previously shown biological activity. Even more experimental effort is required for the determination of pharmacokinetic properties such as oral bioavailability. Therefore, these experiments are typically done in the later stages of lead optimization. This has consequences for the availability of training data, which for pharmacokinetic properties is often available only for known drug compounds and chemical series that have entered lead optimization. The experimental values for pharmacokinetic properties and more complex drug-like properties can vary considerably with the experimental procedure used. For example, solubility and permeability measurements are frequently used to guide the medicinal chemistry decisions throughout lead optimization. Measurements of solubility give different results depending whether the extrapolated solubility of the neutral species, the solubility in a buffer of specified pH or the solubility in unbuffered water is measured. Especially when collecting historical literature data for the purpose of assembling a training set

Table 2.1 Machine learning algorithms used for the prediction of ADME properties.

Algorithm	Property	Type	Linear	Reference
Least squares (LS)	log P	Quantitative	Yes	[9, 10]
Partial least squares (PLS)	Aqueous solubility	Quantitative	Yes	[11]
Neural network (NN)	Aqueous solubility	Quantitative	No	[12]
Associative neural networks (ASNN)	Aqueous solubility, octanol–water partition (logP, logD)	Quantitative ± Error	No	[13–15]
Neural network/ genetic algorithm feature selection	Aqueous solubility	Quantitative	No	[8]
Decision trees	Intestinal absorption	Classifier	No	[16]
k-Nearest neighbors	Intestinal absorption	Quantitative	No	[6]
Neural network/ genetic algorithm feature selection	Intestinal absorption	Quantitative	No	[7]
Naïve Bayesian classifier	Intestinal absorption (passive), blood–brain barrier penetration, serum protein binding	Classifier	No	[17]
Support vector machines (SVM)	Intestinal absorption	Quantitative	No	[18]
Kernel-based method directly working on chemical graph	Intestinal absorption	Quantitative	No	[5]

it is necessary to assert that all included values are derived from equivalent measurements. The absorption rate of a lead candidate across the intestinal epithelial cell barrier is often modeled using a Caco-2 cell line. Such a model includes both active and passive transport; however the experiment has a limited throughput. Parallel artificial membrane permeability assay (PAMPA), despite being limited to passive transport is often utilized as a cost-effective approach to model permeability.

Thus it is often advisable to train a model on the data derived by one experimental protocol only, which further limits the amount of training data. Because of this limitation of training data, it cannot be taken for granted that such models are globally valid. It is of particular interest to determine whether the prediction of a new test structure is still in the applicability domain of the model covered by the training data and whether the prediction can be expected to be reasonably accurate [15, 19, 20]. However, only very few models give this kind of information. It has also been pointed out that the value range covered in the training data of early models is often very large. For example, in aqueous solubility logS values between -12 and $+2$ yield a good overall correlation of the model with the training data. But the area of interest for drug discovery is often much smaller. Focusing on a narrower range (e.g., $-6 < \log S < -3$) reveals that the prediction accuracy of these models is often unsatisfactory [19].

2.2.2
Empirical Rules and Their Basis

Given the difficulties of developing global statistical models for ADME properties, it is understandable that simple empirical rules are used to predict drug-likeness and to filter unwanted compounds in the lead finding phase of drug discovery. The most prominent rule set is the "rule of five" of Lipinski [21] but other variants also exist. Such rules have been derived from the analysis of the properties of known drugs, or drug candidates which have been successfully developed into drugs. In contrast to models derived by machine learning, these rules typically use very few properties which are typically chemically intuitive and interpretable such as molecular weight. Certain properties like the octanol–water partition coefficient (logP) are derived from statistical models [9, 10]. However, the models used to calculate those properties are well established and are typically based on a wide range of chemotypes. During their history of practical application, their limitations and shortcomings have become well understood. Other properties like molecular polar surface area (PSA) are calculated properties. PSA as a property was originally derived from the 3D structure and is therefore a conformation dependent calculation. However, it has been shown that PSA can be calculated with almost no loss in accuracy from 2D fragment contributions by dividing the query molecule into substructures and adding up their individual contributions [22].

Reviewing these empirical rules on Table 2.2, it appears that two properties play an important role: logP and PSA. The relationship between PSA and intestinal absorption has been recognized for over a decade [27–29]. For intestinal absorption the compounds need to pass the cell membranes of the gut cells. If it is assumed that this happens by passive transport, then two possible rate limiting steps can be envisaged, namely the desolvation of the molecule when entering the membrane from the aqueous phase and secondly its diffusion through the membrane. In a study on pyridine derivatives, desolvation was shown to be the rate-limiting step [30]. This makes the influence of the PSA easily understandable: the more polar groups there are on the surface of the molecule, the more energy is needed for desolvation. Since H-bonding contributes to a large extent to solvation, the count of H-bond donors and acceptors (as used in Lipinski's rule of five) could also be understood as a descriptor of the cost for desolvation. In the calculation of PSA from fragments, Ertl *et al.* [22] suggested scaling the contributions of polar fragments by the strength of the H-bonds which they form. There is a general consensus that passive transport, the mechanism for which these empirical rules are valid, is for the majority of drugs the predominant mechanism for the membrane penetration [31], despite the claims of individual authors that the role of active transport has been underestimated so far [32].

The other term frequently occurring in such equations is the octanol–water partition coefficient, logP. It describes the lipophilicity of the compound. It is related to water solubility by Yalkowski's general solubility equation (GSE) [33, 34]:

$$\log S_W = 0.5 - 0.01(T_m - 298) - \log P \tag{2.1}$$

Table 2.2 Empirical rules used to predict drug-likeness.

Purpose	Name	Rule	Reference
Estimate whether a compound's absorption and membrane permeation is good enough to be orally bioavailable	Rule of five	At maximum one of the following conditions *may be* violated MW ≤ 500 Da ClogP ≤ 5 HBD ≤ 5 HBA ≤ 10	[21]
	Egan egg	Ellipse defined in the ClogP and PSA space	[23]
	Veber	PSA ≤ 140 Å² AND RTB ≤ 10	[24]
	ABS	Predominant charge state at physiological pH: Anionic: PSA < 150 Å² Non-anionic: according to the rule of five	[25]
Identify compounds which have the potential to be successful leads	Lead-likeness	MW ≤ 460 Da AND −4 ≤ C log P ≤ 4.2 AND Log S$_w$ ≥ −5 AND RTB ≤ 5 AND RNG ≤ 4 AND HBD ≤ 5 AND HBA ≤ 9	[26]

ClogP, computed logP (octanol–water partition coefficient of neutral species); HBA, number of H-bond acceptors; HBD, number of H-bond donors; MW, molecular weight; PSA, polar surface area; RNG, number of rings; RTB, number of rotatable bonds.

Where T_m is the melting point, used to describe the energy needed for breaking down the crystal lattice. The GSE is valid only for organic non-electrolytes. It includes some simplifying assumptions: The melting entropy for all organic compounds is an identical constant and the octanol–water distribution coefficient, logP, describes adequately the distribution of the compound between an "ideal solvent" with the same polarity of the compound and water. The cost to dissolve the crystal lattice is described by the term $0.01(T_m - 298)$. Even if the melting point, which is difficult to calculate, is not available, the logP value can be used to estimate the upper boundary for water solubility. logP itself can then be substituted by clogP, a predicted logP value calculated from fragment contributions [9, 10].

The most important shortcoming of GSE is that it is valid only for non-electrolytes, whereas many drug compounds and compounds in screening libraries are acidic or basic. In this case the solubility is pH-dependent. If one assumes for simplicity's sake that the ionized form is infinitely soluble in water, then the Henderson–Hasselbalch equation can be used to calculate the solubility at a given pH when the intrinsic solubility is known – which in turn could be estimated by the GSE.

$$\log S_{pH} = \log S_i + \log [1 + 10^{(pH-pKa)\delta i}] \quad \text{where } \delta i = 1 \text{ for acids and} \quad (2.2)$$
$$\delta i = -1 \text{ for bases}$$

This adds pKa prediction as an additional complication to the prediction of aqueous solubility. While there are numerous models to predict pKa [35–37], most of them rely on a "knowledge base" of known ionizable centers which are used to compute the pKa of these centers based on their chemical neighborhood. This usage of a knowledge base means that these prediction methods are not truly global and do not predict properly the ionization states and pKa of ionizable hetero-cycle or functional groups not included in the knowledgebase. Therefore, water solubility remains a challenging property to predict [38] and the usage of clogP as an estimator for it neglects important contributions.

Water solubility and membrane permeability are competing objectives: whereas membrane permeability requires that the energy required for desolvation is low, this contradicts the requirements for good water solubility, unless solubility is limited by high crystal lattice energy. The same is true for their related parameters clogP and PSA. These properties are becoming even more difficult to reconcile as molecular weight increases. ClogP is calculated by fragment contribution and is determined by the ratio of lipophilic versus hydrophilic fragments – with lipophilic fragments giving positive contributions and hydrophilic fragments giving negative contributions. Lowering clogP by adding solubilizing groups increases the PSA, which is calculated as the sum of contributions from polar fragments. In turn, lowering clogP by removing lipophilic fragments does not affect PSA – to which lipophilic fragments do not contribute – but means that the molecule becomes smaller. Thus, a requirement for low clogP and low PSA also implies a constraint on the molecular weight. Therefore the requirement for low clogP and PSA at the same time biases the library towards low molecular weight compounds. Since the probability of finding compounds in random screening is expected to be higher (more promiscuous) when smaller molecules are screened [39], and the space of small molecules can be more efficiently sampled than the space of larger molecules [26], this bias is also beneficial for the probability of identifying hits in the absence of prior knowledge.

2.2.3
Drug-Likeness of Natural Products

Drug-likeness is a self-fulfilling prophecy where medicinal chemists are expected to design and synthesize compounds that comply with drug-like rules during lead optimization. These compounds are later added to the HTS deck and assayed in future projects. As a result, the screening collection evolve to be drug-like. Compounds outside the drug-like space, namely natural products such as cyclosporine

(1202 Da) would not be discovered by HTS. Natural products may have a higher molecular weight and be more complex (e.g., more chiral centers) although this is not always the case and many natural products are in fact drug-like [40]. Many biopharmaceutical companies do value natural products which, unlike synthetic compounds, were optimized during the course of evolution. Natural products explore parts of chemical space that synthetic drug-like compounds do not essentially cover and, for example, can serve as an excellent source for novel antibiotics. Many antibiotics target complex and essential machinery in bacterial cells, such as protein synthesis, nucleic acid replication and cell wall synthesis. The bacteria cannot easily modify or bypass this machinery to develop resistance. Complex molecules such as natural products are often needed to inhibit such complex targets. For example, vancomycin (1449 Da) – the cell wall synthesis inhibitor in Gram-positive bacteria is a complex molecule with 18 chiral centers. Due to its size and hydrophilicity vancomycin creates a five-point H-bond interaction with N-acetylmuramic acid (NAM)- and N-acetylglucosamine (NAG)-peptide subunits. This interaction inhibits the incorporation of the NAM/NAG-peptide subunits into the cell wall. Neomycine (615 Da; five chiral centers) binds to different complex machinery, the 30S subunit of the bacterial ribosome and 16S rRNA, interrupting protein synthesis. In a recent review by GSK scientists, [41] the authors described more than 70 unsuccessful high-throughput screening campaigns against antibacterial targets using a standard "drug-like" screening deck. Indeed, the optimal starting point for an antibacterial drug may be a novel natural product and not a traditional HTS on a "drug-like" screening deck. A recent paper [42] contains a useful analysis of the physicochemical properties of antibacterial compounds and clearly demonstrates that general empirical rules such as Lipinski's rule of five do not apply here. The authors identified substantial differences between compounds with Gram-positive activity, Gram-negative activity, and non-antibacterial drugs. Average molecular weights are usually higher for antibacterials than drug-like compounds, especially for the group with Gram-positive activity such as azithromycin (749 Da) and polymyxin B1 (1203 Da). Antibacterial compounds are also more polar. The average logP value for Gram-negative antibacterials is more than four log units lower (more hydrophilic) compared to the compounds in the comprehensive medicinal chemistry (CMC) database. Similarly, the number of H-donors and acceptors, and relative PSA all render the antibacterial drugs more hydrophilic. This does not mean that the oral bioavailability of such natural product drugs is necessarily high, but the high potency such natural product drugs often have means that only a relatively low plasma concentration level needs to be maintained, and thus a relatively low bioavailability is tolerable. It has also been hypothesized that in the more complex natural product molecules the PSA calculated by additive group contributions might not be any more predictive for the desolvation energy, since these molecules might adopt for the purpose of membrane penetration conformations with intra-molecular H-bonds. These conformations would then have a lower desolvation energy than predicted with a simple additive model which assumes that all H-bond donors and acceptors are exposed to the solvent [43].

2.2.4
Do Ligands of Different Target Classes Differ in Their Drug-Like Properties?

An analysis of the properties of ligands by target family showed that the ligands differ in molecular weight and clogP [44]. The target families included in this study were: protein kinases, peptide GPCRs, aminergic GPCRs, nuclear hormone receptors, serine proteases, metalloproteases, phosphodieterases and ligand-gated ion channels. With the GPCR peptide ligands, protein–protein interactions are also partially covered in this analysis. GPCR peptide ligands have a higher molecular weight than the other activity classes. Whereas in the other classes a molecular weight limit of 600 covered at least 90% of the ligands, in peptide GPCRs this molecular weight limit was 750. The nuclear receptor activity class included the most lipophilic ligands. More specifically, the clogP values for nuclear receptor binders covered 90% at an upper clogP limit of 7.5, and for all classes except peptide GPCR, 90% of the ligands were covered at a clogP upper limit of about 6.0. This trend may be explained by the high lipophilicity of the endogenous nuclear receptor binders. Unlike the GPCRs, which are on the surface of the cell, the nuclear receptor binders must pass through cell membranes. The rule of five limit of ≤ 10 H-bond acceptors was satisfied by 90% of the ligands for each class, and the same was true for the criterion of ≤ 5 H-bond donors, where the peptide GPCRs are the only exception with a limit of 7 H-bond donors covering 90% of the ligands. In general, if a binding pocket is rather shallow, such as in the case of protein–protein interactions, it can be expected that large ligands are necessary to make enough attractive interactions to generate the required binding compared to the case where smaller ligands are often sufficient for deeper binding pockets.

2.2.5
Unwanted Structural Elements

Substructure filtering is a way to address problems caused by chemical reactivity, which is often related to well defined functional groups such as Michael acceptors, epoxides and acid chlorides [45]. Chemical reactivity often causes low stability – especially when stored as a solution over long periods of time – and hence causes technology compatibility problems. At the same time some toxic effects are related to chemical reactivity. Most important here is the reactivity towards DNA which may cause mutagenicity of the compound. Several sets of non-drug-like substructures have been published and they show a large degree of overlap [45, 46]. When implementing substructure filters based on structural elements shown in these papers, care needs to be taken to formulate the substructure query in a way that does not exclude substructures not originally intended. Typically this requires the use of advanced query features such as those defined in the MDLmolfile standard, or SMARTS. When using a substructure filtering tool, it must be verified that this tool correctly implements the set of query features which were intended. Problems can especially occur in the interpretation of aromaticity, which varies significantly between different chemoinformatics tools. For the prediction of individual toxicological endpoints there exist specific software packages. An example of this is DEREK [47], which not only provides a substructure alert, but also background information about liable compounds triggering the alerts and the literature references responsible for the alert.

Since the formulation of precise and well defined substructure queries is not trivial, other approaches to identify unwanted substructures are used as well. If the decisions made by medicinal chemists whether to accept or reject individual screening hits based on purely structural criteria has been captured, this can be used to train a statistical model predicting medicinal chemists' judgment on chemical structures. The consensus among medicinal chemists has been demonstrated to be limited [48]. Therefore, this exercise must be based on the decision of a larger group of chemists in order not to bias the model towards the preferences of any individual chemist. In a similar way such models can be trained on experimental toxicity data for an individual experimentally determined toxicological endpoint. An example of commercial software for using such models for toxicity prediction is MULTICASE [49].

In contrast to toxicity caused by chemical reactivity that may be non-target-specific, other toxic effects are caused by an off-target effect, namely the undesirable interaction between the compound and an unintended target. A good example is the hERG (human ether-a-go-go related gene) channel. Blocking this potassium channel can lead to fatal cardiac arrhythmia. This type of toxicity cannot be reliably predicted with substructure filters. Although there is usually a basic amine and an aromatic group present in hERG blockers, it is not possible to attribute the activity to a more specific substructure. Pharmacophore-based models have usually a higher predictivity [50]. Difficulty in defining a precise substructure also arises with the cytochrome P450 superfamily, which oxidizes a plethora of both exogenous and endogenous compounds.

2.3
What is the Best Practice in Utilizing Drug-Likeness in Drug Discovery?

Filters for drug-likeness can be applied at several stages of lead discovery:

1. Before synthesis or acquisition of the compound.
2. Before inclusion of an existing compound in a focused screening set for an individual target.
3. After the HTS primary screening but before cherry picking (individually selecting) compounds for dose–response measurements.
4. During the validation of the HTS hits in secondary assays.

The question that needs to be addressed is at what stage is filtering for drug-likeness truly beneficial and how should the filters be used? In early lead discovery there are some specific requirements regarding the predictive models used. Since they should be applied to many compounds, their application must be reasonably fast. This typically excludes all models involving pharmacophore matching, force field calculations or higher levels of complexity. It is mandatory that the calculation can be executed in a batch mode or precomputed and stored in a database without being tied to graphical user interface. The model output is required to support filtering – typically one single number or a yes/no flag. More complex information will usually not be used. As the purpose is filtering alone, the tradeoff – that some of the models may be less intuitive and the results are not easily interpretable – may be tolerated. Models need to be as global as possible, since the aim of lead discovery is to discover active compounds in new areas of the chemistry space.

Synthesizing libraries or purchasing compounds to enhance a screening collection is a costly endeavor. For each library synthesized, resources are consumed that are not then available for other activities (opportunity costs). The question as to whether there are enough interesting drug-like compounds to build up a diverse, non-redundant screening collection can clearly be answered with yes, as the size of the likely available chemistry space is vast [51]. However, if one intends to purchase screening compounds from enumerated catalogs alone, then the choices of what is available off the shelf seems to be limited. Over time though, vendors have learned to adapt themselves to the requirements of their regular customers and are starting to offer more drug-like compounds. Since some target families require larger or more lipophilic compounds, care must be taken not to apply drug-likeness filters too rigorously at this stage, especially for compounds designed as ligands for antibacterial projects, targets involving protein–protein interactions or nuclear hormone receptors, where exceptions need to be made. If a library is actively designed and synthesized or compounds are searched in a database for a specific target or target family, it is recommended to incorporate relaxed rules for such compounds, leaving the strict rules in place for diversity-based selections without a specific anticipated target.

Ideally it would be desirable to define the selection criteria for each primary screen individually based on the knowledge about the target class and the required lead criteria. In such a scenario the screening costs for compounds not appropriate for a particular target would be saved. However, the logistics effort to individually assemble screening sets in this way is high. A typical practice is to screen the full deck and then apply filtering after the primary screening. After the primary HTS, compounds with significant activity are cherry-picked for confirmation assays and dose response curve measurement as well as for chemical analytics to verify the integrity and chemical identity of the screening solution. This is a decision point at which drug-likeness filters customized to the specific target could be applied. Removing unwanted compounds at this step does not only save costs for dose–response curve measurement, but also reduces the load on cherry picking and chemical analytics systems. Compounds with other liabilities that the substructure filters did not capture are somewhat tolerated in early lead discovery (HTS), where the throughput of the assays is generally high. In contrast, removal of an attractive compound is unacceptable (a potential missed opportunity, such as a viable starting point for a chemistry program). In HTS primary hit list triaging, the outcome of the HTS is still unknown. It is difficult to predict the specificity, selectivity and the potency of the hits. There is a limitation on the number of compounds that could be followed up in secondary assays and biophysical measurements. Therefore, the objective at this stage is to *balance* the number of hits and their quality. For less tractable targets (e.g., protein–protein interactions) it is acceptable to lower the bar and cherry pick non-drug-like compounds. However, for targets where hit finding is easier (e.g., kinases) the bar should be raised, and compounds with liabilities should be deprioritized. Drug-likeness criteria have to be more stringent in the later stages of drug discovery, namely during lead optimization where synthesizing compounds is a costly endeavor, and should be based on experimental data obtained for the chemical series studied. At that stage drug-likeness is used to guide the medicinal chemistry efforts in solving certain liabilities associated with the chemical series at hand, such as hERG or cytochrome P450 inhibition. In contrast to the requirement for global models in the hit-finding stage, local models limited to a few chemical series of interest are perfectly acceptable at the lead optimization stage.

2.4 Concluding Discussions

As we have shown above, it is not trivial to set up drug-likeness filtering rules that are globally valid for chemical structures and all targets. However the application of clogP, PSA and molecular weight filters are synergistically beneficial for technology compatibility, the probability of ligands to match the target and bias towards an oral bioavailability. Therefore, the application of such filters during the assembly of the screening collection is generally recommended, provided the flexibility to relax or even waive such filtering criteria for compounds designed or selected for targets with special ligand requirements is retained. If more elaborated statistical models are used to identify compounds with low solubility, low permeability or toxicity, it is necessary to be aware of the applicability domain of such models. They are helpful in detecting structural elements known to be associated with unwanted properties, but should not be expected to be globally valid. Whenever possible, models giving an estimate of the reliability of the prediction, together with predicted property values or class, should be preferred, and structures where the prediction is indicated to have low reliability should be given the benefit of doubt.

Abbreviations

ADME	Absorption, distribution, metabolism and excretion
BCS	Biopharmaceutical classification system
clogP	Calculated octanol water partition coefficient
GPCR	G Protein-cooupled receptor
GSE	Yalkowski's general solubility equation
hERG	Human ether-a-go-go related gene
HTS	High-throughput screening

MDLmolfile   Standardized file format for chemical structures including substructure query features (initially defined by Molecular Design Ltd)
PSA   Polar surface area
SMARTS   Substructure query language (developed by Daylight Inc.)

References

1 Davies, J.W., Glick, M. and Jenkins, J.L. (2006) Streamlining lead discovery by aligning in silico and high-throughput screening. *Current Opinion in Chemical Biology*, **10**, 343–351.

2 McGovern, S.L., Helfand, B.T., Feng, B. and Shoichet, B.K. (2003) A Specific Mechanism of Nonspecific Inhibition. *Journal of Medicinal Chemistry*, **46**, 4265–4272.

3 Gleeson, M.P. (2008) Generation of a set of simple, interpretable ADMET rules of thumb. *Journal of Medicinal Chemistry*, **51**, 817–834.

4 Hastie, T., Tibshirani, I. and Friedman, J.R. (eds) (2003) *The elements of statistical learning*, 3rd edn, Springer, Berlin. ISBN 978-0387952840.

5 Froehlich, H., Wegner, J.K., Sieker, F. and Zell, A. (2006) Kernel functions for attributed molecular graphs – a new similarity-based approach to ADME prediction in classification and regression. *QSAR Combinatorial Science*, **25**, 317–326.

6 Gunturi, S.B. and Narayanan, R. (2007) In Silico ADME Modeling 3: Computational Models to Predict Human Intestinal Absorption Using Sphere Exclusion and kNN QSAR Methods. *QSAR Combinatorial Science*, **5**, 653–668.

7 Wessel, M.D., Jurs, P.C., Tolan, J.W. and Muskal, S.M. (1998) Prediction of human intestinal absorption of drug compounds from molecular structure. *Journal of Chemical Information and Computer Sciences*, **38**, 726–735.

8 Wegener, J.K. and Zell, A. (2003) Prediction of aqueous solubility and partition coefficient optimized by a genetic algorithm based descriptor selection method. *Journal of Chemical Information and Computer Sciences*, **43**, 1077–1084.

9 Leo, A.J. (1993) Calculating log Poct from structures. *Chemical Reviews*, **93**, 1281–1306.

10 Ghose, A.K., Viswanadhan, V.N. and Wendoloski, J.J. (1998) Prediction of hydrophobic (lipophilic) properties of small organic molecules using fragmental methods: An analysis of AlogP and ClogP methods. *Journal of Physical Chemistry A*, **102**, 3762–3772.

11 Bergström, C.A.S., Wassvik, C.M., Norinder, U., Luthman, K. and Artursson, P. (2004) Global and local computational models for aqueous solubility: Prediction of drug-like molecules. *Journal of Chemical Information and Computer Sciences*, **44**, 1477–1488.

12 Huuskonen, J. (2000) Estimation of aequeous solubility for a diverse set of organic compounds based on molecular topology. *Journal of Chemical Information and Computer Sciences*, **40**, 773–777.

13 Tetko, I.V. and Tanchuk, V.Y. (2002) Application of associative neuronal networks for the prediction of Lipophilicity in ALOGPS 2.1 program. *Journal of Chemical Information and Computer Sciences*, **42**, 1136–1145.

14 Tetko, I.V. and Poda, G.I. (2004) Application of ALOGPS 2.1 to predict logD distribution coefficients for Pfizer proprietary compounds. *Journal of Medicinal Chemistry*, **47**, 5601–5604.

15 Tetko, I.V., Bruneau, P., Mewes, H.-W., Rohrer, D.C. and Poda, G.I. (2006) Can we estimate the accuracy of ADME-Tox predictions? *Drug Discovery Today*, **11**, 700–707.

16 Hou, T., Wang, J., Zhan, W. and Xu, X. (2007) ADME Evaluation in drug discovery 7. Prediction of oral absorption by correlation and classification. *Journal of Chemical Information and Modeling*, **47**, 208–218.

17 Klon, A.E., Lowrie, J.F. and Diller, D.J. (2006) Improved naive Bayesian modeling of numerical data for absorption, distribution, metabolism and excretion (ADME) property prediction. *Journal of Chemical Information and Modeling*, **46**, 1945–1956.

18 Liu, H.X., Hu, R.J., Zhang, R.S., Yao, X.J., Liu, M.C., Hu, Z.D. and Fan, B.T. (2005) *Journal of Computer-Aided Molecular Design*, **19**, 33–46.

19 Norinder, U. (2006) Bergström CAS prediction of ADMET properties. *ChemMedChem*, **1**, 920–937.

20 Weaver, S. and Gleeson, M.P. (2008) The importance of the domain of applicability in QSAR modeling. *Journal of Molecular Graphics & Modelling*, **26**, 1315.

21 Lipinski, C.A., Lombardo, F., Dominy, B.W. and Feeney, P.J. (1997) Experimental and computational approaches to estimate solubility and permeability in drug discovery and development settings. *Advanced Drug Delivery Reviews*, **23**, 3–25.

22 Ertl, P., Rohde, B. and Selzer, P. (2000) Fast calculation of molecular polar surface area as a sum of fragment-based contributions and its application to the prediction of drug transport properties. *Journal of Medicinal Chemistry*, **43**, 3714–3717.

23 Egan, W.J., Merz, K.M. and Baldwin, J.J. (2000) Prediction of drug absorption using multivariate statistics. *Journal of Medicinal Chemistry*, **43**, 3867–3877.

24 Veber, D.F., Johnson, S.R., Cheng, H.-Y., Smith, B.R., Ward, K.W. and Kopple, K.D. (2002) Molecular properties that influence the oral bioavailability of drug candidates. *Journal of Medicinal Chemistry*, **45**, 2615–2623.

25 Martin, Y.C. (2005) A bioavailability score. *Journal of Medicinal Chemistry*, **48**, 3164–3170.

26 Hann, M.M. and Oprea, T.I. (2004) Pursuing the leadlikeness concept in pharmaceutical research. *Current Opinion in Chemical Biology*, **8**, 255–263.

27 Van der Waterbeemd, H., Smith, D.A., Beaumont, K. and Walker, D.K. (2001) Property-based design: optimization of drug absorption and pharmacokinetics. *Journal of Medicinal Chemistry*, **44**, 1313–1333.

28 Palm, K., Luthman, K., Ungell, A.L., Strandlund, G., Beigi, F., Lundahl, P. and Artursson, P. (1998) Evaluation of dynamic polar molecular surface area as predictor of drug absorption: comparison with other computational and experimental predictors. *Journal of Medicinal Chemistry*, **41**, 5382–5392.

29 Clark, D.E. (1999) Rapid calculation of polar molecular surface area and its application to the prediction of transport phenomena. 1. Prediction of intestinal absorption. *Journal of Pharmaceutical Sciences*, **88**, 807–814.

30 Chen, I.J., Taneja, R., Yin, D., Seo, P.R., Young, D., MacKerell, A.D. and Polli, J.E. (2006) Chemical substituent effect on pyridine permeability and mechanistic insight from computational molecular descriptors. *Molecular Pharmacology*, **3**, 745–755.

31 Avdeef, A., Artursson, P., Bendels, S., Di, L., Ecker, G.F., Faller, B., Fischer, H., Gerebtzoff, G., Kansy, M., Lennernaes, H., Senner, F. and Sugano, K. (2009) Coexistence of passive and active carrier-mediated uptake processes in drug transport: a more balanced view, in press.

32 Dobson, P.D. and Kell, D.B. (2008) Carrier-mediated cellular uptake of pharmaceutical drugs: an exception or the rule? *Nature Reviews. Drug Discovery*, **7**, 205–220.

33 Ran, Y. and Yalkowsky, S.H. (2001) Prediction of drug solubility by the general solubility equation (GSE). *Journal of Chemical Information and Computer Sciences*, **41**, 354–357.

34 Jain, N. and Yalkowski, S.H. (2001) Estimation of aqueous solubility I: Application to organic nonelectrolytes. *Journal of Pharmaceutical Sciences*, **90**, 234–252.

35 Jelfs, S., Ertl, P. and Selzer, P. (2007) Estimation of pKa for drug-like compounds using semiempirical and information-based descriptors. *Journal of Chemical Information and Modeling*, **47**, 450–459.

36 Shelley, J.C., Cholleti, A., Frye, L.L., Greenwood, J.R., Timlin, M.R. and Uchimaya, M. (2007) Epik: a software program for pKa prediction and protonation state generation for drug-like molecules. *Journal of Computer-Aided Molecular Design*, **21**, 681–691.

37 Milletti, F., Storchi, L., Sforna, G. and Cruciani, G. (2007) New and original pKa prediction method using grid molecular interaction fields. *Journal of Chemical Information and Modeling*, **47**, 2172–2181.

38 Delaney, J.S. (2005) Predicting aqueous solubility from structure. *Drug Discovery Today*, **10**, 289–295.

39 Hann, M.M., Leach, A.R. and Harper, G. (2001) Molecular complexity and its impact on the probability of finding leads for drug discovery. *Journal of Chemical Information and Computer Sciences*, **41**, 856–864.

40 Ertl, P., Roggo, S. and Schuffenhauer, A. (2008) Natural product-likeness score and its application for prioritization of compound libraries. *Journal of Chemical Information and Modeling*, **48**, 68–74.

41 Payne, D.J., Gwynn, M.N., Holmes, D.J. and Pompliano, D.L. (2007) Drugs for bad bugs: confronting the challenges of antibacterial discovery. *Nature Reviews. Drug Discovery*, **6**, 29–40.

42 O'Shea, R. and Moser, H.E. (2008) Physicochemical properties of antibacterial compounds: implications for drug discovery. *Journal of Medicinal Chemistry*, **51**, 2871–2878.

43 Ganesan, A. (2008) The impact of natural products upon modern drug discovery. *Current Opinion in Chemical Biology*, **12**, 306–317.

44 Paolini, G.V., Shapland, R.H.B., van Hoorn, W.P., Mason, J.S. and Hopkins, A.L. (2006) Global mapping of pharmacological space. *Nature Biotechnology*, **24**, 805–815.

45 Rishton, G.M. (2002) Nonleadlikeness and leadlikeness in biochemical screening. *Drug Discovery Today*, **8**, 86–96.

46 Charifson, P.S. and Walters, W.P. (2002) Filtering databases and chemical libraries. *Journal of Computer-Aided Molecular Design*, **16**, 311–323.

47 Greene, N., Judson, P.N., Langowski, J.J. and Marchant, C.A. (1999) Knowledge-based expert systems for toxicity and metabolism prediction: DEREK, StAR and METEOR. *SAR and QSAR in Environmental Research*, **10**, 299–314.

48 Lajiness, M.S., Maggiora, G.M. and Shanmugasundaram, V. (2004) Assessment of the consistency of medicinal chemists in reviewing sets of compounds. *Journal of Medicinal Chemistry*, **47**, 4891–4896.

49 Rosenkranz, H.S. (2003) SAR in the assessment of carcinogenesis: the MultiCASE approach. *QSAR*, **2003**, 175–206.

50 Thai, K.-M. and Ecker, G.F. (2007) Predictive models for hERG channel blockers: ligand-based and structure-based approaches. *Current Medicinal Chemistry*, **14**, 3003–3026.

51 Fink, T. and Reymond, J.-L. (2007) Virtual exploration of the chemical universe up to 11 atoms of C, N, O, F: assembly of 26.4 million structures (110.9 million stereoisomers) and analysis for new ring systems, stereochemistry, physicochemical properties, compound classes, and drug discovery. *Journal of Chemical Information and Computer Sciences*, **47**, 342–353.

3
Integrative Risk Assessment
Bernard Faller and Laszlo Urban

3.1
The Target Compound Profile

3.1.1
Introduction

One of the most important elements in drug discovery is to design a target compound profile (TCP) for a particular clinical indication. In addition to target validation, drug discovery teams consider drug-like properties which ensure efficacious exposure at the expected site of action without any major safety issues for the patients (safety profiling plan). Thus, the definition of the TCP is essential for the design of a meaningful flowchart for a drug discovery project. The TCP is impacted by factors linked to the target itself (i.e., peripheral vs. central), the type/class of chemical structure, the projected therapeutic dose, the route of administration, metabolism, the likelihood of co-medications and the potential on- and off-target side effects which can be anticipated even at early stages of the project. Most of these factors also need to be balanced with respect to the medical value of the treatment or severity of the disease.

Optimization of pharmacokinetics, addressing metabolism and drug–drug interactions are now integrated into very early phases of drug discovery [1, 2]. This requires teams of scientists with diverse skills, ranging from theoretical chemistry to medical expertise. While this is complex enough, one has to take into consideration the performance of competitor compounds designed for the same target or disease, social aspects such as administering the medicine in an institutionalized environment or in outpatient care.

The focus of this book is on methods and processes designed to predict drug-like properties, exposure and safety during hit and lead discovery. We do not intend to cover specific cultural considerations and marketing aspects [3]. What we will highlight is the need of a "risk aware" environment for drug discovery, where data-based integrated risk assessment is part of daily life of the team and drives the projects towards molecules with features fit for the description of an efficacious and safe medicine.

Hit and Lead Profiling. Edited by Bernard Faller and Laszlo Urban
Copyright © 2009 WILEY-VCH Verlag GmbH & Co. KGaA, Weinheim
ISBN: 978-3-527-32331-9

When we talked with a new generation of medicinal chemists, fresh out of college and asked them about their "dream drug", they enthusiastically described wonderful orally available molecules, extremely potent at the target, once daily dose, no side effects, certainly blockbusters. When we talked about how to avoid compounds with poor solubility and poor permeability or how to optimize such molecules, they were sure that this was not going to be a major issue. Still, we lose a lot of molecules during late phases of drug discovery because difficult BCS class III–IV compounds cannot be evaluated for a safe therapeutic index (TI) due to inadequate exposure. Is this due to poor planning or is this the result of unfounded optimism, based on a previous culture of "high potency rules" philosophy?

The same group of chemists were asked to look at the side effect profile (*in vitro* data) of an, to them unknown, successful anticancer drug (we took out hair loss, just to make the indication less obvious). The majority guessed that this was a failed compound, with horrendous side effects, which should not be allowed into the clinic. This example shows how scientists look at adverse effects in early drug discovery. We tend to be more risk aversive rather than risk aware. No medicine is absolutely safe, side effects are common and should be well managed. We have to learn to take risk and measure the risk–benefit ratio during drug development to be able to compete and develop more and more efficacious medicines. The important thing is that we take the right risk and calculate the benefit, based on integrated analysis and interpretation of data. In a simple way, profiling of compounds along the rough route of drug discovery is to interpret "the right data at the right time".

In this chapter we make a humble attempt to explain how one might achieve this objective.

3.1.2
The Importance of the Projected Clinical Compound Profile in Early Drug Discovery

There is rarely a case where a disease can be managed or cured by affecting a single and only target. Blocking the function of a protein could have a significant effect on a whole pathway while inhibiting its neighbors might produce no or minor change due to redundancy or compensatory mechanisms. Furthermore, diseases could involve multiple proteins in different pathways differently expressed in various tissues and organs, thus the same target involved in the generation of pain in a dorsal root ganglion might be responsible for a rate limiting or life-threatening adverse effect in the heart. No wonder that "well defined" targets often fail during clinical trials and the pharmaceutical industry lose an estimated 30–45% of compounds due to lack of efficacy [4] partly because a poor or nonexistent therapeutic index (TI) does not allow to reach efficacious concentration. Thus, selection of a good target for a disease is crucial for any drug discovery project. Knowledge of human pathophysiology and genetic background of certain diseases are essential, but not enough. To start with, the project team has to look into possible on-target adverse reactions. For example, all calcium channel inhibitors cause dizziness to various degrees [5]. While this might not be a major roadblock for development, selecting a different target for hypertension devoid of this side effect might create an advantage in the clinic. Difficult targets, such as those

Table 3.1 Dependence of the target compound profile (TCP) on minimum solubility at neutral pH for an oral agent.

Oral dose (mg/kg)	Permeability		
	High	Medium	Low
0.1	0.001	0.005	0.02
1	0.01	0.05	0.2
10	0.1	0.5	2

Numerical values represent minimum required equilibrium solubility (g/L) of the agent under various permeability conditions and dosing regimen. (Adapted from Lipinski [14].)

interfering with protein–protein interactions require unconventional resources, extended timelines and carry a higher degree of risk for successful completion [6, 7].

Once the target is selected and agreed, the project team needs to explore requirements for the specific disease area: medical need versus possible adverse effects, preferred dosing regimen, route of administration and target patient population.

At the beginning of the project, it is often difficult to have a precise idea of the projected therapeutic dose. Projects usually start with an estimated average potency of 1 mg/kg, once daily dose as an optimal approach. When initial pharmacokinetic/pharmacodynamic (PK/PD) data becomes available one can better refine the TCP. Table 3.1 gives some guidelines on how to adjust the solubility requirement depending on the therapeutic dose and compound permeability.

The efficacious plasma or tissue concentration largely defines the course of ADME optimization. Pharmacokinetic features have a significant impact on safety. Off-target effects often limit the use of efficacious doses, as they make safety margins too narrow. Thus, the combination of PK characteristics and off-target activities are largely responsible for an acceptable TI.

It is also important to define the expected clinical profile with present or expected competitors in mind. Compounds with inferior PK and/or pharmacokinetics in comparison to marketed drugs certainly do not have much chance of market capitalization. There is a strong belief that first to the clinic gives a clear competitive edge and ensures success. However, analysis of competitor performance revealed that the case is more complex and depending on the circumstances, follow-up drugs can take over those first in market. Cohen [3] suggested that "... sustained growth of treatment-eligible population, quality-dominant (homogeneous) consumer expectations of product and exploitable quality deficiencies of early entrants ..." can be considered when planning innovation strategies to maximize the return on investment of late entrants.

3.1.3
The Impact of Delivery On the Design of the Drug Discovery Process

Most compounds are designed for single (acute) or regular (chronic) oral application with a well defined route of absorption within the GI tract and with a consideration of first pass metabolism in the liver. Absorption and hepatic metabolism will play a very important role in the plasma level for all of these molecules. Therefore optimization for these parameters is required at the earliest possible phase of drug discovery. *In vitro* profiling assays which can help predict absorption and metabolic stability are broadly used in pharmaceutical industry [8, 9].

While oral administration is by far the preferred route of administration, other routes can also be considered and in some cases provide advantage over the oral route. For example, topical application is attractive for highly potent compounds and/or if the target is in the skin. This route of administration largely reduces the impact of metabolism (no first pass) and usually improves the side effect profile. One such case is Exelon (rivastigmine), which in a formulation of a slow-release transdermal patch that ensures steady supply of the active ingredient, diminishes side effects and greatly improves compliance of patients suffering from mild or moderate Alzheimer's disease [10].

There are special conditions such as septic shock or stroke, when the time window for successful intervention is very narrow and quick effect is needed. Considering the general condition of these patients, the preferred route of administration in the emergency situation is parenteral. Bolus injections carry the danger of very high C_{max}, which might create safety issues. In addition, when the target is in the central nervous system (e.g., stroke), one needs to address blood–brain barrier (BBB) penetration. These requirements have a significant effect on the way drug discovery projects address specific parameters which determine the right pharmacokinetic profile.

Severe, life-threatening diseases, such as cancer require a different drug discovery approach. Safety requirements in most oncology targets tolerate more side effects, which otherwise would severely limit the use of a medicine in other indications. For example, in addition to hair loss, a common side effect of cancer treatment, compounds which affect cell cycle, cell proliferation and apoptosis pathways also cause other serious side effects and make the patient endure severe adverse drug reactions (ADRs).

Another important consideration associated with specific diseases is co-morbidity, which often complicates chronic diseases such as diabetes or congestive cardiac disease. For example, medicines which could be perfectly safe in the early phase of type II diabetes could cause serious side effects if nephropathy develops. This could be the consequence of the impaired route of elimination or by direct effect on the damaged kidney.

Equally important is to determine the target patient population, for example, sex, age or race, as it could have significant influence on the design of drugs. Some genetic disorders are associated with ethnic groups (e.g., Gaucher disease) which could predispose for decreased tolerance of certain drugs (particularly if liver enzymes are affected in hereditary diseases).

Polymorphism also adds more variability to safety margins. Polymorphism of CYP enzymes is particularly important as it may have a profound effect on the pharmacokinetic features of a drug. For example, the benzodiazepine etizolam is almost exclusively metabolized by CYP2C19 and its deficiency could lead to toxicity [11].

A number of parameters need to be adjusted depending on the target location, route of administration and expected dose. Let us take the case of compounds for central nervous system (CNS) targets which need to cross the blood–brain barrier. As this is usually achieved by trans-cellular passive diffusion, CNS-penetrating compounds are relatively lipophilic, characterized by logP values in the range of 3–6 as opposed to 1–3 for peripherally acting compounds. The blood–brain barrier is not only a physical but also a biochemical barrier which is able to efflux compounds out of the brain tissue. The best known efflux transporter is the P-glycoprotein. While efflux is an obstacle in the development of CNS drugs it can also be used to eliminate side effects. One example is the antidiarrheral compound loperamide (an opioid) for which CNS-related adverse effects (e.g., sedation, dependence) are removed as the compound is effectively "effluxed" from the brain [12]. Sedation associated with the first generation of anti-histaminic compounds (diphenhydramine, hydroxyzine) has been removed with the development of compounds that do not penetrate into the brain (i.e., fexofenadine) due to a lower permeability and/or efflux mechanism [13].

Plasma protein binding has an impact on drug distribution which can significantly influence efficacy and safety profile. High plasma protein binding typically reduces the volume of distribution and this feature may or may not be desired depending on the nature of the target. Human serum albumin binding is driven by lipophilicity and the acidic/basic nature of the compound (acids are significantly more tightly bound at equal lipophilicity). Their generally poor permeability at neutral pH explains why there are very few acids successfully developed for central targets. Drug distribution properties are further affected by transporters, in particular for compounds characterized by a low passive permeability (see Section 3.3).

There are many more examples for specific considerations in various disease conditions and patient population. However, the examples above highlight sufficiently the influence of medical indication on drug design and the many elements of risks to be considered at the beginning of the drug discovery process.

3.2
The Concept of Hierarchical Testing in Primary and Follow-Up Assays

As demonstrated above, there is a large and diverse array of issues which one needs to address during drug discovery. The question is where to start? What should drug discovery teams look at first? Is there a general recipe or should one use diagnostic tools to define testing priorities? First, we need to take account of the most important, basic elements of drug discovery and define associated tools and assays to address them. We can divide these roughly into two areas: ADME (exposure) and safety aspects.

It is easy to understand that one cannot profile each synthesized compound for all characteristics within the frame of a parallel process accomplished for every synthetic cycle. This approach would be neither economically viable nor a large fraction of the data used for decision making. However, a fully customized approach would make each individual study relatively expensive and to great extent incompatible with short cycle times. One way to capitalize on the strengths of both approaches is to define assay packages which are suited for testing less optimized compounds, but fit the early objective: "get to know your scaffold".

A profiling package can be defined as a group of assays which run at the same stage of drug discovery and which together address a common scientific question. For example, a primary absorption package includes solubility, passive permeability and oxidative metabolism assays. A parallel, early safety package might check for the frequency and potency of hERG inhibition, basic mutagenic potential and general cytotoxicity. A more detailed view on this package is given in Table 3.2.

Let us take the exposure packages as an example: technically, most of these assays are highly automated, require small amount of compounds and have a brief cycle time. Scientifically, they fulfill requirements to predict exposure by addressing the three major contributing factors: solubility, passive permeability and metabolic (hepatic) clearance. These type of packages are ideal to explore or diagnose scaffold characteristics and define project flowcharts. They can be used repeatedly to test newly synthesized compounds and guide SAR. A number of compounds within a

Table 3.2 The concept of hierarchical testing.

	Exposure	Safety
Primary Broad profiling to annotate risk	Absorption package Solubility in buffer medium Passive permeability Phase I metabolism in PK species	hERG RLB (cardiac) micro-Ames (genotoxicity) cytotoxicity profile
Secondary Advanced compounds only refined analysis	Active transports and efflux Phase I metabolism in additional species CYP-450 inhibition CYP-450 inactivation pKa/logP Solubility pH-profile	hERG patch clamp Nav1.5 Cav1.2 KCNQ In vitro safety pharmacology Micronucleus test Organ-specific toxicity Phototoxicity
Tertiary Hypothesis testing Requires in-vivo data	Plasma protein binding Plasma stability Biliary excretion Phase II metablolism	hERG trafficking Isolated heart (Langendorf) Purkinje fibre assay In vivo safety pharmacology

A simplified view on the introduction of profiling assays as compounds progress through drug discovery. Primary assays are usually used during lead selection and lead optimization, while more complex assays might be limited to later phase profiling. This scheme works only when (1) assays have a high predictive value for the downstream tests and (2) primary assays address the most frequent liabilities.

chemical series with reasonable diversity uniformly showing very poor solubility and low permeability would indicate difficulties in optimizing the series for absorption. These assays are able to detect and confirm the expected effects of modifications to enhance solubility and absorption. However, they need to be supplemented by further, more sophisticated tests which address further components of absorption (e.g., efflux) and validated with early *in vivo* pharmacokinetic experiments before being used to optimize the compound series. Furthermore, the package discussed above has an important influence on other assays: (i) it can decide whether a compound can be tested in an other package (e.g., soluble in the assay buffer) or (ii) information from the data generated by the package can influence the interpretation of data obtained in other assays (e.g., low permeability might explain lack of activity of compounds which require access to intracellular targets in cellular assays).

3.2.1
Impact of Turn-Around Time

Cycle time is defined as the time between the test request and the availability of data to the submitter. During lead optimization, short turn-around times are critical as this might determine the number of optimization cycles (or number of MedChem decisions) per time unit. A good practice is a one week turn-around time for primary assays, two weeks for follow-up (secondary) assays and two or three weeks for hypothesis-based studies (tertiary assays).

3.2.2
Assay Validation and Reference Compounds

It is highly important to choose the right compounds to validate assays. In most cases generic drugs are used for this purpose. These drugs have a large volume of relevant data, published and confirmed. However, one has to keep in mind that generic drugs are already optimized molecules (e.g., they are usually relatively soluble) while lead optimization compounds are likely to be more difficult to be measured reliably under the same conditions. The selected compounds should cover the assays' dynamic range (positives/negatives; low/medium/high) as well as a reasonable physicochemical property space. In most cases, at least 30 well chosen compounds are necessary to validate an *in vitro* assay. In addition to generic drugs, assay validation should include less optimized compounds which are taken from drug discovery phases. They should be highly representative for the test compounds the assay will handle when fully implemented. The best examples are those which have been extensively tested in similar assays or downstream tests but abandoned for reasons irrelevant to the assay in validation. Testing of this compound set gives the best estimate of the dynamic range and limitations of the assay.

The choice of reference compound(s) which can serve as internal standards is also crucial. It is important to choose a reference compound, which has the right physicochemical properties and its readout or affinity is in the mid-range of the expected values. For example, most active compounds in a functional hERG assay are in the range of 2–15 µM IC_{50}. Thus, a very weak or an extremely active molecule would not be representative for the test set. The choice of molecule should inhibit hERG at $IC_{50} = 2$–5 µM.

Finally, as profiling assays run repeatedly in cycles, unlike HTS campaigns, it is wise to create a "reference plate" with well characterized, diverse compounds to be tested at a frequency of 3–4 months. This test set ensures that any shift in dynamic range, technical fault associated with plate outlay, alteration of reagent quality or liquid handling is detected.

Once the assay is validated by these two sets of compounds, it can be used to test a larger group of marketed compounds, which will reveal the performance of the assay with an unbiased set of diverse, already well characterized compounds. False positive and false negative rates can be often defined with this validation.

3.2.3
Requirements of Profiling Assay Quality

Assay robustness is essential as compounds are often tested in various format of an assay or tested in related assays at various time-points. There are many factors influencing assay robustness (e.g., reproducibility, dynamic range, specificity and sensitivity in correlation to *in vivo* assays and clinical predictive power). It starts with compound logistics where one needs to minimize the risk that samples (batches) are being mixed up during the assay process steps. Next, high quality liquid handling is essential to get good reproducibility. For example, it is best to avoid pushing robotic systems close to their specification limits. A number of other factors which are partially linked to the compound itself are also potential source of data scattering: How is the assay readout affected by potential synthesis byproducts, residual particles (from chromatography) or simply dust in the solid material? This is particularly important when toxicity testing is performed which requires high concentrations. How is the assay performing with low soluble compounds? What is the assay intra- and inter-day variability? All these aspects need to be considered within the assay validation phase. When data are reported, care needs to be taken to avoid over-interpretation of the results: sometimes, it is preferable to simply bin compounds rather than reporting a numeric value. When numeric values are reported one needs to make clear what is the standard deviation associated with the number, to avoid erroneous ranking or false conclusions.

3.2.4
The Importance of Follow-Up Assays

Primary assays are referred sometimes as "sentinels". A good example is the hERG radioligand binding assay for cardiac safety testing which addresses a single, nevertheless highly important aspect of cardiac safety. The channel is very promiscuous and attracts a large proportion of small molecules which block it and could potentially cause QT prolongation and arrhythmia. This is the reason, while hERG inhibition is addressed as the first-line test in cardiac safety. The radioligand assay is highly reliable, inexpensive and fast. However, a functional follow-up is necessary to confirm positive findings because temperature- and activity-dependence or lack of permeability could alter hERG inhibition. In a flowchart, the radioligand binding provides the power of testing a large volume of molecules and reliably supports SAR, and the follow-up (secondary) patch clamp assays are used to spot-check whether hERG binding translates into cellular function (see Table 3.2). While these assays together are predictive for arrhythmia caused by hERG inhibition, one has to test other components of cardiac safety which might influence hERG channel expression and effects at other cardiac channels and receptors. However, the likelihood of positive findings in these later assays is significantly diminished. Thus, the two steps of early cardiac safety testing are: (i) confirm hERG effect by the primary and secondary assays and (ii) use tertiary assays to describe further components of cardiac safety.

The definition of secondary and follow-up assays is not straightforward. It really depends on the quality and economics of the assays. For example, functional ion channel assays are mostly used as a second line during the early phase of drug discovery. However, technological advances, such as the introduction of microfluidics and improved detection technologies make them more and more suitable for first-line profiling.

The relevance of *in vitro* assays to downstream *in vivo* assays is a matter of extensive discussion. For example, positive findings in a high quality *in vitro* genotoxicity assay, such as the high-content micronucleus assay do not always translate into positive findings *in vivo*. It is recommended to use a combination of three different *in vitro* genotoxicity assays to achieve a higher level of prediction. While early profiling assays try to focus on single targets, more system-based assays in later phase development include multiple targets, which can complicate or modify interpretation. While hERG channel inhibition is a serious flag for long QT and arrhythmias, it might prove a "false positive prediction" if compensatory mechanisms interfere in the animal (e.g., effect of the compound on other cardiac channels). The opposite can be true, when a compound is negative in the hERG assay but because of a hERG-positive metabolite can induce arrhythmia. However, the above discrepancies can be flagged by integrated risk assessment, when data from metabolic stability measured in liver microsomes and data from other cardiac ion channel assays are available and considered together.

3.3
Exposure Assays

3.3.1
Basic Absorption Assays

Solubility and permeability, which together largely define absorption, are the two pillars of the Biopharmaceutics Classification Scheme (BCS).

3.3.1.1 Solubility Assays

We distinguish between two families of solubility assays based on their use for different purposes:

- **Kinetic solubility:** This pragmatic approach starts with a concentrated compound solution in pure DMSO further diluted in a buffer medium. The amount of compound in solution is measured after a few minutes incubation either by recording its UV absorbance (with or without a chromatographic step) or precipitate formation using an optical method (turbidimetry, nephelometry or flow cytometry). This approach mimics the typical path of the compound in biochemical, cellular assays or *in vivo* animal models. Kinetic solubility usually serves as a quality filter prior to cell based assays (see paragraphs on solubility, permeability and cellular assays).

- **Equilibrium solubility:** This approach is considered a first attempt to characterize the true thermodynamic solubility of the compound. It is used to rank-order compounds and to extract a structure–solubility relationship within the chemical series. In this assay, compounds are usually equilibrated for 24 h before analysis. One can start from powder, but this is a quite labor-intensive step. In most cases one starts from DMSO stock solutions (usually 10 mM) because it is much more efficient from a compound logistics viewpoint. The solvent is then usually removed and the compound is dried before addition of the buffer medium [15, 16].

In the early phase the solid state of discovery compounds is usually not characterized and powders are often not crystalline. When starting with stock solutions the solid material obtained after evaporation of DMSO is mostly amorphous. However, there is evidence of crystallization upon incubation in the aqueous medium if the incubation time is long enough [17]. It has been reported that solubility data obtained from DMSO stock solutions are getting close to the values obtained from crystalline material after 20 h equilibration [17]. Quantitative aspects of solubility/dissolution are discussed in details in Chapter 4.

3.3.1.2 Permeability Assays

Basic permeability assays address passive permeability only. In this respect, parallel artificial membrane permeability assays (PAMPAs) have gained popularity among industry during the past decade due to their advantageous cost/throughput ratio and assay versatility (membrane composition, iso- and pH gradient possible). Various versions of this assay have been reported [15, 18–20]. PAMPA assays allow an estimation of compound permeability across a wide range of pH values which improves the characterization of ionizable compounds. While a well functioning PAMPA assay mimics trans-cellular permeability only, it is possible to add a paracellular component mathematically [21]. A detailed overview of permeability assays is given in Chapter 6.

3.3.2
Active Transports and Efflux

Cell-based models represent the next level of sophistication of permeability assays as they address both the physical and the biochemical barrier aspects. The most commonly used systems are the Caco-2 and P-glycoprotein transfected MDCK monolayer models. While the importance of transporters in GI tract absorption is probably not major (unless a low dose is considered) there is growing evidence of their importance in drug elimination and distribution properties. The impact of P-glycoprotein on brain exposure is well documented in the literature. Perhaps less well known is the organ-specific distribution induced by transporters: in some cases this transporter-driven organ-specific accumulation of drug is beneficial as in the case of statins [22] while in other cases it can lead to deleterious effects such as the renal accumulation of beta lactams in tubular cells [23], both mediated by organic anion transporter uptake.

3.3.3
Metabolism

Drug metabolism is the main cause for the absence of correlation between permeability and bioavailability in low dose PK experiments, as illustrated in Figure 3.1. Refined aspects of metabolism are presented in Chapter 7. As a first approach one can use the following relation to connect the fraction bioavailable with its basic components:

$$\text{Fraction bioavailable} = F_a \times F_g \times F_h$$

F_a, F_g and F_h being the fraction absorbed, fraction metabolized in the gut and fraction metabolized in the liver, respectively. F_g and F_h represents the metabolic barriers for drug absorption. For most compounds liver metabolism is the main metabolic barrier. Gastro-intestinal passive permeability is the main nonmetabolic barrier for oral absorption but not the only one. Counter-absorptive mechanisms or efflux mechanisms such as P-glycoprotein (P-gp) can also limit oral bioavailability. Furthermore, these elements can act in a synergistic manner. For example, several authors have reported that CYP-3A4 and P-gp can act in a concerted way to limit drug absorption in the gut. In this scenario, the P-gp activity facilitates CYP-3A4 to metabolize xenobiotics. This synergistic mechanism is particularly effective due to the co-localization of the proteins in the gut and their overlapping substrate specificity. This concerted mechanism largely determines the bioavailability of cyclosporine A, but in general P-gp efflux is not considered as a major obstacle for oral absorption.

3.3.4
Distribution and Elimination

Drug distribution and elimination are important factors influencing the PK/PD relationship. Models and latest advances in drug distribution prediction are reviewed in Chapter 9. Metabolism is a major route of elimination for xenobiotics and

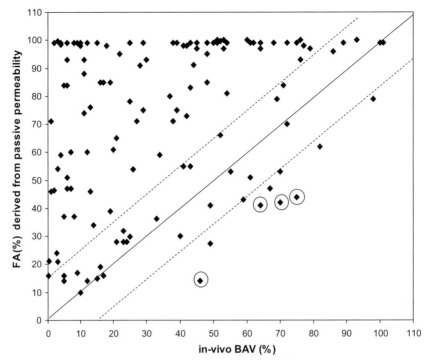

Figure 3.1 Correlation between passive permeability and *in vivo* BAV in Sprague Dawley rats ($N = 128$). The PAMPA F(%) values in the y-axis were derived from the passive permeability measurements in a PAMPA assay [19] using a calibration curve with reference compounds of known fraction absorbed. The *in vivo* BAV were values (x-axis) were calculated from AUC ratios from experiments done at 1 mg/kg iv vs. 3 mg/kg po. The solid line is the unity line between the fraction absorbed (%F) predicted from the *in vitro* passive permeability model and the *in vivo* measured BAV. The dotted line represents a 15% deviation to take into account the variability of the measurements.

the aspects of metabolic clearance and bioactivation are discussed in detail in Chapter 7.

What makes prediction of drug elimination complex are the multiple possible pathways involved which explain why there is no simple *in vitro* clearance assay which predicts *in vivo* clearance. Because oxidative metabolism plays a major role in drug elimination, microsomal clearance assays are often used as a first line screen with the assumption that if clearance is high in this *in vitro* assay it is likely to be high *in vivo*. This assumption is often, but not always true because, for example, plasma protein binding can limit the rate of *in vivo* metabolism. However, compounds which have a low clearance in hepatic microsomes can be cleared *in vivo* via other mechanisms (phase II metabolism, plasmatic enzymes). Occasionally, elimination is limited by hepatic blood flow, and other processes like biliary excretion are then involved. The conclusion is that the value of *in vitro* assays needs to be established for each chemical series before it can be used for compound optimization.

3.3.5
Drug–Drug Interactions

Drug–drug interactions (DDIs) can lead to significant variations in exposure, potentially moving compounds from an efficacious to a toxic concentration. DDI risk assessment is reviewed in Chapter 8. DDI risks need to be analyzed taking into account the elimination pathway of the drug as well as the therapeutic dose and potential co-medications. The clinically relevant interaction between gemfibrosil and cerivastatin (fivefold increase in exposure) appears to be related to the inhibition of CYP2C8 by the glucuronide metabolite of gemfibrosil [24]. While DDIs typically involve CYP450 enzymes, other transporters like OATP and Pgp have also been reported to cause clinically relevant DDIs (we recommend the excellent review on the impact of transporters on pharmacokinetics and safety by Ward [25]). Co-administration of rosuvastatin with cyclosporine A led to a sevenfold increase of the statin exposure due to OATP2 inhibition [26]. Important variations in brain exposure have been observed in mdr1(−/−) knockout animal models with the pain killer asimadoline and the antipsychotic risperidone, (both being P-glycoprotein substrates) affecting their brain levels (10-fold increase or more) [27, 28].

3.3.6
iviv Correlations

The analysis of the correlation between molecular descriptors, *in vitro* data and PK/PD is essential to get a meaningful SAR. As every *in vitro* assay has inherent limitations it is important to confirm the predictive power of the assay using *in vivo* data obtained with a representative molecule for the scaffold. Figure 3.1 show the relationship between the fraction absorbed derived from passive permeability measurements and *in vivo* bioavailability. These data show that when passive permeability is low in the passive permeability assay, the oral bioavailability is almost always low (lower right corner poorly populated). When the passive permeability assay predicts high absorption, the *in vivo* BAV can be high or low, depending on other factors influencing BAV like metabolism. The 4/128 compounds circled below the dotted line have all PSA values >100 $Å^2$ and could therefore be absorbed using a facilitated or active transport process.

As modern screening technologies produce a large amount of data, the challenge is often to extract relevant information from a pool of metadata of different dimensions and possibly partially inter-correlated. In this respect, principal component analysis (PCA) has proven a useful approach to handle data in a multidimensional space. Figure 3.2 shows a PCA loading plot obtained with project data (local model). One can see that in this project there is a tight IVIV correlation between the systemic exposure and the PD readout as blood levels are close to the percent inhibition. Proper interpretation of the data requires knowledge of the project itself, how *in vitro* assays are connected to each other and what they can and cannot predict. For example, the apparent inverse relation between the efflux ratio (ER) and the ClogD(7.4) parameter is misleading if taken without additional knowledge, as increasing ClogD(7.4) does not necessarily reduce the probability of the drug to be a P-glycoprotein substrate.

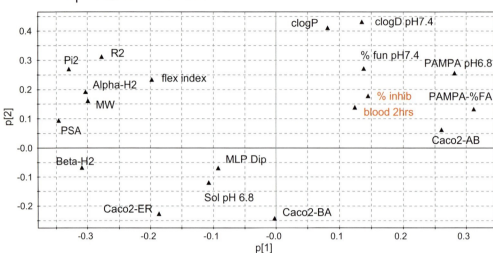

Figure 3.2 iviv correlation analysis using a PCA loading plot. This PCA plot was done using SIMCA P v. 11 using a set of 59 compounds. Pi2, R2, Alpha-H2, Beta-H2 are the parameters defined by Abraham [43] and calculated with the ABSOLV module of the ADME Boxes software [http://pharma-algorithms.com/adme_boxes.htm]. flex index is the number of rotatable bonds/molecular weight, MLP Dip represents the lipophilicity dipole moment. Sol pH6.8 is the aqueous solubility at pH6.8, Caco2-AB, Caco2BA and Caco2-ER are the Caco-2 permeability values in the apical to basolateral, basoletaral to apical and the Caco-2 efflux ratio respectively. ClogP and ClogD values are the calculated logP and D (at pH7.4) values. % fun pH 7.4 is the fraction unionized at pH7.4. PAMPA pH6.8 is the effective permeability measured in a PAMPA assay [19] and PAMPA%FA is the fraction absorbed extrapolated from the PAMPA permeability assay. Blood 2hrs is the blood concentration 2 hours after p.o. administration of the compound and % inhibition is the functional readout.

Looking at the situation in more depth one can see that the fraction of compounds for which a significant efflux ratio is observed is quantitatively linked to passive permeability, as shown in Figure 3.3. This observation largely explains the inverse correlation with logD. Therefore, it would be an erroneous conclusion to conclude than increasing logD(7.4) directly allows to escape P-glycoprotein efflux, although these two parameters are symmetric in the PCA loading plot.

The compound property distribution also impacts the analysis. For example, in Figure 3.2, solubility appears to have a relatively low weight (close to the center): this is not because solubility does not impact exposure but is due to the fact that all compounds tested had a low solubility and therefore this parameter could not discriminate compounds.

3.4
Iterative Assays: Link Between Assays

The outcome of one assay can affect the design of another assay or requires a follow-up assay. Low solubility can influence the result of other assays, and

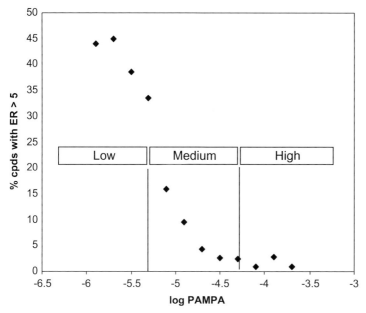

Figure 3.3 Impact of passive permeability on the efflux ratio (ER). Passive permeability (x-axis) was measured in a PAMPA assay [19]. Efflux ratios were derived from permeability measurements in a Caco-2 monolayer assay [44] and are expressed as the basolateral to apical/apical to basolateral permeability ratios. The loading concentration was 5 µM in the PAMPA assay and 10 µM in the Caco assay. LC-MS/MS readout was used for both assays. The y-axis represents the fraction of compounds with an ER>5. The study was done with 1404 compounds from 24 chemical series which were binned in 12 equally populated passive permeability categories (mean = 117, SD = 25). The low, medium and high labels refer to the permeability classes defined in PAMPA assay based on the correlation between permeability and fraction absorbed *in vivo* (low: <20%, high >80%) when absorption is limited by permeability.

among those, permeability assays are the most affected because there are generally few ingredients tolerated in the buffer medium which significantly improve solubility without altering the integrity of the membrane. When the loading concentration is significantly above the solubility limit, the compound precipitates in the donor compartment and leads to an underestimation of the true permeability. For this reason, kinetic solubility is sometimes used as a filter for permeability assays.

Low permeability can itself be the cause of apparent discrepancies between biochemical and cell-based assays and may or may not have physiological relevance. Independent of the solubility limitation mentioned above, the selection of an appropriate loading concentration in cell-based permeability assays impacts on the assay outcome and depends on what information one wants to extract from the measurement: loading at high concentration (i.e., 100 µM) will essentially cancel the effect of active transports unless passive diffusion is low. When high loading concentrations are used, poor recovery and bioanalytics are usually not an issue.

Loading at low concentration (i.e., 5 µM) will increase the sensitivity to active transports but make recovery and bioanalytical aspects more challenging.

Although the impact of transporters on absorption appears to be moderate there is increasing evidence showing that transporters can significantly affect drug distribution, in particular for low permeable compounds. In this context transporter assays need to be prioritized for compounds with medium to low passive permeability.

Data generated from metabolic clearance measurements using liver microsomes can lead to an overestimation of the true *in vivo* clearance if the free versus bound fraction is not considered. A useful follow-up assay is therefore plasma protein binding measurement. The impact of cytochrome P-450 inhibition on metabolic clearance of the parent (and thus exposure) is more complicated and it remains rather difficult to make quantitative predictions from *in vitro* data alone. The reason is that there are generally multiple clearance pathways involved and genetic polymorphism needs to be considered as well.

3.5
Specific Safety Profiling Assays

Profiling for toxic effects of compounds at early phase is one of the most debated territories of drug discovery. Many traditional toxicologists still maintain that this is mission impossible. There are two main arguments to support their views:

1. Classic toxicology is to a great extent retrospective. Histopathology performed on animals from acute and chronic toxic dosing gives guidance for further, mechanism-based studies, concentrating on a single molecule. Until recently, this approach has rarely involved chemical structural considerations (SAR).
2. *In vitro* toxicology assays are often of poor quality: they lack the complexity of the organism, cultures cannot be maintained long enough in a correct "phenotypic state", and they are often too expensive. Cellular assays are performed often on genetically engineered cells which do not express crucial targets the same way as the native cell, therefore their performance might be different.

However, recent developments in genetics and molecular biology have provided more reliable *in vitro* tools which are also predictive for clinical performance [8, 9]. Classic organ toxicity is broken down into distinct mechanisms with identified targets, such as the hERG potassium channel which is an important component of the repolarization phase of the cardiac action potential (see details in Chapter 16). A large amount of new genes and proteins are identified which are responsible for various side effects, such as transport proteins in the bile ducts for cholestasis [29], or agonism at the 5HT2B receptor causing cardiac valvulopathy [30]. Specific assays which measure inhibition of the transporter or the 5HT2B receptor can be high throughput, inexpensive, reliable and most importantly predictive for cholestasis and cardiac valvulopathy, respectively.

Another area of advance includes the miniaturization of existing assays by introducing automated systems with precise liquid handling and altered experimental conditions. A miniaturized version of the Ames test [31, 32] provides early access to genetic toxicity testing of large number of compounds. The emphasis is not only on the increased capacity of these assays to support SAR, but also the decrease of compound demand which can assure the project teams that small amounts of compounds can be tested in a fairly large variety of assays without conducting animal experiments. It is worth mentioning that this can be done as early as lead nomination and could save significant expenses by avoiding toxic molecules during lead optimization.

It is important to decide what to test at an early phase of drug discovery. As miniaturized assays become available it is more and more tempting to test as much as possible. Earlier, we took cardiac safety to demonstrate a reasonable and logical approach to address early testing for possible arrhythmogenesis, considering inhibition of hERG and other cardiac ion channels. Cardiac safety profiling is addressed in detail in Chapter 16.

While cardiac safety testing is relatively well established and early profiling assays are based on defined targets, it remains a challenge to address other organ-specific toxicities. For example, hepatotoxicity occurs relatively frequently and is responsible for several withdrawals and the black box label [33]. The problem is that hepatotoxicity is complex and multifactorial, and it is difficult to maintain native, dissociated hepatocytes in culture long enough. More importantly they undergo phenotypic changes and lose their specific functions, such as expression of functional liver enzymes and transporters responsible for bile production. In short, novel assay conditions, such as sandwich technology [34] and microscale assay environment [35] might help to rectify this problem and provide more reliable hepatocyte-specific cultures. This advance with the combination of high content imaging of distinct physiological effects, such as oxidative stress, specific mitochondrial or lysosomal damage gives us a hope to establish early screening for hepatotoxicity and avoid or limit drug-induced liver injury (DILI). Various aspects of hepatotoxicity can be investigated by using a "systems biology" approach [36] which provides a more refined and predictive combination score derived from multiple readouts. Hepatotoxicity is addressed in detail in Chapter 15.

More and more biomarkers and gene arrays have been identified and getting ready to enter the profiling portfolio to address organotypic toxicity. We refrain from detailed analysis here and refer the reader to the specific chapter addressing hepatotoxicity and hematotoxicity (Chapter 17).

Two more important areas of non-organ toxicity should be discussed: genetic toxicity (Chapter 11) and phototoxicity (Chapter 19). While genetic toxicity is addressed by the Ames test and its higher throughput variants with clear go/no go endpoints, the early phototoxicity 3T3 NRU PT is much less decisive largely due to a higher level of false positives. Furthermore, accumulation in the eye and/or skin of potentially photosensitive molecules or photochemically induced genotoxicity is considered necessary to have high alert for potential phototoxicity and trigger more decisive preclinical studies such as the UV-local lymph node assay (UV-LNNA). Also, while no compounds enter clinical application with a positive Ames result, compounds causing phototoxicity are in clinical use with the appropriate caution. Chapter 19 provides detailed information on phototoxicity testing.

Finally, we would like to comment on the application of *in vitro* safety (off-target) pharmacology profiling [37]. It is recognized that some targets associated with adverse drug reactions (ADRs) are highly promiscuous and attract many compounds. However, some chemical structures are attracted to many targets. This was described as target hit rate (THR) which is defined in Chapter 12. Briefly, the higher the THR is, the most likely that the molecule will cause side effects in clinical settings. Assay panels to test THR have been constructed, partially with the aid of *in silico* tools and are used to diminish pharmacological promiscuity and widen the therapeutic index (TI) of clinical candidates. While this effort is considered for derivative purposes, sometimes it can also identify advantageous properties due to off-target effects. It has been used successfully to identify "bait" compounds for specific targets, which have to be absolutely clear of off-target effects. *In vitro* safety pharmacology panels differ in minor details, but agree in that they cover a large chemistry and pharmaceutics space and they are mostly based on fast and robust biochemical assays. However, recently functional, cellular assays were also used as first-line screening, particularly when either an agonist or an antagonist effect was associated with the ADR and the opposite effect was considered to be silent.

3.5.1
Sensitivity and Specificity of Safety Assays should be Adjusted to the Phase of Drug Discovery

At the early stage of drug discovery, a variety of compounds are often considered and chemists usually look at several chemical scaffolds for parallel optimization. While it is important to identify molecules or scaffolds with "bad behavior", it is essential not to mislead the chemists with false positive findings. Thus, the selection of the assay with the right sensitivity and specificity is important. While Ames positive structures would fail to reach clinical phase, other early genotoxicity assays might produce high positive rates with no further consequence. Therefore highly specific but less sensitive assays could do a good job, by weeding out the worst compounds and not throwing out others by labeling them false positives. These assays might miss some positive compounds (false negatives) as their sensitivity is set at a higher level. This scenario is allowed in early phase drug discovery for two reasons: (i) a large number of compounds could be tested and the probability of false negatives is diminished and (ii) more sophisticated follow-up assays are used on compounds of "great importance" to test whether the project is on the right track.

3.5.2
Addressing Species Specificity in Early *In Vitro* Assays

It is often argued by fellow toxicologists that early assays should focus on targets aligned with those of "tox. species", such as rat and dog. The simple reasoning behind this is that the next stage after *in vitro* profiling in drug discovery is the extensive safety analysis in these species. However, some of the animal studies have limited relevance to human conditions while the early assays carry the advantage that they can relatively easily use human targets. For example, there are well documented discrepancies between primate, human, rodent and canine metabolism [38]. It is often necessary to test compounds in parallel in different species. For metabolism, most laboratories test compounds on microsomes and hepatocytes from various species. While the targets might be the same, the role of the target protein could be different in non-human species. Neurokinin antagonists are very potent in blocking airway irritation, broncho-constriction in guinea-pigs, while their importance in human airways seems to be less significant. The same is true for some teratogenic effects, when administration to rats might produce positive findings, irrelevant for primates. These cases have to be carefully considered on individual base which is not within the scope of this book.

3.6
Data Reporting and Data Mining

Pharmaceutical companies are making significant investment to mine data, transfer old, nonstructured, often report-based data into central data warehouses for common access. The rapid change in IT infrastructure and technologies for data storage has created a very difficult environment where access to data can be cumbersome and requires enormous efforts and investment.

Today, most data are entered into corporate databases which consider the need of the user and the purpose of data. They are structured, searchable, contain both raw and metadata. Decision-making tools can mine these databases and if necessary combine data from various sources, including genetic, proteomic, clinical and chemical databases.

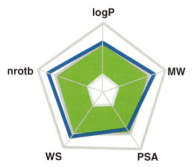

Figure 3.4 Radar plot to demonstrate the physicochemical characteristics of Lipitor. The simple plot demonstrates that two parameters fall within the optimal zone (logP and PSA), while three others slightly exceed the boundaries: molecular weight, water solubility and number of rotatable bonds.

During lead selection and lead optimization, SAR is a determinant component which drives the discovery process. Therefore any database should link chemical structures with various physicochemical and biological data. However, too many data on a large number of compounds could be very difficult to visualize and analyze. Therefore many tools cluster data and use heat maps, graphs and radar plots. A simple example is given in Figure 3.4 for a data cluster generated for a single compound for addressing basic physicochemical properties (largely based on Lipinski's rule of five [14]). As in many cases, the cluster is generated against "ideal" conditions, which are within the boundaries marked in green. In the case where any of the measured parameters of the compound are less optimal, the radar plot expands out of the "green zone". This visualized profile can easily be put together with other simple profiles for data analysis and characterization of compounds by parameters closely involved in absorption, metabolism and various aspects of pharmacokinetics and safety. Scores and categories are also often used to address exposure (e.g., the Biopharmaceutical Classification System; BCS) or safety (Redfern's approach to analyze the effects of hERG channel inhibition on cardiac safety [39]).

While this demonstration gives some characteristics of a single compound, other tools are needed to visualize compound series, trends of biological data within the series or for comparison between series. Many decision-making tools use SpotFire or PipelinePilot for data mining. An important element of comparative studies is the introduction of marketed drugs. This approach links together data generated by the profiling portfolio and published clinical information. This combination is essential for several reasons: (i) it can be used for validation of profiling assays, (ii) it can aid competitor intelligence and (iii) it can guide drug discovery projects to achieve a desired clinical profile by alerting to side effects and PK properties linked with comparable *in vitro* characteristics. The best known effort to implement this strategy is BioPrint [40] which can analyze large number of compounds by their performance in *in vitro* assays and compare the data to those obtained from compounds in clinical use and hence fully characterized for correlation between their *in vitro* and clinical performance.

3.6.1
Decision Making: Trend Analysis, Go/No Go Decisions

How do we approach early preclinical integrative risk assessment and what are the prerequisites of success? First, we need to look at the validity and precision of *in vitro* profiling data. As discussed before, any compound feature which could compromise the performance of an assay should be noted and the dynamic range of the assays considered. Often, the combination of "bad" physicochemical properties such as the coincidence of high logP and low solubility with hERG inhibition could cause serious problems and prolong time to success. When one reviews *in vitro* profiling data, it is essential to know whether the compounds are "sticky" or poorly soluble, as both of these features might affect data in such a way that activity is underestimated. While these features might not have a major effect on the assays which measure activity at the primary target (usually activity in the nanomolar range), profiling assays are more affected, as they deal with much higher concentrations of compounds. This is particularly true for assays related to safety, as we need to look for relatively high concentrations (a minimum is $30\,\mu M$ in most assays). The picture is further complicated with cellular assays, which only tolerate low co-solvent concentrations and with intracellular targets, permeability is a further major determinant (e.g., hERG channel inhibition).

Early ADMET profiling has relatively little power to provide data for go/no go decisions, at least based on a single assay result. For example, physicochemical properties such as solubility and permeability might be poor and the compounds tested might not qualify for further investigation, but collective data obtained from several compounds from the same chemical series might give clues for consequent modifications and require the testing of further compounds synthesized based on the clues. This common early profiling scenario is the basis for trend analysis, which is often used to define a collective feature of molecules from the same chemical series and SAR.

Assays addressing safety usually follow optimization of basic physicochemical properties and come on board with some delay. Early profiling of hepatotoxicity, genotoxicity, bone marrow toxicity (or hematotoxicity) and phototoxicity are used in various combinations during lead selection and optimization. With few exceptions, these assays are "sentinels" which trigger more mechanistic studies to find targets, associated with the signaled toxic effects. Modern drug discovery has invested a significant effort to develop *in vitro* safety testing protocols; however they are by far not perfect. However, the implementation of genomic, metabonomic and proteomic approaches gives hope that fast, relatively inexpensive tests will enter drug discovery to deal with safety aspects early.

3.7
Integrative Risk Assessment

At early phases of drug discovery, such as lead selection, project teams should define or update their target compound profile and consider possible liabilities associated with the selected structure and measure them against activity at the primary target. This is very rarely a single component, and in some cases could be a combination of unwanted features which significantly limits progress. As discussed previously, risk identification is possible by using first line, primary assays for many drug-like features and safety factors. Furthermore, the profiling portfolio should define follow-up assays to reveal underlying mechanisms, particularly in case of assays addressing phenomena, such as organ toxicity with possible multiple targets. In addition to the profiling plan, early integrative risk assessment can force teams to make early decisions. For example, overlap between a primary target pharmacophore with that of a major liability-target could provide an insurmountable difficulty and is very likely to be a "no go" sign. Many compounds suffer from low bioavailability, which seriously compromises efficacious plasma concentration and cripples the establishment of a safe therapeutic index. Teams should do some SAR analysis based on absorption risk and make sure that enhancing very poor solubility and permeability does not evoke other liabilities. The "brickdust" feature of early phase molecules predicts a rocky road and big obstacles towards clinical application. Liabilities associated with a parent compound could be carried over to its metabolites, to a lesser or greater extent, and could modify the TI. Unknown species-specific metabolites could cause serious hiccups by producing species related side effects, which would not appear in clinical setting. However, human-specific metabolites might surprise clinical teams by producing side effects never seen in animal studies. Therefore, testing of these metabolites separately in different species could avoid bad surprises and delays in development, or in the worst case scenario the nomination of the wrong compound.

Once we understand the individual data or data sets, the next step is integration of data from various assays. For example, early data on liver microsomal stability can alert the team to look for possible metabolites and get their profile (see above reference to species differences in metabolism). The poster child for this scenario is terfenadine, which has an active metabolite, fexofenadine (a safe drug), while the parent compound is a potent hERG channel blocker [41]. A retrospective, integrated risk assessment of terfenadine based on present, routine *in vitro* profiling clearly alerts to hERG inhibition, but equally importantly also shows the predicted high metabolism of this compound. Early analysis of the predicted metabolites in the *in vitro* profiling assays would have pointed directly towards the development of the safer compound, fexofenadine (Table 3.3).

Once the drug is in clinical trials and therapeutic exposure is established, the most important question is whether it comes with a "clean sheet" in terms of safety. This is the time to find out how good was the prediction of the therapeutic index from preclinical studies, particularly from *in vivo* experiments. However, before we know the PK profile in humans, we have to rely on the results generated in the *in vitro* and *in vivo* assays. Equivalent affinity to on- and off-target site(s) has a very high possibility to translate into the side effect anticipated from the off-target functionality. The Bioprint approach [40] goes one step further and proves that relatively low affinity (IC_{50} values between 1.0 and 10.0 µM), based on the analysis of metadata, could manifest in side effects, even somewhat disconnected from the activity at the primary target.

This often overlooked aspect originates from the frequent belief that high affinity to a target will require low systemic exposure, which will avoid off-target effects. In

Table 3.3 Hepatic metabolism, measured in liver microsomes and hERG IC_{50} (patch clamp data) of terfenadine and fexofenadine, determined and compared in early, routinely used *in vitro* profiling assays.

Compound	*In vitro* hepatic extraction ratio	hERG radioligand binding (IC_{50}; uM)	hERG electrophysiology (IC_{50}; uM)
Terfenadine	90%	0.16	0.4
Fexofenadine	15%	>30	>30

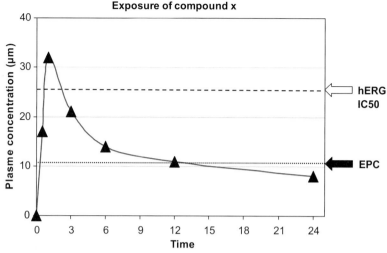

Figure 3.5 PK profile of a compound with hERG inhibition with an IC$_{50}$ between 20–30 μM. The effective plasma concentration is 10 μM. The single dose produced a spike of over 30 μM plasma concentration, not required for therapeutic effect but for a sufficient level 12 hours after administration. However, the C$_{max}$ associated with this dose/formulation reached the level when hERG inhibition occurs.

spite of their high affinity to the primary target, many compounds require high plasma levels to ensure therapeutic efficacy. The reasons for this discrepancy could be due to poor BBB permeability in case of drugs with central nervous system targets, compound distribution in the body, high C$_{max}$ which might accompany the AUC required for therapeutic effects. Figure 3.5 demonstrates this later scenario. The compound represented in this graph requires a minimum 10 μM concentration to maintain therapeutic effect at a b.i.d. dosing regimen. However, the formulation used in this case produced a high initial exposure, which would exceed the hERG IC$_{50}$, measured *in vitro* by patch clamp. It is an important element, that inhibition of the hERG channel has an imminent functional effect on the heart by causing modification of the repolarizing phase of the cardiomyocyte action potential which could trigger early after-depolarization. Thus, this compound, at least with the demonstrated PK profile, carries a risk to produce arrhythmia. One possible solution could be to modify formulation and prevent the high C$_{max}$ while ensuring that the required therapeutic level is maintained between doses.

In addition to possible high therapeutic plasma levels, accumulation in target organs also complicates the side effect picture. Thus, early estimates of safety margins should be approached with a "pinch of salt" and predicted adverse reactions should be carefully monitored during late phase *in vivo* studies and clinical trials.

In summary, this book is an attempt to collect ADMET profiling approaches suitable for early use during drug discovery, when a large number of compounds need to be tested to aid SAR for lead selection and optimization. It has been recognized that drug-like properties are equally important to the primary activity and should be taken into consideration early. Recent developments provide an arsenal of assays, in silico tools and processes together with more refined analysis of data to aid this strategy and weed out compounds by their most common and least compatible features towards clinical use.

There are various ways to do this and this book reflects on the many alternatives. Certainly, return on investment is an important matter when it comes to build early ADMET profiling. In these regards, we would like to close this chapter with an excerpt from Chris Lipinski, whose contribution was a milestone on the road to modern drug discovery: "The 'rule of five' deals with physicochemical properties and then the computational approaches deal with the metabolism and elimination parts of ADME, so they are both part of trying to filter things early. But I don't think these fail early approaches are going to get the 200% increase in productivity that senior executives in big Pharma are talking about. It's going to take something more than that, and the problem is that fail early approaches only deal with the things that we know about. I would say that if we implement things sufficiently and screen early then we might get a 25–35% increase in productivity, because it's the things you don't know about that kill you in drug development, toxicity in particular" [42].

Acknowledgments

The authors wish to thank Dr. Giorgio Ottaviani for providing project data analysis to illustrate the IVIV correlation section, Steven Whitebread, Drs. Jianling Wang and Xueying Cao for the data presented in Table 3.3 and Dr. Alfred Zimmerlin for useful discussions on metabolism and drug–drug interaction aspects.

References

1 Kola, I. and Landis, J. (2004) Can the pharmaceutical industry reduce attrition rates? *Nature Review*, **3**, 711–715.

2 Smith, D., Schmid, E. and Jones, B. (2002) Do drug metabolism and pharmacokinetic departments make any contribution to drug discovery? *Clinical Pharmacokinetics*, **41**, 1005–1019.

3 Cohen, J.P. (2006) Cost-effectiveness and resource allocation. *JAMA*, **295**, 2723–2724.

4 Schuster, D., Laggner, C. and Langer, T. (2005) Why drugs fail – a study on side effects in new chemical entities. *Current Pharmaceutical Design*, **11**, 3545–3549.

5 Mason, J.S., Migeon, J., Dupuis, P. and Otto-Bruc, A. (2008) Use of broad biological profiling as a relevant descriptor to describe and differentiate compounds: structure – *in vitro* (pharmacology-ADME) – *in vivo* (safety) relationships, in *Antitargets*, (eds R.J. Vaz and T. Klabunde), Springer, Heidelberg, pp. 23–50.

6 Gerrard, J.A., Hutton, C.A. and Perugini, M.A. (2007) Inhibiting protein-protein interactions as an emerging paradigm for

drug discovery. *Mini-Reviews in Medicinal Chemistry*, **7**, 151–157.

7 Michnick, S.W., Ear, P.H., Manderson, E.N., Remy, I. and Stefan, E. (2007) Universal strategies in research and drug discovery based on protein-fragment complementation assays. *Nature Reviews. Drug Discovery*, **6**, 569–582.

8 Faller, B., Wang, J., Zimmerlin, A., Bell, L., Hamon, J., Whitebread, S., Azzaoui, K., Bojanic, D. and Urban, L. (2006) High-throughput *in vitro* profiling assays: lessons learnt from experiences at Novartis. *Expert Opinion on Drug Metabolism and Toxicology*, **2**, 823–833.

9 Wang, J., Urban, L. and Bojanic, D. (2007) Maximising use of *in vitro* ADMET tools to predict *in vivo* bioavailability and safety. *Expert Opinion on Drug Metabolism and Toxicology*, **3**, 641–665.

10 Lefèvre, G., Pommier, F., Sedek, G., Allison, M., Huang, H.L., Kiese, B., Ho, Y.Y. and Appel-Dingemanse, S. (2008) Pharmacokinetics and bioavailability of the novel rivastigmine transdermal patch versus rivastigmine oral solution in healthy elderly subjects. *Journal of Clinical Pharmacology*, **48**, 246–252.

11 Fukasawa, T., Suzuki, A. and Otani, K. (2007) Effects of genetic polymorphism of cytochrome P450 enzymes on the pharmacokinetics of benzodiazepines. *Journal of Clinical Pharmacy and Therapeutics*, **32**, 333–341.

12 Zoghbi, S.S., Liow, J.S., Yasuno, F., Hong, J., Tuan, E., Lazarova, N., Gladding, R.L., Pike, V.W. and Innis, R.B. (2008) 11C-loperamide and its N-desmethyl radiometabolite are avid substrates for brain permeability-glycoprotein efflux. *Journal of Nuclear Medicine*, **49**, 649–656.

13 Obradovic, T., Dobson, G.G., Shingaki, T., Kungu, T. and Hidalgo, I.J. (2006) Assessment of the first and second generation antihistamines brain penetration and role of P-glycoprotein. *Pharmaceutical Research*, **24**, 318–327.

14 Lipinski, C.A. (2000) Drug-like properties and the causes of poor solubility and poor permeability. *Journal of Pharmacological and Toxicological Methods*, **44**, 235–249.

15 Kansy, M., Senner, F. and Gubernator, K. (1998) Physicochemical High Throughput Screening: Parallel Artificial Membrane Permeation Assay in the Description of Passive Absorption Processes. *Journal of Medicinal Chemistry*, **41**, 1007–1010.

16 Zhou, L., Yang, L., Tilton, S. and Wang, J. (2007) Development of a high throughput equilibrium solubility assay using miniaturized shake-flask method in early drug discovery. *Journal of Pharmaceutical Sciences*, **96**, 3052–3071.

17 Sugano, K., Kato, T., Suzuki, K., Keiko, K., Sujaku, T. and Mano, T. (2006) High throughput solubility measurement with automated polarized light microscopy analysis. *Journal of Pharmaceutical Sciences*, **95**, 2115–2122.

18 Avdeef, A., Strafford, M., Block, E., Balogh, M.P., Chambliss, W. and Khan, I. (2001) Drug absorption *in vitro* model: filter-immobilized artificial membranes 2. Studies of the permeability properties of lactones in Piper methysticum Forst. *European Journal of Pharmaceutical Sciences*, **14**, 271–280.

19 Wohnsland, F. and Faller, B. (2001) High-Throughput Permeability pH Profile and High-Throughput Alkane/Water log P with Artificial Membranes. *Journal of Medicinal Chemistry*, **44**, 923–930.

20 Zhu, C., Jiang, L., Chen, T.-M. and Hwang, K.-K. (2002) A comparative study of artificial membrane permeability assay for high throughput profiling of drug absorption potential. *European Journal of Medicinal Chemistry*, **37**, 399–407.

21 Sugano, K., Takata, N., Machida, M., Saitoh, K. and Terada, K. (2002) Prediction of passive intestinal absorption using biomimetic artificial membrane permeation assay and the paracellular pathway model. *International Journal of Pharmaceutics*, **241**, 241–251.

22 Deng, J.W., Song, I.-S., Shin, F H.J., Yeo, C.-W., Cho, D.-Y., Shon, J.-H. and

Shin, J.-G. (2008) The effect of SLCO1B1*15 on the disposition of pravastatin and pitavastatin is substrate dependent: the contribution of transporting activity changes by SLCO1B1*15. *Pharmacogenetics and Genomics*, **18** (5), 424–433.

23 Westphal, K., Weinbrenner, A., Zschiesche, M., Franke, G., Knoke, M., Oertel, R., Fritz, P., von Richter, O., Warzok, R., Hachenberg, T., Kauffmann, H.-M., Schrenk, D., Terhaag, B., Kroemer, H.K. and Siegmund, W. (2000) Induction of P-glycoprotein by rifampin increases intestinal secretion of talinolol in human beings: a new type of drug/drug interaction. *Clinical Pharmacology and Therapeutics (St. Louis)*, **68** (4), 345–355.

24 Shitara, Y., Hirano, M., Sato, H. and Sugiyama, Y. (2004) Gemfibrozil and its glucuronide inhibit the organic anion transporting polypeptide 2 (OATP2/OATP1B1:SLC21A6)-mediated hepatic uptake and CYP2C8-mediated metabolism of cerivastatin: Analysis of the mechanism of the clinically relevant drug-drug interaction between cerivastatin and gemfibrozil. *Journal of Pharmacology and Experimental Therapeutics*, **311**, 228–236.

25 Ward, P. (2008) Importance of drug transporters in pharmacokinetics and drug safety. *Toxicology Mechanisms and Methods*, **18**, 1–10.

26 Simonson, S.G., Raza, A., Martin, P.D., Mitchell, P.D., Jarcho, J.A., Brown, C.D.A., Windass, A.S. and Schneck, D.W. (2004) Rosuvastatin pharmacokinetics in heart transplant recipients administered an antirejection regimen including cyclosporine. *Clinical Pharmacology and Therapeutics (St. Louis)*, **76**, 167–177.

27 Jonker, J.W., Wagenaar, E., Van Deemter, L., Gottschlich, R., Bender, H.M., Dasenbrock, J. and Schinkel, A.H. (1999) Role of blood-brain barrier P-glycoprotein in limiting brain accumulation and sedative side-effects of asimadoline, a peripherally acting analgesic drug. *British Journal of Pharmacology*, **127**, 43–50.

28 Wang, J.-S., Ruan, Y., Taylor, R.M., Donovan, J.L., Markowitz, J.S. and DeVane, C.L. (2004) The brain entry of risperidone and 9-hydroxyrisperidone is greatly limited by P-glycoprotein. *International Journal of Neuropsychopharmacology*, **7**, 415–419.

29 Sakurai, A., Kurata, A., Onishi, Y., Hirano, H. and Ishikawa, T. (2007) Prediction of drug-induced intrahepatic cholestasis: in vitro screening and QSAR analysis of drugs inhibiting the human bile salt export pump. *Expert Opinion on Drug Safety*, **6**, 71–86.

30 Elangbam, C.S., Job, L.E., Zadrozny, L.M., Barton, J.C., Yoon, L.W., Gates, L.D. and Slocum, N. (2008) 5-Hydroxytryptamine (5HT)-induced valvulopathy: Compositional valvular alterations are associated with 5HT2B receptor and 5HT transporter transcript changes in Sprague-Dawley rats. *Experimental and Toxicologic Pathology*, **60**, 253–262.

31 Ames, B.N., Lee, F.D. and Durston, W.E. (1973) An improved bacterial test system for the detection and classification of mutagens and carcinogens. *Proceedings of the National Academy of Sciences of the United States of America*, **70**, 782–786.

32 Flamand, N., Meunier, J., Meunier, P. and Agapakis-Caussé, C. (2001) Mini mutagenicity test: a miniaturized version of the Ames test used in a prescreening assay for point mutagenesis assessment. *Toxicology In Vitro: An International Journal Published in Association with BIBRA*, **15**, 105–114.

33 Lammert, C., Einarsson, S., Saha, C., Niklasson, A., Bjornsson, E. and Chalasani, N. (2008) Relationship between daily dose of oral medications and idiosyncratic drug-induced liver injury: search for signals. *Hepatology (Baltimore, Md)*, **47**, 2003–2009.

34 Berthiaume, F., Moghe, P.V., Toner, M. and Yarmush, M.L. (1996) Effect of extracellular matrix topology on cell structure, function, and physiological responsiveness: hepatocytes cultured in a

sandwich configuration. *FASEB Journal*, **10**, 1471–1484.

35 Khetani, S.R. and Bhatia, S.N. (2008) Microscale culture of human liver cells for drug development. *Nature Biotechnology*, **26**, 120–126.

36 Giuliano, K.A., Johnston, P.A., Gough, A. and Taylor, D.L. (2006) Systems cell biology based on high-content screening. *Methods in Enzymology*, **414**, 601–619.

37 Whitebread, S., Hamon, J., Bojanic, D. and Urban, L. (2005) Keynote review: *in vitro* safety pharmacology profiling: an essential tool for successful drug development. *Drug Discovery Today*, **10**, 1421–1433.

38 Martignoni, M., Groothuis, G.M. and de Kanter, R. (2006) Species differences between mouse, rat, dog, monkey and human CYP-mediated drug metabolism, inhibition and induction. *Expert Opinion on Drug Metabolism and Toxicology*, **2**, 875–894.

39 Redfern, W.S., Carlsson, L., Davis, A.S., Lynch, W.G., MacKenzie, I., Palethorpe, S., Siegl, P.K., Strang, I., Sullivan, A.T., Wallis, R., Camm, A.J. and Hammond, T.G. (2003) Relationships between preclinical cardiac electrophysiology, clinical QT interval prolongation and torsade de pointes for a broad range of drugs: evidence for a provisional safety margin in drug development. *Cardiovascular Research*, **58**, 32–45.

40 Krejsa, C.M., Horvath, D., Rogalski, S.L., Penzotti, J.E., Mao, B., Barbosa, F. and Migeon, J.C. (2003) Predicting ADME properties and side effects: the BioPrint approach. *Current Opinion in Drug Discovery and Development*, **6**, 470–480.

41 Scherer, C.R., Lerche, C., Decher, N., Dennis, A.T., Maier, P., Ficker, E., Busch, A.E., Wollnik, B. and Steinmeyer, K. (2002) The antihistamine fexofenadine does not affect I(Kr) currents in a case report of drug-induced cardiac arrhythmia. *British Journal of Pharmacology*, **137**, 892–900.

42 Lipinski, C.A. (2003) Chris Lipinski discusses life and chemistry after the Rule of Five. *Drug Discovery Today*, **8**, 876–877.

43 Abraham, M.H. (1993) Scales of solute hydrogen-bonding: their construction and application to physicochemical and biochemical processes. *Chemical Society Reviews*, **22** (2), 73–83.

44 Artursson, P. and Karlsson, J. (1991) Correlation between oral drug absorption in humans and apparent drug permeability coefficients in human intestinal epithelial (Caco-2) cells. *Biochemical and Biophysical Research Communications*, **175** (3), 880–885.

Part II

4
Solubility and Aggregation

William H. Streng

4.1
Importance of Solubility

During the development of pharmaceutically important compounds, the question is often asked: "what is the solubility of the compound?" While the question appears to be simple and not too demanding, it can upon further contemplation be very difficult to answer. Not only is it necessary to know from what perspective the question is being asked, but it is also necessary to know to what depth of understanding the questioner expects an answer. If the questioner is someone who has spent much time and energy determining the solubility of compounds, then the question more than likely will be required to include much more detail than if the questioner is someone who is involved in high throughput screening and is anxious to receive an "it is" or "it is not" soluble response. Having to answer the question can be very disconcerting.

Why is it necessary to ask this question? At what time during the development of a compound should the question be asked? How correct does the answer need to be? Who is best able to answer the question? There are not necessarily simple or definitive answers to these questions.

Considerable effort is spent trying to synthesize new compounds. The focus of the chemist should be on modifying the structures of compounds in ways which will increase the pharmacological response for a specific activity while minimizing the side effects. Today, chemists need to know about the human genome and the sites at which a specific activity can be achieved. In addition they must be able to modify the structures of the compounds in ways that will permit the compounds to dock at these active sites. Almost of equal importance is an understanding of the effect that specific functional groups will have on the solubility, stability and ability of the compounds to distribute between different phases. This last aspect is related to the ability of the compounds to be transported between, or through, membranes. Addressing the solubility, if a compound is very insoluble in a series of compounds being considered (even though it might have a much greater absolute pharmacological response), it can

Hit and Lead Profiling. Edited by Bernard Faller and Laszlo Urban
Copyright © 2009 WILEY-VCH Verlag GmbH & Co. KGaA, Weinheim
ISBN: 978-3-527-32331-9

exhibit a lower response than one which has a smaller absolute pharmacological response but is more soluble. Conversely, if a compound is extremely soluble and if its route of absorption is transcellular passive diffusion, it might not be easily transported through membranes to arrive at the active site and therefore very large doses might be required even though the absolute activity is reasonably good. Therefore, solubility does play an important role in selecting a compound for continued development.

The question is asked: "how accurately does the solubility need to be determined?" Here again, the answer is not easy to give. During the early stages of development, any reasonable answer is better than none. It is at this time that testing is frequently being conducted using solvents other than water. It might be acceptable to indicate in a series of compounds that all of the compounds were dissolved in order to obtain a good comparison of their relative activities. Later on during development it is important to have a good determination of the solubility. The solubility should be determined in a variety of solvents and under different conditions, such as pH and temperature.

There is no specific person who can best answer the question concerning the solubility. At first a more qualitative answer might be obtained from the discovery chemist who needed to dissolve the compound in the different solvents used in the synthesis and purification of the compound. Later it should be determined by someone who is familiar with the nuances of measuring the solubility and those factors which can influence the final result.

4.2
Factors Influencing Solubility

If a compound is ideal and is placed in an ideal solvent, the solubility of the compound can be shown to be simply related to the heat of fusion of the compound. As will be shown, the ideal solubility relationship is given by the van't Hoff equation and relates the solubility to the heat of fusion of the compound, the melting point of the compound and the temperature of interest. Because of this simple relationship, there is nothing relating to the solvent in which the compound is dissolved. It can therefore be concluded that the solubility should be the same in all solvents. Everyone knows that this just is not the case. Anything which contributes to the solubility and which is not the heat of fusion of the compound or its melting point become clumped together in the non-ideal part of the solubility. This non-ideal part is formally given by the heat of mixing of the compound with the solvent and has several contributing factors. When someone says that the solubility has heat of mixing contributions, unless they have done much more work to clarify, they are not making the job of understanding the solubility behavior any easier, because there can be many factors which need to be included in this term.

What are some of the factors which are included in this term heat of mixing? When a compound is dissolved a hole must be made in the solvent. This hole must be made between the solvent molecules and if the solvent lacks a dipole and is not polarizable, little work should be needed to introduce the compound. The closer the molecular volume of the compound is to that of the solvent, the less work that is done. However, if there is much solvent–solvent interaction and the solvent has a dipole or is polarizable, much more work is required to make the hole in the solvent to introduce the compound. A solvent which has little solvent–solvent interaction and does not have a dipole is benzene. Conversely, a solvent which has considerable solvent–solvent interactions and has a dipole is the common solvent water. With this in mind, what is the solvent that is most frequently used in the pharmaceutical industry? Water.

Solvent–solvent interactions have already been mentioned as a possible factor which can contribute to the heat of mixing. Two other interactions which can be present in solution are solute–solvent and solute–solute interactions. In aqueous solutions these types of interactions are almost always present when considering the structures of the molecules of interest in the pharmaceutical industry. These molecules usually possess a dipole or can be polarized and therefore form, at the very least, weak long-range interactions with other molecules and/or with water. This is not to say that they form a more strongly bonded associated aggregate in solution, but weaker interactions do exist which contribute to the heat of mixing. Because the functional parts associated with a pharmaceutically active molecule usually possess a dipole or are polarizable, they orient the water molecules around themselves. By orienting the water molecules, they are forming solute–solvent interactions which affect the heat of mixing.

As is well known, different solvents can have profoundly different abilities to dissolve or solubilize a specific compound. There are many different classification schemes used to classify solvents based on their properties. Each one meets a specific need. The properties used in a specific scheme normally do not have an abrupt change in their value and in fact change over a wide range. It is therefore somewhat disconcerting to realize that there is a sense of arbitrary assignment of a value at which point the solvent changes from one type to another. Even in the same classification scheme there can be overlap of values from one type to another. One classification scheme uses dielectric constant, relative acidity and relative basicity and considers solvents to be: (i) amphiprotic, capable of accepting or donating a proton; (ii) protogenic, acidic; (iii) protophilic, basic; (iv) aprotic, incapable of proton transfer; and (v) non-polar, not possessing a dipole. As a result of using three properties where each property can have one of two values, there are a total of eight (2^3) different classifications for the solvents. Where is this taking us? By knowing something about the structure of the molecule and whether it is a base or acid or has a relatively high or relatively low dielectric constant, some sense of the ability of a solvent to solubilize the compound can be realized. A very rough rule which is used to help in identifying how well a solvent will solubilize a compound is, "like dissolves like". While there are many exceptions to this rule, it can be used as a first estimation.

If a molecule is an acid or base it will take on either a positive or negative charge upon its ionization. The type of solvent used will significantly influence the observed solubility of the charged species. If the solvent is aprotic or non-polar, the solubility of the charged species will be much less than if the solvent is amphiprotic, protogenic or protophilic. The same effects will be observed if the compound is present as a salt. The enhanced solubilities are due to the solute–solvent charge-dipole type interactions. It is important to understand, when trying to decide on an appropriate solvent to select, whether the conditions are such that the compound will be present as a charged species.

It is safe to say that almost all, if not all, compounds which are of pharmaceutical importance possess multiple dipoles. These dipoles interact with any solvent dipoles, resulting in an enhanced solubility in these solvents. These dipoles act in the microenvironment surrounding the individual components more so than the molecule as a whole (the net dipole for the molecule). The dipoles alter the solvent structure depending on the orientation of the partial charges associated with the dipole. If the charge on the dipole oriented towards the solvent is positive, the negative end of the solvent dipole orients towards the molecule. If another component has the negative charge oriented towards the solvent, then the positive end of the solvent molecule orients towards the molecule. When there are several components which are orienting the solvent molecules differently, there can be a significant de-structuring effect upon the solvent. Similarly, if a solvent has a sufficiently high dipole it can induce or enhance a dipole. This effect not only influences the solubility of the compound but can also alter its stability.

4.3
Methods Used to Determine Solubility

During the development of a compound, different methods can be used to determine the solubility. Because the degree of accuracy of the different methods is not the same, it is important to recognize how the reported values were determined. The methods can be divided into screening tests and conclusive tests but this does not imply that each type does not have its own merit and importance. Either type can be done using a range of solvents and can include buffers to establish solubilities at specific pH values. Some of the commercially available instruments adjust the total ionic strength to a specific value. When this is done it must be remembered that the standard state for these solubilities is not the same as the conventional standard state of zero total ionic strength. While these differences are usually not critically important and the values at a non-zero total ionic strength can be corrected to zero ionic strength, these are real differences. Although it is not the purpose of this chapter, the use of these types of instruments to determine the pK_a also results in the same difference in standard states, which can be corrected if needed.

Screening tests are those which are used because there is little compound, little time, or many different compounds to be tested. Many compounds can be synthesized using high throughput screening techniques. During this stage biological tests are conducted to ascertain the activity of the compounds. The compounds are synthesized using 96 well or larger plates. The solubility of the compounds can be estimated using a method in which a known volume of solvent is placed in the wells and a light passed through the cell. By the reflection of the light, or lack thereof, an estimation of its solubility can be made. If there is considerable turbidity or light scattering, the compound is not dissolved. Additional solvent can be added until there is no turbidity. Another technique that can be used is to take a sample of the solution and using microtechniques obtain a UV visible spectrum of the dissolved material. From the spectra a concentration can be estimated using a Beer's law plot in which a specific functional group is used to quantitate the amount of compound dissolved. Both of these methods require small quantities of compound, can be done rapidly, many compounds can be tested within a short period of time and are for the most part independent of the solvent used, therefore meeting the restraints for this stage of development. Some problems associated with these testing procedures include: (i) not having a stable polymorph or a crystalline form of the compound; (ii) having different particle sizes which can influence the rate of dissolution; (iii) not having a good or representative chromophore which is used to quantitate the spectral measurement, chemical stability problems; (iv) not having relatively pure compounds; or (v) having a residual solvent present in the test solution which is used in the experimental procedure (e.g., DMSO). These problems notwithstanding, these methods are valid during this stage of development.

More conclusive tests for the solubility usually use traditional procedures in which the compound is placed in a container along with a solvent and the system equilibrated for a period of time. As a consequence, these experiments often require more amounts of compound and take more time to complete. Depending on the ultimate use of the data, these procedures are at times modified to use less amounts of compound and/or less time. For instance, if someone wants to know how much compound can be dissolved in a certain period of time, a time restriction can be placed on the experiment. For example, this is done when the interest is in knowing how best to prepare a dosage form. If a time restriction is placed on the experiment, it must be realized that independent variables such as particle size and the particular polymorph used can have significant effects on the final results. Another question sometimes asked is similar but not exactly the same. When a solution of a specific concentration is required, then a specific amount of the compound is placed in the container and a quantity of solvent added which usually results in a solution concentration less than saturated. Again, the same concerns dealing with what particle size and polymorph is being used are important.

When restrictions are not placed on the amount of time or the amount of material, different solvents or different quantities of acid or base are usually used as variables. It is not only important to know the solubility of the compounds in aqueous solutions but also in other solvents to which the compound might be exposed during synthesis and formulation. The solvents usually have a wide range of dielectric constants and the experimental results provide a solubility profile which can be utilized in the selection of appropriate solvents to use during the development of the compound. Since the compounds almost always selected for development are either weak acids or weak bases, the solubilities of the compounds will be pH-dependent. The use of different amounts of acid or base with an excess amount of compound permits the determination of a pH-solubility profile.

Mention was made of the effects of particle size on the observed solubility. It may seem strange but different solubilities can be obtained when different particle sizes are used. If experimentally a long time is used to equilibrate the solutions, then the effect of particle size is not significant; but when short equilibration times are utilized, then the size of the particles can have an effect on the results. The reason for this is because the surface energy on a particle is related to the size of the particle. The energy increases with a decrease in the particle size. Therefore enhanced dissolution rates are observed when smaller particle sizes are used. It is observed that smaller particles dissolve faster than larger particle sizes. If an excess of compound is present, the smaller particles dissolve and can supersaturate the solution. When the supersaturated solution comes out of solution, the size of the larger particles increases. If the solution is not at equilibrium, the solubility results obtained can be higher than the actual solubility due to this supersaturation.

Different polymorphs or pseudo-polymorphs will have different solubilities. The definition of a polymorph is a compound which has exactly the same molecular formula and arrangement of functional groups but the solid state configuration of the molecules is different. This includes the solvation of the compound. Often compounds with different solvates are compared, for example, a mono-hydrate and a tri-hydrate, and are listed as polymorphs but they are not according to the above definition. When comparing a compound with different solvates of this type they are sometimes referred to as pseudo-polymorphs. Because polymorphic composition is a solid state property and relates to the arrangement of the molecules in the crystal, different polymorphs have different solubilities due to their different crystal energies. Therefore it is important to be sure to know what polymorph is being used in the experiment and understanding what the effects will be if the solvation is changed.

Another factor which can result in different solubilities is the isomeric composition of a compound. When a compound contains an asymmetric carbon atom, the four different groups attached to the carbon can be in different arrangements. These different arrangements result in the stereochemical behavior of the compound. When there is one asymmetric carbon atom there are two isomeric configurations. These configurations are mirror images of each other. Because the arrangement of the groups is different, there can be different intramolecular and intermolecular interactions. This results in different solute–solute and solute–solvent interactions. The net result of this is that, during the early stages of development, a single isomer is not always available and therefore the solubilities reported can be different than later when a relatively pure isomer is available. While this is not something that needs to be of concern with many of the compounds being developed, it must be recognized when a compound does have an asymmetric carbon atom.

4.4
Approaches to Solubility

Several different approaches have been made to theoretically determine the solubilities of compounds. Before discussing two of these, a brief review of what is meant by ideal solubility is presented.

4.4 Approaches to Solubility

The van't Hoff equation can be used to represent the solubility of a compound.

$$\frac{d \ln x_2}{dT} = \frac{\Delta H_s}{RT^2} \qquad (4.1)$$

Where: X_2 = mole fraction solubility; ΔH_S = heat of solution of the solute; T = temperature; R = gas law constant.

The heat of solution is related to the heat of fusion and heat of mixing according to:

$$\Delta H_S = \Delta H_f + \Delta H_{mix} \qquad (4.2)$$

For an ideal solution the heat of mixing is zero and therefore Equation (4.1) after integrating becomes:

$$\ln x_2 = -\frac{\Delta H_f}{R}\left(\frac{T_m - T}{T_m T}\right) \qquad (4.3)$$

Where: T_m is the melting temperature of the compound. Also, the heat of fusion is a function of temperature given by:

$$\Delta H_f = \Delta H_{f,m} - \Delta C_P (T_m - T) \qquad (4.4)$$

Where: ΔC_P = heat capacity difference between the solid and supercooled liquid; $\Delta H_{f,m}$ = heat of fusion at the melting point.

Substituting Equation (4.4) into Equation (4.1) and integrating results in:

$$\ln x_2 = -\frac{\Delta H_{f,m}}{R}\left(\frac{T_m - T}{T_m T}\right) + \frac{\Delta C_P}{R}\left(\frac{T_m - T}{T}\right) - \frac{\Delta C_P}{R} \ln \frac{T_m}{T} \qquad (4.5)$$

According to Equation (4.5) the ideal solubility of a compound is only dependent upon the heat of fusion, the difference in heat capacity of the solid and supercooled liquid and the melting point of the compound. Since there are no properties of the solvent included in the ideal solubility equation, the solubility of a compound should be the same in all solvents. This equation overlooks all solute–solvent and solvent–solvent interactions.

One of the approaches to calculating the solubility of compounds was developed by Hildebrand. In his approach, a "regular" solution involves no entropy change when a small amount of one of its components is transferred to it from an ideal solution of the same composition when the total volume remains the same. In other words, a regular solution can have a non-ideal enthalpy of formation but must have an ideal entropy of formation. In this theory, a quantity called the Hildebrand parameter is defined as:

$$\delta = \frac{\Delta U_i}{V_i} \qquad (4.6)$$

Where: δ = Hildebrand parameter; ΔU_i = molar energy of vaporization of i; V_i = molar volume of i.

With this definition, an expression for the activity coefficient can be derived which is:

$$\ln \gamma_2 = \frac{V_2 \phi_1^2 (\delta_1 - \delta_2)^2}{RT} \qquad (4.7)$$

Where: ϕ_1 = the volume fraction of the solvent $\phi_1 = \frac{V_1 x_1}{V_1 x_1 + V_2 x_2}$.

Equation (4.7) is the non-ideal part of the solubility and can be added to Equation (4.3) to obtain an expression for the solubility of a regular solution.

$$\ln x_2 = -\frac{\Delta H_f}{R}\left(\frac{T_m - T}{T_m T}\right) - \frac{V_2 \phi_1^2 (\delta_1 - \delta_2)^2}{RT} \quad (4.8)$$

Because the entropy of formation in Hildebrand theory is ideal, this approach should be restricted to those systems in which there are no structure effects due to solute–solvent and solvent–solvent interactions. The implication of this is that the solute should be non-ionic and not have functional groups which can interact with the solvent. According to Equation (4.8), the maximum solubility occurs when the Hildebrand parameter of the solvent is equal to the Hildebrand parameter of the solute. That is, when plotting the solubility versus the Hildebrand parameter, the solubility exhibits a maximum when the solubility parameter of the solvent is equal to the solubility parameter of the solute.

Utilizing this same type of approach but incorporating a non-ideal entropy is a theory called the molecular group surface area approach (MGSA). Instead of using the internal energy, ΔU, the MGSA uses reversible work, W, to represent the molecular pair interactions. An equation for the activity coefficient can be derived and is given by:

$$\ln \gamma_2 = \frac{\sigma_{12}^h A_2^h + \sigma_{12}^p A_2^p}{kT} \quad (4.9)$$

Where: σ = the surface free energy or surface tension; k = Boltzmann constant; A = the molecular surface area of the solute.

The superscripts h and p refer to group contributions due to hydrocarbon and polar groups, respectively. The polar term is often found to be small while the shape of the cavity occupied by the solute molecule is irregular and requires a shape factor. Equation (4.9) then becomes:

$$\ln \gamma_2 \cong \frac{c\sigma_{12}^h A_2^h}{kT} \quad (4.10)$$

Where: c is the shape factor.

Adding Equation (4.10) to Equation (4.3) results in:

$$\ln x_2 = -\frac{\Delta H_f}{R}\left(\frac{T_m - T}{T_m T}\right) - \frac{c\sigma_{12}^h A_2^h}{kT} \quad (4.11)$$

Equation (4.11) includes both non-ideal entropy and non-ideal enthalpy and therefore can be applied to solutions which contain electrolytes and systems which have solute–solvent and/or solvent–solvent interactions.

4.5
Solubility in Non-Aqueous Solvents and Co-Solvents

None of the material presented in the last section was restricted to a specific solvent system. In fact, the use of the Hildebrand theory should be limited to those systems in which there are no significant structure effects related to solute–solvent and solvent–solvent interactions and is therefore better suited for non-aqueous solvents. Both the Hildebrand and MGSA theory can be applied to co-solvent systems by modifying the interaction parameters.

The Hildebrand parameter for the solvent in Equation (4.8), $\delta 1$, needs to be replaced by the value for the mixture determined by multiplying the pure solvent values by their volume fractions as given below for a two-solvent system.

$$\delta_{mix} = \frac{\phi_i \delta_i + \phi_j \delta_j}{\phi_i + \phi_j} \qquad (4.12)$$

Where: i and j represent the two solvents. In addition, the volume fraction of the solvent needs to be replaced with the sum of the volume fractions of all solvents, therefore Equation (4.8) becomes:

$$\ln x_2 = -\frac{\Delta H_f}{R}\left(\frac{T_m - T}{T_m T}\right) - \frac{V_2 \left(\sum_i^n \phi_i\right)^2 (\delta_{mix} - \delta_2)^2}{RT} \qquad (4.13)$$

Additional terms can be added to this equation in order to correlate with experimental data.

When considering the MGSA model, a similar approach can be made. Starting with Equation (4.11) the mole fraction solubility of a single solvent system can be calculated and labeled $x_{2,1}$. The mole fraction solubility of a two solvent system can be given as $x_{2,mix}$. A linear function of the solubility in the mixed solvent system can be calculated according to:

$$\ln X_{2,mix} = \ln X_{2,1} + k_2 \phi_2 \qquad (4.14)$$

Where: k_2 = a constant and is obtained by correlating with experimental data.

Many systems have been found to correlate with this function but for those which do not a polynomial expression can be used instead of k_2.

Even though Hildebrand theory should not apply to solvent systems having considerable solvent–solvent or solute–solvent interactions, the solubility of compounds in co-solvent systems have been found to correlate with the Hildebrand parameter and dielectric constant of the solvent mixture. Often the solubility exhibits a maximum when plotting the solubility versus either the mixed solvent Hildebrand parameter or the solvent dielectric constant. When comparing different solvent systems of similar solvents, such as a series of alcohols and water, the maximum solubility occurs at approximately the same dielectric constant or Hildebrand parameter. This does not mean that the solubilities exhibit the same maximum solubility.

4.6
Solubility as a Function of pH

The solubilities of weak acids and bases are dependent upon the pK_a value(s) of the compound, the pH of the solution and the concentration of any counter ions to the

80 | *4 Solubility and Aggregation*

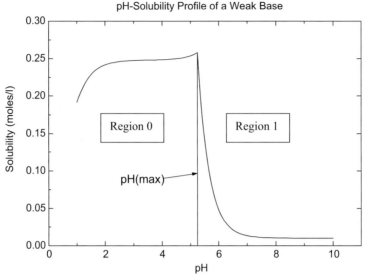

Figure 4.1 Solubility versus pH for a monoprotic weak base. A constant amount of weak base is considered and the pH is adjusted with a strong acid or strong base.

charged species of the weak acid or base. Figure 4.1 is a solubility versus pH profile obtained for a monoprotic weak base, when different amounts of strong acid or strong base have been added to a constant amount of weak base. In this figure it can be seen that there are two regions: one at pH values less than the pH value labeled pH$_{max}$, designated region 0, and the second at pH values greater than pH$_{max}$, designated region 1. It can be shown that for a monoprotic weak base, the solubility in region 0 is controlled by the solubility product (pK$_{sp}$) of the charged weak base species with the counter ion present in the solution and the pK$_a$ of the compound, while in region 1 the solubility is controlled by the neutral species intrinsic solubility and the pK$_a$. The downturn in the profile at low pH is due to the solubility product effect of adding more strong acid counter ion to the solution as the pH is decreased.

Equations can be derived which can be used to calculate the pK$_a$, pK$_{sp}$ and intrinsic solubility of the neutral species of a weak base. Because the solubility is controlled by the solubility product in region 0 and the intrinsic solubility of the neutral species in region 1, two equations are required to represent the entire profile.

Region 0:

$$S_{1,0} = \frac{-\left([M^+] + \frac{\{H^+\}}{\gamma_{H^+}} - \frac{K_w}{\{H^+\}\gamma_{OH^-}}\right) \left(\left([M^+] + \frac{\{H^+\}}{\gamma_{H^+}} - \frac{K_w}{\{H^+\}\gamma_{OH^-}}\right)^2 + \frac{4K_{sp}}{\gamma_{X^-}\gamma_{HB^+}}\right)^{1/2}}{2\left(\frac{\{H^+\}\gamma_B}{\{H^+\}\gamma_B + K_a\gamma_{HB^+}}\right)}$$

(4.15)

Region 1:

$$S_{1,1} = \left(\frac{1}{\gamma_B} + \frac{\{H^+\}}{K_a \gamma_{HB^+}}\right) \{B\}_S \qquad (4.16)$$

Where: $S_{1,0}$ and $S_{1,1}$ represent the solubility of a monoprotic compound in region 0 and region 1 respectively; [M$^+$] is the molar concentration of strong base cation; { } represents the activity of the indicated species; K_w, K_{sp}, K_a are the ionization constant of water (w), the solubility product of the weak base with its counter ion (sp) and a weak base dissociation constant (a), respectively; y_i is the activity coefficient of the indicated species.

The pH at which the profile changes from region 0 to region 1 is designated as pH$_{max}$. This pH can be calculated for a monoprotic weak base according to Equation (4.17)

$$\{H_{max}^+\} = \frac{-[M^+] + \left([M^+]^2 + 4\left(\frac{1}{\gamma_{H^+}} + \frac{\{B\}_S}{K_a \gamma_{HB^+}}\right)\left(\frac{K_w}{\gamma_{OH^-}} + \frac{K_a K_{sp}}{\{B\}_S \gamma_{X^-}}\right)\right)^{1/2}}{2\left(\frac{1}{\gamma_{H^+}} + \frac{\{B\}_S}{K_a \gamma_{HB^+}}\right)} \qquad (4.17)$$

Figure 4.1 shows that the solubility is a maximum at pH$_{max}$. This occurs because, at this pH, the solution is saturated in both the weak base salt species and the neutral species; that is, the solubility is controlled by both the solubility product and the neutral species intrinsic solubility. According to Equation (4.17) an increase in cation concentration gives an increase in the pH of maximum solubility (a decrease in $\{H_{max}\}$).

Similar to a weak base, the solubility pH profile for a weak acid is shown in Figure 4.2. This figure is a mirror image of the profile for a weak base.

Again, the profile can be divided into two regions. The region where the pH is less than pH$_{max}$ is designated region 0 while that region where the pH is greater than pH$_{max}$ is designated as region 1. For a weak acid, the intrinsic neutral species solubility is controlling the solubility in region 0 and the solubility product of the anionic species of the weak acid with its cationic counter ion is controlling the solubility in region 1. Although the downturn in the profile is not shown in this simulation, if the calculations had been made at higher pH values, a decrease in the solubility would have been calculated. This decrease is due to the solubility product effect which accompanies an increase in the counter ion concentration because of the additional strong base present. Equations can be derived which can be used to calculate the pK$_a$, pK$_{sp}$ and intrinsic solubility of the neutral species of a weak acid. Because the solubility is controlled by the intrinsic solubility of the neutral species in region 0 and the solubility product in region 1, two equations are required to represent the entire profile.

Region 0:

$$S_{1,0} = \left(\frac{1}{\gamma_{HA}} + \frac{K_a}{\{H^+\}\gamma_{A^-}}\right) \{HA\}_S \qquad (4.18)$$

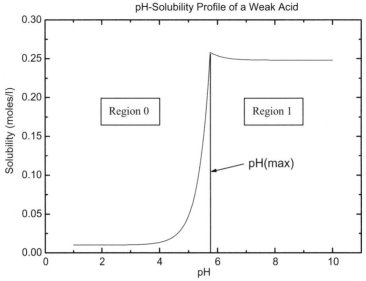

Figure 4.2 Solubility versus pH for a monoprotic weak aid. A constant amount of weak base is considered and the pH is adjusted with a strong acid or strong base.

Region 1:

$$S_{1,1} = \frac{-\left([X^-] + \frac{\{H^+\}}{\gamma_{H^+}} - \frac{K_w}{\{H^+\}\gamma_{OH^-}}\right) \left(\left([X^-] + \frac{\{H^+\}}{\gamma_{H^+}} - \frac{K_w}{\{H^+\}\gamma_{OH^-}}\right)^2 + \frac{4K_{sp}}{\gamma_M + \gamma_{A^-}}\right)^{1/2}}{2\left(\frac{K_a \gamma_{HA}}{\{H^+\}\gamma_{A^-} + K_a \gamma_{HA}}\right)}$$

(4.19)

The pH at which the profile changes from region 0 to region 1 is designated as pH$_{max}$. This pH can be calculated for a monoprotic weak base according to Equation (4.20)

$$\{H^+_{max}\} = \frac{[X^-] + \left([X^-]^2 + 4\left(\frac{K_{sp}}{K_a\{HA\}_s \gamma_{M^+}} + \frac{1}{\gamma_{H^+}}\right)\left(\frac{K_a\{HA\}_s}{\gamma_{A^-}} + \frac{K_w}{\gamma_{OH^-}}\right)\right)^{1/2}}{2\left(\frac{K_{sp}}{K_a\{HA\}_s \gamma_{M^+}} + \frac{1}{\gamma_{H^+}}\right)}$$

(4.20)

Figure 4.2 shows that the solubility is a maximum at pH$_{max}$. This occurs because, at this pH, the solubility is controlled by both the solubility product and the neutral species intrinsic solubility. According to Equation (4.20), an increase in anion concentration gives a decrease in the pH of maximum solubility (an increase in $\{H_{max}\}$).

4.7
Effect of Aggregation Upon Solubility

The self-association of a compound in solution is an effect which should always be considered when conducting solubility studies. It is recognized that surfactant type molecules require this property in order to form micelles. Not as well known is the fact that aggregation also occurs with the organic compounds of interest to the pharmaceutical industry. There are many different types of studies which can be used to determine the aggregation number of a compound which does form aggregates in solution. Some of these are conductivity, calorimetry, osmometry, pH and solubility. In fact, any type of experiment can be used which is measuring a colligative property of the solution; that is, measuring a property which is dependent upon the total number of particles in the solution.

The solubility profiles obtained for a compound which aggregates have the different regions as described previously, but the mathematical functions describing the change in solubility with pH are much more complex. The additional equilibrium for a monoprotic weak base when the charged species is aggregating is:

$$n\mathrm{HB}^+ + p\mathrm{X}^- \rightleftharpoons (\mathrm{HB}^+)_n(\mathrm{X}^-)_p \tag{4.21}$$

The equilibrium given by Equation (4.21) has the equilibrium constant:

$$K_{\mathrm{assoc}} = \frac{\{(\mathrm{HB}^+)_n(\mathrm{X}^-)_p\}}{\{\mathrm{HB}^+\}^n \{\mathrm{X}^-\}^p} \tag{4.22}$$

The solubility of the weak base is then given by the equation:

$$S = [\mathrm{HB}^+] + [\mathrm{B}] + n[(\mathrm{HB}^+)_n(\mathrm{X}^-)_p] \tag{4.23}$$

This scheme assumes that aggregation is only occurring with the charged species. When this equilibrium is taken into consideration, the equations which describe the solubility in the two regions become:

Region 0:

$$S_{1,0} = \left(\frac{1}{\gamma_{\mathrm{HB}^+}} + \frac{K_a}{\{\mathrm{H}^+\}\gamma_\mathrm{B}}\right)\frac{K_{sp}}{\{\mathrm{X}^-\}} + n\left(\frac{K_{\mathrm{assoc}}}{\gamma_{(\mathrm{HB}^+)_n(\mathrm{X}^-)_p}}\right)\{\mathrm{X}^-\}^p\left(\frac{K_{sp}}{\{\mathrm{X}^-\}}\right)^n \tag{4.24}$$

Region 1:

$$S_{1,1} = \left(\frac{1}{\gamma_\mathrm{B}} + \frac{\{\mathrm{H}^+\}}{K_a \gamma_{\mathrm{HB}^+}}\right)\{\mathrm{B}\}_s + n\left(\frac{K_{\mathrm{assoc}}}{\gamma_{(\mathrm{HB}^+)_n(\mathrm{X}^-)_p}}\right)\{\mathrm{X}^-\}^p\left(\frac{\{\mathrm{H}^+\}}{K_a}\right)^n \{\mathrm{B}\}_s^n \tag{4.25}$$

The contribution of the aggregation to the solubility is given by the last terms in Equations (4.24) and (4.25). Similarly an equation can be derived which gives the pH of maximum solubility, $\mathrm{pH}_{\mathrm{max}}$.

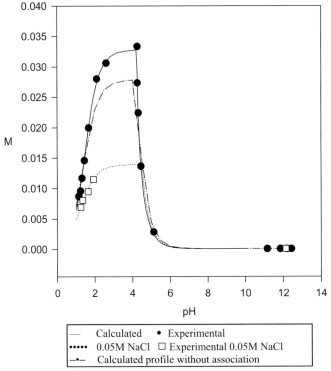

Figure 4.3 Solubility versus pH for a compound which forms aggregates in solution.

$$(n-p)\left(\left(\frac{K_{assoc}}{\gamma_{(HB^+)_n(X^-)_p}}\right)K_{sp}^p\left(\frac{K_a}{\{B\}_s}\right)^{(p-n)}\{H_{max}^+\}^{(n-p+1)}\right) \quad (4.26)$$

$$+ \{H_{max}^+\}^2\left(\frac{1}{\gamma_{H^+}} + \frac{\{B\}_s}{K_a\gamma_{HB^+}}\right) + \{H_{max}^+\}[M^+] - \left(\frac{K_a K_{sp}}{\{B\}_s\gamma_{X^-}} + \frac{K_w}{\gamma_{OH^-}}\right) = 0$$

An example of a compound which forms aggregates in the aqueous phase is shown in Figure 4.3. In this figure the data were first treated without assuming aggregate formation and the curve calculated is given by the dash-dot-dash line. The figure shows that there is little correlation between the experimental data and the calculated curve particularly for the higher concentration data. Fitting the data to Equations (4.24) through (4.26) resulted in the solid line curve and the dotted curve. It can be seen that there is very good correlation between the data and the calculated curves.

The data were fit to a model which had an aggregate species with the formula $(BH^+)_2(X^-)$. Additional studies were conducted using different techniques which confirmed an aggregate of this composition is present in the solution. In this figure the dotted line is the calculated curve for which the solution had an additional 0.05 M NaCl added. The significant decrease in the solubility when a salt is present having a common ion with the strong acid or base used to adjust the pH is not restricted to solutions for which aggregates are present. In fact, this is observed with all solutions over the pH range where the solubility is controlled by the solubility product between the charged species of the weak acid or base and a counter ion. According to the derivation, the assumption was made that the monomeric species controls the solubility through its solubility product (K_{sp}) in Region 0 when aggregation occurs. This follows the convention that the solubility product is written as the lowest common ratio of the species involved. However, when there are significant quantities of an aggregate in the solution, it might be more correct to express the controlling solubility product in terms of the aggregate. This would change the interpretation of the calculated parameters but it should not have an effect on the equations used to determine the solubility.

The total solubility of a monoprotic weak acid, when the negative species is aggregating, is given in the following equation.

$$S = [HA] + [A^-] + p[(M^+)_n(A^-)_p] \tag{4.27}$$

The equations for the pH dependency of the solubility in the two regions for a weak acid are given as follows:

Region 0:

$$S_{1,0} = \left(\frac{1}{\gamma_{HA}} + \frac{K_a}{\{H^+\}\gamma_A}\right)\{HA\}_s + p\left(\frac{K_{assoc}}{\gamma_{(M^+)_n(A^-)_p}}\right)\{M^+\}^n\left(\frac{K_a}{\{H^+\}}\right)^p\{HA\}_s^p \tag{4.28}$$

Region 1:

$$S_{1,1} = \left(\frac{\{H^+\}}{K_a\gamma_{HA}} + \frac{1}{\gamma_A}\right)\frac{K_{sp}}{\{M^+\}} + p\left(\frac{K_{assoc}}{\gamma_{(M^+)_n(A^-)_p}}\right)\{M^+\}^n\left(\frac{K_{sp}}{\{M^+\}}\right)^p \tag{4.29}$$

An equation can be derived which results in the pH of maximum solubility, pH_{max}, for a weak acid.

$$\{H^+\}_{max}^2\left(\frac{K_{sp}}{K_a\{HA\}_s\gamma_{M^+}} + \frac{1}{\gamma_{H^+}}\right) - \{H^+\}_{max}[X^-] - \left(\frac{K_a\{HA\}_s}{\gamma_{A^-}} + \frac{K_w}{\gamma_{OH^-}}\right)$$

$$-\frac{(n-p)K_{assoc}K_{sp}^n(K_a\{HA\}_s)^{(p-n)}(\{H^+\}_{max})^{(n-p+1)}}{\gamma_{M_nA_p}} = 0 \tag{4.30}$$

The above equilibria were restricted to aggregate formation involving the charged species of the weak acid or base. As with the weak base equations, the assumption was also made that the monomeric species is controlling the solubility through its solubility product. A similar approach can be made when an aggregate is formed with the neutral species. In addition to these cases, it is possible that both the charged and neutral species could form aggregates and then the equations would need to include both terms. A major assumption in deriving these equations is that there is only one aggregate species present; that is, all of the aggregates have the same number of weak acid or base molecules. This is usually safe to assume and it is very uncommon for there to be a significant concentration of more than one aggregate species with a specific weak acid or weak base species. Another type of interaction that can occur is the formation of complexes when a complexing agent has been added to the solution. For this case, the same type of approach can be made by substituting into the equations the ligand for the common ion species of the strong acid or base. With the necessary equations, it becomes possible to determine the aggregation numbers and equilibrium constants through the use of solubility data. In the case of solubility data, when the experimental data cannot be fit to the known expressions assuming no aggregation, there is a high probability that aggregation is occurring.

4.8
Dependence of Dissolution upon Solubility

The rate at which a compound dissolves is dependent upon its surface area, solubility, solution concentration, rate of reaction and transport rate. These quantities are defined as follows: surface area – the surface area of the individual particles if the compound is not compressed or the surface area of a disk if the compound is compressed; solubility – the solubility of the polymorphic form in the solid phase; solution concentration – the concentration of the compound in the bulk of the solution; rate of reaction – the rate at which the solid surface reacts with the solvent or dissolution medium; transport rate – the rate at which the compound travels through the diffusion layer. The rate of dissolution, or flux, of a compound can be given as:

$$J = k_{r,t}(C_s - C_b) \tag{4.31}$$

Where: J is the dissolution rate; $k_{r,t}$ is the rate of reaction or transport rate; C_s is the solubility of the compound; C_b is the concentration in the bulk of the solution.

In Equation (4.31) the rate constant is either the reaction rate constant or the transport rate constant, depending on which rate controls the dissolution process. If the reaction rate controls the dissolution process, then $k_{r,t}$ becomes the rate of the reaction; while if the dissolution process is controlled by the diffusion rate, then $k_{r,t}$ becomes the diffusion coefficient (diffusivity) divided by the thickness of the diffusion layer. It is interesting to note that both dissolution processes result in the same form of expression. From this equation the dependence on the solubility can be seen. The closer the bulk concentration is to the saturation solubility the slower the dissolution rate will become. Therefore, if the compound has a low solubility in the dissolution medium, the rate of dissolution will be measurably slower than if the compound has a high solubility in the same medium.

It was mentioned that the solubility is that of the polymorph used to prepare the solid phase. It is possible to achieve higher dissolution rates by using unstable polymorphic forms of the compound. For example, if a hydrate is the stable polymorphic form in the presence of water, an anhydrous form would be more soluble and therefore exhibit a faster dissolution rate. If the most stable form of a compound is a hydrate, then the dissolution rate can potentially be increased by using the anhydrous polymorphic form. Related to this is the fact that if the compound is amorphous, the dissolution rate is higher than if a crystalline material is used. Another factor which influences the dissolution rate and is related to the solubility is the form of the compound when the compound is a weak acid or base. If the neutral form of the compound is used for the solid phase the dissolution rate is slower than when a salt form is used, assuming all other factors remain the same.

4.9
Partitioning and the Effect of Aggregation

When two immiscible solvents are placed in contact with each other and a non-ionizable compound is dissolved in one of the solvents, the compound distributes itself between the two solvents. This distribution is referred to as partitioning. The ratio of the concentrations of the compound in each phase is a constant for a specific set of solvents, pH, buffers, buffer concentrations, ionic strength and temperature. This ratio is referred to as a partition coefficient or distribution coefficient and is equal to the ratio of the solubilities in the two solvents. When the compound is a weak acid or base, the distribution of the compound can be shown to be given by the following equation for a monoprotic compound:

$$k_{ow} = \frac{k_0 + k_1 \left(\frac{K_a}{[H]}\right)}{1 + \left(\frac{K_a}{[H]}\right)} \qquad (4.32)$$

Where: k_{ow} is the distribution coefficient; k_0 and k_1 are the intrinsic partition coefficient for species 0 and 1 where species 0 is the most protonated.

If aggregation occurs in one of the phases, Equation (4.32) needs to be modified. Let the aggregation be represented by:

$$nC_1 \rightleftharpoons C_n \qquad (4.33)$$

Where: n is the number of monomers in the aggregate; C_1 is the concentration of the monomer; C_n is the concentration of the aggregate.

For the condition in which there is only one primary monomeric species present in the aqueous phase and in which the aggregation occurs in the organic phase the following equation can be derived:

$$k_{ow} = nK_n k_1^n (C_{1(w)})^{(n-1)} \qquad (4.34)$$

Where: K_n is the equilibrium constant for the formation of the aggregate.

$$K_n = \frac{C_n}{(C_1)^n}$$

Where: k_1 is the intrinsic partition coefficient for the monomeric species; $C_{1(w)}$ is the concentration of the monomer in the aqueous phase.

The following relationship holds when there is only one primary species in the aqueous phase:

$$\log C_{T(O)} = \log n\, K_n k_1^n + n \log C_{T(w)} \tag{4.35}$$

Where: $C_{T(O)}$ is the total concentration in the organic phase; $C_{T(w)}$ is the total concentration in the aqueous phase.

If the aggregation occurs in the aqueous phase the following equation can be derived when there is only one primary monomeric species present in the organic phase:

$$k_{ow} = \left(n \frac{K_n}{k_1^n} \left(C_{1(O)}^{(n-1)} \right) \right)^{-1} \tag{4.36}$$

The following relationship holds when there is only one primary monomeric species in the organic phase:

$$\log C_{T(O)} = \log k_1 - \frac{1}{n}\log n\, K_n + \frac{1}{n}\log C_{T(w)} \tag{4.37}$$

It can be seen in Equations (4.35) and (4.37) that a log–log plot of the total concentration in the aqueous phase versus the total concentration in the organic phase should be linear with a slope >1 if aggregation occurs in the organic phase and a slope <1 if aggregation occurs in the aqueous phase. Furthermore, the slope of the line is equal to the number of monomeric molecules forming the aggregate in the organic phase and is the reciprocal of the number of monomeric molecules forming the aggregate in the aqueous phase.

The assumption made in these derivations is that the aggregate is only present in one phase and therefore does not partition between the two phases to any appreciable extent. If the aggregate should partition between the two phases, then this approach would not work and the slope of the line would be close to one. It would be expected that highly charged aggregates could form in the aqueous phase and not the organic phase and uncharged aggregates would be more apt to form in the organic phase.

An example of this can be seen in Figure 4.4. This is a zwitterionic compound with two pK_a values, the first about 4.25 and the second at about 9.0, and therefore over the pH range of the study there were three possible species which could form. The measured $\log k_i$ values for the three species were 0.4, 0.3 and 0.74 for the cationic, zwitterionic and anionic species, respectively, when not considering aggregation. Experimentally, three pH were chosen where there was only one monomeric species present: pH 2, pH 7 and pH 11. Four different concentrations of the compound were studied: 1.55×10^{-4} M, 1.01×10^{-4} M, 4.96×10^{-5} M and 1.84×10^{-5} M. It can be seen that the slopes of two of the curves are similar while one is different. The slopes at pH 2 and 7 are 0.86 and 0.97, respectively, while the slope at pH 11 is 0.37. There does not appear to be any aggregation in the organic phase at any pH, but at pH 11 the compound appears to be aggregating in the aqueous phase with an aggregation number of three.

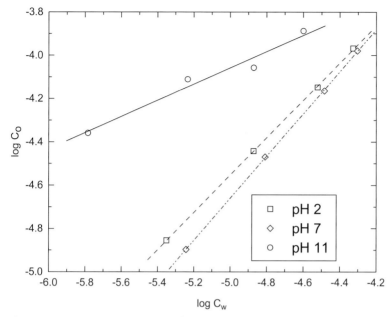

Figure 4.4 Concentration dependence of the partitioning of a compound that forms an aggregate. In this figure, C_0 and C_w are $C_{T(0)}$ and $C_{T(w)}$ in Equation (4.35).

4.10
Solubility in Simulated Biological Fluids

As already mentioned, the solubility of compounds can be influenced by the presence of other compounds in the solution. This can simply be an ionic strength effect which results in changes to the activity coefficients; or the additional compounds can directly interact with the compound of interest and result in complexes or aggregates being formed or salts having lower solubility. The use of simulated biological fluids in the determination of solubilities has not been done extensively. The potential for some type of interaction increases as the solubility of the compound decreases. While these interactions result in an increase in the overall solubility of the compound, it can also have the effect of reducing the transport rate through pharmacological membranes. Some compounds which are used to simulate biological fluids are bile acid salts such as sodium taurocholate. These salts are present in intestinal fluids and are therefore a logical choice to use when trying to simulate intestinal fluids and determine the effect biological fluids might have on the overall solubility.

Simulated intestinal fluid is associated more with dissolution rate determination than solubility measurements. Sometimes when a compound has particularly low solubility the dissolution is studied in simulated fluids. The intent is to try and produce an increased dissolution rate. If there is an increased rate it would be due to an interaction between the compound and the dissolution fluid. Sometimes this increased rate is due simply to an increase in the wettability of the compound and therefore not a specific increase in the solubility; but for poorly soluble compounds any increase in dissolution rate is often due to specific interactions.

Whenever a compound has an increase in solubility when using simulated biological fluids, some concern should be raised because it can be a forebearer of changes to the transport properties. If a compound strongly interacts with something in the fluid there is a good chance that the transport rate across the pharmacological membranes decreases. While this decrease might not be bad, it is something that needs to be understood and investigated.

At other times the compound is found to have significant protein binding. Again this can lead to an increase in the solubility of the compound. If the binding occurs in the blood, it could lead to reduced elimination rate constants. Whenever the pharmacology studies indicate some type of interaction is happening additional studies should be conducted to try and elucidate the interactions. If the compound has a particularly low solubility it can lend itself to solubility studies which can be used to determine the interaction equilibrium constants and effect on the overall solubility.

References

For further reading, the following texts can be used to obtain a more detailed understanding of the material discussed in this chapter.

1 Avdeef, A. (2007) Solubility of sparingly-soluble drugs. In: Special issue. Dressman, J., Reppas, C. (eds) The importance of drug solubility. *Advanced Drug Delivery Reviews*, **59**, 568–590.
2 Avdeef, A., Bendels, S., Tsinman, O., Tsinman, K. and Kansy, M. (2007) Solubility-excipient classification gradient maps. *Pharmaceutical Research*, **24**, 530–545.
3 Avdeef, A., Voloboy, D. and Forman, A. (2006) Dissolution and solubility, in *Comprehensive Medicinal Chemistry II*, Vol. 5, ADME-TOX Approaches (eds B. Testa and H. van de Waterbeemd), Elsevier, Oxford.
4 Avdeef, A. (2001) High-throughput measurements of solubility profiles, in *Pharmacokinetic Optimization in Drug Research* (eds B. Testa, H. van de Waterbeemd, G. Folkers and R. Guy), Wiley-VCH, Weinheim.
5 Avdeef, A. (2003) *Absorption and Drug Development, Solubility, Permeability, and Charge State*, John Wiley & Sons, Hoboken, New Jersey.
6 Connors, K.A. (1987) *Binding Constants, The measurement of Molecular Complex Stability*, John Wiley & Sons, New York.
7 Grant, D.J.W. and Higuchi, T. (1990) Solubility Behavior of Organic Compounds, in *Techniques of Chemistry*, Vol. XXI (ed. W.H. Saunders), John Wiley & Sons, New York.
8 Lewis, G.N., Randall, M., Pitzer, K.S. and Brewer, L. (1961) *Thermodynamics*, McGraw-Hill Book Company, New York.
9 Popovych, O. and Tomkins, R.P.T. (1981) *Nonaqueous Solution Chemistry*, John Wiley & Sons, New York.
10 Shinoda, K. (1978) Translated by P. Becher *Principles of Solution and Solubility*, Marcel Dekker, New York.
11 Streng, W.H. (2001) *Characterization of Compounds in Solution, Theory and Practice*, Kluwer Academic, Plenum.
12 Yalkowsky, S.H. and Banerjee, S. (1992) *Aqueous Solubility, Methods of Estimation for Organic Compounds*, Marcel Dekker.

5
In Silico Tools and In Vitro HTS Approaches to Determine Lipophilicity During the Drug Discovery Process

Sophie Martel, Vincent Gasparik, and Pierre-Alain Carrupt

5.1
Introduction

Advances in rational drug design and combinatorial chemistry increased drastically the number of newly promising active compounds. As inappropriate pharmacokinetics (PK) was recognized as one of the major factors leading to the withdrawal of new chemical entities (NCEs) from drug development [1, 2], efficient *in silico* and *in vitro* models were developed to replace *in vivo* studies for absorption, distribution, metabolism, excretion (ADME) and toxicity (T) in the early phases of drug research [3]. The large number of approaches offering suitable estimates of ADMET properties in the early stages of drug discovery has been extensively reviewed [4–11]. These approaches used largely (Q)SAR models based on physicochemical parameters such as solubility, ionization and lipophilicity. Thus these fundamental physicochemical properties have to be estimated early in drug discovery programs to filter out unsuitable compounds and to rank validated hits in order to select the most promising compounds according to their pharmacodynamic and pharmacokinetic profiles. As the paradigms of hit-like [12, 13], lead-like [13–16] or drug-like properties [17–24] are governing the research, considerable efforts are still carried out to develop efficient virtual and experimental filters to reduce large chemical databases to smaller collections of compounds with suitable PK properties for an *in vivo* high therapeutic potency [25].

Among the physicochemical properties involved in ADMET profiling, lipophilicity has a place of choice as the major contributor to solubility, membrane permeation and protein binding [26, 27], metabolism and the ability to reach and to bind the targeted receptors [28]. This predominant position is well illustrated by numerous papers devoted to this topic (for recent reviews, see [6, 11, 29, 30]). To overcome the limitations of the time-consuming traditional methods such as the shake-flask, potentiometry (for ionizable compounds) and cyclic voltammetry (for ions only), a number of *in silico* and experimental high-throughput techniques

Hit and Lead Profiling. Edited by Bernard Faller and Laszlo Urban
Copyright © 2009 WILEY-VCH Verlag GmbH & Co. KGaA, Weinheim
ISBN: 978-3-527-32331-9

emerged. The scope of this chapter is to review these HTS methods for log P and log D determination in the 1-octanol/water system and in other solvent/water systems useful in the early stages of drug discovery.

5.2
Virtual Filtering: *In Silico* Prediction of log P and log D

Among the large number of existing lipophilicity parameters [31], the descriptor frequently estimated by *in silico* methods is the partition coefficient of a solute between 1-octanol and water, expressed as log P_{oct} [32]. However, lipophilicity determination in different solvent systems, such as alkane/water system, proved its utility in (Q)SAR studies and therefore some predictive methods also emerged in this field. Many publically available databases include numerous experimental values collected through the literature; the quality of the experimental data represents the cornerstone of most of the models developed to predict lipophilicity.

This section presents the different methods employed as virtual filters to predict log P in the 1-octanol/water system and in other solvent systems. In Table 5.1, one can find a list of useful softwares which use one of the reviewed methods (Table 5.1).

5.2.1
Lipophilicity of Neutral Substances: *In Silico* Methods to Predict log P_{oct}^{N}

Medicinal chemists have numerous fast *in silico* tools to evaluate the log P_{oct} of NCEs prior to synthesis. These different methods can be divided in two main classes according to the level of description of molecular structure, namely *2D fragmental methods* which cut the molecule in typical atomic or multiatomic fragments possessing their own lipophilicity coefficients and *3D global methods* which code explicitly the principal intermolecular interactions potential of a 3D molecule. This section presents only an outline of the principal *in silico* methods since this subject was recently reviewed in detail [33, 34].

5.2.1.1 2D Fragmental Approaches
These methods model the log P by adding the specific contributions of elementary building blocks of a molecule, that is, the chemical monoatomic or multiatomic fragments. The geometrical and topological effects that operate in such a case mean that several correction factors have to be added to the additivity scheme.

π-Constant Method The precursor method of Hansch and Fujita [35] consisted in the definition of a hydrophobic substituent constant, π_X, for a fragment X, obtained by a comparison between the lipophilicity of the compound R-X and its hydrogenated parent compound R-H, according to Equation (5.1):

$$\pi_X = \log P_{R-X} - \log P_{R-H} \qquad (5.1)$$

Table 5.1 Non-exhaustive list of software packages which use one of the methods described.

Method/software	Web address[a]
Fragment-based	
CLOGP	www.biobyte.com or http://www.daylight.com/
KLOGP	http://www.multicase.com/
KOWWIN	http://www.epa.gov/oppt/exposure/pubs/episuite.htm
AB/LogP	http://pharma-algorithms.com/
Mi_logP	http://www.molinspiration.com/
ACD/LogP	http://www.acdlabs.com/ilab/
Atom-based Methods	
Spartan	www.wavefun.com
XLOGP	http://fulcrum.physbio.mssm.edu/docs/molmod/xlogp/index.html
Tsar	http://accelrys.com/
Marvin	http://www.chemaxon.com/marvin/help/index.html
MOLCAD	http://www.tripos.com
SLOGP	http://www.chemcomp.com/
Property explorer	www.actelion.com
PrologP	www.compudrug.com
AlogP98	http://accelrys.com/
3D Structure Representation	
QLOGP	www.q-pharm.com
Absolv	http://pharma-algorithms.com/
Chemprop	http://www.ufz.de/index.php?en=10684
SPARC	http://ibmlc2.chem.uga.edu/sparc/
COSMO_therm	http://www.cosmologic.de/
GBLOGP	http://www.molsoft.com/mprop/
HINT	http://www.edusoft-lc.com/hint/
CLIP	http://129.194.54.222/site_lct_gp/sous_sites/clip/docs/main_clip.html
ALOGPS	http://www.vcclab.org/lab/alogps/
VLOGP	www.accelrys.com
VolSurf	http://www.moldiscovery.com/soft_volsurf.php
TLOGP	http://upstream.ch/products/tlogp.html
CS-logP	http://www.chemsilico.com/

[a] All the Internet sites were last visited on June 2009.

Thus, π_X represents the lipophilicity contribution of the fragment X. This π_X constant takes different values according to the aliphatic or aromatic nature of the considered compound. This method, not implemented in any software, is limited by the necessity to have good log P measurements for the parent compounds for tested solutes.

Σf Method This method developed by Rekker and Mannhold [36] uses fragmental hydrophobicity coefficients and correction factors obtained via a "reductionist" approach, deriving the constants for each fragment from Free–Wilson type regression analysis of a large set of experimental log P_{oct} data. The estimated log P is thus calculated using Equation (5.2):

$$\log P_{oct} = \sum_{i=1}^{n} a_i \cdot f_i + \sum_{j=1}^{m} b_j \cdot k_j \cdot C_M \qquad (5.2)$$

where f_i is the hydrophobic fragmental constant of fragment i; a_i is the number of fragment i in the molecule; b is the occurrence of the correction factor j characterized by the product of the coefficient k by the magic constant C_M; n and m are the total number of different fragments and correction factors, respectively [37]. The magic constant (originally 0.289, then revised to 0.219) was derived from the diverse chemical features identified as correction factors which are simple multiples of this constant. This method is still under development and was recently adapted to the alkane/water system [37, 38].

Clog P This method developed by Leo and Hansch presents some similarities with the method of Rekker, since the log P of a molecule is calculated by adding lipophilicity values attributed to multiatomic fragments and numerous corrections factors which take into account not only geometrical and topological effects but also electronic and steric effects (Equation 5.3) [39–41].

$$\log P_{oct} = \sum_{i=1}^{n} a_i \cdot f_i + \sum_{j=1}^{m} b_j \cdot F_j \qquad (5.3)$$

where f_i is the hydrophobic constant of fragment i; a_i is the number of fragment i in the molecule; b is the occurrence of the correction factor j characterized by its lipophilicity contribution F_j; n and m are the total number of different fragments and correction factors, respectively. The way to define the fragments contribution differs from the former method depicted by Rekker since the principles of "constructionism" by deriving fragmental values from a carefully measured log P of a small set of simple molecules was applied [41].

Atom-based Methods As for fragmental methods, the molecule is considered as composed of fragments, but these latter are single atoms instead of functional groups. Each atom is characterized by its own lipophilicity constant and the global lipophilicity is then a sum of each contribution (Equation 5.4).

$$\log P_{oct} = \sum_{i=1}^{n} a_i \cdot f_i^A \qquad (5.4)$$

where f^A is the atomic fragmental constant; a_i indicates the occurrence of a given atom i and n the total number of different atoms in the molecule. Geometrical and topological effects are implicitly encoded in the definition of the different atoms which reflect their hybridization and their chemical environment. Thus a large number of atom types is needed to describe large data set of compounds. The most widely used atom-based approaches are the methods of Ghose and Crippen [42, 43] and Broto and Moreau [44].

5.2.1.2 Prediction Methods Based on 3-D Molecular Structure

These methods were developed to avoid the definition and parameterization of numerous fragments or atomic types and to allow the prediction of lipophilicity for stereoisomers or conformers. Only a selection of methods are highlighted here, since an excellent extensive review was recently published [34].

Use of Modified Atomic Contributions Some variations were made on the atom-based methods by considering the solvent-accessible surface area (SASA) [45, 46].

Villar et al. developed an atomic hydrophobicity contribution that depends on the molecular conformation. The hydrophobicity parameters were calculated by including charge densities, atomic contributions to the total molecular surface area and the molecular dipole moment [47, 48]. This method is implemented in the SPARTAN software.

A modification of the atomic approach was also proposed by Gaillard et al. using molecular lipophilicity potential (MLP) as a 3D source of two lipophilicity parameters calculated from the water-accessible surface, namely a hydrophobic parameter expressed as the sum of the positive lipophilicity potential (ΣMLP+) and a polar parameter expressed as the sum of the negative lipophilicity potential (ΣMLP−) [49, 50]. The lipophilicity of the 3D structure (virtual log P_{oct}) is calculated using Equation (5.5).

$$\log P_{oct} = c_1 \cdot \sum_{i=1}^{n} \mathrm{MLP}_i + + c_2 \cdot \sum_{j=1}^{m} \mathrm{MLP}_j - + c_3 \tag{5.5}$$

where c_1, c_2 and c_3 are regression coefficients, n and m the total number of water-accessible surface points i respectively; with, respectively, a positive and a negative lipophilicity potential.

Cruciani et al., used a dynamic physicochemical interaction model to evaluate the interaction energies between a water probe and the hydrophilic and hydrophobic regions of the solute with the GRID force field. The VolSurf program was used to generate a PLS model able to predict log P_{oct} [51] from the 3D molecular structure.

Use of Topological Descriptors Some in silico tools used topological descriptors calculated from the 3D molecular structure to predict log P_{oct}. For example, MLOGP method [52] which considered atomic contributions to differentiate hydrophobic and hydrophilic atoms and thirteen descriptors such as intramolecular hydrogen bonds abilities and proximity effects, TLOGP which used uniform-length molecular descriptors generated from 3D structures [53]. A "molecular size-based approach" was also published by Bodor and Buchwald using a 3D estimation of molecular size and an algorithm combining analytical and numerical techniques to compute van der Waals molecular volume and surface area [54].

Use of E-state Descriptors A method that is still growing is the use of electro-topological state indices (E-state indices) for the prediction of log P. These E-state indices express both topological and electronic valence status of each atom type in a molecule (atom-type E-state indices). In the same way, such indices describe well specific bonds connecting atoms (bond-type E-state indices) [55]. ALOGPS used linear and neural networks schemes to calculate log P and offered good prediction of log P [34, 56]. VLOGP, included in Topkat (Discovery Studio by Accelrys), also used E-state descriptors treated by the linear free energy relationship (LFER) [57].

Use of Solvatochromic Equations Solvatochromic analysis for log P calculations appears to be one of the more useful approach built using linear free energy relationship (LFER) described by the general Equation (5.6) [58]:

$$\log P = v \cdot V_W + p \cdot \pi^* + a \cdot \alpha + b \cdot \beta + c \quad (5.6)$$

where V_w is the van der Waals volume; π^* is the polarity/polarisability; α and β are the H-bond acidity and basicity respectively; v, p, a, b and c are the multilinear regression parameters. This equation was later modified [59] leading to a new Equation (5.7):

$$\log P = v \cdot V + e \cdot E + s \cdot S + a \cdot A + b \cdot B + c \quad (5.7)$$

where V is the McGowan characteristic volume; E is the solute excess molar refractivity; S is the solute dipolarity/polarizability; A and B are the overall molecule hydrogen bond acidity and basicity respectively. The coefficients v, e, s, a, b, and c are obtained by multiple linear regression analysis and they characterize the balance of intermolecular forces governing the property analyzed (here the log P).

Partitioning in 1-octanol/water system has been characterized from a data set of 600 experimental log P_{oct} values by the following LFER equation (Equation 5.8) [60, 61]:

$$\log P_{oct} = 3.814 \cdot V + 0.562 \cdot E + 1.054 \cdot S - 0.032 \cdot A - 3.460 \cdot B + 0.088 \quad (5.8)$$

which clearly shows that octanol/water partition coefficient are predominantly governed by the volume and the H-bond basicity of the solute.

5.2.1.3 General Comments on the Prediction of log P_{oct}

Several attempts were performed to determine the accuracy of *in silico* prediction tools developed for lipophilicity (for a recent review, see [34]). The main factor limiting the accuracy of all predictive methods is the training sets used to generate the models, in terms of population and quality of the experimental data they contain. Since most of the methods proposed in commercial software were built with data available in the public domain, their accuracy can be expected to be comparable. Thus, in order to select the most suitable prediction tool, other criteria than accuracy have to be used such as the speed of the calculation for large databases, the price of commercial software or the application domain of the model.

Despite the good results obtained in some accuracy tests, one have to keep in mind that fragmental methods suffers from the absence of peculiar fragments that could limit their applicability domain. The prediction performance of fragmental methods also largely depends on the chemical diversity of the molecular structures used to develop the model.

Methods based on molecular properties attempt to avoid the drawbacks of the fragmental methods, such as their failure to calculate log P for structures with missing fragments. However, in some cases, models were derived from sets of compounds with moderate chemical diversity limiting the accuracy of predicted log P.

An interesting solution recently emerged to enhance the accuracy of predictive tools which is the use of several methods and the generation of consensus results. This strategy was successfully applied in QSAR [62] and preliminary results have demonstrated an increased accuracy in log P_{oct} prediction when consensus models were derived by neural network using as input eight well known prediction values [63].

5.2.2
Prediction Models for log P in Other Solvent/Water Systems of Neutral Compounds

Different balance between intermolecular forces can be accessible *via* partition coefficients measured in solvents systems other than the traditional 1-octanol/water. Therefore there was a growing interest in the partition processes in several solvent/water systems [64, 65] and in particular the "critical quartet" of solvents which was designed to merge the main information about a solute concerning its partition and transport. Only a few studies have been performed to characterize the lipophilicity profile of new chemical entities in different solvent/water systems and consequently the number of methods attempting to model such partitioning systems is limited.

Since the $\Delta \log P_{oct-alk}$ is a useful parameter to characterize the polarity of a compounds [31] and to estimate brain permeation [26], the prediction of log P_{alk} retained the attention of researchers. The fragmental approach of Rekker was first used to derive fragment constants for the alkane/water system [36, 38]. Another way to access *in silico* log P_{alk} was derived from LFER equations [60]. By close analogy with the work of Cruciani *et al.* for the prediction of log P_{oct} [51], a method was described for log P_{alk} prediction using Volsurf and a combination of molecular interaction fields descriptors obtained with GRID [66]. Recently, an original work was reported to predict the $\Delta \log P_{oct-alk}$ as a function of the minimized molecular electrostatic potential (V_{min}) that describes the H-bonding capacity of solutes [67].

The LFER approach of Abraham was the most powerful method to predict partition coefficients in varied experimental conditions (for example, see [68–72]). In particular, since 1,2-dichloroethane and *o*-nitrophenyl octyl ether are good experimental substitutes for alkane, *in silico* tools were developed with LFER equations to predict log P_{DCE} [73] or log P_{NPOE} [74, 75].

5.2.3
Prediction Models for log P of Ionic Species (log P^i)

All the previous prediction methods outlined above only deal with the partitioning of the neutral form of the solute. However, most of therapeutic compounds possess ionizable functions and therefore dissociation equilibria in solution have to be considered for their partitioning in biphasic media. The importance of partitioning of ionized species is emphasized in the literature since the prediction of either a distribution coefficient (log D^{pH}) at a given pH or lipophilicity profiles (log D as a function of pH) increases the early physicochemical description of NCEs [76–78]. The pH partition theory links the distribution coefficient of ionizable molecule to the partition coefficients of its electric species by Equation (5.9):

$$D^{pH} = f^N \cdot P^N + \sum f^I \cdot P^I \qquad (5.9)$$

where f is the molar fraction of a given electrical species (neutral or ionized); P is the corresponding partition coefficient. Thus a good prediction of distribution coefficients [79–81] requires not only good models to calculate log P of ionized and unionized species but also good models to estimate the pK_a [82, 83] of ionizable functions and thus their molar fractions at any pH value. The task is more difficult when complex chemical equilibria such as competitive microionization and ion pairing which may differ in aqueous or organic media occur. Thus now *in silico* predictions of log D^{pH} offer only a first ranking of NCEs requiring careful experimental validation (for a recent review, see [27]).

5.3
Experimental Filtering: the ADMET Characterization of a Hit Collection

Among the number of recognized methods to measure partition coefficients, the shake-flask method remains the "gold standard" technique still in use, in particular during new methods validation. However, it suffers from time-consuming steps and a number of parameters have to be seriously controlled to avoid erroneous values [84]. In early discovery, a crucial step is the ADMET characterization of a large number of NCEs to rapidly characterize hit compounds. At this step, experimental methods with an acceptable accuracy, a low sample consumption and above all a high-throughput are required. That is why efforts are still carried out to develop new HTS approaches to cover these needs. The following section rapidly describes methods which have been recently reviewed, while concentrating on methods that are more recent.

5.3.1
HTS log P/log D Determination Based on Microtiterplate Format

Methods have been proposed to miniaturize, speed up and automate the shake-flask approach. The main difficulties in this challenge are the number of time-consuming steps which cannot be totally eliminated and the persistence of well known drawbacks. For example, the mutual saturation and decantation of organic and aqueous phases, or the crucial separation of the two phases after shaking which multiplies the manipulations. Automation of the process is also difficult due to several compound-dependent parameters which have to be rigorously controlled, such as the volume ratio between organic solvent and aqueous phase according to the estimated log P, or the sample concentration.

In general, the great advantage of methods based on the 96-well plate is the decrease in sample amount and the large number of compounds tested simultaneously (parallel process). However, to offer a good throughput, the method has to be as generic as possible.

In 2000, Hitzel et al. [85] proposed an automated and HTS shake-flask method for the determination of distribution coefficients at a fixed pH (log D) [85]. Applying this technique to log D measurements instead of log P limits the number of different buffer solutions in a given plate and therefore simplifies automation. Furthermore, three log D values were determined for each compound, using different loading concentrations and after shaking sample concentrations were determined in the two phases by direct injection in HPLC system, without separation of the two phases. Even if the log D range accessible remains in the range from -2 to $+4$, this miniaturization of the original shake-flask allows for a significant drop in compound quantity and a gain of time. Furthermore, to increase the throughput, the authors encourage the use of a fast gradient liquid chromatography analysis which drastically reduces the analysis time. In practice, a 96-well microtiterplate with 48 compounds (in duplicate) could be prepared, shaked and analyzed in one day using an automated pipeting system for the addition of the two immiscible phases. More recently, HSLogD was developed more specifically for lipophilic compounds ($0 < \log D < +5$) [86]. For such compounds usually highly soluble in 1-octanol, the direct injection and analysis of the lower phase (aqueous phase) could lead to contamination since the concentration in 1-octanol is higher than in water and the presence of a small amount of 1-octanol inside and around the needle cannot be excluded (due to its viscosity). Therefore, a sampling method was adapted to avoid such contamination consisting in an aspiration of water before aspiration of sample, and a thorough needle wash before HPLC injection. Furthermore, after the shaking process, a part of the organic phase was taken and diluted 2500-fold in 1-octanol before analysis. The advantage also lies in the final detection by LC-MS and the use of sample solution stock in DMSO which can be an advantage in the early stage of drug development.

Based on the 96-well format, OCT-PAMPA was proposed and has proved its ability to determine (indirectly) log P_{oct} [87]. PAMPA is a method, first developed for permeability measurements, where a filter supports an artificial membrane (an organic solvent or phospholipids) [88, 89]. With this method, the apparent permeability coefficient (log P_a) of the neutral form of tested compounds is derived from the measurement of the diffusion between two aqueous phases separated by 1-octanol layer (immobilized on a filter). A bilinear correlation was found between log P_a and log P_{oct}, therefore log P_{oct} of unknown compounds can be determined from log P_a using a calibration curve. Depending on the detection method used a range of log P within -2 to $+5$ (with UV detection) and within -2 to $+8$ (with LC-MS detection) was successfully explored. This method requires low compound amounts (300 μl of 0.04 mM test compound) and, as for the previous method, samples can be prepared in DMSO stock solutions. For these experiments, an incubation time of 4 h was determined as the best compromise in term of discrimination. The limitation of the technique lies in the lower accuracy values obtained for compounds with log P within 0 to 2 where the curve flattens, and for the lipophilicity determination of compounds which are never entirely in their neutral form throughout the pH range 2–11.

In the same way, o-nitrophenyl octyl ether (o-NPOE) was immobilized on polycarbonate (PC) filters and the apparent permeability measured after 5 h incubation time was correlated to log P_{NPOE} for a series of reference compounds (log P_{NPOE} ranging from -1 to 3.6) [90]. Lipophilicity values in the alkane/water system were also determined using PAMPA with hexadecane-PC coated filters [89]. In this case, a correlation was found between intrinsic permeability (log P_0, permeability corrected for ionization and for unstirred water layer contribution, which particularly affects permeability of lipophilic compounds) and log P_{alk}. However, log P_0 is obtained from the knowledge of the pK_a value(s) and the permeability pH profile and therefore requires the full permeability pH profile to be measured for each compound, which negatively impacts the assay throughput.

An indirect method for the determination of log P_{oct} was also proposed by Chen et al. [91]. The method is based on the partitioning of solutes between a plasticized PVC film (PVC/dioctyl sebacate) and water (log P_{pw}) in 96-well microtiterplates. For a series of 15 reference compounds with log P_{oct} ranging from 0.5 to 3.2, the authors showed that log P_{oct} was related to log P_{pw} by Equation (5.10):

$$\log P_{pw} = 0.933(\pm 0.054) \cdot \log P_{oct} + 0.185(\pm 0.108)$$
$$n = 15; \; r^2 = 0.95; \; se = 0.170; \; p < 0.0001 \quad (5.10)$$

Therefore, using a calibration curve, log P_{oct} of an unknown compound can be deduced from log P_{pw}. Interestingly, the regression coefficients obtained (slope close to 1 and intercept close to 0) indicate a similarity with the 1-octanol system. However, there are differences between the two systems in term of H-bond donor and acceptor abilities, suggesting a lower efficiency of the approach for compounds with high H-bond capacity.

5.3.2
Chromatographic Methods

The great advantage of chromatography for lipophilicity determination is its ability to estimate log P or log D with a relative accuracy for non-pure samples, with a limited quantity of compound. Furthermore, these methods are relatively easily to automate and they only require an HPLC or UPLC apparatus. Many approaches have been described and this topic was recently reviewed [5, 27]. That is why the focus of the following section is on strategies developed to increase the throughput and the assay dynamic range.

5.3.2.1 Reverse-Phase Liquid Chromatography
Numerous recent reviews and guidelines have been published in this field [5, 84, 92]. Therefore, in this part, we summarize the basic principles only. Briefly, lipophilicity determination by RP-LC is based on the partitioning of the solute between an apolar stationary phase and a polar mobile phase. The experimental retention factor (log k)

can be correlated to log P using the general Equation (5.11):

$$\log P = a \cdot \log k + b \tag{5.11}$$

In practice the regression coefficients a and b have to be determined for every couple of stationary and mobile phases, by measuring the log k values for a series of reference compounds with known log P values. The calibration equation obtained then allows the determination of log P of new compounds.

Numerous stationary phases were studied for their potential to determine lipophilicity [5, 27, 84, 92]. Their ability to predict log P was often limited to congeneric series of compounds, due to the difference in molecular interactions governing both partitioning in 1-octanol/water system and chromatographic retention, and due to specific interactions with silanol groups. Finally only few columns were retained for their real interest [93, 94], in particular the Supelcosil LC-ABZ [95], the Supelcosil LC-ABZ+ and the Discovery RP Amide C16 [94]. The general logP range explored with this technique is from -1 to $+5$, and the pH range recommended is between 2 and 7 for such silica-based stationary phases and therefore remains a limitation for strongly basic compounds. These methods require the use of an organic modifier (methanol or acetonitrile) to avoid the collapse of hydrophobic chains and associated decreased elution time. It has often been considered that $\log k_w$ (extrapolated value obtained from four or five log k values measured for different percentages of organic modifier) was a better predictor of the lipophilicity of solutes compared to log k obtained at a fixed percentage of organic modifier. Therefore, the throughput and the accuracy become lower and lower in particular for highly lipophilic compounds due to their strong retention, the peaks broadening and the long distance extrapolation to 0% of organic modifier from isocratic $\log k_i$ measured.

Recently, short columns have been used to: (i) decrease analysis time; (ii) decrease the percentage of organic modifier used (decreasing the uncertainty due to long distance extrapolation); (iii) enlarge lipophilicity range to values up to 8 [96, 97]. The use of short columns packed with small particles ($< 2\,\mu m$), and working under very high pressures (ultra performance liquid chromatography) also allows a great diminution of analysis time, as recently demonstrated using an Acquity BEH Shield RP18 stationary phase [118].

Furthermore it was shown that the addition of 1-octanol in mobile phase often enhances the correlation between log P_{oct} and log k [97–99]. In the same way the coating of a 0.8 cm HiChrom H5SAS C1 cadridge with 1-octanol recently proved its interest for the determination of log P_{oct} of neutral pharmaceutical compounds ranging from 1 to 4 with a flow gradient mode [100].

To speed up the lipophilicity determination it was also proposed to use gradient elution procedures (for a review and guidelines, see references [5, 101]). This generic approach is particularly useful when series of compounds with a broad lipophilicity range have to be tested since both polar and non-polar solutes can be retained with a reasonable elution time.

As in isocratic mode, the variation in the percentage of organic modifier in the mobile phase can be described by the linear Soczewinski–Snyder model

(Equation 5.12):

$$\log k = \log k_w + S \cdot \varphi \qquad (5.12)$$

where log k_w is the retention factor extrapolated to 100% water as mobile phase; S is a constant for a given solute and a given LC system; φ is the organic modifier percentage in the mobile phase. According to the linear solvent strength (LSS) approach [102], log k_w can be determined with a single gradient [102] run or two gradient runs (more accurate) [93].

The second approach using gradient mode to assess log P values first proposed by Valko et al. is the use of the chromatographic hydrophobicity index (CHI) obtained from a single fast gradient run (<15 min) [103]. Since CHI is considered as a relevant parameter for QSAR studies, it was demonstrated using LSER that differences occur between CHI parameters and true log P because CHI (and log k) are sensitive to H-bond acidity ability whereas log P is not [104]. Thus, CHIs have to be used with precaution.

Nevertheless, even if the accuracy of the gradient methods is slightly lower than with isocratic conditions [105], it offers the ability to extend lipophilicity range determination without too high a loss in resolution. Therefore, it was recommended to preferentially use isocratic mode for expected log P between 0 to 4 and to use gradient mode for more lipophilic compounds [105].

For cost reasons, UV detection is usually used with chromatographic methods. However, MS detection is increasingly more appreciated since several compounds can be analyzed simultaneously, thus greatly increasing the assay throughput [106, 107]

5.3.2.2 Immobilized Artificial Membranes

Due to their better biomimetic properties, phospholipids have been proposed as an alternative to 1-octanol for lipophilicity studies. The use of immobilized artificial membranes (IAM) in lipophilicity determination was recently reviewed and we thus only briefly summarize the main conclusions [108]. IAM phases are silica-based columns with phospholipids bounded covalently. IAM are based on phosphatidylcholine (PC) linked to a silica propylamine surface. Most lipophilicity studies with IAM were carried out using an aqueous mobile phase with pH values from 7.0 to 7.4 (log D measurements). Therefore, tested compounds were neutral, totally or partially ionized in these conditions. It was shown that the lipophilicity parameters obtained on IAM stationary phases and the partition coefficients in 1-octanol/water system were governed by different balance of intermolecular interactions [109]. Therefore the relationships between log k_{IAM} and log P_{oct} varied with the class of compounds studied [110]. However, it was shown that, for neutral compounds with log $P_{oct} > 1$, a correspondence existed between the two parameters when "double-chain" IAM phases (i.e., IAM.PC.MG and IAM.PC.DD2) were used [111]. In contrast, in the case of ionized compounds, retention on IAM columns and partitioning in 1-octanol/water system were significantly different due to ionic interactions expressed in IAM retention but not in 1-octanol/water system and due to acidic and basic compounds behaving differently in these two systems.

Finally the relation between log k_{IAM} and partition in liposomes depends on analytes and was observed only for hydrophilic compounds [110].

5.3.2.3 Hydrophilic Interaction Chromatography

For strong basic compounds, a new approach recently emerged, based on hydrophilic interaction liquid chromatography (HILIC) [112]. Since relative instability at high pH of conventional silica-based stationary phases restricts the lipophilicity determination of basic compounds under their neutral form [110, 113–116], the solution was to measure a retention factor for the cationic form (more hydrophilic), related to lipophilicity of the neutral form. A ZIC p-HILIC column was tested with a series of 40 strong basic compounds (pK_a from 7.6 to 10.8), including β-blockers and local anesthetics with log P_{oct} values ranging from -1.3 to 4.6. The mechanisms governing retention in HILIC mode are complex, namely mainly hydrophilic at high percentages of organic modifier, "reverse phase-like" retention at high proportions of water and ion exchange on the whole scale of the organic modifier (Figure 5.1). Depending on the experimental conditions, the two components of lipophilicity parameter (i.e., polarity and hydrophobicity) can be extracted.

Two retention indices are then measured, log k_{95} (log k obtained with a mobile phase containing 95% of acetonitrile and 5% of buffer solution) and log k_0 (retention factor obtained with a pure aqueous mobile phase). The difference between these two values (log k_{0-95}) is correlated to the 1-octanol/water partition coefficient of the neutral form of tested compounds (Equation 5.13):

$$\log k_{0-95} = 0.87(\pm 0.04) \cdot \log P^N_{oct} - 0.45(\pm 0.09)$$
$$n = 40; \; r^2 = 0.93; \; s = 0.34; \; F = 480 \quad (5.13)$$

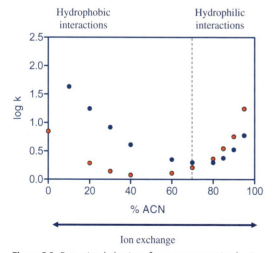

Figure 5.1 Retention behavior of two representative basic compounds (atenolol in red and pindolol in blue) on ZIC p-HILIC stationary phase for different percentages of acetonitrile in mobile phase.

As electrostatic interactions exist between the HILIC zwitterionic stationary phase and charged solutes, particular attention has to be paid to the rigorous control of experimental conditions such as pH, buffer type and ionic strength.

Hydrophilic interaction chromatography was also applied to determine log P in alkane/water system for highly polar compounds (calculated log P_{alk} ranging from 0 to −10) [117]. The retention factor log k_{90} (retention factor obtained with a mobile phase containing 90% of acetonitrile and 10% of buffer solution) measured on a ZIC p-HILIC stationary phase was related to log P_{alk} calculated using the LSER model built on 74 compounds having measured log P_{alk}. It was also demonstrated that the predominant parameters influencing the retention of compounds on ZIC p-HILIC (i.e., volume, hydrogen-bond donor and acceptor capacities) were similar to those involved in the partitioning of solutes in alkane/water system.

5.3.2.4 Capillary Electrophoresis

Lipophilicity determination (log P_{oct}) by capillary electrophoresis (CE) has been extensively published because of its high throughput and low sample consumption compared to liquid chromatography. Four approaches are documented depending on the pseudo-stationary phase considered: (i) MEKC (CE mode based on the partitioning of solute between an aqueous phase and a micellar phase); (ii) MEEKC (with microemulsion as pseudo-stationary phase); (iii) VEKC (with vesicles as pseudo-stationary phase); (iv) LEKC (with liposomes as pseudo-stationary phase) [120–122]. However, it was demonstrated that LEKC was a better predictor for membrane permeability than for 1-octanol/water lipophilicity determination [123]. Also the use of MEKC for log P_{oct} determination remains limited since a congeneric behavior was observed and confirmed by LSER analysis showing a difference in H-bond donor capacity and dipolarity/polarizability between the two processes (i.e., partitioning in water 1-octanol system and retention times measured by CE) [124, 125]. Finally it is now well established that MEEKC provides the best way to evaluate log P_{oct} due to a better stability and reliability, a good reproducibility and an enlarged migration window compared to MEKC or LEKC/VEKC, allowing a dynamic range from −1 to 6.6 [121, 122]. Furthermore, several strategies were reported to increase the throughput, such as pressure-assisted MEEKC where air pressure and voltage were applied to the capillary [126, 127]. Recently, 96-capillary multiplexed MEEKC was developed to meet the demand of the drug discovery process, and further applications to the estimation of log P were published [128–131]. This last methodology allows the determination of up to 46 compounds per hour with a high reproducibility and good precision [132].

5.3.3
A Global View On *In Vitro* HTS Methods to Measure log P/log D

In early discovery, new chemical entities of interest can be either polar compounds (e.g., peptides, nucleotides, sugars) or non-polar compounds (e.g., ligands or inhibitors maximizing hydrophobic interactions with therapeutic targets). Thus ideal HTS *in vitro* methods must be able to cover a large range of lipophilicity values. This goal

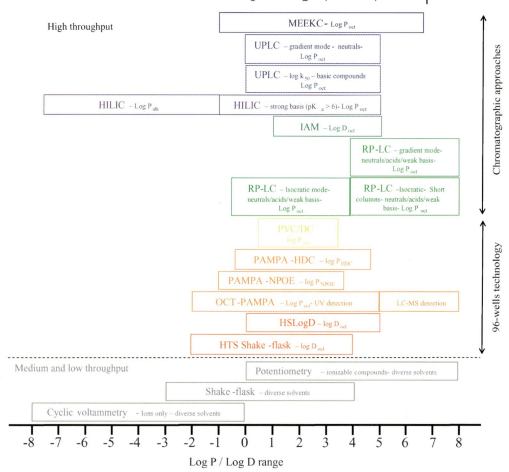

Figure 5.2 The domain of application of *in vitro* techniques used to measure partition coefficients in 1-octanol/water system and in other biphasic systems. In gray: medium- or low-throughput methods not described in this chapter.

cannot be reached with an unique approach but recent developments demonstrated that a combination of different techniques offers the access to a very large range of log P values ($-8 < \log P < 8$), as illustrated on Figure 5.2.

5.4
Concluding Remarks: Efficacy or Accuracy Dilemma

In the drug discovery process, several complementary methods are applied to speed up the identification of compounds with marked therapeutic benefits and to enrich the pharmacokinetic profiles of selected lead compounds. Since the number of potentially interested compounds has largely increased in recent years, information

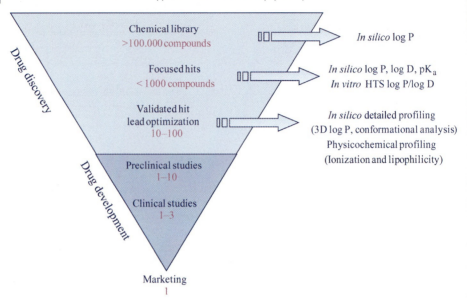

Figure 5.3 Proposed strategy to select the adequate tools to characterize lipophilicity of new chemical entities.

about PK must be obtained as fast and as early as possible in order to select the best possible candidate and decrease attrition during drug development. It is well established that high-quality and precise methods are required to extract the most pertinent information about lipophilicity and ionization from the 3D structure of compounds of therapeutic interest [49, 133–138]. However, the quest for speed is not always compatible with the quality and precision of the method. Thus, the number of compounds to be analyzed frequently governs the choice of method, following the possible strategy described in Figure 5.3.

Briefly, two categories of large chemical databases can be identified, namely commercial available or in-house collections of existing compounds from synthetic or natural origin and collections of virtual compounds generated by virtual combinatorial chemistry or *de novo* design. The very large number of chemical structures composing these databases excludes the use of complex models to estimate their physicochemical or pharmacokinetic profiles. Thus fast *in silico* technologies have to be used to estimate log P from only a 2D description of chemical structure [139]. Since commercial predictive tools are constructed with publicly available log P values of relatively small and mostly neutral molecules, their accuracy on in-house compounds of pharmaceutical companies remains relatively low [30, 56, 140, 141]. In particular, it is not yet feasible to have a good estimation of log D values for these large databases, since precise lipophilicity estimation carries cumulative errors which affect the pK_a predictive tools [82, 83]. In order to increase the accuracy of predicted log P several fast predictive methods can be used and consensus values can be obtained [142].

In contrast fast *in silico* predictive tools for log P and log D (using estimated pK_a values) from the 2D molecular structures can be very useful to enrich the molecular description of hits focused by their predicted (virtual screening) or measured (high-throughput screening) activities on identified targets associated with a given disease. At this stage, *in silico* predictive tools using 3D molecular structures can also be used but their use is restricted to an arbitrary conformation for each compound generally generated by automated tools like Corina [143, 144] or Concord [145]. When these focused chemical libraries are used as a source of validated hits, an early deeper knowledge of their physicochemical properties certainly allows for a better selection of lead candidates. In this context, any improvement of fast high-throughput *in vitro* methods for physiochemical measurement is warmly welcomed, since the molecular complexity of focused hits always represents a problem for theoretical tools.

When a validated hit is selected as a promising lead compound, its physicochemical profile must be studied in detail. Sophisticated *in silico* approaches such as 3D lipophilicity predictions coupled with extensive conformational analysis [49, 50, 135, 146] and molecular field interactions (MIFs) [147–150] could be helpful to better interpret the detailed experimental investigations of their ionization constants by capillary electrophoresis or potentiometric titrations [151, 152] and their lipophilicity profiles by potentiometry [153]. However, these complex approaches cannot be performed easily on large number of compounds and are generally applied only on the most promising compounds.

Acknowledgments

The authors warmly thanks all the co-workers involved in the development of some *in silico* or *in vitro* tools presented here for their enthusiasm and the quality of their research.

References

1 Kennedy, T. (1997) Managing the drug discovery/development interface. *Drug Discovery Today*, 2, 436–444.
2 Hou, T.J. and Xu, X.J. (2003) ADME evaluation in drug discovery. 3. Modeling blood-brain barrier partitioning using simple molecular descriptors. *Journal of Chemical Information and Computer Sciences*, 43, 2137–2152.
3 van de Waterbeemd, H. and Gifford, E. (2003) ADMET in silico modelling: Towards prediction paradise? *Nature Reviews. Drug Discovery*, 2, 192–204.
4 Reist, M., Novaroli, L., Daina, A., Martel, S. and Carrupt, P.A. (2005) The medicinal chemist's dream: faster design of better and safer drug candidates. *Chimia*, 59, 295–298.
5 Martel, S., Guillarme, D., Henchoz, Y., Galland, A., Veuthey, J.L., Rudaz, S. and Carrupt, P.A. (2008) Chromatographic approaches for measuring log P, in *Drug Properties: Measurement and Computation* (ed. R. Mannhold), Wiley-VCH, Weinheim, pp. 331–356.
6 Efremov, R.G., Chugunov, A.O., Pyrkov, T.V., Priestle, J.P., Arseniev, A.S. and Jacoby, E. (2007) Molecular lipophilicity in protein modeling and drug design. *Current Medicinal Chemistry*, 14, 393–415.

7 Verma, R.P., Hansch, C. and Selassie, C.D. (2007) Comparative QSAR studies on PAMPA/modified PAMPA for high throughput profiling of drug absorption potential with respect to Caco-2 cells and human intestinal absorption. *Journal of Computer-Aided Molecular Design*, **21**, 3–22.

8 Davies, J.W., Glick, M. and Jenkins, J.L. (2006) Streamlining lead discovery by aligning in silico and high-throughput screening. *Current Opinion in Chemical Biology*, **10**, 343–351.

9 Wunberg, T., Hendrix, M., Hillisch, A., Lobell, M., Meier, H., Schmeck, C., Wild, H. and Hinzen, B. (2006) Improving the hit-to-lead process: data-driven assessment of drug-like and lead-like screening hits. *Drug Discovery Today*, **11**, 175–180.

10 Gleeson, M.P. (2008) Generation of a set of simple, interpretable ADMET rules of thumb. *Journal of Medicinal Chemistry*, **51**, 817–834.

11 Mannhold, R. (2008) *Molecular Drug Properties*, Wiley-VCH Verlag GmbH & Co, KGaA, Weinheim, pp. 1–471.

12 Roche, O., Schneider, P., Zuegge, J., Guba, W., Kansy, M., Alanine, A., Bleicher, K., Danel, F., Gutknecht, E.M., Rogers-Evans, M., Neidhart, W., Stalder, H., Dillon, M., Sjögren, E., Fotouhi, N., Gillespie, P., Goodnow, R., Harris, W., Jones, P., Taniguchi, M., Tsujii, S., von der Saal, W., Zimmermann, G. and Schneider, G. (2002) Development of a virtual screening method for identification of "frequent hitters" in compound libraries. *Journal of Medicinal Chemistry*, **45**, 137–142.

13 Wunberg, T., Hendrix, M., Hillisch, A., Lobell, M., Meier, H., Schmeck, C., Wild, H. and Hinzen, B. (2006) Improving the hit-to-lead process: data-driven assessment of drug-like and lead-like screening hits. *Drug Discovery Today*, **11**, 175–180.

14 Hann, M.M. and Oprea, T.I. (2004) Pursuing the leadlikeness concept in pharmaceutical research. *Current Opinion in Chemical Biology*, **8**, 255–263.

15 Horio, K., Muta, H., Goto, J. and Noriaki, H. (2007) A simple method to improve the odds in finding "Lead-Like" compounds from chemical libraries. *Chemical & Pharmaceutical Bulletin*, **55**, 980–984.

16 Rees, D.C., Congreve, M., Murray, C.W. and Carr, R. (2004) Fragment-based lead discovery. *Nature Reviews. Drug Discovery*, **3**, 660–672.

17 Andres, C. and Hutter, M.C. (2006) CNS permeability of drugs predicted by a decision tree. *QSAR Combinatorial Science*, **25**, 305–309.

18 Gunturi, S.B., Narayanan, R. and Khandelwal, A. (2006) In silico ADME modelling 2: Computational models to predict human serum albumin binding affinity using ant colony systems. *Bioorganic and Medicinal Chemistry*, **14**, 4118–4129.

19 Kortagere, S., Chekmarev, D., Welsh, W.J. and Ekins, S. (2008) New predictive models for blood-brain barrier permeability of drug-like molecules. *Pharmaceutical Research*, **25**, 1836–1845.

20 Jenwitheesuk, E., Horst, J.A., Rivas, K.L., Van Voorhis, W.C. and Samudrala, R. (2008) Novel paradigms for drug discovery: computational multitarget screening. *Trends in Pharmacological Sciences*, **29**, 62–71.

21 McInnes, C. (2007) Virtual screening strategies in drug discovery. *Current Opinion in Chemical Biology*, **11**, 494–502.

22 Leeson, P.D. and Springthorpe, B. (2007) The influence of drug-like concepts on decision-making in medicinal chemistry. *Nature Reviews. Drug Discovery*, **6**, 881–890.

23 Mohan, C.G., Gandhi, T., Garg, D. and Shinde, R. (2007) Computer-assisted methods in chemical toxicity prediction. *Mini-Reviews in Medicinal Chemistry*, **7**, 499–507.

24 Cheng, A.C., Coleman, R.G., Smyth, K.T., Cao, Q., Soulard, P., Caffrey, D.R.,

Salzberg, A.C. and Huang, E.S. (2007) Structure-based maximal affinity model predicts small-molecule druggability. *Nature Biotechnology*, **25**, 71–75.

25 Brenk, R., Schipani, A., James, D., Krasowski, A., Gilbert, I.H., Frearson, J. and Wyatt, P.G. (2008) Lessons learnt from assembling screening libraries for drug discovery for neglected diseases. *ChemMedChem*, **3**, 435–444.

26 Testa, B., Crivori, P., Reist, M. and Carrupt, P.A. (2000) The influence of lipophilicity on the pharmacokinetic behavior of drugs: concepts and examples. *Perspectives in Drug Discovery and Design*, **19**, 179–211.

27 Lombardo, F., Faller, B., Shalaeva, M., Tetko, I.V. and Tilton, S. (2008) The good, the bad and the ugly of distribution coefficients: current status, views and outlook, in *Molecular Drug Properties. Measurement and Prediction* (eds R. Mannhold, H. Kubinyi and G. Folkers), Wiley-VCH, Weinheim, pp. 407–437.

28 Pliska, V., Testa, B. and van de Waterbeemd, H. (1996) *Lipophilicity in Drug Action and Toxicology*, VCH, Weinheim.

29 Bhal, S.K., Kassam, K., Peirson, I.G. and Pearl, G.M. (2007) The rule of five revisited: Applying log D in place of log p in drug-likeness filters. *Molecular Pharmaceutics*, **4**, 556–560.

30 Schroeter, T., Schwaighofer, A., Mika, S., Ter Laak, A., Suelzle, D., Ganzer, U., Heinrich, N. and Muller, K.R. (2007) Machine learning models for lipophilicity and their domain of applicability. *Molecular Pharmaceutics*, **4**, 524–538.

31 Caron, G., Reymond, F., Carrupt, P.A., Girault, H.H. and Testa, B. (1999) Combined molecular lipophilicity descriptors and their role in understanding intramolecular effects. *Pharmaceutical Science & Technology Today*, **2**, 327–335.

32 Leo, A., Hansch, C. and Elkins, D. (1971) Partition coefficients and their uses. *Chemical Reviews*, **71**, 525–616.

33 Mannhold, R. and Ostermann, C. (2008) Prediction of log P with substructure-based methods, in *Molecular Drug Properties. Measurement and Prediction* (eds R. Mannhold, H. Kubinyi and G. Folkers), Wiley-VCH, Weinheim, pp. 357–380.

34 Tetko, I.V. and Poda, G.I. (2008) Prediction of log P with property-based methods, in *Molecular Drug Properties. Measurement and Prediction* (eds R. Mannhold, H. Kubinyi and G. Folkers), Wiley-VCH, Weinheim, pp. 381–406.

35 Fujita, T., Iwasa, J. and Hansch, C. (1964) A new substituent constant, p, derived from partition coefficients. *Journal of the American Chemical Society*, **86**, 5175–5180.

36 Rekker, R.F. and Mannhold, R. (1992) *Calculation of Drug Lipophilicity*, VCH, Weinheim.

37 Mannhold, R., Rekker, R.F., Dross, K., Bijloo, G.J. and de Vries, G. (1998) The lipophilic behaviour of organic compounds: 1. An updating of the hydrophobic fragmental constant approach. *Quantitative Structure-Activity Relationships*, **17**, 517–536.

38 Rekker, R.F., Mannhold, R., Biljoo, G., de Vries, G. and Dross, K. (1998) The lipophilic behaviour of organic compounds: 2. The development of an aliphatic hydrocarbon/water fragmental system via interconnection with octanol-water partitioning data. *Quantitative Structure-Activity Relationships*, **17**, 537–548.

39 Leo, A.J. (1993) Calculating log Poct from structures. *Chemical Reviews*, **93**, 1281–1306.

40 Leo, A.J. (1996) The future of log P calculation, in *Lipophilicity in Drug Action and Toxicology* (eds V. Pliska, B. Testa and H. van de Waterbeemd), VCH, Weinheim, pp. 157–172.

41 Leo, A.J. and Hoekman, D. (2000) Calculating log P(oct) with no missing fragments; the problem of estimating new interaction parameters. *Perspectives*

in *Drug Discovery and Design*, **18**, 19–38.
42 Ghose, A.K., Pritchett, A. and Crippen, G.M. (1988) Atomic physicochemical parameters for three-dimensional structure-directed quantitative structure-activity relationships. 3. Modeling hydrophobic interactions. *Journal of Computational Chemistry*, **9**, 180.
43 Viswanadhan, V.N., Ghose, A.K., Revankar, G.R. and Robins, R.K. (1989) Atomic physicochemical parameters for three dimensional structure directed quantitative structure-activity relationships. 4. Additional parameters for hydrophobic and dispersive interactions and their application for an automated superposition of certain naturally occuring nucleoside antibiotics. *Journal of Chemical Information and Computer Sciences*, **29**, 163–172.
44 Broto, P., Moreau, G. and Vandycke, C. (1984) Molecular structures: perception, autocorrelation descriptor and SAR studies. System of atomic contributions for the calculation of the n-octanol/water coefficients. *European Journal of Medicinal Chemistry*, **19**, 71–78.
45 Iwase, K., Komatsu, K., Hirono, S., Nakagawa, S. and Moriguchi, I. (1985) Estimation of hydrophobicity based on the solvent-accessible surface area of molecules. *Chemical & Pharmaceutical Bulletin*, **33**, 2114–2121.
46 Masuda, T., Jikihara, T., Nakamura, K., Kimura, A., Takagi, T. and Fujiwara, H. (1997) Introduction of solvent-accessible surface area in the calculation of the hydrophobicity parameter log P from an atomistic approach. *Journal of Pharmaceutical Sciences*, **86**, 57–63.
47 Kantola, A., Villar, H.O. and Loew, G.H. (1991) Atom based parametrization for a conformationally dependent hydrophobic index. *Journal of Computational Chemistry*, **12**, 681–689.
48 Alkorta, I. and Villar, H.O. (1992) Quantum-mechanical parametrization of a conformationally dependent hydrophobic index. *International Journal of Quantum Chemistry*, **44**, 203–218.
49 Gaillard, P., Carrupt, P.A. and Testa, B. (1994) The conformational-dependent lipophilicity of morphine glucuronides as calculated from their molecular lipophilicity potential. *Bioorganic & Medicinal Chemistry Letters*, **4**, 737–742.
50 Gaillard, P., Carrupt, P.A., Testa, B. and Boudon, A. (1994) Molecular lipophilicity potential, a tool in 3D-QSAR. Method and applications. *Journal of Computer-Aided Molecular Design*, **8**, 83–96.
51 Mannhold, R., Cruciani, G., Dross, K. and Rekker, R. (1998) Multivariate analysis of experimental and computational descriptors of molecular lipophilicity. *Journal of Computer-Aided Molecular Design*, **12**, 573–581.
52 Moriguchi, I., Hirono, S., Liu, Q., Nakagome, I. and Matsushita, Y. (1992) Simple method of calculating octanol/water partition coefficient. *Chemical & Pharmaceutical Bulletin*, **40**, 127–130.
53 Junghans, M. and Pretsch, E. (1997) Estimation of partition coefficients of organic compounds: local database modeling with uniform-length structure descriptors. *Fresenius Journal of Analytical Chemistry*, **359**, 88–92.
54 Bodor, N. and Buchwald, P. (1997) Molecular size based approach to estimate partition properties for organic solutes. *Journal of Physical Chemistry. B*, **101**, 3404–3412.
55 Hall, L.H. and Kier, L.B. (1995) Electrotopological state indices for atom types: a novel combination of electronic, topological, and valence state information. *Journal of Chemical Information and Computer Sciences*, **35**, 1039–1045.
56 Tetko, I.V. and Bruneau, P. (2004) Application of ALOGPS to predict 1-octanol/water distribution coefficients, logP, and logD, of AstraZeneca in-house database. *Journal of Pharmaceutical Sciences*, **93**, 3103–3110.
57 Gombar, V.K. and Enslein, K. (1996) Assessment of n-octanol/water partition

58 Kamlet, M.J., Doherty, R.M., Abraham, M.H., Marcus, Y. and Taft, R.W. (1988) Linear solvation energy relationships. 46. An improved equation for correlation and prediction of octanol/water partition coefficients of organic nonelectrolytes (including strong hydrogen bond donor solutes). *Journal of Physical Chemistry,* **92**, 5244–5255.

59 Abraham, M.H., Ibrahim, A. and Zissimos, A.M. (1037) Determination of sets of solute descriptors from chromatographic measurements. *Journal of Chromatography. A,* **2004**, 29–47.

60 Abraham, M.H., Chadha, H.S., Whiting, G.S. and Mitchell, R.C. (1994) Hydrogen bonding. 32. An analysis of water-octanol and water-alkane partitioning and the dlog P parameter of Seiler. *Journal of Pharmaceutical Sciences,* **83**, 1085–1100.

61 Platts, J.A., Abraham, M.H., Butina, D. and Hersey, A. (2000) Estimations of molecular linear free energy relationship descriptors by a group contribution approach. 2. Prediction of partition coefficients. *Journal of Chemical Information and Computer Sciences,* **40**, 71–80.

62 Zhu, H., Tropsha, A., Fourches, D., Varnek, A., Papa, E., Gramatica, P., Oberg, T., Dao, P., Cherkasov, A. and Tetko, I.V. (2008) Combinatorial QSAR modeling of chemical toxicants tested against Tetrahymena pyriformis. *Journal of Chemical Information and Computer Sciences,* **48**, 766–784.

63 Zuaboni, D., Cleva, C. and Carrupt, P.A. (2009) Consensus models and meta-models for the log P using neural networks. Private communication.

64 Leahy, D.E., Morris, J.J., Taylor, P.J. and Wait, A.R. (1992) Model solvent systems for QSAR. Part 2. Fragment values ('f- Values') for the "critical quartet". *Journal of the Chemical Society-Perkin Transactions 2,* 723–731.

65 Leahy, D.E., Morris, J.J., Taylor, P.J. and Wait, A.R. (1992) Model solvent systems for QSAR. Part 3. An LSER analysis of the "critical quartet". New light on hydrogen bond strength and directionality. *Journal of the Chemical Society-Perkin Transactions 2,* 705–722.

66 Caron, G. and Ermondi, G. (2005) Calculating virtual log P in the alkane/water system (log PNalk) and its derived parameters Dlog PNoct-alk and log DpHalk. *Journal of Medicinal Chemistry,* **48**, 3269–3279.

67 Toulmin, A., Wood, J.M. and Kenny, P.W. (2008) Toward prediction of alkane/water partition coefficients. *Journal of Medicinal Chemistry,* **51**, 3720–3730.

68 Abraham, M.H. and Ibrahim, A. (2006) Gas to olive oil partition coefficients: a linear free energy analysis. *Journal of Chemical Information and Modeling,* **46**, 1735–1741.

69 Abraham, M.H. and Acree, W.E. Jr. (2005) Characterisation of the water-isopropyl myristate system. *International Journal of Pharmaceutics,* **294**, 121–128.

70 Torres-Lapasio, J.R., Garcia-Alvarez-Coque, M.C., Roses, M., Bosch, E., Zissimos, A.M. and Abraham, M.H. (2004) Analysis of a solute polarity parameter in reversed-phase liquid chromatography on a linear solvation relationship basis. *Analytica Chimica Acta,* **515**, 209–227.

71 Zissimos, A.M., Abraham, M.H., Barker, M.C., Box, K.J. and Tam, K.Y. (2002) Calculation of Abraham descriptors from solvent-water partition coefficients in four different systems; evaluation of different methods of calculation. *Journal of the Chemical Society,* **3**, 470–477.

72 Valko, K., Du, C.M., Bevan, C.D., Reynolds, D.P. and Abraham, M.H. (2000) Rapid-gradient HPLC method for measuring drug interactions with immobilized artificial membrane: comparison with other lipophilicity measures. *Journal of Pharmaceutical Sciences,* **89**, 1085–1096.

73 Steyaert, G., Lisa, G., Gaillard, P., Boss, G., Reymond, F., Girault, H.H., Carrupt, P.A. and Testa, B. (1997) Intermolecular forces expressed in 1,2-dichloroethane/water partition coefficient: a solvatochromic analysis. *Journal of the Chemical Society-Faraday Transactions*, **93**, 401–406.

74 Liu, X., Bouchard, G., Girault, H.H., Testa, B. and Carrupt, P.A. (2003) Partition coefficients of ionizable compounds in o-nitrophenyl octyl ether/water measured by the potentiometric method. *Analytical Chemistry*, **75**, 7036–7039.

75 Abraham, M.H. and Zhao, Y.H. (2005) Characterisation of the water/o-nitrophenyl octyl ether system in terms of the partition of nonelectrolytes and of ions. *Physical Chemistry Chemical Physics*, **7**, 2418–2422.

76 Reymond, F., Carrupt, P.A., Testa, B. and Girault, H.H. (1999) Charge and delocalisation effects on the lipophilicity of protonable drugs. *Chemistry – A European Journal*, **5**, 39–47.

77 Bouchard, G., Carrupt, P.A., Testa, B., Gobry, V. and Girault, H.H. (2001) The apparent lipophilicity of quaternary ammonium ions is influenced by galvani potential difference, not ion-pairing: a cyclic voltammetry study. *Pharmaceutical Research*, **18**, 702–708.

78 Bouchard, G., Galland, A., Carrupt, P.A., Gulaboski, R., Mirceski, V., Scholz, F. and Girault, H.H. (2003) Standard partition coefficients of anionic drugs in the n-octanol/water system determined by voltammetry at three-phase electrode. *Physical Chemistry Chemical Physics*, **5**, 3748–3751.

79 Scherrer, R.A. and Howard, S.M. (1977) Use of distribution coefficients in quantitative structure-activity relationships. *Journal of Medicinal Chemistry*, **20**, 53–58.

80 Clarke, F.H. and Cahoon, N.M. (1987) Ionization constants by curve fitting: determination of partition and distribution coefficients of acids and bases and their ions. *Journal of Pharmaceutical Sciences*, **76**, 611–620.

81 Manners, C.N., Payling, D.W. and Smith, D.A. (1988) Distribution coefficient, a convenient term for the relation of predictable physico-chemical properties to metabolic processes. *Xenobiotica*, **18**, 331–350.

82 Milletti, F., Storchi, L., Sforna, G. and Cruciani, G. (2007) New and original pKa prediction method using grid molecular interaction fields. *Journal of Chemical Information and Modeling*, **47**, 2172–2181.

83 Meloun, M. and Bordovska, S. (2007) Benchmarking and validating algorithms that estimate pKa values of drugs based on their molecular structures. *Analytical and Bioanalytical Chemistry*, **2007**, 1–15.

84 Gocan, S., Cimpan, G. and Comer, J. (2006) Lipophilicity measurements by liquid chromatography, in *Advances in Chromatography* (eds E. Grushka and N. Grinberg), Taylor & Francis Group, Boca Raton, pp. 79–176.

85 Hitzel, L., Watt, A.P. and Locker, K.L. (2000) An increased throughput method for the determination of partition coefficients. *Pharmaceutical Research*, **17**, 1389–1395.

86 Dohta, Y., Yamashita, T., Horiike, S., Nakamura, T. and Kukami, T. (2007) A system for logD screening of 96-well plates using a water-plug aspiration/injection method combined with high-performance liquid chromatography-mass spectrometry. *Analytical Chemistry*, **79**, 8312–8315.

87 Faller, B., Grimm, H.P., Loeuillet-Ritzler, F., Arnold, S. and Briand, X. (2005) High-throughput lipophilicity measurement with immobilized artificial membranes. *Journal of Medicinal Chemistry*, **48**, 2571–2576.

88 Kansy, M., Senner, F. and Gubernator, K. (1998) Physicochemical high throughput screening: parallel artificial membrane permeation assay in the description of passive absorption

processes. *Journal of Medicinal Chemistry*, **41**, 1007–1010.

89 Wohnsland, F. and Faller, B. (2001) High-throughput permeability pH profile and high-throughput alkane/water log P with artificial membranes. *Journal of Medicinal Chemistry*, **44**, 923–930.

90 Ottaviani, G., Martel, S., Escalara, C., Nicolle, E. and Carrupt, P.A. (2008) The PAMPA technique as a HTS tool for partition coefficients determination in different solvent/water systems. *European Journal of Pharmaceutical Sciences*, **35**, 68–75.

91 Chen, Z. and Weber, S.G. (2007) High-throughput method for lipophilicity measurement. *Analytical Chemistry*, **79**, 1043–1049.

92 Nasal, A. and Kaliszan, R. (2006) Progress in the use of HPLC for evaluation of lipophilicity. *Current Computer-Aided Drug Design*, **2**, 327–340.

93 Poole, S.K. and Poole, C.F. (2003) Separation methods for estimating octanol-water coefficients. *Journal of Chromatography B*, **797**, 3–19.

94 Stella, C., Galland, A., Liu, X., Testa, B., Rudaz, S., Veuthey, J.L. and Carrupt, P.A. (2005) Novel RPLC stationary phases for lipophilicity measurement: solvatochromic analysis of retention mechanisms for neutral and basic compounds. *Journal of Separation Science*, **28**, 2350–2362.

95 Pagliara, A., Khamis, E., Trinh, A., Carrupt, P.A., Tsai, R.S. and Testa, B. (1995) Structural properties governing retention mechanisms on RP-HPLC stationary phase used for lipophilicity measurements. *Journal of Liquid Chromatography*, **18**, 1721–1745.

96 Donovan, S.F. and Pescatore, M.C. (2002) Method for measuring the logarithm of the octanol-water partition coefficient by using short octadecyl-poly (vinyl alcohol) high-performance liquid chromatography columns. *Journal of Chromatography. A*, **952**, 47–61.

97 Lombardo, F., Shalaeva, M.Y., Tupper, K.A., Gao, F. and Abraham, M.H. (2000) ElogPoct: a tool for lipophilicity determination in drug discovery. *Journal of Medicinal Chemistry*, **43**, 2922–2928.

98 Minick, D.J., Frenz, J.H., Patrick, M.A. and Brent, D.A. (1988) A comprehensive method for determining hydrophobicity constants by reversed-phase high-performance liquid chromatography. *Journal of Medicinal Chemistry*, **31**, 1923–1933.

99 Ayouni, L., Cazorla, G., Chaillou, D., Herbreteau, B., Rudaz, S., Lanteri, P. and Carrupt, P.A. (2005) Fast determination of lipophilicity by HPLC. *Chromatographia*, **62**, 251–255.

100 Demare, S., Slater, B., Lacombe, G., Breuzin, D. and Dini, C. (2007) Accurate automated log P-o/w measurement by gradient-flow liquid-liquid partition chromatography Part 1. Neutral compounds. *Journal of Chromatography A*, **1175**, 16–23.

101 Kaliszan, R. (2007) QSRR: quantitative structure-(chromatographic) retention relationships. *Chemical Reviews*, **107**, 3212–3246.

102 Snyder, L.R. and Dolan, J.W. (1996) Initial experiments in high-performance liquid chromatographic method development. I. Use of a starting gradient run. *Journal of Chromatography. A*, **721**, 3–14.

103 Valko, K., Bevan, C. and Reynolds, D. (1997) Chromatographic hydrophobicity index by fast-gradient RP-HPLC: a high-throughput alternative to log P/log D. *Analytical Chemistry*, **69**, 2022–2029.

104 Du, C.M., Valko, K., Bevan, C., Reynolds, D. and Abraham, M.H. (1998) Rapid gradient RP-HPLC method for lipophilicity determination: a solvation equation based comparison with isocratic methods. *Analytical Chemistry*, **70**, 4228–4234.

105 Dias, N.C., Nawas, M.I. and Poole, C.F. (2003) Evaluation of a reversed-phase column (Supelcosil LC-ABZ) under

isocratic and gradient elution conditions for estimating octanol-water partition coefficients. *Analyst*, **128**, 427–433.

106 Zhao, Y., Jona, J., Chow, D.T., Rong, H., Semin, D., Xia, X., Zanon, R., Spancake, C. and Maliski, E. (2002) High-throughput logP measurement using paralell liquid chromatography/ultraviolet/mass spectrometry and sample-pooling. *Rapid Communications in Mass Spectrometry*, **16**, 1548–1555.

107 Camurri, G. and Zaramella, A. (2001) High-throughput liquid chromatography/Mass spectrometry method for the determination of the chromatographic hydrophobicity index. *Analytical Chemistry*, **73**, 3716–3722.

108 Barbato, F. (2006) The use of immobilised artificial membrane (IAM) chromatography for determination of lipophilicity. *Current Computer-Aided Drug Design*, **2**, 341–352.

109 Taillardat-Bertschinger, A., Marca-Martinet, C., Carrupt, P.A., Reist, M., Caron, G., Fruttero, R. and Testa, B. (2002) Molecular factors influencing retention on immobilized artificial membranes (IAM) compared to partitioning in liposomes and n-octanol. *Pharmaceutical Research*, **19**, 729–737.

110 Taillardat-Bertschinger, A., Carrupt, P.A., Barbato, F. and Testa, B. (2003) Immobilized artificial membrane (IAM)-HPLC in drug research. *Journal of Medicinal Chemistry*, **46**, 655–665.

111 Taillardat-Bertschinger, A., Barbato, F., Quercia, M.T., Carrupt, P.A., Reist, M., La Rotonda, M.I. and Testa, B. (2002) Structural properties governing retention mechanisms on immobilized artificial membrane (IAM) HPLC-columns. *Helvetica Chimica Acta*, **85**, 519–532.

112 Bard, B., Carrupt, P.A. and Martel, S. (2009) Determination of partition coefficients of basic drugs using hydrophilic interaction chromatography. *Journal of Medicinal Chemistry*, **52**, 3416–3419.

113 Nawrocki, J. (1997) The silanol group and its role in liquid chromatography. *Journal of Chromatography A*, **779**, 29–71.

114 Stella, C., Seuret, P., Rudaz, S., Carrupt, P.A., Gauvrit, J.Y., Lanteri, P. and Veuthey, J.L. (2002) Characterization of chromatographic supports for the analysis of basic compounds. *Journal of Separation Science*, **25**, 1351–1363.

115 Stella, C., Rudaz, S., Veuthey, J.L. and Tchapla, A. (2001) Silica and other materials as supports in liquid chromatography. Chromatographic tests and their importance for evaluating these supports. Part I. *Chromatographia*, **53**, S-113–S-131.

116 Giaginis, C. and Tsantili-Kakoulidou, A. (2008) Current state of the art in HPLC methodology for lipophilicity assessment of basic drugs. A review. *Journal of Liquid Chromatography & Related Technologies*, **31**, 79–96.

117 Bard, B., Martel, S. and Carrupt, P.A. (2009) Determination of alkane/water partition coefficients of polar compounds using hydrophilic interaction chromatography. *Journal of Chromatography A*, submitted.

118 Henchoz, Y., Guillarme, D., Rudaz, S., Veuthey, J.L. and Carrupt, P.A. (2008) High-throughput log P determination by ultraperformance liquid chromatography: a convenient tool for medicinal chemists. *Journal of Medicinal Chemistry*, **51**, 396–399.

119 Henchoz, Y., Guillarme, D., Martel, S., Rudaz, S., Veuthey, J.L. and Carrupt, P.A. (2009) Fast log P determination by ultra performance liquid chromatography coupled with UV and mass spectrometry detections. *Analytical and Bioanalytical Chemistry*, in press.

120 Jia, Z. (2005) Physicochemical profiling by capillary electrophoresis. *Current Pharmaceutical Analysis*, **1**, 41–56.

121 Huie, C.W. (2006) Recent applications of microemulsion electrokinetic chromatography. *Electrophoresis*, **27**, 60–75.

122 McEvoy, E., Marsh, A., Altria, K., Donegan, S. and Power, J. (2007) Recent advances in the development and application of microemulsion EKC. *Electrophoresis*, **28**, 193–207.

123 Örnskov, E., Gottfries, J., Erickson, M. and Folestad, S. (2005) Experimental modelling of drug membrane permeability by capillary electrophoresis using liposomes, micelles and microemulsions. *Journal of Pharmacy and Pharmacology*, **57**, 435–442.

124 Trone, M.D., Leonard, M.S. and Khaledi, M.G. (2000) Congeneric behavior in estimations of octanol-water partition coefficients by micellar electrokinetic chromatography. *Analytical Chemistry*, **72**, 1228–1235.

125 Trone, M.D. and Khaledi, M.G. (2000) Statistical evaluation of linear solvation energy relationship models used to characterize chemical selectivity in micellar electrokinetic chromatography. *Journal of Chromatography. A*, **886**, 245–257.

126 Jia, Z., Mei, L., Lin, F., Huang, S. and Killion, R.B. (1007) Screening of octanol-water partition coefficients for pharmaceuticals by pressure-assisted microemulsion electrokinetic chromatography. *Journal of Chromatography A*, **2003**, 203–208.

127 Poole, S.K., Durham, D. and Kibbey, C. (2000) Rapid method for estimating the octanol–water partition coefficient (log P ow) by microemulsion electrokinetic chromatography. *Journal of Chromatography B, Biomedical Sciences and Applications*, **745**, 117–126.

128 Tu, J., Halsall, H.B., Seliskar, C.J., Limbach, P.A., Arias, F., Wehmeyer, K.R. and Heineman, W.R. (2005) Estimation of logP(ow) values for neutral and basic compounds by microchip microemulsion electrokinetic chromatography with indirect fluorimetric detection (muMEEKC-IFD). *Journal of Pharmaceutical and Biomedical Analysis*, **38**, 1–7.

129 Wehmeyer, K.R., Tu, J., Jin, Y., King, S., Stella, M., Stanton, D.T., Kenseth, J. and Wong, K.S. (2003) The application of multiplexed microemulsion electrokinetic chromatography for the rapid determination of log Pow values for neutral and basic compounds. *Liquid Chromatography and Gas Chromatography of North America*, **21**, 1078–1088.

130 Wong, K.S., Kenseth, J. and Strasburg, R. (2004) Validation long-term assessment of an approach for the high throughput determination of lipophilicity (log POW) values using multiplexed, absorbance-based capillary electrophoresis. *Journal of Pharmaceutical Sciences*, **93**, 916–931.

131 Marsh, A. and Altria, K. (2006) Use of multiplexed CE for pharmaceutical analysis. *Chromatographia*, **64**, 327–333.

132 Krishna, M.V., Srinath, M. and Sankar, D.G. (2008) Principles and applications of capillary electrophoresis in new drug discovery. *Current Trends in Biotechnology and Pharmacy*, **2**, 142–155.

133 Testa, B., Carrupt, P.A., Gaillard, P., Billois, F. and Weber, P. (1996) Lipophilicity in molecular modeling. *Pharmaceutical Research*, **13**, 335–343.

134 Pagliara, A., Carrupt, P.A., Caron, G., Gaillard, P. and Testa, B. (1997) Lipophilicity profiles of ampholytes. *Chemical Reviews*, **97**, 3385–3400.

135 Carrupt, P.A., Testa, B. and Gaillard, P. (1997) Computational approaches to lipophilicity: methods and applications, in *Reviews in Computational Chemistry* (eds D.B. Boyd and K.B. Lipkowitz), Wiley-VCH, New York, pp. 241–315.

136 Pagliara, A., Testa, B., Carrupt, P.A., Jolliet, P., Morin, C., Morin, D., Urien, S., Tillement, J.P. and Rihoux, J.P. (1998) Molecular properties and pharmacokinetic behavior of cetirizine, a zwitterionic H1-receptor antagonist. *Journal of Medicinal Chemistry*, **41**, 853–863.

137 Tosco, P., Rolando, B., Fruttero, R., Henchoz, Y., Martel, S., Carrupt, P.A. and Gasco, A. (2008) Physicochemical profiling of sartans: A detailed study of ionization constants and distribution

coefficients. *Helvetica Chimica Acta*, **91**, 468–482.

138 Du, Q.S., Huang, R.B., Wei, Y.T., Du, L.Q. and Chou, K.C. (2008) Multiple field three dimensional quantitative structure-activity relationship (MF-3D-QSAR). *Journal of Computational Chemistry*, **29**, 211–219.

139 Oprea, T.I. (2001) Rapid estimation of hydrophobicity for virtual combinatorial library analysis. *SAR and QSAR in Environmental Research*, **12**, 129–141.

140 Tetko, I.V., Bruneau, P., Mewes, H.W., Rohrer, D.C. and Poda, G.I. (2006) Can we estimate the accuracy of ADME-Tox predictions? *Drug Discovery Today*, **11**, 700–707.

141 Bruneau, P. and McElroy, N.R. (2006) logD(7.4) modeling using Bayesian regularized neural networks. Assessment and correction of the errors of prediction. *Journal of Chemical Information and Modeling*, **46**, 1379–1387.

142 Abshear, T., Banik, G.M., D'Souza, M.L., Nedwed, K. and Peng, C. (2006) A model validation and consensus building environment. *SAR and QSAR in Environmental Research*, **17**, 311–321.

143 Sadowski, J., Gasteiger, J. and Klebe, G. (1994) Comparison of Automatic 3-Dimensional Model Builders Using 639 X-Ray Structures. *Journal of Chemical Information and Computer Sciences*, **34**, 1000–1008.

144 Sadowski, J. and Gasteiger, J. (1993) From atoms and bonds to 3-dimensional atomic coordinates – Automatic model builders. *Chemical Reviews*, **93**, 2567–2581.

145 Pearlman, R.S. (1993) 3D molecular structures: generation and use in 3D searching, in *3D QSAR in Drug Design. Theory Methods and Applications*, 1st edn (ed. H. Kubinyi), ESCOM Science Publishers, Leiden, pp. 41–79.

146 Ermondi, G., Caron, G., Bouchard, G., Plemper van Balen, G., Pagliara, A., Grandi, T., Carrupt, P.A., Fruttero, R. and Testa, B. (2001) Molecular dynamics and NMR exploration of the property space of the zwitterionic antihistamine cetirizine. *Helvetica Chimica Acta*, **84**, 360–374.

147 Cruciani, G., Crivori, P., Carrupt, P.A. and Testa, B. (2000) Molecular fields in quantitative structure permeation relationships: the VolSurf approach. *Journal of Molecular Structure*, **503**, 17–30.

148 Cruciani, G., Clementi, S., Crivori, P., Carrupt, P.A. and Testa, B. (2001) VolSurf and its interest in structure-disposition relations, in *Pharmacokinetic Optimization in Drug Research: Biological, Physicochemical and Computational Strategies* (eds B. Testa, H. van de Waterbeemd, G. Folkers and R.H. Guy), Wiley-VCH, Weinheim, pp. 539–550.

149 Cruciani, G. (2006) *Molecular Interaction Fields*, Wiley-VCH, Weinheim, pp. 1–307.

150 Mannhold, R., Berellini, G., Carosati, E. and Benedetti, P. (2006) Use of MIF-based VolSurf descriptors in physicochemical and pharmacokinetic studies, in *Molecular Interaction Fields* (ed. G. Cruciani), Wiley-VCH, Weinheim, pp. 173–196.

151 Geiser, L., Henchoz, Y., Galland, A., Carrupt, P.A. and Veuthey, J.L. (2005) Determination of pKa values by capillary zone electrophoresis with a dynamic coating procedure. *Journal of Separation Science*, **28**, 2374–2380.

152 Henchoz, Y., Schappler, J., Geiser, L., Prat, J., Carrupt, P.A. and Veuthey, J.L. (2007) Rapid determination of pKa values of 20 amino acids by CZE with UV and capacitively coupled contactless conductivity detections. *Analytical and Bioanalytical Chemistry*, **389**, 1869–1878.

153 Avdeef, A. (2001) Physicochemical profiling (solubility, permeability and charge state). *Current Topics in Medicinal Chemistry*, **1**, 277–351.

6
Membrane Permeability – Measurement and Prediction in Drug Discovery

Kiyohiko Sugano, Lourdes Cucurull-Sanchez, and Joanne Bennett

6.1
Overview of Membrane Permeation

Membrane permeability is one of the most important determinants of pharmacokinetics, not only for oral absorption, but also for renal re-absorption, biliary excretion, skin permeation, distribution to a specific organ and so on. In addition, modification of membrane permeability by formulation is rarely successful. Therefore, membrane permeability should be optimized during the structure optimization process in drug discovery. In this chapter, we give an overview of the physiology and chemistry of the membranes, *in vitro* permeability models and *in silico* predictions. This chapter focuses on progress in recent years in intestinal and blood–brain barrier (BBB) membrane permeation. There are a number of useful reviews summarizing earlier work [1–5].

6.1.1
Structure, Physiology and Chemistry of the Membrane

The epithelial cells lining the gut wall provide the main barrier to drug permeation. The surface area for absorption is enhanced by microvilli, villi and folding of the epithelial membrane (Figure 6.1). Drug molecules can pass through the epithelial membrane by: (i) passive transcellular pathway; (ii) passive paracellular route; (iii) active transports (influx and efflux; Figure 6.1). The majority of lipophilic drugs are mainly absorbed via the passive transcellular pathway. However, more hydrophilic drugs are absorbed via pathways (ii) and (iii). The epithelial cellular membrane mainly consists of phospholipids, cholesterol and membrane proteins. The membrane is negatively charged by anionic phospholipids such as phosphatidylserine and phosphatidylinositol. In addition, the intestinal epithelial membrane is covered by a mucus layer which maintains an unstirred water layer (UWL). A drug molecule has to diffuse through the UWL before reaching the epithelial membrane.

Hit and Lead Profiling. Edited by Bernard Faller and Laszlo Urban
Copyright © 2009 WILEY-VCH Verlag GmbH & Co. KGaA, Weinheim
ISBN: 978-3-527-32331-9

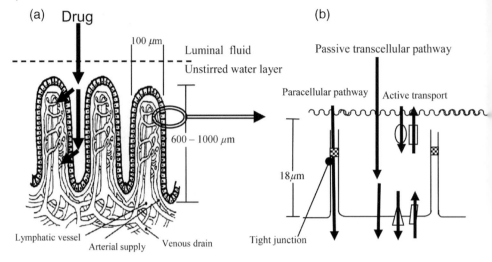

Figure 6.1 Schematic representation of the intestinal membrane structure. The singlet arrow in the figure illustrate the permeation pathways. (a) Villous structure of intestine. Unstirred water layer is adjacent to villi. (b) Permeation pathways of compounds across the intestinal epithelial membrane. (Adapted from [14] and modified from Bentham Science Publishers, Ltd.)

The BBB separates cerebral capillary blood from brain parenchymal tissue. The BBB is formed by endothelial cells lining the blood capillaries in the brain. Unlike the intestinal membrane, BBB has little UWL. The paracellular pathway is negligible for most compounds under physiological conditions.

6.1.2
Passive Transcellular Pathway: pH Partition Theory as the Basis of Understanding Membrane Permeability

The cellular membrane is largely hydrophobic consisting of phospholipids and cholesterol. Therefore, it is the major permeation barrier for hydrophilic molecules. In the case of weak acids and bases, the uncharged species are much more lipophilic than charged species and more easily permeate the cell membrane. The fraction of uncharged species depends on the pH near the membrane surface and the pK_a of a drug. The pH at the intestinal membrane surface is 6.0–6.5. When only the uncharged species are assumed to permeate the membrane and the permeation of charged species are assumed to be negligible, the membrane permeability can be expressed as:

$$P_{trans} = P_{trans,n}/(1+10^{pH-pK_a}) \quad \text{for acidic compounds}$$

$$P_{trans} = P_{trans,n}/(1+10^{pK_a-pH}) \quad \text{for basic compounds}$$

where P_{trans} is the passive transcellular permeability (cm/sec); $P_{trans,n}$ is that of uncharged species. Therefore pK_a is one of the most important physicochemical properties which affect the apparent membrane permeability. Since the apparent passive membrane permeability is determined by $P_{trans,n}$ and pK_a, the structure permeability relationship should be derived for $P_{trans,n}$, independently from pK_a (cf. Section 6.5).

6.1.3
Paracellular Pathway

Small (<200–400 MW) and cationic drugs can pass through the tight junction (TJ) between intestinal epithelial cells. Since TJ is negatively charged, this route is more favorable for cationic molecules. The effective pore size of TJ is 8–13 Å in humans and rats and much larger in dogs [6]. A number of hydrophilic drugs are known to be absorbed via this pathway. In contrast, the TJs of BBB endothelial cells are severely restrictive to paracellular drug permeation [4].

6.1.4
Active Transporters

Active transporters are thought to play an important role in the pharmacokinetics of drugs, not only because they can regulate the permeability of drugs as substrate-specific efflux or influx pumps, but also because of their widespread presence across *in vivo* membrane systems, from the intestinal epithelia to the BBB. Generally speaking, the absorption direction transporters tend to have narrower substrate specificity than the excretion direction transporters. Active transporters also play a significant role in biliary and renal excretion.

6.1.5
In Vitro–In Vivo Extrapolation

The presence of folds and villi structures on the surface area is not taken into account for the *in vivo* effective intestinal membrane permeability (P_{eff}; when extrapolated from a perfusion experiment, a smooth tube is usually assumed). In humans, the fold expansion (FE) of the surface area is about threefold, and villi expansion (VE) is about 10-fold [7]. In the case of high epithelial membrane permeability (P_{ep}) absorption occurs at the top of the villi before diffusing down the villi channels, whereas low P_{ep} compound may diffuse down the villi channels to the crypts (Figure 6.1). Therefore, accessibility (Acc) to the surface depends on P_{ep} and diffusion coefficient [7, 8]. The effective membrane permeability can be expressed as:

$$\frac{1}{P_{eff}} = \left(\frac{1}{P_{UWL}} + \frac{1}{VE \cdot Acc \cdot P_{ep}} \right) \cdot \frac{1}{FE} \quad (6.1)$$

$$P_{ep} = P_{trans} + P_{para} + P_{active} \quad (6.2)$$

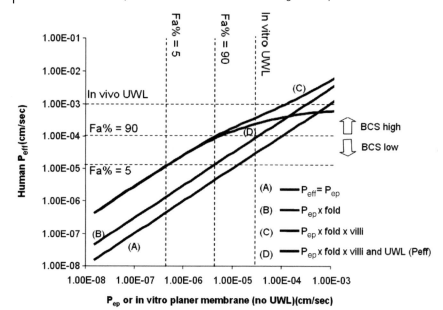

Figure 6.2 Relationship between the epithelial membrane permeability and the effective intestinal membrane permeability in humans. Based on [6] an recalculated including fold expansion and UWL effect.

P_{para}, P_{active} and P_{UWL} are *paracellular*, *active* transport and *UWL* permeability, respectively. P_{eff} can be further converted to Fa% as [9]:

$$Fa\% = \left(1-\exp\left(-\frac{S_{SI}}{V_{SI}} \cdot P_{eff} \cdot T_{si}\right)\right) \times 100$$

$$= \left(1-\exp\left(-DF \cdot \frac{2}{r_{GI}} \cdot P_{eff} \cdot T_{si}\right)\right) \times 100 \tag{6.3}$$

where T_{si} is the transit time through the absorption region (for the human small intestine, about 3.0–3.5 h); S_{SI} is the effective intestinal surface area (as smooth tube); V_{SI} is the effective intestinal fluid volume; Fa% is the fraction of a dose absorbed. The S_{SI}/V_{SI} ratio is related to the degree of flatness (DF) and the intestinal radius (r_{GI}). DF obtained by P_{eff} – Fa% curve is about 2.8 (r_{GI} = 1.75 cm, T_{si} = 3 h) [9], which is higher than the theoretical value for the cylinder (= 1), suggesting that intestinal tubing is rather flat [10]. Figure 6.2 shows the relationship between P_{ep} and P_{eff}. The biopharmaceutical classification system criterion for high permeability is Fa% = 90%, which theoretically corresponds to P_{eff} = about 1×10^{-4} cm/s. If the lack of folds and villous structures in *in vitro* systems are taken into consideration, the theoretical *in vitro* permeability which corresponds to P_{eff} = 1×10^{-4} cm/s is likely to be reduced by about 10- to 30-fold [11] and corresponds to about 5–10×10^{-6} cm/s, assuming that the *in vivo* epithelial cell is to be similar to the *in vitro* cell models

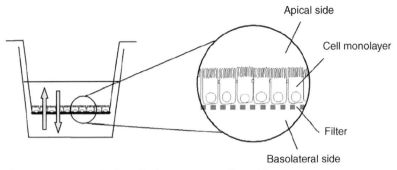

Figure 6.3 Diagram of *in vitro* cell culture system used in studying bidirectional transport. (Modified from [13]).

(Figure 6.3). Metoprolol permeability is often regarded as a borderline between high and low permeability and is used as a standard compound for *in vitro* cell models.

Furthermore, the P_{eff} data can be integrated with solubility/dissolution data to predict the oral absorption from the solid dosage form (see Chapter 10). Gastrointestinal transit absorption model (GITA) [12, 13], advanced compartmental absorption and transit model (ACAT, GastroPlus), advanced drug absorption and metabolism model (ADAM, SimCYP) and so on have been reported as useful integration models (see Chapter 10).

6.2
In Vitro Cell Models

Cell culture models are routinely used to assess permeability of new potential drug candidates. The simplicity and higher throughput of these models makes them a useful alternative to *in vivo* studies. These models are used to predict absorption *in vivo*, rank order compounds and examine absorption mechanism. Transcellular, paracellular, active uptake and efflux mechanisms can be studied with these models.

Cells are grown on a permeable filter support inserted on a 12-, 24- or 96-well plate. This forms a two-compartment system with an apical and basolateral chamber [14]. Absorptive flux is determined by adding drug to the apical compartment and measuring transport across the cell monolayer into the basolateral compartment. Secretory flux may also be measured by adding drug to the basolateral compartment and measuring transport into the apical compartment.

6.2.1
Intestinal Cell Culture Models

There are a number of cell culture models available that mimic human epithelia *in vivo* (Caco-2, HT29, T84, IEC 18, TC7, LLCPK1, MDCK). Some of these cells are derived from human colon carcinomas (e.g., Caco-2, T84, HT29) and have many properties of the normal intestinal epithelium. The Caco-2 cell model is one of the most widely studied and used in the pharmaceutical industry. When grown on permeable filter supports they spontaneously differentiate to form polarized cell monolayers with well defined TJs and microvilli. They express a number of intestinal enzymes (e.g., aminopeptidases, esterases, sulfatases, UDP-glucuronyl transferase, CYPs) and transporters (e.g., bile acid transporter, LNAA, HPT1, PEPT1, Pgp, MRP2 (cMOAT), BCRP) [15, 16]. Cell lines which have some of these transporters or enzymes induced or overexpressed have been developed to enable their study and overcome problems with low expression [17–21].

Conventional Caco-2 cells require long culturing times (>15 days). Alternative app-roaches have been sought to reduce regular maintenance and feeding requirements. Manipulation of the growth media and extracellular matrix for Caco-2 was shown to reduce time to confluency and effect transporter expression. An alternative epithelial cell line commonly used for assessing permeability is the Madin–Darby canine kidney(MDCK) cell line, which has a much shorter culturing time (2–6 days). MDCK permeability was shown to correlate well with Caco-2 permeability ($r^2 = 0.79$) [15, 22, 23].

The paracellular permeation pathway in the intestinal cell monolayer models is often limited. Therefore these models are not suitable for predicting permeability of paracellularly absorbed compounds. The average pore radius in Caco-2 cells (<6 Å) is more representative of the colon than the small intestine (8–13 Å) and paracellular transport can be up to 100-fold lower in Caco-2 cells than in the small intestine. Investigation of a rat intestinal cell line 2/4/A1, which forms polarized cell monolayers and has an average pore radius (9 Å) more representative of the small intestine, showed improved prediction of oral absorption for incompletely absorbed drugs [24, 25].

It should also be noted that many of the cell lines used to predict intestinal permeability lack the mucin-producing goblet cells and therefore the mucus layer. *In vivo* the mucus layer may alter permeability through stabilization of the UWL or by directly interacting with the drug molecule or formulation. Some studies were undertaken in cell models to examine the effects of mucus on permeability. HT29-MTX and HT29-H cells were developed from the HT29 parental line to express the morphological and mucin-producing characteristics of goblet cells. The mucus layer may not be that important in limiting the transport of small hydrophilic molecules, however it may be relevant in restricting the diffusion of highly lipophilic molecules. Permeability of testosterone was shown to be limited by mucus in HT29-MTX but not in HT29-H. It is hypothesized that differences in the mucus secreted by these two cell lines may explain the discrepancy [26, 27]. Mucus may also be relevant in limiting the transport of macromolecules due to the restriction of diffusion in the matrix [28].

6.2.2
BBB Cell Culture Models

There are a number of cell-based models available which were developed using endothelial cells from cow, pig, rat and even human brain tissue. There are a number of immortalized cell lines derived from the BBB available, for example, RBE 4 (rat) and SV-HCEC (human); however none of the cell lines exhibit the necessary restrictive paracellular properties for them to be suitable for drug screening.

Primary cultures developed from pig and cow tissue are the best studied [29–32]. These models closely resemble the BBB, exhibiting many of the key biological properties. However isolation of blood–brain endothelial cells requires relatively complex cell isolation procedures which are labor-intensive and not ideal for screening purposes. Other cell types have been shown or proposed to induce barrier function, for example, astrocytes/pericytes. Significant improvements in barrier function was achieved in these primary culture models by including astrocyte conditioned media or co-culturing with astrocytes [33]. The complexity of primary cultures led to the use of epithelial cell lines not derived from the BBB (e.g., MDCK, MDCK-MDR1 or LLC-PK1) [33].

6.2.3
Cell Models to Study Active Transporters

A lot of effort focused recently on the identification and understanding of the role of active transport mechanisms in permeability. There are a large number of active transporters expressed in the gut and brain which are increasingly being shown to be relevant to drug transport both in the active uptake of drugs (e.g., PepT1, OATP) and the efflux of drugs (e.g., P-gp, MRP2, BCRP) [2, 5, 34].

Studies were undertaken to quantify transporters and examine regional expression in the intestine. mRNA levels in the gut were studied by Englund et al. [35]. Nine transporters were examined and eight were shown to have significant regional differences in expression. In addition, up to a 20-fold difference in expression was observed for certain transporters between intestinal tissue and Caco-2 cells. Expression of transporters in cell models compared to normal tissue can be markedly different, depending on the age of the cells, passage number and culture conditions [35]. Cell models may under- or overexpress transporters. In addition cell lines may express transporters which may not be relevant in vivo.

There is a lot of interest in P-gp and its role in limiting absorption of drugs. However, there is increasing evidence P-gp may not impact on the intestinal permeability of some drugs identified as substrates. In the case of compounds with high passive permeability, the effect of P-gp may be small due to the rapid permeation of the drug, which minimizes interaction with the transporter [36]. In addition, higher concentration in the in vivo GI tract relative to in vitro studies saturates the transporter [37]. However with the increasing number of poorly soluble, potent compounds and modified release dosage forms, this should be considered on a case by case basis.

The relevance of P-gp at the BBB is considered highly important due to the low drug concentrations in the systemic circulation. The interest in transporters led to development of cell lines that overexpress them, for example, MDCK-MDR1 and MDCK-MDR2. MDCK-MDR1, which overexpresses P-gp, is one of the most widely used models in early drug discovery screening [38, 39].

In addition it was also suggested that cell lines that have limited expression of transporters (e.g., 2/4/A1) are of use in understanding passive permeability. Saturation of transporters or inhibition can also be used to understand the contribution of passive permeation and active transport.

6.2.4
Correlation of in Vitro Models to Human P_{eff} and Fraction Absorbed Data

Correlation of *in vitro* data with human P_{eff} and Fa% was undertaken with a number of models [25, 27]. Although Fa% data is useful and more broadly available, the introduction of the Loc-I-Gut model by Lennernas allowed direct measurement of P_{eff}. In the Loc-I-Gut model, a segment of the small intestine in humans is isolated using a balloon catheter, disappearance of the drug is measured and the P_{eff} can be generated [40].

The availability of human P_{eff} data is more limited than Fa% data and is biased towards highly absorbed compounds. Therefore, the use of *in vivo* P_{eff} data is more limited for understanding incompletely absorbed compounds which may be subject to paracellular transport or active uptake and efflux mechanisms.

The use of *in vitro* models for prediction of compounds that are predominantly absorbed passively by the transcellular route is generally good with these models. Predicting compounds which are absorbed paracellularly or via active uptake or efflux mechanisms is more difficult. There is a lack of understanding of expression levels of transporters in the gut, which makes *in vivo* predictions difficult.

6.2.5
Correlation of Cell Culture Models with In Vivo Brain Penetration

There are a number of *in vivo* methods used to assess brain penetration each with their own benefits and limitations [41]. Much of the *in vivo* data comes from the brain: blood ratio, which is not a direct measure of permeability and therefore is not directly comparable to *in vitro* permeability values [4].

Recently Carrara *et al.* looked at the utility of optimized PAMPA and MDCK-MDR1 cells in predicting brain penetration for known CNS-penetrating and nonpenetrating drugs. The MDCK-MDR1 cells correctly predicted 29 out of the 34 compounds (85%) which had known CNS penetration [42].

Garberg *et al.* compared a number of *in vitro* cell models of the BBB with *in vivo* data (including primary cow and human brain endothelial cells co-cultured with astrocytes, MDCK, MDCK-MDR1, Caco-2, ECV304/C6, MBEC4, SV-ARBEC co-cultured with astrocytes). The best correlation, although poor, was seen with cow brain endothelial cells (r^2 0.43) and MDCK (r^2 0.46). The correlation was improved with Caco-2 when only passively transported compounds were included in the analysis ($r^2 = 0.86$), BBEC showing a similar correlation [39].

Further understanding of active transporters in the brain and in *in vitro* models is required to improve predictability of these models.

6.3
Artificial Membranes

The octanol/water partition coefficient (log P_{oct}) is used as a surrogate of the passive transcellular permeation. However, it has two drawbacks: (i) low to moderate correlation with *in vivo* absorption; (ii) time-consuming assay. Therefore, various artificial membrane assays were extensively investigated as alternative approaches with better predictive power and allowing for higher throughput.

6.3.1
Partition and Permeation

Physicochemical tools can be categorized into two types: membrane binding experiments and permeation experiments (Figure 6.4) [3]. The permeation barrier of a phospholipid bilayer is heterogeneous in nature and the rate-limiting barrier

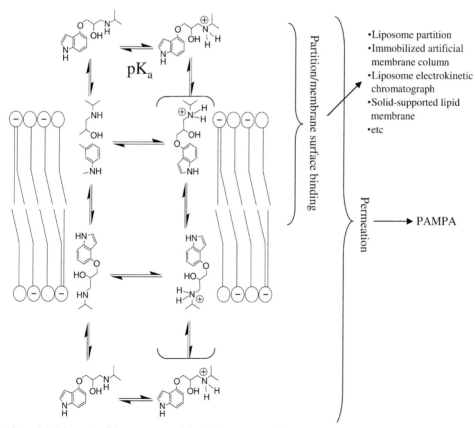

Figure 6.4 Schematic of the two step model and the categories of physicochemical tools. (Adapted from [3]).

differs, depending on the chemical structure of the permeant. According to the barrier solubility diffusion theory (BDSD) [43, 44], the membrane permeability solely depends on the partition coefficient of a solute from water to the hydrophobic central region of the membrane (not from the polar head group interface). Therefore, membrane surface binding is not directly relevant to permeability. However, there are many reports suggesting that membrane binding correlates with the *in vivo* absorption. A two-step model (flip-flop model) was proposed to describe the transmembrane movement of a substrate, especially that of large amphiphilic molecules or peptide mimetic molecules [45]. Some compounds do not permeate the membrane though they strongly bind to the membrane, probably because the polar part of the molecule (e.g., the amidine group) cannot penetrate into the hydrophobic region of the membrane, whereas the lipophilic part can insert into the hydrophobic region [46].

6.3.2
Parallel Artificial Membrane Permeation Assay: Recent Progress

One decade has passed since the parallel artificial membrane permeation assay (PAMPA) was first introduced in 1998 [47]. Since then, PAMPA rapidly gained wide popularity in drug discovery [3, 48–51]. Today, PAMPA is the most widely used physicochemical membrane permeation model. The term "PAMPA" is now used as the general name for a plate-based (HTS enabled), filter-supported (filter immobilized) artificial membrane. Typically, phospholipids dissolved in an organic solvent are impregnated into the filter to construct a PAMPA membrane.

Recently, there is some negativity towards PAMPA [52], seemingly due to an over-expectation and misunderstanding of PAMPA and the science of passive membrane permeation [53]. PAMPA is a refined descendant of log P_{oct} and is an improved surrogate measurement for passive transcellular permeation. PAMPA permeability usually correlates well with passive transcellular permeation. It is important to correctly understand the pros and cons of this tool and to use it appropriately in drug discovery.

6.3.2.1 Understanding PAMPA

PAMPA membranes typically consist of phospholipids dissolved in an organic solvent. Both of them affect chemical selectivity. Phospholipids facilitate the permeability of moderately hydrophilic molecules by ionic or hydrogen-bonding interactions (phopholipids are hydrogen bond acceptors). This allows permeation of moderately lipophilic compounds. Recently, it was shown that anionic phospholipid(s) increases the permeation of basic compounds by ion pair mechanism [54–56]. Many PAMPA variants (and other artificial membrane tools) add anionic phospholipid(s) to increase the *in vivo* predictability.

Though phospholipids may add some similarity to the biological membrane, the organic solvent remaining in the membrane largely affects its permeability. The BDSD theory would support the use of an alkane or alkyldiene [43].

6.3.2.2 Variation of PAMPA: Recent Progress

Composition of the PAMPA membrane varies from a purely organic solvent membrane to a purely phospholipid membrane. At the first international conference of PAMPA in 2002 (www.pampa2002.com/), it was agreed that these variations would be notated as initials or a short adjective at the head of PAMPA (e.g., BM-PAMPA for biomimetic PAMPA). The original PAMPA (Egg-PAMPA) [47], hexadecane membrane PAMPA (HDM-PAMPA) [48], BM-PAMPA [49], double sink PAMPA (DS-PAMPA) and blood–brain barrier PAMPA (BBB-PAMPA) [51] are reviewed elsewhere [3].

6.3.2.3 Phospholipid Vesicle PAMPA

Falten et al. recently reported that phospholipid membrane vesicles can be constructed on a filter scaffold without any organic solvent [57–60]. In this system, the phospholipid vesicle occupies the filter pores to form a permeation barrier. This is more relevant to the cellular membrane than PAMPA membranes with organic solvent. The membrane can be stored up to two weeks without significant change and is stable at pH 2–8. The Fa% predictability was compared with BM-PAMPA, DS-PAMPA, Caco-2 and immobilized liposome chromatography, resulting in promising predictability.

6.3.2.4 Phospholipid–Octanol PAMPA

Recently, octanol was used as the organic solvent [61, 62]. Compared to alkanes, octanol is less hydrophobic and may decrease the permeation barrier for hydrophilic compounds. This may avoid the false negative predictions found with the use of alkanes.

6.3.2.5 Tri-Layer PAMPA

Chen et al. reduced the volume of organic solvent (hexadecane) down to $1\,\mu L$ per well (usually 4–5 μL/well) [63]. Phospholipid/hexane solution was applied on both side of the thin hexadecane membrane (40 μg phospholipid). After the evaporation of hexane, phospholipid/hexadecane/phospholipid tri-layer was formed (according to the original article). With the 2% phospholipid/dodecane membrane (4 μL/well) and DS-PAMPA, permeability of some compounds such as caffeine and antipyrine were underestimated, whereas tri-layer PAMPA gave an appropriate estimate.

6.3.2.6 Mucus Layer Adhered PAMPA

The intestinal wall is covered by a mucus layer. This mucus layer prevents direct contact of the lumenal contents with the epithelial membrane. Mucus can be attached onto the lipid membrane by the aid of agar and hydrophilic filter scaffold [64, 65]. This allows the simultaneous assessment of dissolution and permeation. Food effects were adequately predicted using this method. Loftsson et al. used a cellophane membrane as a surrogate for the mucus layer [66].

6.3.3
Application of PAMPA for Drug Discovery

Due to its applicability to high-throughput assays, PAMPA would have most impact when used at early stages of drug discovery. The PAMPA membrane is resistant to high levels of organic solvent (e.g., up to 10–30% AcCN, EtOH, or DMSO) [67] and therefore is less limited in studying low-solubility compounds than biological membranes. Unlike cell systems, PAMPA does not require any pre-maintenance, is reproducible and is easy to assay. Simple UV detection can be used because of no interference from biological contaminants and the use of high concentrations. PAMPA is suited for both automation (>500 compounds/day) and manual procedures.

In addition to screening compounds, PAMPA was recently applied for high-throughput formulation screening. For early *in vivo* toxicity studies, it is often necessary to rapidly develop an effective formulation to increase exposure. Such formulations are usually a combination of several excipients. Simultaneous assessment of solubility and permeability is required since formulation excipients may reduce the apparent permeability by reducing the free fraction of a drug [68].

PAMPA data were also used to understand permeation into the pharmacological and toxicological target cells. A discrepancy between the enzyme level assay and cell-based assay is often observed in drug discovery, resulting in a misreading of the structure–activity relationship [69].

6.4
Limitation of *In Vitro* Assays

It is important to understand some limitations of *in vitro* artificial membrane and cell permeability assays when the data is used for compound selection and structure permeability relationship study. Therefore, before moving into the structure permeability relationship section, limitations of *in vitro* assays are discussed in this section. There are a number of other limitations of *in vitro* models which should be considered [3, 70].

6.4.1
Impact of UWL on Permeability

In *in vitro* permeability studies conducted in static systems, the UWL adjacent to the membrane can be up to 1500–4000 μm thick, whereas *in vivo* the UWL is only 30–300 μm in the GI tract and is negligible for the BBB [71]. The experimental system is often stirred or shaken to minimize the effects of the UWL. An orbital shaker is often not effective and can be modified by adding beads to enhance the agitation. Recently, it has been clearly demonstrated that the quantitative structure activity relationship was interfered if the UWL limited permeation and membrane limited permeation were simultaneously analyzed [53, 72]. Usually, if the *in vitro* permeability is >about 40×10^{-6} cm/s, the UWL has a significant effect on the permeability (membrane permeability would be underestimated).

6.4.2
Membrane Binding

Where a compound is highly lipophilic, membrane binding also retards the permeability [73, 74]. Therefore, it is important to measure the membrane binding at the same time of the permeation assay. *In vivo*, the blood flow removes the compound from the basolateral side [75]. As a rule of thumb, when log D_{oct} (at assay pH) > 1.5, membrane binding may be an issue [73].

6.4.3
Low Solubility

When a compound has a low solubility, precipitation can occur on the apical side of the membrane. In the case of PAMPA, several solubilizer agents can be used, such as DMSO or bile acids. When cyclodextrin, micelle systems and so on are used, it should be recognized that the free fraction of the drug would be reduced. In biological membranes, solubilizers should be selected with care, since it may affect the cell viability. The concentration used with *in vitro* cell models is limited due to toxicity of compounds/formulations/solubilizing solvents at high concentrations. Generally, compounds are evaluated at concentrations below 100 µM and with low levels of solubilizing solvents (e.g., <1% DMSO) to avoid toxicity issues.

6.4.4
Difference of the Paracellular Pathway

Usually, PAMPA does not have any aqueous pores and is therefore not suitable for examining paracellular transport. Some cell models, for example, Caco-2 and MDCK, have a narrower tight junction than the *in vivo* human intestine and may underestimate paracellular transport. However, the contribution of the paracellular pathway can be added using an *in silico* approach [76–78].

6.4.5
Interlaboratory Variability

Significant interlaboratory differences in permeability measurements are observed with cell-based assays. It is important to standardize culture conditions and characterize a cell line within one's own laboratory. Permeability differences can be attributed to a number of factors, for example, heterogenecity of cell line, passage number, culture conditions, characteristics of the filter membrane, age of monolayers and level of differentiation and experimental methodology used. Active transporters have been shown to be expressed differently in different laboratories. For example, P-gp was shown to be expressed consistently from day 6 in one laboratory and only found to be functional from day 17 in another [79]. It should also be noted that some transporters (e.g., PEPT 1) are proton-dependent and therefore optimization of the apical pH may be required [23, 79].

6.5
Computational Approaches/In Silico Modeling

6.5.1
In Vivo Systems

Classically the term "*in silico* modeling" referred to the process of building a model to predict a given endpoint from a set of molecular properties derived purely from the chemical structure of a number of compounds of which the endpoint of interest is known.

However, in recent years the term "*in silico*" expanded its meaning to any type of modeling performed with the use of a computer. This includes the use of experimentally measured *in vitro* and/or *in vivo* data for the prediction of *in vivo* pharmacokinetics, as well as the construction and analysis of molecular databases.

This is a reflection of the increasing knowledge of the complexity of *in vivo* systems, and also the current powerful computational resources to capture, analyze, interpret and model those systems. In view of this complexity, not only the development of genomics, proteomics and metabonomics databases, but also the development of systems biology methods helps us to understand the underlying mechanisms in any given ADME process [80].

In this respect, the *in silico* modeling of membrane permeation is one of the most advanced ADME areas. The reason is that it became apparent that, whilst physicochemical properties and QSAR models are useful compound selection tools, these methods alone cannot provide a good estimate of the *in vivo* permeability and understanding of the mechanism behind it. Some mechanistic knowledge needs to be incorporated in the equation in order to achieve the desired prediction power. Therefore in recent years, a number of *mechanism-based approaches* emerged, either for predicting *in vivo* membrane absorption, or for understanding the mechanisms involved in permeation processes and understanding interactions between drugs and biological molecules.

In a recent review of pharmacokinetics in drug discovery, Ruiz-Garcia *et al.* [81] compiled an exhaustive list of software resources for absorption prediction. The main topic in the described databases is transporters, in particular the ATP-binding cassette, of which the efflux transporter P-gp and the peptide transporter PEPT1 are well known examples. These examples show that science is moving away from the simplistic passive transport view of permeability and towards an all-inclusive, mechanism-understanding model of absorption, which takes account of all the interactions between the agents involved in the specific permeation process, including the levels of gene expression at different tissues, species and individual patients.

Mechanism-based approaches for passive permeation have been used to model passive intestinal absorption, explicitly taking into account the paracellular and transcellular pathways [82–84]. The transcellular model was based on the pH partition theory (explicitly considers pK_a, see Section 6.1.2). Log P_{oct} was simply used to represent the permeation of non-ionized and ionized molecules. The paracellular pathway was modeled as permeation through a charged aqueous pore [21, 22]. A consideration of the permeation mechanism increased the predictive power and mechanistic understanding, with less risk of over-fitting. The *in silico* intestinal device (ISID) approach by Garmire *et al.* further progressed this direction [85–88]. ISID consists of a mechanistic model developed within the Swarm platform (www.swarm.org) that combines passive transcellular, paracellular, P-gp efflux and intestinal P450 metabolism. By adjusting the model parameters to the mean transit time of a test compound, and simulating different levels of expression of P-gp and CYPs, the authors are able to rule out synergy between those proteins and detect a significant amount of antagonism between them.

Another promising approach is the recently launched "ADMET Predictor" (http://www.simulations-plus.com/products.html), also mentioned in Ruiz-Garcia's review [81]. This software package complements the "GastroPlus" package [89], which is not an *in silico* predictor in the classic sense, but uses "physiologically based pharmaco-kinetics (PBPK)" models to translate information derived from *in vitro* assays into pharmacokinetic profiles and parameters, including intestinal absorption. The advantage of this method is that it enables the integration of mechanistic knowledge about the compound into the predictions, such as, for example, the involvement of a transporter in the intestinal absorption process [90]. Given the focus of this chapter on *in silico* methods, the description of PBPK modeling and simulation methods is out of scope in this section – however, a whole chapter is devoted to this methodology elsewhere in this volume. The ADME-Predictor is a classic *in silico* predictor that was designed to generate estimates for all the *in vitro* endpoints that "GastroPlus" needs as input, such as solubility, PAMPA, MDR1, Caco-2 permeability, fraction unbound of the compound in plasma and so on. The relevant aspect of this new approach is that it allows the prediction of pharmaco-kinetic parameters directly from the molecular structure of the compound(s) of interest, without having to perform any *in vitro* assay. This highlights the importance of achieving accurate *in silico* predictions of *in vitro* permeability assay endpoints, which is covered in the next section.

Of course traditional *in silico* approaches are still being applied to the permeability/absorption problem, although the applicability of these models is confined to compounds that are most predominantly passively transported across the membranes, which can become a significant limitation if the compounds of interest have a more complex mechanism of absorption. The general observation is that hydrogen bonding, also a heavy component in Lipinski's rule of five, has a strong effect on intestinal passive permeability [91]. However, as Johnson and Zheng point out [92], the number and the chemical diversity of the examples on which the models or the rules are based is limited [93], so the statistics describing the scope of the training set and the model performance should be inspected carefully.

It is important to understand the limitations of each type of data used in the modeling: effective intestinal permeability, human intestinal absorption and bioavailability, although intimately related to intestinal endothelial penetration processes, encompass different levels of complexity and are not equivalent. Similarly, when inspecting brain penetration models, care should be taken about whether the measurements correspond to partitioning of drugs from blood (or plasma) into whole brain, or into the aqueous phase of the CNS. For an overview of the most recent classical *in silico* modeling and SAR rule-derivation efforts on *in vivo* permeability, the reader is encouraged to examine the review by Hou *et al.* [94], which covers blood–brain partitioning as well as intestinal penetration.

Unfortunately the number of *in silico* modeling studies on brain membrane permeability is significantly smaller than for human intestinal absorption, resulting in a lack of consensus about how to assess brain penetration (both *in vitro* and *in vivo*) and the intrinsic difficulty of measuring this particular endpoint, which overall results in a low turnover of data generation that could be used to build *in silico* models [95, 96]. For this reason, the *in silico* models used to assess brain permeability in the discovery process focus normally on P-gp efflux and some measure of *in vitro* membrane permeability, methods which are reviewed in the next section.

An area that has not drawn much attention from *in silico* modelers is ocular permeability, where higher aqueous solubility rather than in intestinal permeability is required, yet without compromising the corneal membrane permeability. Usually this type of penetration is optimized by introducing slight changes to the formulation and molecular structure of orally administered compounds and then using animal models to assess the pharmacokinetic profile of the modified drug. The lack of *in silico* models can be ascribed to the small amount of ocular drugs being developed in comparison with targets in other organs and to the good correlations generally observed between animal and human corneal permeability [97].

6.5.2
In Vitro Cellular Membrane Systems

One of the main *in vitro* permeability assays used in the pharmaceutical industry has been for many years the Caco-2 monolayer. Therefore, most of the *in silico* models developed to predict permeability were based on Caco-2 data. Hou and Johnson produced a couple of reviews that comprehensibly summarizes the recent efforts using Caco-2 permeability data [92, 94]. All those models are designed to predict the influx or apparent permeability of drugs in the same direction as intestinal absorption occurs, that is, from the apical to the basal side of the cell line, regardless of the extent of active transport involved in the permeation process.

An interesting and more mechanistic approach was taken by Stoner *et al.* [98] who collected the largest self-consistent Caco-2 data set known to date and used the efflux ratio values (i.e., the basal to apical divided by the apical to basal apparent permeability) to exclude compounds subject to any active transport, thus focusing the modeling process exclusively onto passive permeability.

The known variability associated to the behavior of Caco-2 cell lines, together with the need to find a more robust and easy to grow type of culture led the pharmaceutical industry to substitute this system by, for example, MDCK cell cultures. So *in silico* modelers have also turned towards this new kind of *in vitro* cell data, although to a lesser extent than with Caco-2 systems. Perhaps the only notable example of the use of MDCK data is Refsgaard's categorical model, where a dataset of Caco-2 permeability values was enriched with MDCK permeability data [99].

Although the main assumption in the hit-to-lead process is that membrane permeation is mainly driven by passive diffusion processes (i.e., dependent on the extent of concentration gradient), it becomes increasingly clear that the effect of transporters also needs to be understood. Although the amount of data available is still sparse, *in silico* modeling has also impacted this area, in particular in the development of models for efflux pumps such as P-glycoprotein/MDR1, MRP and BCRP, which not only reduce intestinal or brain permeation significantly, but may also originate drug–drug interaction problems.

The most recent example of *in silico* efflux modeling has been based on Caco-2 permeability measured in the basal to apical direction [100]. This model can be very effective at ruling out compounds that most likely will show low *in vivo* intestinal absorption – however it cannot indicate which efflux pump(s) is/are responsible for that, making it more difficult for designers to circumvent the problem. Johnson [92] also included in his review an excellent summary of QSAR models and rules of thumb developed for P-gp substrates and inhibitors. These models are normally based on efflux ratios from MDCK/MDR1 or Caco-2 cell lines – in the latter case it is important to notice that the data is combined with inhibition values from the calcein-AM assay, as the observed efflux might not be exclusively due to P-gp.

A publication that nicely complements this review is Chang's account of pharmacophore-based *in silico* models [101] which, in addition to P-gp, is dedicated to the other two major efflux pumps: MRP1 and BCRP. Unfortunately the most recent nonpharmacophoric *in silico* modeling efforts around the latter transporters are solely based on flavonoid compounds, which limits the applicability of their conclusions [102, 103].

The only other major transporter that has been a matter of study by *in silico* modelers is PEPT1, probably as a result of its successful inclusion in the drug design process in the 1990s. The most recent publication in this field is a comparison of several *in silico* classification models based on inhibition data and using fast-calculated 2D molecular descriptors [104]. Previous to that, Biegel [105] developed a pharmacophoric 3D QSAR model using a "conformational analysis and molecular alignment (CoMSIA)" approach, which was subsequently used to design a new compound that was recognized by PEPT1. This work was later complemented by comparison to the structural requirements for substrates of PEPT2, using their respective CoMSIA contour plots [106]. Chang and Ekins also include a pharmacophore model for PEPT1 in their review [101].

There are no recent improvement in the paracellular pathway permeation models, probably because there is no specific *in vitro* or *in vivo* system to measure the paracellular pathway contribution. The paracellular pathway models was constructed using very hydrophilic compounds [107] or subtracting the contribution of transcellular pathway from the total passive permeation [78]. Paracellular pathway was modeled as permeation through a charged aqueous pore. A combination of size sieving function and electric field function was found to model the paracellular pathway [78, 87, 88].

6.5.3
Artificial Membranes

In silico models for artificial membrane basically corresponds to a model for the transcellular passive permeability pathway. Probably the most popular permeability assay given its robustness, its high throughput and its low cost, is the PAMPA. Consequently, this system has also inspired a number of *in silico* modeling groups. In general, the transmembrane diffusion process of undissociated molecule is determined by the lipophilicity and hydrogen bonding ability of the compounds, expressed as either polar surface area or counts of hydrogen bond donors and acceptors. That still is the case, as a recent work by Fujikawa shows [72] where, in an attempt to extend a previous QSAR model [108] to highly hydrophobic compounds, a new bi-linear *in silico* model is built to predict PAMPA permeability.

An alternative approach and perhaps more applicable to drug designers was taken by Verma and co-workers [109]. They estimated several PAMPA systems as a function of calculated logP and a number of what they call "indicator variables (I_n)". In the presence of specific chemical groups, such as –COOH, –SO_2NH_2, aromatic –OH and –N(CH_3)$_2$, these variables take the value of unity and their positive or negative coefficient in the equation describes whether their effect is favorable or detrimental to membrane permeability.

Kalyanaraman and Jacobson also report very successful results in predicting PAMPA permeability ranking within a series of weakly basic compounds, using molecular mechanics (MM) [110]. The main advantage of their *in silico* method is that it does not require the training of the model with examples of previously measured values – they use MM energy functions to calculate the minimum free energy change involved in the transition from a water to a membrane-solvated conformation.

A similarly "training-independent" strategy, using a mechanism-based compartmental model, was followed by Zhang *et al.* [111] to bin compounds as "high" or "low" permeability in relationship to the reference compound, metoprolol. The interesting outcome of this model is that it allows to define a physico-chemical space within which molecules display the maximal transcellular permeability with minimal intracellular retention, reducing the risk of exhibiting undesirable side effects. The chemical space is described in terms of lipophilicity of the neutral form of the drug, the ionized form and its pK_a.

6.5.4
Perspectives

As the current trends show, the *in silico* modeling of membrane permeability is evolving towards a better integration of the contemporary understanding of absorption pathways in the predictive systems [112]. If the hit-to-lead *in silico* profiling process wants to succeed in the prediction of *in vivo* absorption, *in silico* modeling needs to expand in the following three directions:

1. **Developing qualitative knowledge:** helping to gain an understanding of the pathways and mechanisms involved, gaining qualitative knowledge that can influence strategic decisions in the drug development. At the same time, sharing that information and linking it to genomic and proteomic ontologies is vital, not only to avoid duplication of efforts, but also to effectively build the deep knowledge of targets and pathways that will lead to high quality *in silico* models and eventually to more robust personalized medicines than the mechanism-based approach. This is the realm of *in silico* simulations, text mining, database management, classic *in silico* qualitative SAR modeling and physiology modeling.

2. **Developing quantitative knowledge:** providing the scientific community with different numerical models for each specific mechanism that can occur during any membrane permeation event. This requires a good understanding of the limitations of the data on which the modeling is built, that is, of its variability and also of the assumptions underlying in the data acquisition process. This is the role of classic quantitative SAR *in silico* modeling.

3. **Integrating quantitative and qualitative knowledge:** as more information becomes available from the previous two fronts, a framework that contains the whole picture of the absorption process, as well as the detailed knowledge of pathways needs to be put in place [112]. The scaffold of this system needs to be flexible enough to evolve as new knowledge comes into play, and as this happens the predictions will get closer and closer to the actual *in vivo* measurements. In this case the disciplines involved are systems biology, mechanistic pathway modeling, PBPK and less traditional *in silico* modeling which combines quantitative and qualitative modeling techniques.

In summary, *in silico* needs to embrace the complexity of the several membrane permeation processes that occur *in vivo*, in order to provide the drug developers with a pure *in silico* decision making tool, which can predict *in vivo* endpoints for specific genomic profiles, exclusively from a compound's molecular structure.

6.6
Outlook

Organ-specific permeation of a drug is one area currently extensively investigated. While passive permeation determines the baseline of pharmacokinetics for most cases, active transport would add the organ-specific permeation. From the viewpoint of pharmacology, toxicology and drug delivery, organ-specific permeation is of great interest. Knowledge of the transport proteins are rapidly increasing through the application of genomics, proteomics and bioinformatics. In the future, it may become possible to connect pharmacokinetics and systems biology. This will enable more robust PK/PD analysis and target validation.

Acknowledgment

Sections 6.1–6.4 are attributed to J.B. and K.S. Section 6.5 is attributed to L.C. K.S. and J.B. thank the members of the Drug Delivery Group, Research Formulation, Sandwich, for their kind support.

References

1 Artursson, P. and Matsson, P. (2006) Cell culture absorption models-state of the art, in *Pharmacokinetic Profiling Drug Research* (eds B. Testa, S. Krämer, H. Wunderli-Allenspach and G. Folkers), Wiley-VCH, Zurich, pp. 71–78.

2 Artursson, P., Neuhoff, S., Matsson, P. and Tavelin, S. (2006) Passive permeability and active transport models for, the prediction of oral absorption. *Comprehensive Medicinal Chemistry II*, **5**, 259–278.

3 Sugano, K. (2007) Artificial membrane technologies to assess transfer and permeation of drugs in drug discovery, in *Comprehensive Medicinal Chemistry II, ADME-Tox Approach*, Vol. V (eds B. Testa and H. van de Waterbeemd), Elsevier, Oxford, pp. 453–487.

4 Abbott, N.J. (2006) *In vitro* models for examining and predicting brain uptake of drugs, in *Comprehensive Medicinal Chemistry II, ADME-Tox Approach*, Vol. 5 (eds B. Testa and H. van de Waterbeemd), Elsevier, Oxford, pp. 301–320.

5 Scherrmann, J.M. (2006) The biology and function of transporters, in *Comprehensive Medicinal Chemistry II, ADME-Tox Approach*, Vol. 5 (eds B. Testa and H. van de Waterbeemd), Elsevier, Oxford, pp. 51–85.

6 He, Y., Murby, S., Warhurst, G., Gifford, L., Walker, D., Ayrton, J., Eastmond, R. and Rowland, M. (1998) Species differences in size discrimination in the paracellular pathway refrected by oral bioavailability of poly(ethylene glycol) and D-peptides. *Journal of Pharmaceutical Sciences*, **87**, 626–633.

7 Oliver, R.E., Jones, A.F. and Rowland, M. (1998) What surface of the intestinal epithelium is effectively available to permeating drugs? *Journal of Pharmaceutical Sciences*, **87**, 634–639.

8 Winne, D. (1978) The permeability coefficient of the wall of a villous membrane. *Journal of Mathematical Biology*, **6**, 95–108.

9 Fagerholm, U., Johansson, M. and Lennernaes, H. (1996) Comparison between permeability coefficients in rat and human jejunum. *Pharmaceutical Research*, **13**, 1336–1342.

10 Chiou, W.L. (1994) Effect of "unstirred" water layer in the intestine on the rate and extent of absorption after oral administration. *Biopharmaceutics & Drug Disposition*, **15**, 709–717.

11 DeSesso, J.M. and Jacobson, C.F. (2001) Anatomical and physiological parameters affecting gastrointestinal absorption in humans and rats. *Food and Chemical Toxicology*, **39**, 209–228.

12 Haruta, S., Iwasaki, N., Ogawara, K.-i., Higaki, K. and Kimura, T. (1998) Absorption behavior of orally administered drugs in rats treated with propantheline. *Journal of Pharmaceutical Sciences*, **87**, 1081–1085.

13 Sawamoto, T., Haruta, S., Kurosaki, Y., Higaki, K. and Kimura, T. (1997) Prediction of the plasma concentration profiles of orally administered drugs in rats on the basis of gastrointestinal transit kinetics and absorbability. *Journal of Pharmacy and Pharmacology*, **49**, 450–457.

14 Hubatsch, I., Ragnarsson, E.G.E. and Artursson, P. (2007) Determination of drug permeability and prediction of drug absorption in Caco-2 monolayers. *Nature Protocols*, **2**, 2111–2119.

15 Hidalgo, I.J. (2001) Assessing the absorption of new pharmaceuticals. *Current Topics in Medicinal Chemistry*, **1**, 385–401.

16 Behrens, I., Kamm, W., Dantzig, A.H. and Kissel, T. (2004) Variation of peptide transporter PepT1 and HPT1 expression in Caco-2 cells as a function of cell origin. *Journal of Pharmaceutical Sciences*, **93**, 1743–1754.

17 Tang, F., Horie, K. and Borchardt, R.T. (2002) Are MDCK cells transfected with the human MRP2 gene a good model of the human intestinal mucosa? *Pharmaceutical Research*, **19**, 773–779.

18 Evers, R., Kool, M., Van Deemter, L., Janssen, H., Calafat, J., Oomen, L.C.J.M., Paulusma, C.C., Elferink, R.P.J.O., Baas, F., Schinkel, A.H. and Borst, P. (1998) Drug export activity of the human canalicular multispecific organic anion transporter in polarized kidney MDCK cells expressing cMOAT (MRP2) cDNA. *Journal of Clinical Investigation*, **101**, 1310–1319.

19 Evers, R., Cnubben, N.H.P., Wijnholds, J., van Deemter, L., van Bladeren, P.J. and Borst, P. (1997) Transport of glutathione prostaglandin A conjugates by the multidrug resistance protein 1. *FEBS Letters*, **419**, 112–116.

20 Tang, F., Horie, K. and Borchardt, R.T. (2002) Are MDCK cells transfected with the human MDR1 gene a good model of the human intestinal mucosa? *Pharmaceutical Research*, **19**, 765–772.

21 Benet, L.Z., Cummins, C.L. and Wu, C.Y. (2004) Unmasking the dynamic interplay between efflux transporters and metabolic enzymes. *International Journal of Pharmaceutics*, **277**, 3–9.

22 Irvine, J.D., Takahashi, L., Lockhart, K., Cheong, J., Tolan, J.W., Selick, H.E. and Grove, J.R. (1999) MDCK (Madin-Darby canine kidney) cells: A tool for membrane permeability screening. *Journal of Pharmaceutical Sciences*, **88**, 28–33.

23 Shah, P., Jogani, V., Bagchi, T. and Misra, A. (2006) Role of Caco-2 cell monolayers in prediction of intestinal drug absorption. *Biotechnology Progress*, **22**, 186–198.

24 Tavelin, S., Taipalensuu, J., Hallboeoek, F., Vellonen, K.-S., Moore, V. and Artursson, P. (2003) An improved cell culture model based on 2/4/A1 cell monolayers for studies of intestinal drug transport: characterization of transport routes. *Pharmaceutical Research*, **20**, 373–381.

25 Matsson, P., Bergstroem, C.A.S., Nagahara, N., Tavelin, S., Norinder, U. and Artursson, P. (2005) Exploring the role of different drug transport routes in permeability screening. *Journal of Medicinal Chemistry*, **48**, 604–613.

26 Wikman, A., Karlsson, J., Carlstedt, I. and Artursson, P. (1993) A drug absorption model based on the mucus layer producing human intestinal goblet cell line HT29-H. *Pharmaceutical Research*, **10**, 843–852.

27 Pontier, C., Pachot, J., Botham, R., Lenfant, B. and Arnaud, P. (2001)

HT29-MTX and Caco-2/TC7 monolayers as predictive models for human intestinal absorption: role of the mucus layer. *Journal of Pharmaceutical Sciences*, **90**, 1608–1619.

28 Keely, S., Rullay, A., Wilson, C., Carmichael, A., Carrington, S., Corfield, A., Haddleton, D.M. and Brayden, D.J. (2005) *In vitro* and ex vivo intestinal tissue models to measure mucoadhesion of poly (methacrylate) and N-trimethylated chitosan polymers. *Pharmaceutical Research*, **22**, 38–49.

29 Gumbleton, M. and Audus, K.L. (2001) Progress and limitations in the use of *in vitro* cell cultures to serve as a permeability screen for the blood-brain barrier. *Journal of Pharmaceutical Sciences*, **90**, 1681–1698.

30 Lundquist, S. and Renftel, M. (2002) The use of *in vitro* cell culture models for mechanistic studies and as permeability screens for the blood-brain barrier in the pharmaceutical industry-Background and current status in the drug discovery process. *Vascular Pharmacology*, **38**, 355–364.

31 Breedveld, P., Beijnen, J.H. and Schellens, J.H.M. (2006) Use of P-glycoprotein and BCRP inhibitors to improve oral bioavailability and CNS penetration of anticancer drugs. *Trends in Pharmacological Sciences*, **27**, 17–24.

32 Pardridge, W.M. (2007) Drug targeting to the brain. *Pharmaceutical Research*, **24**, 1733–1744.

33 Cecchelli, R., Dehouck, B., Descamps, L., Fenart, L., Buee-Scherrer, V., Duhem, C., Lundquist, S., Rentfel, M., Torpier, G. and Dehouck, M.P. (1999) *In vitro* model for evaluating drug transport across the blood-brain barrier. *Advanced Drug Delivery Reviews*, **36**, 165–178.

34 Balimane, P.V., Han, Y.-H. and Chong, S. (2006) Current industrial practices of assessing permeability and P-glycoprotein interaction. *AAPS Journal*, **8**, E1–E13.

35 Englund, G., Rorsman, F., Roennblom, A., Karlbom, U., Lazorova, L., Grasjoe, J., Kindmark, A. and Artursson, P. (2006) Regional levels of drug transporters along the human intestinal tract: co-expression of ABC and SLC transporters and comparison with Caco-2 cells. *European Journal of Pharmaceutical Sciences*, **29**, 269–277.

36 Toyobuku, H., Tamai, I., Ueno, K. and Tsuji, A. (2003) Limited influence of P-glycoprotein on small-intestinal absorption of cilostazol, a high absorptive permeability drug. *Journal of Pharmaceutical Sciences*, **92**, 2249–2259.

37 Lennernas, H. (2003) Intestinal drug absorption and bioavailability: Beyond involvement of single transport function. *Journal of Pharmacy and Pharmacology*, **55**, 429–433.

38 Wang, Q., Rager, J.D., Weinstein, K., Kardos, P.S., Dobson, G.L., Li, J. and Hidalgo, I.J. (2005) Evaluation of the MDR-MDCK cell line as a permeability screen for the blood-brain barrier. *International Journal of Pharmaceutics*, **288**, 349–359.

39 Garberg, P., Ball, M., Borg, N., Cecchelli, R., Fenart, L., Hurst, R.D., Lindmark, T., Mabondzo, A., Nilsson, J.E., Raub, T.J., Stanimirovic, D., Terasaki, T., Oeberg, J.O. and Oesterberg, T. (2005) *In vitro* models for the blood-brain barrier. *Toxicology In Vitro: An International Journal Published in Association with BIBRA*, **19**, 299–334.

40 Lennernaes, H. and Abrahamsson, B. (2006) The biopharmaceutics classification system. *Comprehensive Medicinal Chemistry II*, **5**, 971–988.

41 Feng, M.R. (2002) Assessment of blood–brain barrier penetration: *In silico*, *in vitro* and *in vivo*. *Current Drug Metabolism*, **3**, 647–657.

42 Carrara, S., Reali, V., Misiano, P., Dondio, G. and Bigogno, C. (2007) Evaluation of *in vitro* brain penetration: Optimized PAMPA and MDCKII-MDR1 assay comparison. *International Journal of Pharmaceutics*, **345**, 125–133.

43 Xiang, T., Xu, Y. and Anderson, B.D. (1998) The barrier domain for solute permeation varies with lipid bilayer phase structure. *Journal of Membrane Biology*, 165, 77–90.

44 Joguparthi, V., Xiang, T.-X. and Anderson, B.D. (2007) Liposome transport of hydrophobic drugs: gel phase lipid bilayer permeability and partitioning of the lactone form of a hydrophobic camptothecin, DB-67. *Journal of Pharmaceutical Sciences*, 97, 400–420.

45 Burton, P.S., Conradi, R.A. and Hilgers, A.R. (1991) Mechanisms of peptide and protein absorption. (2). Transcellular mechanism of peptide and protein, absorption: passive aspects. *Advanced Drug Delivery Reviews*, 7, 365–386.

46 Sugano, K., Yoshida, S., Takaku, M., Haramura, M., Saitoh, R., Nabuchi, Y. and Ushio, H. (2000) Quantitative structure-intestinal permeability relationship of benzamidine analogue thrombin inhibitor. *Bioorganic & Medicinal Chemistry Letters*, 10, 1939–1942.

47 Kansy, M., Senner, F. and Gubernator, K. (1998) Physicochemical high throughput screening: parallel artificial membrane permeation assay in the description of passive absorption processes. *Journal of Medicinal Chemistry*, 41, 1007–1010.

48 Wohnsland, F. and Faller, B. (2001) High-throughput permeability pH profile and high-throughput alkane/water log P with artificial membranes. *Journal of Medicinal Chemistry*, 44, 923–930.

49 Sugano, K., Hamada, H., Machida, M. and Ushio, H. (2001) High throuput prediction of oral absorption: Improvement of the composition of the lipid solution used in parallel artificial membrane permeation assay. *Journal of Biomolecular Screening*, 6, 189–196.

50 Avdeef, A., Strafford, M., Block, E., Balogh, M.P., Chambliss, W. and Khan, I. (2001) Drug absorption *in vitro* model: filter-immobilized artificial membranes; 2. Studies of the permeability properties of lactones in Piper methysticum Forst. *European Journal of Pharmaceutical Sciences*, 14, 271–280.

51 Di, L., Kerns, E.H., Fan, K., McConnell, O.J. and Carter, G.T. (2003) High throughput artificial membrane permeability assay for blood-brain barrier. *European Journal of Medicinal Chemistry*, 38, 223–232.

52 Galinis-Luciani, D., Nguyen, L. and Yazdanian, M. (2007) Is parallel artificial membrane permeability assay a useful tool for discovery? *Journal of Pharmaceutical Sciences*, 96, 2886–2892.

53 Avdeef, A., Bendels, S., Di, L., Faller, B., Kansy, M., Sugano, K. and Yamauchi, Y. (2007) Parallel artificial membrane permeability assay (PAMPA)-critical factors for better predictions of absorption. *Journal of Pharmaceutical Sciences*, 96, 2893–2909.

54 Sugano, K., Nabuchi, Y., Machida, M. and Asoh, Y. (2004) Permeation characteristics of a hydrophilic basic compound across a bio-mimetic artificial membrane. *International Journal of Pharmaceutics*, 275, 271–278.

55 Seo, P.R., Teksin, Z.S., Kao, J.P.Y. and Polli, J.E. (2006) Lipid composition effect on permeability across PAMPA. *European Journal of Pharmaceutical Sciences*, 29, 259–268.

56 Teksin, Z.S., Hom, K., Balakrishnan, A. and Polli, J.E. (2006) Ion pair-mediated transport of metoprolol across a three lipid-component PAMPA system. *Journal of Controlled Release*, 116, 50–57.

57 Flaten, G.E., Bunjes, H., Luthman, K. and Brandl, M. (2006) Drug permeability across a phospholipid vesicle-based barrier. *European Journal of Pharmaceutical Sciences*, 28, 336–343.

58 Flaten, G.E., Dhanikula, A.B., Luthman, K. and Brandl, M. (2006) Drug permeability across a phospholipid vesicle based barrier: A novel approach for studying passive diffusion. *European Journal of Pharmaceutical Sciences*, 27, 80–90.

59 Flaten, G.E., Luthman, K., Vasskog, T. and Brandl, M. (2008) Drug permeability across a phospholipid vesicle-based barrier. *European Journal of Pharmaceutical Sciences*, **34**, 173–180.

60 Flaten, G.E., Skar, M., Luthman, K. and Brandl, M. (2007) Drug permeability across a phospholipid vesicle based barrier: 3. Characterization of drug-membrane interactions and the, effect of agitation on the barrier integrity and on the permeability. *European Journal of Pharmaceutical Sciences*, **30**, 324–332.

61 Corti, G., Maestrelli, F., Cirri, M., Furlanetto, S. and Mura, P. (2006) Development and evaluation of an *in vitro* method for prediction of human drug absorption. *European Journal of Pharmaceutical Sciences*, **27**, 346–353.

62 Corti, G., Maestrelli, F., Cirri, M., Zerrouk, N. and Mura, P. (2006) Development and evaluation of an *in vitro* method for prediction of human drug absorption. *European Journal of Pharmaceutical Sciences*, **27**, 354–362.

63 Chen, X., Murawski, A., Patel, K., Crespi, C.L. and Balimane, P.V. (2008) A novel design of artificial membrane for improving the parallel artificial membrane permeability assay model. *Pharmaceutical Research*, **25**, 1511–1520.

64 Sugano, K. and Sakai, K. (2004) Mucopolysaccharide-layered lipid membrane, membrane permeability-measuring filter/apparatus/kit, membrane permeability evaluation method, and test substance-screening method. Patents 31362, 2005221442, 20040206.

65 Sugano, K., Okazaki, A., Sugimoto, S., Tavornvipas, S., Omura, A. and Mano, T. (2007) Solubility and dissolution profile assessment in drug, discovery. *DMPK*, **22**, 225–254.

66 Loftsson, T., Konradsdottir, F. and Masson, M. (2006) Development and evaluation of an artificial membrane for determination of drug availability. *International Journal of Pharmaceutics*, **326**, 60–68.

67 Sugano, K., Hamada, H., Machida, M., Ushio, H., Saitoh, K. and Terada, K. (2001) Optimized conditions of bio-mimetic artificial membrane permeation assay. *International Journal of Pharmaceutics*, **228**, 181–188.

68 Bendels, S., Tsinman, O., Wagner, B., Lipp, D., Parrilla, I., Kansy, M. and Avdeef, A. (2006) PAMPA-excipient classification gradient map. *Pharmaceutical Research*, **23**, 2525–2535.

69 Li, C., Nair, L., Liu, T., Li, F., Pichardo, J., Agrawal, S., Chase, R., Tong, X., Uss, A.S., Bogen, S., Njoroge, F.G., Morrison, R.A. and Cheng, K.C. (2008) Correlation between PAMPA permeability and cellular activities of hepatitis C virus protease inhibitors. *Biochemical Pharmacology*, **75**, 1186–1197.

70 Balimane, P.V. and Chong, S. (2005) Cell culture-based models for intestinal permeability: A critique. *Drug Discovery Today*, **10**, 335–343.

71 Youdim, K.A., Avdeef, A. and Abbott, N.J. (2003) *In vitro* trans-monolayer permeability calculations: often forgotten assumptions. *Drug Discovery Today*, **8**, 997–1003.

72 Fujikawa, M., Nakao, K., Shimizu, R. and Akamatsu, M. (2007) QSAR study on permeability of hydrophobic compounds with artificial membranes. *Bioorganic & Medicinal Chemistry*, **15**, 3756–3767.

73 Kansy, M., Fischer, H., Kratzat, K., Senner, F., Wagner, B. and Parrilla, I. (2001) High-throughput artifical membrane permeability studies in early lead discovery and development, in *Pharmacokinetic Optimization in Drug Research*, 3-906390-22-5 ed. (eds B. Testa, H. van de Waterbeemd, G. Folkers and R. Guy), Wiley-VCH, Zürich, pp. 447–464.

74 Krishna, G., Chen, K.-j., Lin, C.-c. and Nomeir, A.A. (2001) Permeability of lipophilic compounds in drug discovery using in-vitro human absorption model, Caco-2. *International Journal of Pharmaceutics*, **222**, 77–89.

75 Yamashita, S., Tanaka, Y., Endoh, Y., Taki, Y., Sakane, T., Nadai, T. and Sezaki, H. (1997) Analysis of drug permeation across Caco-2 monolayer: implication for predicting in vivo drug absorption. *Pharmaceutical Research*, **14**, 486–491.

76 Saitoh, R., Sugano, K., Takata, N., Tachibana, T., Higashida, A., Nabuchi, Y. and Aso, Y. (2004) Correction of permeability with pore radius of tight junctions in Caco-2 monolayers improves the prediction of the dose fraction of hydrophilic drugs absorbed by humans. *Pharmaceutical Research*, **21**, 749.

77 Sugano, K., Nabuchi, Y., Machida, M. and Aso, Y. (2003) Prediction of human intestinal permeability using artificial membrane permeability. *International Journal of Pharmaceutics*, **257**, 245–251.

78 Sugano, K., Takata, N., Machida, M., Saitoh, K. and Terada, K. (2002) Prediction of passive intestinal absorption using bio-mimetic artificial membrane permeation assay and the paracellular pathway model. *International Journal of Pharmaceutics*, **241**, 241–251.

79 Volpe Donna, A. (2008) Variability in Caco-2 and MDCK cell-based intestinal permeability assays. *Journal of Pharmaceutical Sciences*, **97**, 712–725.

80 Ekins, S., Mestres, J. and Testa, B. (2007) In silico pharmacology for drug discovery: methods for virtual ligand screening and profiling. *British Journal of Pharmacology*, **152**, 9–20.

81 Ruiz, G.A., Bermejo, M., Moss, A. and Casabo, V.G. (2008) Pharmacokinetics in drug discovery. *Journal of Pharmaceutical Sciences*, **97**, 654–690.

82 Camenisch, G., Folkers, G. and van de Waterbeemd, H. (1996) Review of theoretical passive drug absorption models: historical background, recent developments and limitations. *Pharmaceutica Acta Helvetiae*, **71**, 309–327.

83 Sugano, K., Obata, K., Saitoh, R., Higashida, A. and Hamada, H. (2006) Processing of biopharmaceutical profiling data in drug discovery, in *Pharmacokinetic Profiling in Drug Research* (eds B. Testa, S. Krämer, H. Wunderli-Allenspach and G. Folkers), Wiley-VCH, Zurich, pp. 441–458.

84 Obata, K., Sugano, K., Saitoh, R., Higashida, A., Nabuchi, Y., Machida, M. and Aso, Y. (2005) Prediction of oral drug absorption in humans by theoretical passive absorption model. *International Journal of Pharmaceutics*, **293**, 183–192.

85 Liu, Y. and Hunt, C.A. (2005) Studies of intestinal drug transport using an in silico epithelio-mimetic device. *BioSystems*, **82**, 154–167.

86 Liu, Y. and Hunt, C.A. (2006) Mechanistic study of the cellular interplay of transport and metabolism using the synthetic modeling method. *Pharmaceutical Research*, **23**, 493–505.

87 Garmire, L.X. and Hunt, C.A. (2008) In silico methods for unraveling the mechanistic complexities of intestinal absorption: metabolism-efflux transport interactions. *Drug Metabolism and Disposition*.

88 Garmire, L.X., Garmire, D.G. and Hunt, C.A. (2007) An in silico transwell device for the study of drug transport and drug-drug interactions. *Pharmaceutical Research*, **24**, 2171–2186.

89 Willmann, S., Lippert, J. and Schmitt, W. (2005) From physicochemistry to absorption and distribution: predictive mechanistic modelling and computational tools. *Expert Opinion on Drug Metabolism and Toxicology*, **1**, 159–168.

90 Tubic, M., Wagner, D., Spahn, L.H., Bolger, M.B. and Langguth, P. (2006) In silico modeling of non-linear drug absorption for the P-gp substrate talinolol and of consequences for the resulting pharmacodynamic effect. *Pharmaceutical Research*, **23**, 1712–1720.

91 Shaikh, S.A., Jain, T., Sandhu, G., Latha, N. and Jayaram, B. (2007) From

drug target to leads–sketching a physicochemical pathway for lead molecule design in silico. *Current Pharmaceutical Design*, **13**, 3454–3470.

92 Johnson, S.R. and Zheng, W. (2006) Recent progress in the computational prediction of aqueous solubility and absorption. *AAPS Journal*, **8**, E27–E30.

93 Gola, J., Obrezanova, O., Champness, E. and Segall, M. (2006) ADMET property prediction: The state of the art and current challenges. *QSAR and Combinatorial Science*, **25**, 1172–1180.

94 Hou, T., Wang, J., Zhang, W., Wang, W. and Xu, X. (2006) Recent advances in computational prediction of drug absorption and permeability in drug discovery. *Current Medicinal Chemistry*, **13**, 2653–2667.

95 Palmer, A.M. and Stephenson, F.A. (2005) CNS drug discovery: challenges and solutions. *Drug News & Perspectives*, **18**, 51–57.

96 Lemaire, M. and Desrayaud, S. (2005) The priorities/needs of the pharmaceutical industry in drug delivery to the brain. *International Congress Series*, **2005**, 32–46.

97 Yoshihisa, S. (2008) Molecular design for enhancement of ocular penetration. *Journal of Pharmaceutical Sciences*, **97**, 2462–2496.

98 Stoner, C.L., Troutman, M., Gao, H., Johnson, K., Stankovic, C., Brodfuehrer, J., Gifford, E. and Chang, M. (2006) Moving in silico screening into practice: A minimalist approach to guide permeability screening! *Letters in Drug Design and Discovery*, **3**, 575–581.

99 Refsgaard, H.H.F., Jensen, B.F., Brockhoff, P.B., Padkjar, S.B., Guldbrandt, M. and Christensen, M.S. (2005) In silico prediction of membrane permeability from calculated molecular parameters. *Journal of Medicinal Chemistry*, **48**, 805–811.

100 Zhang, L., Balimane, P.V., Johnson, S.R. and Chong, S. (2007) Development of an in silico model for predicting efflux substrates in Caco-2 cells. *International Journal of Pharmaceutics*, **343**, 98–105.

101 Chang, C., Ekins, S., Bahadduri, P. and Swaan, P.W. (2006) Pharmacophore-based discovery of ligands for drug transporters. *Advanced Drug Delivery Reviews*, **58**, 1431–1450.

102 van, Z.J.J., Wortelboer, H.M., Bijlsma, S., Punt, A., Usta, M., Bladeren, P.J.v., Rietjens, I.M.C.M. and Cnubben, N.H.P. (2005) Quantitative structure activity relationship studies on the flavonoid mediated inhibition of multidrug resistance proteins 1 and 2. *Biochemical Pharmacology*, **69**, 699–708.

103 Zhang, S., Yang, X., Coburn, R.A. and Morris, M.E. (2005) Structure activity relationships and quantitative structure activity relationships for the flavonoid-mediated inhibition of breast cancer resistance protein. *Biochemical Pharmacology*, **70**, 627–639.

104 Kamphorst, J., Cucurull-Sanchez, L. and Jones, B. (2007) A performance evaluation of multiple classification models of human PEPT1 inhibitors and non-inhibitors. *QSAR & Combinatorial Science*, **26**, 220–226.

105 Biegel, A., Gebauer, S., Hartrodt, B., Brandsch, M., Neubert, K. and Thondorf, I. (2005) Three-dimensional quantitative structure-activity relationship analyses of beta-lactam antibiotics and tripeptides as substrates of the mammalian H+/peptide cotransporter PEPT1. *Journal of Medicinal Chemistry*, **48**, 4410–4419.

106 Biegel, A., Gebauer, S., Brandsch, M., Neubert, K. and Thondorf, I. (2006) Structural requirements for the substrates of the H+/peptide cotransporter PEPT2 determined by three-dimensional quantitative structure-activity relationship analysis. *Journal of Medicinal Chemistry*, **49**, 4286–4296.

107 Adson, A., Ruab, T.J., Burton, P.S., Barsuhn, C.L., Hilgers, A.R., Audus, K.L. and Ho, N.F.H. (1994) Quantitative approaches to delineate paracellular diffusion in cultured epithelial cell monolayers. *Journal of Pharmaceutical Sciences*, **83**, 1529–1530.

108 Fujikawa, M., Ano, R., Nakao, K., Shimizu, R. and Akamatsu, M. (2005) Relationships between structure and high-throughput screening permeability of diverse drugs with artificial membranes: application to prediction of Caco-2 cell permeability. *Bioorganic and Medicinal Chemistry*, **13**, 4721–4732.

109 Verma, R.P., Hansch, C. and Selassie, C.D. (2007) Comparative QSAR studies on PAMPA/modified PAMPA for high throughput profiling of drug absorption potential with respect to Caco-2 cells and human intestinal absorption. *Journal of Computer-Aided Molecular Design*, **21**, 3–22.

110 Kalyanaraman, C. and Jacobson, M.P. (2007) An atomistic model of passive membrane permeability: application to a series of FDA approved drugs. *Journal of Computer-Aided Molecular Design*, **21**, 675–679.

111 Zhang, X., Shedden, K. and Rosania, G.R. (2006) A cell-based molecular transport simulator for pharmacokinetic prediction and cheminformatic exploration. *Molecular Pharmaceutics*, **3**, 704–716.

112 Sugano, K., Obata, K., Saitoh, R., Higashida, A. and Hamada, H. (2006) *Processing of Biopharmaceutical Profiling Data in Drug Discovery*, Wiley-VCH, Zurich, pp. 441–458.

7
Drug Metabolism and Reactive Metabolites
Alan P. Watt

7.1
Introduction to Drug Metabolism

Drug metabolism is central to the understanding of drug therapy and toxicity. On administration of a drug, this has to distribute throughout the body to get to the desired site of action. The pharmacokinetics of the molecule, a mathematical description of how extensively a drug is distributed and how effectively it is cleared, determines the dose amount and the dose frequency. Additionally, dosing has to be appropriately chosen to achieve concentrations within the therapeutic window, that is, the concentration range between biological effect and toxicity. Central to this is the concept of clearance, that is, how the drug is removed from an organism. There are three basic pathways: (i) removal of drug unchanged either in the urine or feces; (ii) biotransformation of the drug by the organism followed by either excretion of conjugation; (iii) conjugation with an amino acid or sugar to create a more water-soluble entity that is subsequently excreted. Consequently, an understanding of the metabolic fate of a compound is critical in understanding its clearance mechanism and the nature of the products that are formed as to whether they possess the desired activity, an alternate pharmacology or perhaps toxicity.

7.1.1
Historical Perspective

The earliest records detailing what could, in modern times, be termed drug metabolism studies were performed in the early to mid-nineteenth century. The conversion of benzoic acid to hippuric acid in dogs was first speculated on but not conclusively proved by Woehler in 1824, then in 1841 Ure ingested benzoic acid and observed hippuric acid in his urine, the first human drug metabolism study [1, 2] (Figure 7.1).

Although the formation of hippuric acid is a conjugation reaction, many metabolic conversions require the ability of living organisms to oxidize compounds; and in

Hit and Lead Profiling. Edited by Bernard Faller and Laszlo Urban
Copyright © 2009 WILEY-VCH Verlag GmbH & Co. KGaA, Weinheim
ISBN: 978-3-527-32331-9

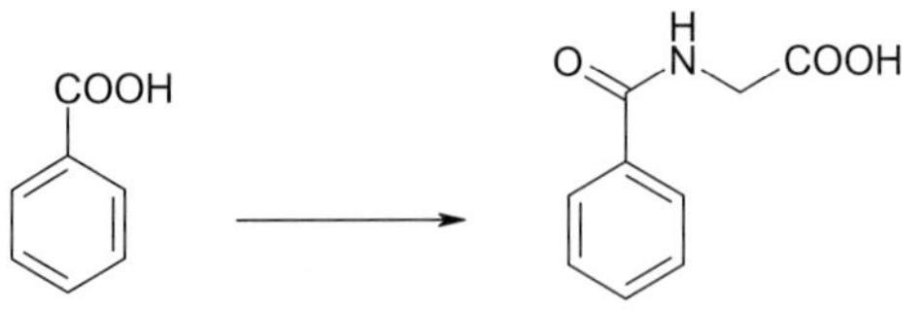

Figure 7.1 Conversion in humans of benzoic acid into hippuric acid, the glycinyl conjugate of benzoic acid.

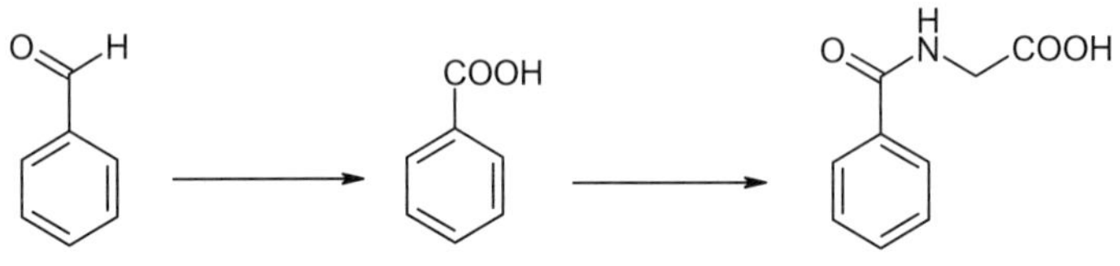

Figure 7.2 The formation of hippuric acid from benzaldehyde in humans, demonstrating oxidative metabolic capabilities.

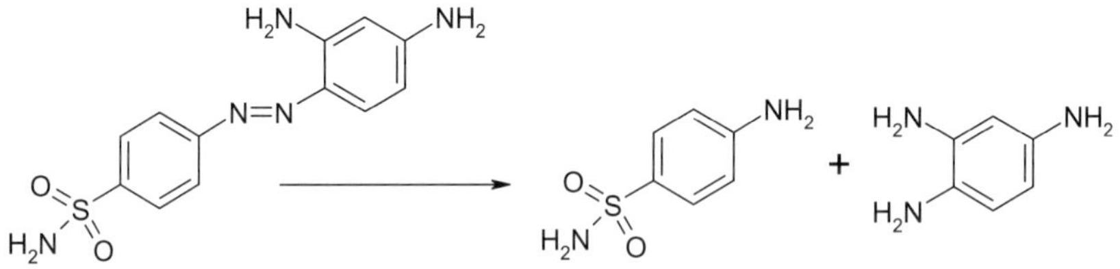

Figure 7.3 Metabolic cleavage of the antibiotic agent prontosil to form the bioactive sulfonamide.

1848 Woehler and Frerichs demonstrated this through the dosing of benzaldehyde to volunteers, which still yielded hippuric acid [2] (Figure 7.2).

By the late nineteenth century, it was clear that organisms possessed a capacity to elicit many chemical reactions on foreign compounds that were not accessible at the time to chemists. In the early twentieth century, the success of the antibacterial agent Prontosil [3] was followed by perhaps an even greater interest when it was demonstrated that the activity was in fact due to metabolic conversion of the diazo linkage to form the sulfonamide (Figure 7.3) [4]. This opened the way for new antibacterial sulfonamide drugs and gave the field of drug metabolism a new importance and credibility.

7.1.2
In Vitro Metabolism

From purely physiological consideration it was clear that the liver, situated between the gastrointestinal tract and the systemic circulation, was likely to play a critical role in drug metabolism. The introduction of non-destructive homogenization techniques and differential centrifugation of subcellular organelles allowed the use of liver homogenates to study the metabolism of the rat carcinogen dimethylaminoazobenzene (DAB; Figure 7.4). The metabolism was shown to be dependant on oxygen and

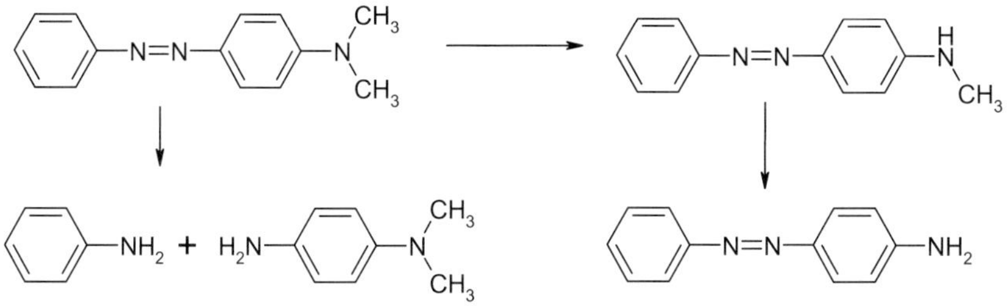

Figure 7.4 Metabolic pathways of 4-dimethylaminoazobenzene (DAB) determined in rat liver microsomes.

the reductant nicotinamide–adenine dinucleotide phosphate (NADPH) [5] and furthermore was shown to be the mechanism responsible for the bioconversion of a wide range of drugs and other chemicals.

The ability to conduct *in vitro* metabolism studies led to investigations on the fate and toxicity of known drugs at the time, as the reason for such toxicities was completely unknown. For example, the analgesic commonly used since the 1880s was acetanilide which, although effective, caused methemoglobinaemia (a breakdown of hemoglobin, causing cyanosis) in a subset of patients [6]. It was demonstrated that acetanilide was metabolized to aniline and that this molecule was responsible for the toxicity [7]. However, it had been known since the nineteenth century that para-hydroxylation led to a metabolite which possessed similar analgesic properties. Since this molecule was without the toxicity of acetanilide, this led to the subsequent re-introduction in the 1950s of the metabolite acetaminophen (paracetamol) as a safe alternative to acetanilide (Figure 7.5). Consequently, not only can an understanding of metabolism lead to an elucidation of toxic process but it may also offer alternative molecules for biological evaluation.

A seminal work in the drug metabolism field by Richard Tecwyn Williams defined xenobiotic metabolism as we know it today, relating metabolic processes to an organic chemistry classification [8, 9]. Importantly, Williams was the first to recognize the two distinct processes of drug metabolism: a first phase consisting of oxidations, reductions and hydrolyses; and a second phase consisting of conjugation reactions. These Phase I and Phase II metabolic process classifications are now used routinely. Furthermore, it became apparent that, far from consistently detoxifying compounds,

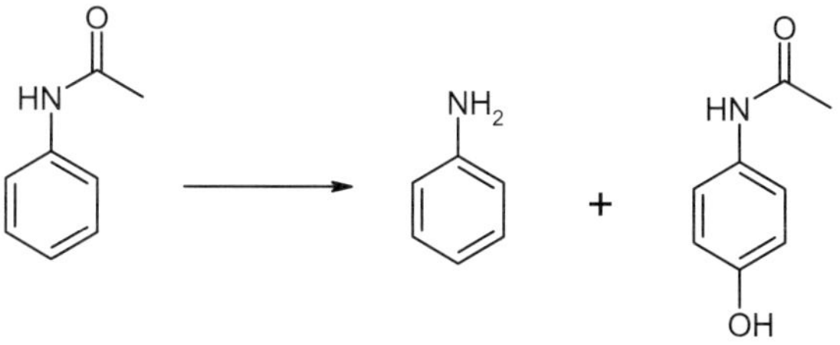

Figure 7.5 Metabolism of (a) acetanilide into the toxic species (b) aniline and the safer analgesic (c) acetaminophen (paracetamol).

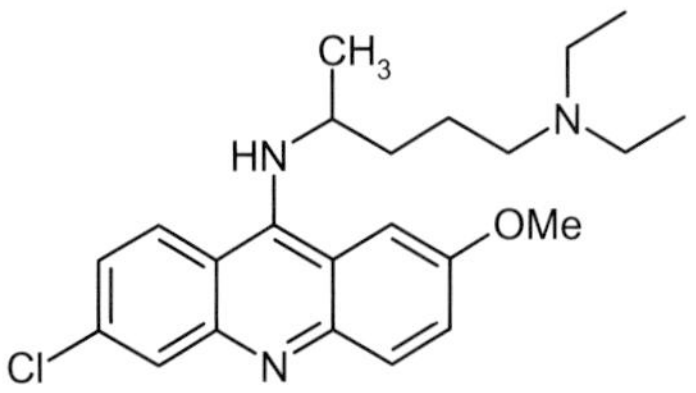

Figure 7.6 Structure of atabrine (quinacrine).

there were many instances where metabolism contributed to an increased toxicity. Williams concluded that Phase I reactions were not true detoxification mechanisms and were often intermediates to allow Phase II reactions, while generally Phase II processes were detoxifying, although exceptions to both these instances existed. Such a general statement holds true today, underlining the importance of this work in defining the metabolism of xenobiotics.

The development of understanding of xenobiotic metabolism is intrinsically linked with improvements in analytical technology. The first clear demonstration of this was the application of state of the art analytical technologies for the separation of atabrine from its metabolites (Figure 7.6) [10]. This allowed for the first time accurate quantification and analysis of the distribution of the parent compound which in turn permitted design of a dosing regime to provide a much needed antimalarial therapy. This has clearly found parallels with each improvement in analytical technology rapidly being applied to further the understanding of drug metabolism; and this has never been more true than for the recent application of modern mass spectrometric techniques [11, 12].

7.1.3
Cytochrome P450

Until the 1950s it was understood that "oxygenases" within liver microsomes, requiring molecular oxygen and NADPH for activity, were responsible for the oxidative metabolism of molecules but the precise nature of the oxygenases was unknown [13]. Since they required both an oxidant and reductant, however, they were trivially referred to as "mixed-function oxidases". The biochemical basis for this stemmed from the discovery of a pigment in liver microsomes that, on binding CO, gave an absorbance spectrum with a λ_{max} at 450 nm [14]. This was characterized as a heme-containing cytochrome enzyme [15]. Subsequent work showed that the cytochrome P-450 enzyme was indeed the component responsible for the delivery of oxygen in the conversions of endogenous steroids as well as drug molecules [16]. From these humble beginnings the field of cytochrome P-450 research has increased markedly as the critical nature of this enzyme superfamily has grown. Although the subcellular location of these enzymes, to the smooth endoplasmic reticula of hepatocytes, was determined and their central importance in the biotransformation of drug molecules recognized, it was not clear until the 1990s that distinct families and subfamilies of these enzymes existed and these were classified on the basis of their sequence homologies [17]. Molecular cloning techniques as well as chemical

Table 7.1 Some advantages and disadvantages of typical *in vitro* metabolism systems.

System	Advantages	Disadvantages
Microsomes	Can be frozen and used on demand	Limited enzyme complement
	Contains major drug metabolizing enzymes	Closed system so may not be representative of *in vivo* situation
	Straighforward to use	
S9 fraction	Can be frozen and used on demand	Closed system so may not be representative of *in vivo* situation
	Contains both cytosolic and membrane-bound enzyme	
	Straighforward to use	
Hepatocytes	Culture methods available	Require fresh tissue
	Full enzyme complement – contain enzymes and enzyme cofactors not present in subcellular fractions	No cell–cell contact
	Full enzyme complement – contain enzymes and enzyme cofactors not present in subcellular fractions	Need collagenase digestion
	Can be used quantitatively	Handling difficult
	Useful for prediction of Phase I and II metabolism	Closed system so may not be representative of *in vivo* situation
Liver slices	Easy to prepare	Require fresh tissue
	Cell–cell contact	Necrosis of slice centre
	No use of proteolytic enzymes	Long-term culture difficult
	All cell types present	Quantitative studies variable
	Phase I and II metabolic processes accessible	

inhibitors and inhibitory monoclonal antibodies have allowed much greater understanding of the contribution of these individual isozymes to the metabolism of drug molecules [18].

7.1.4
Prediction of Drug Metabolism

Whilst the only true measure of the disposition of metabolites in humans is to measure excreted and circulating drug-related material, many systems exist enable the prediction of metabolic pathways *in vitro*, *in vivo* or *in silico*. The advantages and disadvantages of some typical *in vitro* metabolism systems are shown in Table 7.1.

7.2
Adverse Drug Reactions

A major problem in the development of pharmacotherapy is the interperson response to drug treatment. This can lead to either failure of treatment or an adverse response in populations or subpopulations of patients. Serious adverse drug reactions (ADRs) are estimated as high as 6.7%, of which 4.7% resulted in hospitalization [19]. This was confirmed by similar studies in the United Kingdom and Sweden that found that ADRs contributed to 7% and 13% of all hospital admissions, respectively [20, 21]. As well as being a significant cause of morbidity and mortality, ADRs are also one of the most common causes of marketed drug withdrawals. However, most clinically relevant ADRs occur at relatively low levels of incidence with a rate of ~1 in 3000, hence many ADRs are not discovered until postmarketing.

7.2.1
ADR Classification

ADRs can be categorized as either predictable or idiosyncratic. Predictable reactions are common and often related to the primary or secondary pharmacology of a molecule. The relationship with dose is usually good and whilst morbidity is high, mortality is low. These effects may be observed as early as Phase I and are usually reproducible in preclinical species. By contrast, idiosyncratic drug reactions (IDRs) cannot be simply explained on the basis of the pharmacology of the drug, the relationship with dose is poor or non-existent and both morbidity and mortality is high [22]. IDRs are rarer, accounting for only approximately 6–10% of all ADRs [23] and consequently due to their low frequency are only usually detected post-launch. Furthermore it is not possible to model these responses in animals.

7.2.2
Idiosyncratic Drug Reactions

Idiosyncratic drug reactions (IDRs) are most commonly characterized by a reaction involving fever or rash, with or without internal organ involvement. The spectrum of responses ranges from a minor rash, to potentially fatal toxic epidermal necrosis and Stevens–Johnson syndrome. Immunoglobulin E (IgE)-mediated anaphylactic shock, occasional joint pain, hepatotoxicity or nephrotoxicity are also well documented [24]. The frequency of such reactions are unknown but estimated to be between 1 : 1000 and 1 : 10 000 exposures and may be enhanced on re-challenging susceptible individuals with the same drug.

Most idiosyncratic drug reactions cannot, with any certainty, be assigned a mechanism. Indeed, predisposition to reactions of an idiosyncratic nature are not generally ascribable to a single factor but are most likely multifactorial involving both gene defects and environmental risks such as concomitant disease or infection. However, there is substantial circumstantial evidence suggests that drugs associated with the highest incidence of idiosyncratic reactions also tend to form reactive (electrophilic) metabolites which in turn leads to the hypothesis that these reactive species are some way responsible for the observed toxicity.

7.3
Bioactivation

7.3.1
Definition

Drug molecules are cleared from an organism either by elimination of the drug unchanged in urine or feces through biotransformation to usually more polar or water-soluble species that may be eliminated or conjugated, or conjugation with a sugar or amino acid moiety followed by elimination. Whilst it is generally accepted that these processes are detoxifying, occasionally metabolites are formed that are more reactive than the parent compound and electrophilic in nature [25].

7.3.2
Reactions of Electrophilic Metabolites

Since biological systems are rich in nucleophiles (DNA, proteins, etc.) the possibility that electrophilic metabolites may become irreversibly bound to cellular macromolecules exists. Electrophiles and nucleophiles are classified as "hard" or "soft" depending on the electron density, with hard electrophiles generally having more intense charge localization than soft electrophiles in which the charge is more diffuse. Hard electrophiles tend to react preferentially with hard nucleophiles and soft electrophiles with soft nucleophiles.

7.3.3
Glutathione

The intracellular nucleophile glutathione (GSH; γ-Glu-Cys-Gly) acts as a protective mechanism against electrophilic insults and may be present at concentrations of up to 10 mM [26]. The reaction of glutathione with a non-polar compound bearing an electrophilic carbon, nitrogen or sulfur atom may be mediated enzymatically by glutathione-S-transferase (GST), with typical substrates being species such as arene oxides, quinones and α,β-unsaturated carbonyl compounds.

7.3.4
Detection of GSH Conjugates

The detection of glutathione conjugates provides one mechanism for the deduction of the formation of reactive metabolites, since in order for glutathione to react, either the parent compound is electrophilic or it is metabolized to produce an electrophile or the metabolism proceeds through an electrophilic intermediate [27]. Furthermore, glutathione conjugates may be further metabolized by selective peptidases to produce a cysteinyl conjugate which is then acetylated to produce and N-acetyl cysteine conjugate, commonly referred to as a mercapturic acid. Glutathione conjugates tend to be biliary excreted whilst mercapturic acids are excreted renally, hence analysis of these biofluids gives an appropriate starting point for detection of the formation of reactive metabolites *in vivo*. Using an *in vitro* system of hepatocytes in culture or suspension, one may also generate glutathione conjugates since all of the cellular mechanisms are present in these cells. Consequently, the fact that reactive intermediates are formed for a number of drug classes is incontrovertible, as evidenced by the detection of glutathione or mercapturic acid conjugates.

7.3.5
Acyl Glucuronides

Many carboxylic acid containing drugs are cleared through the formation of acyl glucuronide (AG) conjugates and it is widely believed this may pose a toxicological risk through reaction of these conjugates with proteins. Two mechanisms for this are proposed: (i) transacylation in which a protein nucleophile displaces the glucuronic acid moiety through reaction at the carbonyl carbon of the AG; (ii) glycation which proceeds following 2, 3 or 4 migration of the sugar moiety via an Amadori rearrangement to react with protein amines to form stable 1-amino 2-keto adducts [28]. However, these pathways remain theoretical risks and many successful carboxylic acid drugs that are cleared through this pathway do not lead to reactive species hence it would be unwise to advocate a risk simply due to the presence of acyl glucuronides. More recently, publications on diclofenac, zomepirac and tolmetin which all postulated to elicit their toxicity through the reactivity of their acyl-glucuronide metabolites were shown to form reactive species via an oxidative metabolism pathway [29]. Consequently oxidative reactive metabolites as well as reactive acyl glucuronides may be contributors to the anaphylaxis seen with these NSAIDs.

7.3.6
Free Radicals and Oxidative Stress

Free radicals are formed in many biological process, with the key reactive species being superoxide radical, hydrogen peroxide and nitric oxide. Many drugs, particularly those that undergo redox cycling, have been shown to divert cellular electron flow to produce superoxide directly which is controlled through the action of the enzyme superoxide dismutase to produce hydrogen peroxide. This is further metabolized by catalase and glutathione peroxidase. The excessive production or insufficient disposal of reactive oxygen species constitutes oxidative stress. Certain functional groups such as hydroperoxide, oxime, hydrazine, hydrazide and hydroxylamine may be metabolized via one-electron oxidations or reductions to form free radicals which may react with DNA.

As well as the formation of radicals, oxidative stress may also contribute to the toxicity of electrophilic metabolites. This may result from depletion by electrophiles of the glutathione pool, one of the major defenses against damage by reactive oxygen species.

7.4
Reactive Metabolites and Idiosyncratic Toxicity

7.4.1
The Hapten Hypothesis

One proposal to explain the proposed link between idiosyncratic reactions and reactive metabolites is the hapten hypothesis. This suggests that the small molecules such as drugs can be immunogenic (i.e., capable of eliciting an immune response) through a reactive metabolite covalently binding to a protein to form a hapten which is then seen as foreign by the immune system [30]. The types of hypersensitivities that are best understood by this mechanism are those responses mediated by IgE antibodies directed against a drug-hapten conjugated to protein, such as those observed for penicillin. However, the genetic predispositions underlying this rare anaphylactic response are unknown and even the penicillins do not precisely fulfill the criteria of forming a reactive intermediate as the species formed is not metabolically generated but formed due to the reactivity of the beta-lactam ring.

Whilst this may explain potentially explain many cases, this does not represent the full mechanism which is undoubtedly more complex as not all reactions appear to be immunological. For example, paracetamol is known to form reactive intermediates but yet is not involved in idiosyncratic reactions. Indeed, with some notable exceptions such as the penicillins, many drugs involved in idiosyncratic reactions do not mediate their toxicity through a immune response.

7.4.1.1 Immune-Mediated Cutaneous Reactions

Cutaneous reactions such as rash or Stevens–Johnson syndrome are also consist with initiation through protein haptenation, although in this case dendritic cell activation/migration and T-cell propagation are involved [31]. Other immune mediators such as cytokines, nitric oxide and reactive oxygen species which may be linked to the formation of reactive metabolites may also be implicated, as may specific processes occurring at the level of the keratinocyte.

Where drug are shown to form reactive intermediates by specific enzyme systems, it might be expected that the polymorphism or absence of these systems would track idiosyncratic reactions but to date no such link has been established. In fact, the most confounding element of idiosyncratic reactions is their unpredictable nature and whilst reactive intermediates may present a risk factor the true nature of the response is likely to be multifactorial. Changes in drug metabolizing capacity, affecting the balance of bioactivation and bioinactivation processes which may be mediated through concomitant infection may also be a contributory factor.

7.4.2
The Danger Hypothesis

An alternative theory to the hapten hypothesis that goes some way to explain why not all drugs that form reactive intermediates are associated with idiosyncratic reactions is the so-called danger hypothesis [32]. The major difference from the hapten hypothesis assumes that not all foreign antigens are necessarily problematic and that immune response are only triggered by the presence of a "danger" signal, produced when a cell either becomes stressed or dies chaotically in a non-apoptotic controlled manner. Drugs that form reactive intermediates but do not initiate such danger signals would not then be associated with idiosyncratic reactions, but other drugs, particularly those that elicit cellular toxicities in subsets of patients, may also give rise to idiosyncratic reactions due to the presence of danger signals. Other procedures such as surgery can elicit danger signals due to cell damage and is also associated with idiosyncratic reactions.

7.4.3
Alternate Perspectives to Covalent Binding (CB)

It is tempting, given the above, to conclude that any degree of covalent binding of drug species to macromolecules will lead to a toxic response. However, this is clearly not the case as there are plenty of examples where covalent binding has had no toxicological consequence.

7.4.3.1   Non-Toxicological Covalent Binding

An oft-quoted example is that of paracetamol, a compound known to undergo extensive bioactivation to a quinoneimine which is trapped by glutathione. In systems to measure covalent binding especially in the absence of glutathione, paracetamol can be shown to bind extensively to proteins and it is this binding that is believed to mediate its toxicity *in vivo* following overdose and the depletion of the glutathione pool. However, the 3-hydroxy analog of paracetamol also binds to the same extent as paracetamol under the same conditions, yet there are no toxicological consequences associated with this molecule [33]. One can speculate that this is because different proteins are adducted leading to different biological responses, but the reality is that insufficient data is currently available to definitively make this link.

7.4.3.2   Covalent Binding as Detoxification

Whilst it is clear that reactive metabolites and covalent binding of these metabolites to macromolecules are associatively linked with idiosyncratic reactions, unfortunately it is impossible to make the link that covalent binding necessarily leads to idiosyncratic toxicity. Indeed, there are suggestions that some degree of covalent binding may be a detoxification mechanism since, if adducts are not immunogenic, these will be degraded and removed from the organism. Since reactive species including dietary and environmental insults are adequately dealt with through protective mechanisms including the binding of these species to macromolecules, one cannot therefore postulate that all covalent binding is detrimental. However, it is precisely because with the current state of knowledge that it is impossible to delineate "good" from "bad" covalent binding that attempts were made to minimize the exposure of these species as part of a drug development program.

7.5
Measurement of Reactive Metabolites

In discussing the measurement of reactive metabolites, it is important to distinguish between those assays for which qualitative or structural information may be obtained and for assays in which a more quantitative assessment of reactive species may be made. In making decisions about the management of risk in progressing drug candidates, one would clearly wish to have a quantitative evaluation; however it must be recognized that the knowledge around the toxicological predictability of these assays currently is low and that any assessment is unlikely to be able to provide a clear-cut decision based on this data alone.

7.5.1
Trapping Assays

One of the most effective methods of determining whether a reactive metabolite has been formed is to use an *in vitro* system capable of forming metabolites (e.g., liver microsomes with an NADPH cofactor) and fortify this with nucleophilic-trapping agents that will react with an electrophilic species. As stated above, it is important that the nature of the trapping agent be considered since both soft and hard electrophiles may be formed, therefore it is important that appropriate trapping agents are also included. Detection is typically performed by mass spectrometry.

7.5.1.1 Soft Nucleophiles
Given the ubiquity of glutathione as an *in vivo* trapping agent, most attention has been focused on the use of this molecule in *in vitro* systems, particularly as GST enzyme systems are available to facilitate the reactions. This is a straightforward experiment to accomplish and is potentially scalable should larger quantities of conjugates be required. However, although it is the natural nucleophile, it may not always be the best and other soft nucleophiles such as cysteine, *N*-acetyl cysteine and β-mercaptoethanol can all be considered.

7.5.1.2 Hard Nucleophiles
The classic hard nucleophile used in trapping hard metabolite electrophiles is cyanide. Indeed, with modern detection sensitivities it is now often possible to detect cyanide adducts from microsomal incubations that were quenched with acetonitrile, with the residual cyanide in the acetonitrile reacting with the electrophilic species. In an experiment designed specifically to generate and detect cyanide adducts, millimolar concentrations of cyanide may be included in a microsomal incubation with no detrimental effect on the metabolic turnover.

7.5.2
Mass Spectrometric Detection of GSH Conjugates and Mercapturic Acids

Following incubation of a test compound in a system designed to generate trapped conjugates of reactive metabolites (e.g., supplemented microsomes or hepatocytes) or dosing of a compound to preclinical species to generate urine, feces or bile, mass spectrometric analysis of these samples can be conducted and an assessment of the presence or absence of conjugates made. Glutathione conjugates, mercapturic acids and other conjugates may all be detected in an analogous fashion but for simplicity GSH only will be referred to. By knowing the molecular mass of the parent molecule and estimating the mass of a putative glutathione conjugate (addition of the mass of GSH and various oxidations, i.e., +16 amu, +32 amu, etc.) a mass spectrometer can be set up to detect these species specifically. However, with no prior knowledge of the routes of metabolism of a molecule, this is likely to miss any unusual conjugates since the mass will simply neither be sought nor observed.

An alternate methodology is to use a feature of a tandem mass spectrometer to perform a double scanning technique known as constant neutral loss (CNL) [34]. In this, the two mass analyzers of the spectrometer are scanned across a defined mass range, but with a fixed mass offset between the quadrupoles. Molecules are then mass-filtered in the first quadrupole, fragmented in the collision cell (where they typically lose a portion of the molecule as a neutral fragment) and then mass selected again in the third quadrupole. If the first and third quadrupoles are set to scan at, for example, 100 amu apart, only those compound that lose a fragment of 100 amu in the collision cell would be detected. Fortunately, GSH conjugates fragment readily with a typical loss of 129 amu, hence irrespective of the starting mass of the conjugate all GSH conjugates in a sample can be detected. One drawback with this technique however is that it is relatively insensitive since duty cycle is not very effective on quadrupole instruments. Newer quadrupole-TOF instruments, whilst not having true CNL capabilities can reconstruct these in software and are therefore proving somewhat more effective.

The identity of GSH conjugates may be determined to a limited degree by mass spectrometry using product ion scanning techniques. However, these are often quite uninformative as one or two fragment ions tend to dominate the mass spectrum and localization of the conjugate onto either one portion of the molecule or another is all that can be delineated. For further structural work additional techniques are required.

7.5.3
Radiometric Assays

Using LC-MS or other chromatographic techniques with, for example, UV detection one can never fully quantify unknown species since, without an authentic standard it is impossible to know the precise response for the molecule. Currently, the only sure way of quantifying this is to use radiolabeled drug material then track where this material goes as a result of metabolism. However, these are resource-intensive studies since the radiolabeled drug substance must be prepared which is typically not performed until after candidate selection. Currently the capabilities to conduct these syntheses inhouse are limited and the cost of outsourcing high, hence careful consideration needs to be given to where in the cascade one should place these studies.

7.5.3.1 Covalent Binding to Liver Microsomes

Typically, the extent of covalent binding of microsomal protein may be evaluated by incubating ^{14}C- or ^{3}H-labeled drug substance with liver microsomes in the presence of the cofactor NADPH. Following quenching of the reaction, proteins may be precipitated and pelleted then extensively washed to remove any non-covalently bound material. The resulting protein can then be solubilized with SDS and radioactivity associated with protein measured by scintillation counting [35]. Clearly, only material irreversibly bound to protein will still be present and be detected, hence this provides a convenient way of assessing covalent binding to macromolecules. Data is expressed as picomolar equivalents per milligram of protein and is "equivalent" since the exact nature of the species bound at this point is unknown. Typically both human and rat liver microsomes would be used in order to get an estimate of bioactivation, since there may be substantial species differences. The rat data may be correlated with rat *in vivo* data to help contextualize the human data.

An additional and often informative adjunct to this experiment is to include trapping agents within the incubation, such as GSH. With this, one may often observe an amelioration of the binding since reactive species are preferentially deactivated through reaction with the trapping agent rather than protein and therefore this serves as a measure of the extent to which protective mechanisms may contribute. Furthermore, should ambiguous data be generated in microsomes (e.g., if there is a large disconnect between species), or if the metabolic pathways are known to be predominantly Phase II, then it may be informative to conduct a covalent binding experiment in hepatocytes.

7.5.3.2 *Ex Vivo* Covalent Binding

In order to contextualize the *in vitro* data, an assay may be conducted in which the radiolabeled drug substance is dosed into rats and then plasma and tissue are harvested after a defined period and the extent of irreversible binding of this substance to protein is determined. Dose selection is important in such a study, since one could either choose a fixed dose such that the total amount an animal sees is comparable across different studies, or some normalization to either exposure or to no adverse effect level (NOAEL) can be made if this is known. Maintaining exposure in the region of an anticipated therapeutic exposure however would seem prudent to give some indication of the likely risk. Typically liver tissue and blood plasma are taken at fixed time points out to 24 or 48 h and the samples are processed through an exhaustive extraction procedure before solubilization and scintillation counting. Other tissues may be taken but the two main concerns with this assay are binding to liver proteins and the possible link with hepatotoxicity and binding to blood proteins with the potential for an immune response.

7.5.3.3 ^{14}C Cyanide Trapping

An assay using the hard nucleophile cyanide was described in Section 7.5.1.2, where non-radiolabeled KCN was used to detect the presence of cyanide adducts using mass spectrometry. However, by using $K^{14}CN$, it is possible to make this a quantitative assay by assessing the amount of cyanide incorporated into a non-radiolabeled test compound [36]. The assay is conducted by incubating test compound with microsomes in the presence of NADPH and $K^{14}CN$. Following quenching of the reaction, unreacted cyanide is removed by reversed-phase solid-phase extraction since this is unretained, then the parent compound and any potential adducts are eluted prior to scintillation counting. Such an assay may be semiautomated and conducted using microtitre plate technology such that multiple compounds may be evaluated simultaneously.

7.5.3.4 Radiolabeled Soft Nucleophile Trapping

An analogous assay using a radiolabeled soft nucleophile would also be required to complement the hard nucleophile radiolabeled cyanide trapping assay. Investigations into radiolabeled glutathione have proved unsuccessful since the material is unstable due to cross-reactions induced by beta radiation. Alternate soft nucleophiles such as cysteine, N-acetyl cysteine and β-mercaptoethanol all have promise as radiolabeled substances for quantitative trapping experiments since they are more stable than GSH and equally nucleophilic, although clearly these would not be substrates for GST.

7.5.4
Alternate Approaches

Given the availability of radiolabeled material, quantitative whole body autoradiography may be employed to assess long-lived radioactivity, although this does not indicate what is bound versus what is free [37]. More recently, approaches employing modified glutathione species have been reported which may offer alternate non-radiolabeled alternatives to soft-nucleophile trapping. Using a quaternary ammonium derivative of GSH with detection by mass spectrometry, a semiquantitative measure of adduction can be derived, since the MS response is dominated by the quaternary ammonium species [38]. Alternatively, using a dansyl glutathione derivative, detection on the basis of fluorescence can be achieved [39] but clearly all of the drawbacks associated with fluorescent analysis still persist (quenching, background interference, etc.).

Using an 11-amino-acid peptide (ECGHDRKAHYK) containing cysteine and other nucleophilic amino acid residues, reactive metabolites generated using microsomal or recombinant P 450 enzymes can be trapped. The charged residues of the peptide enhance binding to a weak cation exchange chip surface which are then detected using surface-enhanced laser desorption ionization–time of flight mass spectrometry [40].

Electrochemical oxidation is a means of generating reactive metabolites either in the absence of biological nucleophiles or through the addition of nucleophiles under controlled conditions. Mass spectrometric, NMR and IR evaluations can all be performed as described for amodiaquine [41] but recapitulation of microsomal metabolism under electrochemical conditions is not always possible and hence this technique is probably of limited applicability.

LC-MS/MS has also been used to detect adducts to human serum albumin following pronase E digestion and analysis of the resulting Cys-Pro-Phe tripeptide. Modification of this tripeptide was observed for paracetamol and additionally demonstrated using albumin isolated from blood from patients [42].

7.6
Strategies for Minimizing Reactive Metabolite Risk

Although methodologies for the binding of drugs to macromolecules are available as shown above, it is impossible to determine whether observed bioactivation will translate into an idiosyncratic toxicity. As well as the lack of correlation with absolute covalent binding levels to toxicity, other factors influence the amount of risk associated with this phenomenon that one may wish to carry forward; and this varies from molecule to molecule. For example, if a molecule carries a covalent binding risk but is "first in class" in an unprecedented field, it may be worth taking this molecule into a clinical setting to establish whether a dose–efficacy relationship is observed. Conversely, in a backup program in which the lead molecule carries the same risk, it would be prudent to reduce any danger associated with covalent binding as much as possible. An experimental cascade for dealing with a covalent binding liability will therefore depend on a company's attitude to risk for a specific molecule as described above. Nevertheless, some generic points may still be considered.

7.6.1
Dose and Exposure

If there is high confidence that the dose will be low either because of the dose route (e.g., inhaled) or because the target is precedented and similar molecules are known to work at a low dose or exposure, then this is sufficient to proceed at risk to candidate selection since the incidence of idiosyncratic toxicity decreases considerably with dose and few if any examples are present for compounds dosed at 10 mg or less in human. If however a high dose is predicted or there is considerable uncertainty in the prediction then some evaluation of CB risk should be made.

7.6.2
Structural Alerts

If the molecule contains a structural alert then an *in vitro* trapping assay should be used to assess whether hard or soft nucleophiles are able to trap any species formed. If this can be a quantitative or semiquantitative assay then decision making will be clearer. If there are no structural alerts then a standard paradigm of evaluating time-dependent inhibition before nucleophile trapping can be used. A negative result in these assays would suggest minimal risk in proceeding, but should there be a strong positive then it is suggested that it would be helpful to synthesize radiolabeled drug and perform additional studies prior to compound progression.

7.6.3
Cascade for Radiolabeled Covalent Binding Experiments

With radiolabeled drug material, one would first conduct an *in vitro* covalent binding experiment in rat and human liver microsomes. A negative in this (values to be defined) could allow progression, but if the *in vitro* CB results are positive, a rat *in vivo* experiment would be conducted and a positive in this assay would invariably result in the termination of the molecule. However, there is one caveat on progressing a compound that is negative in the *in vitro* CB, which is where the human *in vitro* data is more positive than the rat. In this instance, the rat *in vivo* model may not be representative of the human situation and hence a negative may not completely discharge the risk, so an useful adjunct may be to conduct a human hepatocyte CB study to demonstrate that a protective mechanism is operational for a human system.

7.6.4
Criteria for Progression

Clearly, the success or failure of a compound or program may hinge on how covalent binding criteria are defined. There are plenty of examples where what is considered an acceptable value for progression of a compound for one drug target may prove unacceptable for another, hence any values proffered can only be viewed within the context of guidelines. For example, one might wish to take more risk for oncology than for a non-life-threatening condition or be more concerned over a paediatric indication than an adult one. Merck used a guidance of 50 pmol/mg protein as being approximately 10-fold above background and 5% of the level observed with known hepatotoxins [43] although other companies have worked with somewhat less-exacting criteria. In reality organizations generally tend to place more weight on *in vivo* rather than *in vitro* data and regard the *in vitro* data as a continuum of risk rather than a cut-off value.

7.7
Conclusions

From a purely pragmatic perspective, it is clear that reactive metabolites are linked with toxicity and that a circumstantial link can be made to idiosyncratic toxicities. Consequently, even though the mechanism of this toxicity is not fully understood, since assays are available to measure the potential for bioactivation in an ideal world one would not carry this liability forward. Conversely, it is not an ideal world, all drug molecules have challenges and the definition of therapeutic index (i.e., the ratio between the toxic exposure and the therapeutic exposure) is critical. Covalent binding of reactive metabolites to macromolecules is a crude measure and not a full predictor of toxicity, and it is well known that toxicity can be ameliorated by a lower dose. Furthermore, the so-called "definitive" assays require radiolabeled drug material which is expensive and generally slow to produce.

With the current state of knowledge, it is recommended that at least a surrogate (i.e., non-radioactive) measure of bioactivation be provided early in drug discovery, such that minimization of the potential of a molecules to form reactive metabolites can be factored into the drug design process. It would be unwise to eliminate molecules solely on a covalent binding experiment since other factors such as the indication, the target population and whether the drug is for chronic or acute therapy are important. Finally, all things being equal, risk can be obviated by driving for the lowest efficacious exposure.

References

1 Ure, A. (1841) *Pharmaceutical Journal Transactactions*, **1**, 24.
2 Woehler, F. and Frerichs, F.T. (1848) *Ann. Chem. Pharm.*, **63**, 335; in Conti, A., and Bickel, M.H., (1977) History of drug metabolism: discoveries of the major pathways in the 19th century. *Drug Metabolism Reviews*, **6** (1), 1–50.
3 Domagk, G. (1935) Chemotherapy of bacterial infections. *Deutsche Medizinische Wochenschrift*, **61**, 250–253.
4 Trefouel, J., Nitti, F. and Bovet, D. (1935) Action of p-aminophenylsulfamide in experimental streptococcus infections of mice and rabbits. *Comptes Rendus des Seances de la Societe de Biologie.*, **120**, 756–758.
5 Mueller, G.C. and Miller, J.A. (1949) Reductive cleavage of 4-dimethyl-aminoazobenzene by rat liver tissue. Intracellular distribution of the enzyme system and its requirement for triphosphopyridine nucleotide. *Journal of Biological Chemistry*, **180**, 1125–1136.
6 Smith, P.K. (1940) Change in blood pigments associated with the prolonged administration of large doses of acetanilide and related compounds. *Journal of Pharmacology and Experimental Therapeutics*, **70**, 171–178.
7 Brodie, B.B. and Axelrod, J. (1948) The fate of acetanilide in man. *Journal of Pharmacology and Experimental Therapeutics*, **94**, 29–38.
8 Williams, R.T. (1947) *Detoxication mechanisms: the metabolism and detoxication of drugs, toxic substances and other organic compounds*, Chapman & Hall, London.
9 Williams, R.T. (1959) *Detoxication mechanisms: the metabolism and detoxication of drugs, toxic substances and other organic compounds*, 2nd edn, Chapman & Hall, London.
10 Shannon, J.A., Earle, D.P., Brodie, B.B., Taggart, J. and Berliner, R.W. (1944) The application of analytical technologies for the separation of atabrine from its metabolites. *Journal of Pharmacology and Experimental Therapeutics*, **81**, 307–330.
11 Gilbert, J.D., Hand, E.L., Yuan, A.S., Olah, T.V. and Covey, T.R. (1992) Determination of L-365,260, a new cholecystokinin receptor (CCK-B) antagonist, in plasma by liquid chromatography/atmospheric pressure chemical ionisation mass sectrometry. *Biological Mass Spectrometry*, **21** (2), 63–68.
12 Ma, S., Chowdhury, S.K. and Alton, K.B. (2006) Application of Mass Spectrometry for Metabolite Identification. *Current Drug Metabolism*, **7**, 503–523.
13 Mason, H.S. (1957) Mechanisms of oxygen metabolism. *Advances in Enzymology.*, **19**, 79–233.
14 Garfinkel, D. (1958) Studies on pig liver microsomes. I. Enzymatic and pigment composition of different microsomal fractions. *Archives of Biochemistry*, **77** (2), 493–509.
15 Omura, T. and Sato, R. (1964) The carbon monoxide binding pigment of liver

microsomes. I. Evidence for its hemoprotein nature. *Journal of Biological Chemistry*, **239**, 2370–2378.

16 Estabrook, R.W., Cooper, D.Y. and Rosenthal, O. (1963) The light reversible carbon monoxide inhibition of the stroid C21-hydrolase system of the adrenal cortex. *Biochemische Zeitschrift*, **338**, 741–755.

17 Nebert, D.W. and Nelson, D.R. (1991) P450 gene nomenclature based on evolution. *Methods in Enzymology*, **206**, 3–11.

18 Donato, M.T. and Castell, J.V. (2003) Strategies and molecular probes to investigate the role of cytochrome P450 in drug metabolism: Focus on in vitro studies. *Clinical Pharmacokinetics*, **42**, 153–178.

19 Lazarou, J., Pomeranz, B.H. and Corey, P.N. (1998) Incidence of adverse drug reactions in hospitalized patients: a meta-analysis of prospective studies. *JAMA*, **279** (15), 1200–1205.

20 Wiffen, P., Gill, M., Edwards, J. and Moore, A. (2002) Adverse drug reactions in hospital patients. A systematic review of the prospective and retrospective studies. *Bandolier Extra*, 1–16.

21 Mjörndal, T., Danell Boman, M., Hägg, S., Bäckström, M., Wiholm, B.-E., Wahlin, A. and Dahlqvist, R. (2002) Adverse drug reactions as a cause for admission to a department of internal medicine. *Pharmacoepidemiology and Drug Safety*, **11**, 65–72.

22 Collins, J.M. (2002) Idiosyncratic drug toxicity. *Chemico-Biological Interactions*, **142**, 3–6.

23 Ju, C. and Uetrecht, J.P. (2002) Mechanism of idiosyncratic drug reactions: reactive metabolites formation, protein binding and the regulation of the immune system. *Current Drug Metabolism*, **3**, 367–377.

24 Zaccara, G., Franciotta, D. and Perucca, E. (2007) Idiosyncratic adverse reactions to antiepileptic drugs. *Epilepsia*, **48** (7), 1223–1244.

25 Williams, D.P. and Park, B.K. (2003) Idiosyncratic toxicity: the role of toxicophores and bioactivation. *Drug Discovery Today*, **22**, 1044–1050.

26 Lu, S.C. (1999) Regulation of hepatic glutathione synthesis: current concepts and controversies. *FASEB Journal*, **13**, 1169–1183.

27 Ketterer, B., Coles, B. and Meyer, D.J. (1983) The role of glutathione in detoxication. *Environmental Health Perspectives*, **49**, 59–69.

28 Ding, A., Ojingwa, J.C., McDonagh, A.F., Burlingame, A.L. and Benet, L.Z. (1993) Evidence for covalent binding of acyl glucuronides to serum albumin via an imine mechanism as revealed by tandem mass spectrometry. *Proceedings of the National Academy of Sciences of the United States of America*, **90** (9), 3797–3801.

29 Chen, Q., Doss, G.A., Tung, E.C., Liu, W., Tang, Y.S., Braun, M.P., Didolkar, V., Strauss, J.R., Wang, R.W., Stearns, R.A., Evans, D.C., Baillie, T.A. and Tang, W. (2006) Evidence for the bioactivation of zomepirac and tolmetin by an oxidative pathway: Identification of glutathione adducts *in vitro* in human liver microsomes and *in vivo* in rats. *Drug Metabolism and Disposition: The Biological Fate of Chemicals*, **34** (1), 145–151.

30 Griem, P., Wulferink, M., Sachs, B., Gonzalez, J.B. and Gleichmann, E. (1998) Allergic and autoimmune reactions to xenobiotics: how do they arise? *Immunology Today*, **19** (3), 133–141.

31 Roychowdhury, S. and Svensson, C.K. (2005) Mechanisms of drug-induced delayed-type hypersensitivity reactions in the skin. *AAPS Journal*, **7** (4), E834–E846.

32 Matzinger, P. (1994) Tolerance, danger, and the extended family. *Annual Review of Immunology*, **12**, 991–1045.

33 Roberts, S.A., Veronica, F.P. and Jollow, D.J. (1990) Acetaminophen structure-toxicity studies: *In vitro* covalent binding of a non-hepatotoxic analog, 3-hydroxy-acetanilide. *Toxicology and Applied Pharmacology*, **105**, 195–208.

34 Baillie, T.A. and Davis, M.R. (1993) Mass spectrometry in the analysis of glutathione conjugates. *Biological Mass Spectrometry*, **22**, 319–325.

35 Day, S.H., Mao, A., White, R., Schulz-Utermoehl, T., Miller, R. and Beconi, M.G. (2005) A semi-automated method for measuring the potential for protein covalent binding in drug discovery. *Journal of Pharmacological and Toxicological Methods*, **52** (2), 278–285.

36 Meneses-Lorente, G., Sakatis, M.Z., Schulz-Utermoehl, T., De Nardi, C. and Watt, A.P. (2006) A quantitative high-throughput trapping assay as a measurement of potential for bioactivation. *Analytical Biochemistry*, **351** (2), 266–272.

37 Takakusa, H., Masumoto, H., Yukinaga, H., Makino, C., Nakayama, S., Okazaki, O. and Sudo, K. (2008) Covalent binding and tissue distribution/retention assessment of drugs associated with idiosyncratic drug toxicity. *Drug Metabolism and Disposition: The Biological Fate of Chemicals*, **36** (9), 1770–1779.

38 Soglia, J.R., Contillo, L.G., Kalgutkar, A.S., Zhao, S., Hop, C.E.C.A., Boyd, J.G. and Cole, M.J. (2006) A semiquantitative method for the determination of reactive metabolite conjugate levels *in vitro* utilizing liquid chromatography-tandem mass spectrometry and novel quaternary ammonium glutathione analogs. *Chemical Research in Toxicology*, **19** (3), 480–490.

39 Gan, J., Harper, T.W., Hsueh, M.-M., Qu, Q. and Humphreys, W.G. (2005) Dansyl glutathione as a trapping agent for the quantitative estimation and identification of reactive metabolites. *Chemical Research in Toxicology*, **18** (5), 896–903.

40 Mitchell, M.D., Elrick, M.M., Walgren, J.L., Mueller, R.A., Morris, D.L., David, C. and Thompson, D.C. (2008) Peptide-based *in vitro* assay for the detection of reactive metabolites. *Chemical Research in Toxicology*, **21** (4), 859–868.

41 Jurva, U., Holmén, A., Grönberg, G., Masimirembwa, C. and Weidolf, L. (2008) Electrochemical generation of electrophilic drug metabolites: characterization of amodiaquine quinoneimine and cysteinyl conjugates by MS, IR, and NMR. *Chemical Research in Toxicology*, **21** (4), 928–935.

42 Damsten, M.C., Commandeur, J.N.M., Fidder, A., Hulst, A.G., Touw, D., Noort, D. and Vermeulen, N.P.E. (2007) Liquid chromatography/tandem mass spectrometry detection of covalent binding of acetaminophen to human serum albumin. *Drug Metabolism and Disposition: The Biological Fate of Chemicals*, **35** (8), 1408–1417.

43 Evans, D.C., Watt, A.P., Nicoll-Griffith, D.A. and Baillie, T.A. (2004) Drug-protein adducts: an industry perspective on minimizing the potential for drug bioactivation in drug discovery and development. *Chemical Research in Toxicology*, **17** (1), 3–16.

8
Drug–Drug Interactions: Screening for Liability and Assessment of Risk

Ruth Hyland, R. Scott Obach, Chad Stoner, Michael West, Michael R. Wester, Kuresh Youdim, and Michael Zientek

8.1
Introduction

Drug–drug interactions (DDI) are a major liability for any new drug entering the marketplace. Adverse drug reactions, of which DDI are a significant component, are a leading cause of hospital admissions [1] and drug withdrawals [2]. The simultaneous co-administration of multiple drugs to patients is commonplace, with patients receiving multiple therapies for one disease (e.g., HIV infection) or treatment for several diseases concurrently. Therefore there is greater potential for DDI in this polypharmacy environment. Five of the 12 drugs withdrawn from the United States market between 1997 and 2002 were prone to metabolic drug–drug interactions [3]. For these reasons, pharmaceutical companies are scrupulous in their desire to understand DDI potential.

A DDI is said to occur when co-administration of one drug alters the effects of another. Interactions may be pharmacodynamic-based, where two drugs act on the same or an interrelated receptor, having an additive, synergistic or antagonistic effect, for example, monoamine oxidase inhibitors combined with selective serotonin reuptake inhibitors resulting in serotonin syndrome [4, 5]. Pharmacokinetic interactions arise from a change in absorption, distribution, metabolism or elimination (ADME). In terms of ADME properties and DDI, metabolism is the most important and represents the major mechanism for pharmacokinetic-based interactions. A new drug may be the victim and/or perpetrator of a DDI. Therefore, screening for drug–drug interaction potential needs to be assessed early in the drug discovery phase, to avoid the development of drug candidates with high potential for DDI. Development of compounds with DDI liability is undesirable, as to ensure patient safety a large number of clinical DDI studies will need to be completed in order to convince the regulatory authorities that the new chemical entity (NCE) is approvable. In addition, a DDI will lead to labeling restrictions and warnings that may be seen as a competitive disadvantage.

Understanding DDI through clinical studies is costly, both in terms of dollars and time. Such studies are inevitable if an enzyme inhibitor or inducer is progressed through drug discovery into full drug development. If however, at an early stage, DDI potential can be designed out, then the need for running such studies is negligible. DDI assessments performed during hit-to-lead profiling will inevitably be less rigorous than those studies performed later in drug development, due to the sheer numbers of compounds to be investigated. The drug discovery process evolved significantly in the past 20 years, and now pharmaceutical companies conduct more studies to understand the role of enzymes and transporters in drug–drug interactions at an earlier stage. Combinatorial chemistry/parallel synthesis results in a large amount of substrate for assessment of DDI potential. This leads to a heavier reliance on *in silico* and *in vitro* screening assays in order to cope with the large numbers of compounds processed during this stage. Automation technology enables the generation of large databases of information, from which *in silico* models can be built. *In silico* DDI can now be a first-line screen for virtual compounds and compound libraries, thereby highlighting potential DDI liabilities at a very early stage. In the laboratory condensed studies need to be performed, whilst incorporating all the kinetic principles of the definitive DDI studies (e.g., using a single inhibitor concentration, or a recombinant enzyme system). For these reasons, data from such assays are more often used for ranking purposes as opposed to quantitative DDI predictions for which additional *in vitro* and *in vivo* data would be required.

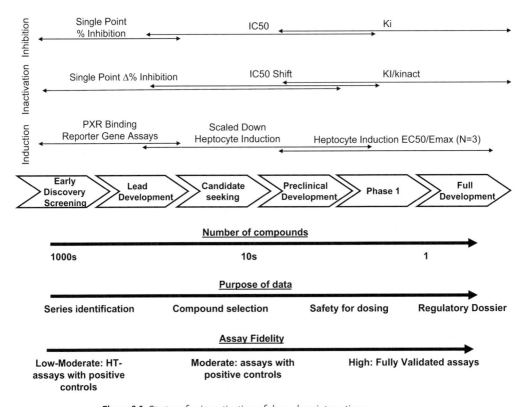

Figure 8.1 Strategy for investigation of drug–drug interactions.

From early discovery through development there is a hierarchical strategy for investigating drug–drug interaction potential (Figure 8.1). The hierarchy is to achieve two things: (i) to provide the greatest amount of quality data early in discovery; (ii) to control overall cost. Early during drug discovery, the emphasis is to determine the potential for a DDI as one of the components used to select and/or optimize molecules for drug development. Therefore, the research effort is focused on a quick assessment and this usually concentrates on an estimation of reversible inhibition. Later in drug development, these studies provide a mechanism-orientated approach that can be further addressed in the clinical plan, as well as satisfying regulatory expectations.

This chapter focuses upon pharmacokinetic-based drug–drug interactions. Since the *in silico* and *in vitro* tools for CYP-based DDI are the most advanced, these enzymes are used as examples. However, similar principles apply for both *in silico* models and *in vitro* as reagents (e.g., recombinant systems, specific/selective inhibitors/substrates, etc.) become available for other enzymes and transporters.

8.2
In Silico Approaches

In silico modeling can be described as using computers to model how chemical structures behave either *in vitro* or *in vivo* via computer-aided simulations. The current *in silico* DDI methodologies generally focus on the main CYP enzymes (CYP3A4, CYP2D6, CYP1A2, CYP2C9). High-throughput data generation yields vast amounts of screening data which enables multiple approaches to computational prediction. Most of these models are based on statistical approaches or molecular and protein modeling. Throughout most industrial drug discovery organizations, quantitative structure activity relationships (QSAR) methods are used to link chemical features with the experimental inhibition data. These models can be applied on large libraries of virtual compounds and aid discovery teams in multiple directions [6]. The first potential impact is to not choose to prosecute libraries that are likely inhibitors of CYPs. The second big impact is in directing the synthesis towards lower risk compounds. A summary of CYP inhibition models and the key descriptors was described by Refsgaard *et al.* [7].

In general the existing models mimic the experimental models providing for a prediction of a yes/no for inhibition based on a predefined experimental cut-off, a percent inhibition or an IC_{50} value. Some models also provide information on the potential for reactive metabolite formation, which may produce a subsequent DDI. The use of *in silico* predictions is a hotly debated topic. In general, when assessing the predictive ability of any new *in silico* model, the end user should consider a number of key factors to aid in the interpretation of the prediction. First, are any of the compounds being predicted part of the original training set of the model? This assessment allows for a direct comparison of measured versus predicted data. If none of the compounds being predicted are part of the training set, how similar is the compound that is being predicted to any compounds used in the training of the model?

For the earliest predictions, it is common to only produce a binary prediction, whereby a compound is predicted as high risk or low risk for DDI against the various CYP enzymes. This simplistic approach flags the risky chemical space and helps the medicinal chemists prioritize which compounds to actually make. *In silico* methodologies can also be used to prioritize which compounds to test earlier to determine the impact or severity of a DDI. Stoner *et al.* [8, 9] described a number of approaches that discovery teams can take to visualize and prioritize *in silico* and *in vitro* data to help aid in multi-parameter optimization (MPO). In general most researchers use an "in combo" approach, whereby *in silico* data is used in combination with *in vitro* data. This approach has been shown to be particularly valuable when trying to make specific design recommendations. By combining wet DDI data along with CYP docking information, specific designs can be proposed that alter interaction with the proteins either through directly blocking the confounding heme interaction, or altering the 3D shape, so as to block or reduce the docking.

Docking methods used to design out of CYP-based DDI metabolism issues also fall under the general category of *in silico* approaches to aid in compound re-design in the face of DDI. These methods are also sometimes referred to as structure-based drug design (SBDD), taking into account specific molecular interactions between compound and the active site of the CYP enzyme and have been made possible by the solution of crystal and co-crystal structures of several key drug-metabolizing CYP enzymes in complex with substrates or inhibitors [10–13]. Currently, however, co-crystallization efforts with CYP enzymes can take several weeks or months. This lag is not compatible with most project timelines and *in silico* approaches have an upper hand in this regard. In order to successfully initiate and interpret docking experiments designed to address DDI problems, data identifying the CYP enzyme involved as well as site of metabolism or reactive species generated are generally necessary. While computational methods are being developed to obtain some of this information (e.g., CypScore, isoCyp), most modern drug metabolism laboratories can easily determine this experimentally, making the exercise often a joint effort by computational and traditional biochemists. In addition, spectral binding assays performed in the laboratory can also often offer insight into the inhibitory binding mode of the ligand [14], particularly in the case of nitrogen containing type II inhibitors.

A successful *in silico* docking experiment can identify the binding mode of a specific ligand in the active site of the CYP enzyme that affords the ligand inhibitory potency or that is compatible with the generation of the reactive metabolite responsible for the mechanism-based inhibitor. One of the most notable complicating factors is the known conformational flexibility of these enzymes in response to ligand binding, making it a challenge to identify the proper static model into which to initiate the docking [15]. It is anticipated that rapidly increasing computing power will ultimately allow dynamic docking simulations which allow realtime flexibility of the protein backbone to be computationally reasonable, but static docking methods are currently necessary for useful throughput.

The knowledge gained from the docking studies in elucidating a number of the structural fragments that are most likely to cause a specific DDI are becoming increasingly understood. Kalgutkar *et al.* [16] provide a nice summary of many of the known "structural alerts" that are likely to contribute to a DDI. A number of approaches exist for identifying these components of structures. Many recent presentations have been made showing how tools such as Pipeline Pilot, from Accelerys, can be used to search through large numbers of compounds and identify those structural features that may have a propensity for bioactivation and subsequent interaction with CYP enzymes, either through interaction with the heme or apoprotein.

The key descriptors used to predict the likelihood of a CYP inhibition are incredibly vast. Descriptors can, for example, be defined as spatial, electronic or conformational. Some of the key structural properties include lipophilicity, pK_a and PSA and are relatively easy to interpret, while others are more complex. For further information on descriptors used in DDI modeling, please refer to De Groot et al. [6].

A number of reports also describe the prediction of mechanism-based inhibition (MBI) [17, 18]. In this type of model, MBI is determined in part by spectral shift and inactivation kinetics. Jones et al. applied computational pharmacophores, recursive partitioning and logistic regression in attempts to predict metabolic intermediate complex (MIC) formation from structural inputs [17]. The development of models that accurately predict MIC formation will provide another tool to help reduce the overall risk of DDI [19].

In summary, *in silico* approaches to aid in removing DDI should be actively applied in early lead development. The application of these models in early drug discovery will reduce the frequency and cost of drug candidates that require clinical DDI studies. In the future, it is possible that a great majority of CYP-based DDI issues will be removed during lead development.

8.3
Perpetrators of Drug–Drug Interactions: Enzyme Inhibition

8.3.1
Competitive Inhibition

A competitive inhibition screen is often the first step in understanding the DDI potential of a NCE. The definitive assessment of inhibition is the inhibition constant (K_i), which provides not only the inhibition potency but also information on the mechanism of inhibition (competitive, non-competitive). However in the hit to lead profiling environment this approach is over-complex for the question being asked, and generates far too many samples to enable rapid screening of compound series. DDI assays based upon the IC_{50} principle are therefore favored. The relationship between K_i and IC_{50} for a competitive inhibitor is:

$$IC_{50} = K_i \left(1 + \frac{[S]}{K_M}\right) \tag{8.1}$$

Under assay conditions whereby the concentration of the probe substrate is equivalent to K_M, an IC_{50} estimate is equivalent to twofold K_i. For non-competitive inhibition, K_i is equivalent to IC_{50} since inhibitor and substrate binding are independent.

Simplifying the experimental system even further by using a single point concentration rather than a concentration range for a full IC_{50} determination reduces the number of samples further. Typically the five major enzymes are investigated (CYP1A2, CYP2C9, CYP2C19, CYP2D6, CYP3A4), accounting for greater than 90% of total hepatic CYPs [20, 21] and 70% of metabolism of all marketed drugs [22]. The two DDI screens most commonly used are the conventional inhibition screen and the fluorescent inhibition screen.

For any inhibition assay, be it screening or definitive, there are criteria that should be adhered to which will enable reliable data:

1. The probe substrate should be specific/selective and the concentration should be at or below K_M. See Table 8.1 for a list of recommended CYP substrates.

2. Low microsomal protein concentrations of 0.1 mg/mL or below reduce effects of microsomal binding.

3. No more than 10–30% substrate or inhibitor depletion should occur during the reaction.

4. Incubation conditions should be established whereby there is a linear relationship between time and product formation and between amount of enzyme and product formation.

5. Positive controls for inhibition should be employed (see Table 8.1 for CYP inhibitors)

6. Low concentrations of organic solvent ($\leq$1%, v/v; preferably <0.1%) should be used to dissolve substrates and NCEs which may lead to compound solubility issues. Higher percentages of organic solvents in the final reaction volume can inhibit enzyme activity [23–25]. No inhibitor control samples, reflecting 100% activity, should be solvent-matched with the test incubations.

7. Water baths or thermocylers give a more consistent incubation than dry-heat incubation, as does using tubes or microplates with free access to individual wells. Microplates without access to individual wells incubate from the outside to the middle of the plate, such that wells on the outside have higher turnover rates than the inside wells.

8.3.2
Conventional CYP Inhibition Screen

The DDI conventional inhibition screen is moderate throughput and can range from a few compounds per week to a few hundred per week depending on the amount of inhibitor concentrations, inhibition curve replicates and analytical methods used. This screen typically uses 96- or 384-well formats. The reaction components (HLM, 100 mM potassium phosphate buffer, specific probe substrate, NCE, NADPH cofactor or NADPH-regenerating system) are pre-warmed to 37 °C and are mixed together to initiate the reaction, then incubated at 37 °C for the appropriate length of

Table 8.1 Recommended CYP specific inhibitors and concentrations.

CYP	Conventional probe[a]		Fluorescent probe[b]			Inhibitor	Inhibitor concentration	Comments
	Substrate	K_M	Substrate	Recommended screening concentration				
CYP1A2	Phenacetin O-deethylation	1.7–152	CEC	5		Furafylline	10 μM	Inactivator, peincubation for 15 min with NADPH + microsomes will yield better inhibition.
CYP2B6	Tacrine 1-hydroxylation	2.8, 16	Vivid EOMCC	3		Methyl-phenyl-ethyl piperidine (MPEP)	10 μM	
	Bupropion hydroxylation	61–168	EFC	2.5				
CYP2C8	Efavirenz hydroxylase	17–23	Vivid BOMCC	5		Montelukast	0.1 μM	Potency decreases upon increased incubation protein concentration.
	Taxol 6-hydroxylation	5.4–19	DBF	1				
	Amodiaquine N-deethylation	2.4						
CYP2C9	Diclofenac 4'-hydroxylation	3.4–32	MFC	75		Sulfaphenazole	10 μM	
	S-warfarin 7-hydroxylation	1.5–4.5	Vivid BOMCC	10				
CYP2C19	S-mephenytoin 4'-hydroxylation	13–35	CEC	25		(+)N-benzylnirvanol	10 μM	
	Omeprazole 5-hydroxylation	17–26	Vivid EOMCC	10				
CYP2D6	Dextromethorphan O-demethylation	0.44–8.5	AMMC	1.5		Quinidine	1 μM	Higher concentrations can affect CYP3A (inhibit or activate)
	(+/−)Bufuralol 1'-hydroxylation	9–15	Vivid EOMCC	10				
CYP3A4/5	Midazolam 1-hydroxylation	1–14	7-BQ	40		Ketoconazole	0.1 μM	Ketoconazole also inhibits CYP2C8 and 1A1
	Testosterone 6b-hydroxylation	52–94	Vivid BOMCC	10				
	Nifedipine oxidation	5.1–47						
PAN-CYP						Miconazole	10 μM	

Abbreviations: CEC: 3-cyano-7-ethoxycoumarin; EFC: 7-ethoxy-4-trifluoro-methyl-coumarin; DBF: Dibenzylfluorescein; 7-MFC: 7-methoxy-4-trifluoro-methyl-coumarin; AMMC: 3-[2-(N,N-diethyl-N-methylamino)ethyl]-7-methoxy-4-methyl-coumarin; 7-BQ: 7-Benzyloxyquinone.
[a] FDA website.
[b] BD Bioscience website, Invitrogen website.

time according to the specific CYP assay conditions. The reaction is quenched with solvent and centrifuged at 3000 rpm for 10 min. HPLC, LC/UV and LC/MS/MS are analytical detection methods for this screen. The amount of metabolite formed from the probe substrate is measured relative to the uninhibited wells. LC/MS/MS detection is faster, more accurate and has less interference than HPLC or LC/UV. However, LC/MS/MS of a single substrate reaction is more expensive and time-consuming than a screen with fluorescent detection.

8.3.3
Fluorescent Inhibition Screen

The DDI fluorescent inhibition screen is a high-throughput screen, primarily as a result of reduced analysis time, and can range from a few hundred compounds per week to a thousand per week. The assay uses recombinant microsomes prepared from insect cells infected with recombinant baculovirus containing a human CYP enzyme and individual fluorogenic substrates. In this instance the substrates are not specific and hence cannot be used in a mixed enzyme system such as HLM. In addition, this assay is more prone than the conventional inhibition screen (Section 8.3.2) to NCE interferences within the assay (i.e., inherently fluorescent NCEs, fluorescent quenching by the NCE).

This screen typically uses 96- or 384-well formats. The plate is ideally incubated within the fluorescent plate reader such that readings are taken at timed intervals across the incubation period. Most plate readers are equipped with plate shakers and an incubator chamber with temperature control. Monitoring metabolism of the probe in real time provides a metabolic rate. The ratio of the rate in presence of NCE to that in control incubations yields the percentage control activity. The DDI fluorescent screen has the benefit of being relatively simple and inexpensive, with the ability to bin compounds (low, medium, high risk). Caution does need to be taken when fluorescent data is used to drive decision making for DDI due to known differences in inhibitory potencies which can be observed between the fluorescent screen and the conventional screen [26]. Understanding the limitations of any approach and the rates of false positives and negatives compared to the conventional screen is vital. The fluorescent assay has most value in screening out potent CYP inhibitors from within a large data set, with the risk of potentially throwing away some good compounds. Compounds that are brought forward as being weak inhibitors in this assay should be followed up using the conventional approach.

8.3.4
DDI Single Point versus IC$_{50}$ Determinations

In early discovery determination of percent inhibition at a single concentration is sufficient to compare compounds within a chemical series. Typically concentrations in the 1–5 μM range are used [27, 28]. Test compounds and vehicle control are incubated with the probe substrate and the amount of metabolite formation from the probe substrate determined. The metabolic rate can then be expressed as a percentage of the control (uninhibited activity) and a percent inhibition value determined by subtraction from 100%. The analytical methods most widely used are LC/MS/MS detection for the DDI conventional inhibition screen and fluorescence detection for the DDI fluorescence inhibition screen. An estimated IC_{50} can be determined by fitting the average percent control activity into a model [28, 29]. The data from this screen can be used primarily as a flag for DDI inhibition and binned into three categories:

- Inhibition greater than 50% = high risk
- Inhibition between 30–50% = moderate risk
- Inhibition less than 30% = low risk

Flagged compounds of interest may be followed up with the DDI multi-point determination to verify the results with more definitive data. The DDI multi-point determination uses a serial dilution of concentrations of the NCE spanning over a few orders of magnitude of a third-log scale. An IC_{50} is determined by plotting the percent control activity (y-axis) to the inhibitor concentration (x-axis) and using statistical software to fit the sigmoid dose response derived from the Hill equation [28–30] to get the concentration at which there is 50% depletion of the control. The DDI multi-point inhibition screen is a lower-throughput assay, but can be used at a higher capacity by using a substrate cocktail approach.

8.3.5
DDI Cocktail Assay

As mentioned previously there is a disconnect between data generated in the high-throughput fluorescent probe assay and the moderate-throughput conventional assay. Therefore, the substrate cocktail approach was developed to provide a balance of sufficient throughput without compromising data relevance. This method was made possible due to advances in chromatographic methods and mass spectrometry sensitivity, in addition to further understanding into specific clinically relevant probes for each CYP isoform [28, 31–40]. Immediate benefits seen from a cocktail or cassette method is a complete evaluation of the major metabolizing enzyme in a single reaction under the same conditions and the number of compounds that can be assessed by such a reaction. Chemical series modifications can be assessed providing information on minor changes in SAR revealing shifts in potency toward or away from one or many isoforms.

Certainly there are compromises that need to be made when adding complexity to an already complicated system.

1. The enzyme concentration should coincide to the measurable rates of metabolism, taking into account the highest and lowest rates of metabolism seen for each enzyme. At the same time, protein content should still be kept low to minimize the compound binding [41–43].

2. An appropriate incubation time should also be evaluated to measure initial rate kinetics (depletion) of the most extensively metabolized substrate while maintaining sensitivity of the least metabolized substrate.

3. Potential competition of individual isoforms for cytochrome b5 and NADPH reductase may limit the electron transport and thus metabolic rate [44, 45].

It has been shown that such issues can be overcome and in an acceptable range to provide an appropriate level of quality data [25, 46].

8.3.6
Mechanism-Based Inhibition

In addition to the assessment of reversible inhibition, the role played by mechanism-based inhibitors (irreversible inhibitors) provides a focus during lead development, as it can result in a more profound and prolonged effect than that suggested by the therapeutic dose or exposure. Mechanism-based inhibition (MBI) occurs as a result of the CYP generating reactive intermediates that bind to the enzyme causing irreversible loss of activity. Oxidative metabolism via that CYP is only restored upon re-synthesis of that enzyme. Three mechanisms have been reported showing how intermediate species act as mechanism-based inhibitors:

1. reacting with nucleophilic amino acids in the active site;
2. reacting with the heme nitrogen atoms;
3. co-ordination of the heme iron to form a metabolite-intermediate complex (MIC).

A comprehensive overview of MBI chemistry is not within the scope of this section, but the reader is referred to recent reviews that discuss this topic in more detail [47–50].

The most commonly used approach in assessing MBI is through the use of specific CYP probes in conjunction with HLM or individually expressed recombinant CYPs [51–54]. One approach is a simplified experiment based on the enzyme inactivation constant (K_I) and the maximum rate if inactivation (k_{inact}). The assay determines enzyme inactivation using a pre-incubation of the enzyme (at 37 °C), NADPH (by definition reactive intermediates are only produced by CYP in the presence of NADPH added directly or generated *in situ* by a NADPH-regenerating system) and a NCE for varying time-points, followed by dilution into a further activity mix containing the probe substrate. During early screening an initial assay can be used using human liver microsomes normally at sufficiently high enough concentrations (ideally 1–2 mg/mL) to provide catalytic activity following dilution into the activity mixture, with one or two inhibitor concentrations. The pre-incubation step is normally performed for 30 min (to ensure identification of weak inhibitors, avoiding false negatives), after which an aliquot of the pre-incubation mix is added to the activity mix containing probe substrate, and further incubated. Figure 8.2 depicts the approach used in the authors' laboratories.

This further incubation should be sufficiently long enough to observe measurable metabolite formation. There is some debate as to the most ideal dilution scheme that should be followed, but the general consensus is that a higher dilution (e.g., >10-fold) reduces the influence of competitive inhibition. Also the concentration of probe substrate should ideally be at least 5 K_M, the purpose being that the high probe concentration together with the dilution step minimizes competitive inhibition of

1) Inactivation / "Inhibitor preincubation" Assay

NADPH (1mM) regeneration sys.

Protein: 1 mg/mL HLM

Prewarm: 5 min

Inhibitor: 0, 10 & 60 μM

Inhibitor incubation: 0 & 30 min

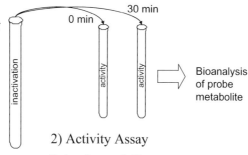

2) Activity Assay

Probe substrate: 5x Km

NADPH (1mM) regeneration sys.

Substrate and NADPH prewarmed

Protein: start reaction with 15 μl aliquot from Inactivation assay: final carried over protein conc 0.05 mg/mL

Perform substrate incubation

Final carried over inhibitor conc (0.5 and 3 μM)

Figure 8.2 Schematic representation of the steps involved in the dilution approach used to determine a crude potency of compounds as mechanism-based inhibitors.

the CYP by the compound being investigated. However, this is not exclusively the case, as recently reported by Kent et al. [55, 56] and Polasek et al. [55, 56], who found that certain substrates for CYP2C9 and CYP3A4 accelerate inactivation, indicative of multiple substrate binding sites. A representation of the results obtained from these studies is shown in Figure 8.3(a). These various approaches have gained continued favor in light of their amenability to automation and or use with recombinant CYPs [57, 58], allowing assessment of larger numbers of compounds earlier on during discovery to better guide projects around potential DDIs. A similar approach to that above can be followed except with addition of probe directly into pre-incubation mix, thus omitting any dilution step [59]. This all in one approach using progress curve analysis allows the investigation of both reversible (K_{iapp}) and irreversible (K_I, k_{inact}) features of the reaction mechanism. Fairman and co-workers [59] demonstrated that this alternative approach yielded data comparable with the conventional dilution approach against CYP1A2 MBIs.

For the aforementioned studies, the decreases in the natural logarithm of activity over time should be plotted for each inhibitor concentration. The negative slopes of each line represent the k_{obs} values, and should be plotted against inhibitor concentration, from which the K_I and k_{inact} are generated using non-linear regression of the data (Figure 8.3b). The values can then be used to assess the relative clinical risk of the inhibitor [50]. The k_{inact}/K_I ratio can be used to compare enzyme efficiency. IC_{50} shift studies have also been used to investigate MBI [60]. Typically, multiple concentrations of inhibitors are pre-incubated for up to 30 min, covering a range 10× the IC_{50} measured for reversible inhibition. Hence after dilution (10-fold) into the activity

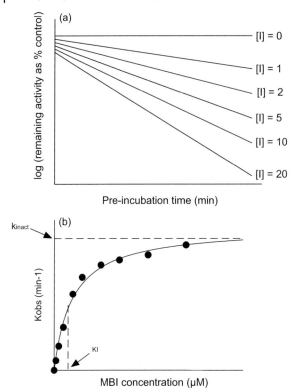

Figure 8.3 Graphical representations relevant to the dilution approach for characterizing mechanism-based inhibitors. (a) Time- and concentration-dependant inactivation of enzyme by a mechanism-based inhibitor (slopes of each line represent Kobs). Fewer inactivator concentrations required during early screening, but at least six concentrations should be used to determine enzyme inactivation constant (K_I) and the maximum rate of inactivation (k_{inact}) (b).

mix, the concentrations span the IC_{50}. Pre-incubations are performed in the presence and absence of NADPH with substrate concentrations proximal to the K_M (see Table 8.1). Obach and co-workers [61] showed a good correlation between the shifted IC_{50} and k_{inact}/K_I and also the K_I, indicating that the shifted IC_{50} contains elements of the inactivator potency. As such the fold-change in IC_{50} alone is not the most important predictor of the efficiency of an inactivator but rather the potency after conducting 30 min incubation before measuring activity. Although this approach is empirical, the shifted IC_{50} can be used to identify MBI [61].

8.4
Perpetrators of Drug–Drug Interactions: Enzyme Induction

Induction of drug metabolizing enzymes by xenobiotics is an important factor in understanding variations in drug response. Drug-mediated increases in these enzymes can result in DDI as a result of inefficacy of drug treatment. In clinical practice, enzyme induction can enhance clearance of the drug itself or a co-administered drug, which could lead to loss of therapeutic effect. The number of clinically relevant CYP inducers is small, and there is no structure–activity relationship reported. Yasuda *et al.* report that *in silico* and *in vitro* studies can help prioritize potential for CYP3A4 induction within series [62]. The common denominator amongst CYP inducers is dose size, with the majority of clinically significant CYP3A4 inducers being administered at doses of 500–1000 mg/day [63]. Nevertheless some assessment of CYP induction, be it *in vitro* or *in vivo* is important for DDI predictions. The "gold standard" measurement of CYP induction is considered to be induction of enzyme activity in human hepatocyte cultures [64]. In a drug discovery program, induction screening may be relevant. For example, in a research program for a female-specific indication, in a compound series where dose is unlikely to be low, there may be a concern with regards to ineffective oral contraceptive (OC) cover, due to enzyme induction [65], which could be de-risked early.

Due to the high cost of human hepatocytes and length of experiments this system cannot be utilized early in a drug discovery program. Other screening systems are therefore used. Since induction is generally as a result of activation in gene transcription there is the opportunity for *in vitro* ligand binding assays and reporter gene assays to be utilized as an early screening approach. CYP induction is most often mediated through the orphan nuclear receptors pregnane X receptor (PXR), constitutive androstane receptor (CAR) and aryl hydrocarbon receptor (AhR) [66, 67]. One notable exception is CYP2E1 where protein stabilization and mRNA stabilization are important mechanisms for induction [66, 68]. For PXR, the relationship between ligand binding, receptor activation and target gene induction is well established [69].

8.4.1
Ligand Binding Assay

Jones *et al.* [70] have described in detail a binding assay utilizing the displacement of a high-affinity PXR ligand SR12 813. By radiolabeling and using scintillation proximity assays (SPA) this ligand assay is more amenable to an automated, high-throughput format. Assessment of several SPA bead types identified poly(vinyltoluene) streptavidin beads as most suitable for high-throughput format due to the better compatibility with liquid handling devices, low background binding of the radioligand and easy coupling of the receptor to the SPA bead [70]. Briefly, the purified biotinylated PXR receptor is allowed to couple to the SPA beads which are then resuspended in buffer, and radioligand added at 10 nM. This is then added to wells containing test compounds 0.5 nM to 10 µM. Additional wells contain DMSO alone for total binding and 1 mM clotrimazole to determine non-specific binding. Plates are sealed, mixed and counted after 1–2 h at room temperature. The percent radioligand bound values, corrected for non-specific binding are plotted against log test compound concentration to calculate an IC_{50}.

It should be noted that receptor affinity does not always correlate to downstream response, for example, a compound may bind to the receptor as an antagonist rather than an agonist. Zhu et al. have developed and validated a high-throughput binding assay utilizing a single concentration of test compound (10 µM) [71]. In a data set of 616 compounds a non-linear relationship was observed between the binding and reporter gene assay (see below for details of reporter gene assays). 9% of compounds demonstrated high binding but low transactivation which would constitute a false positive in an induction screen, whilst only 1% of compounds would be considered false negatives. Hence the probability of missing an inducer is low, though more compounds than actual inducers would be taken through to transactivation assays.

8.4.2
Reporter Gene (Transactivation) Assays

Cell-based assays utilizing transiently expressed reporter genes have been widely used to investigate induction [72–74]. The method is of lower throughput than the binding assay already discussed, but offers the benefit of measuring activation rather than simple binding. Two plasmids are typically used in these studies, a reporter plasmid and an expression plasmid. The reporter plasmid contains the reporter gene such as chloramphenicol acetyltransferase (CAT) or luciferase and a control element of the gene of interest. The expression plasmid contains the sequence needed to transiently express the nuclear receptor of interest. The two plasmids are transfected into the host cells which are usually cell types which do not express PXR themselves, for example, CV-1 cells (monkey) or HepG2 and HuH7 (human hepatoma cell lines). Often an expression vector as an internal control for transfections is also used (e.g., alkaline phosphatase; AP). Test compounds are presented to cells in media in which endogenous AP activity has been removed and incubated for 18 h at 37 °C. Following this AP and the reporter gene activities are measured. Reporter activity is normalized to the AP activity and then the normalized values used to calculate fold activation over vehicle control. An increase in reporter gene activity will be detected if the compound is a nuclear receptor ligand which is directly proportional to increased nuclear receptor activation. Fold activation versus log test compound concentration are plotted and used to calculate EC_{50} and V_{max} values.

The majority of reporter gene assays utilize a transient transfection, however stable expression cell lines are also being developed [75–77]. Such systems offer advantages in terms of ease of use and the opportunity to develop standardized screens. In one study, a stably transfected AhR reporter gene assay and a PXR reporter gene assay were evaluated for their ability to predict clinical induction [78]. For PXR activation, ranking compounds based upon AUC_{total}/EC_{50} clustered all but one of the inducers, with a cut-off of 3 indicating a potential for clinically relevant induction. For AhR activation, whilst compounds were identified as activators, the authors were unable to identify any drugs that induce CYP1A in vivo in humans at therapeutic doses. Sinz et al. evaluated 170 known drugs and natural products in a PXR reporter gene assay and 54% demonstrated some level of transactivation, which is significantly higher than the number of clinically relevant inducers [79]. A number of interpretation criteria related to cell culture conditions (compound solubility, cytotoxicity, drug concentration in media vs liver concentration and non-specific binding) and the *in vivo* ADME properties of the drug (including, route of administration, dosing regimen, efficacious concentration, compounds that induce and inhibit) reduced this to 5% of compounds predicted as inducers. The reader is directed to the full publication for more detail on these criteria and how they were applied [79].

8.4.3
Overall Evaluation of High-Throughput Induction Assays

Ligand binding assays are high throughput and will indicate the ability for a test compound to bind to the receptor of interest, but provide no information on the functional consequence of binding (agonist or antagonist). The reporter gene assay allows a large number of compounds to be evaluated in a relatively quick and inexpensive manner, and measurement of PXR activation by this method is a reliable method for assessing CYP3A4 induction potential [73]. However the method is only able to assess one mechanism at a time, unlike the primary hepatocyte which contains all the response elements. In addition due to different mechanisms of activation some nuclear receptors are more difficult to adapt to reporter gene assays. For example, whilst PXR ligands directly activate the PXR located in the nucleus, activation of CAR occurs via an unknown indirect mechanism. CAR is located in the cytoplasm until drugs trigger a cytoplasm–nucleus translocation of the receptor [80]. The mode of receptor modulation in the cytoplasm and nucleus are different. Harmesen and co-workers [81] recently evaluated PXR and CAR reporter gene assays in two immortalized cell lines (HepG2 and LS180). The LS180 cell line was more sensitive to transactivation and a good correlation was observed between the PXR reporter gene assay and CYP3A4 protein expression, whilst no correlation was observed for CAR and CYP3A4 protein expression. No validated systems are available to screen compounds for their ability to activate CAR. Therefore a reporter gene assay as an induction screen runs the risk of false-negative results due to the multiple mechanisms (e.g., non-PXR activation) that may contribute to induction. For this reason, there has been much interest in immortalized human hepatocyte cell lines, as source of human hepatocytes that would be readily available and would not be associated with donor to donor variability. The assays utilizing these systems would not be considered high throughput, require days of cell culture, are more complex analytics than reporter gene assays and are therefore outside of the scope of this chapter. Interested readers are referred to recent publications describing one such cell line (Fa2N-4, a simian virus 40 immortalized human hepatocyte cell line) [82–84].

8.5
Drug–Drug Interactions; Victims of Interaction; Reaction Phenotyping

Reaction phenotyping is the semi-quantitative *in vitro* estimation of the relative contributions of specific drug-metabolizing enzymes to the metabolism of a test compound. It has been well documented that approximately two-thirds of marketed drugs are metabolized by members of the CYP superfamily, in particular the subfamilies CYP1, 2 and 3 [85]. This has ultimately resulted in greater emphasis being paid towards the design of studies aimed at identifying which specific CYP form(s) is (are) involved in the metabolism of a given compound. However, while such approaches are well defined for some specific CYP enzymes (CYP1A2, 2C8, 2C9, 2C19, 2D6, 2E1, 3A) a similar level of appreciation does not yet exist for other CYPs such as CYP1A1, 1B1, 2A6 and 2B6. In addition the science behind non-CYP drug-metabolizing enzymes, such as flavin-containing monooxygenases, monoamine oxidases (MAOS), glucuronosyltransferases (UGTs), sulfotransferases (ST), molybdenum-containing oxidases (Mo-CO), methyltransferases, acetyltransferases and glutathione-S-transferases (GSTs), generally lags behind that of the CYPs [86]. The current section aims to focus on the major studies performed during early discovery, and the reader is referred to some recent review articles describing reaction phenotyping studies for development compounds [87–90], the information from which is included in regulatory documents, product labels, as well as recommendations for dose adjustments [37, 91].

A number of different approaches, have been designed to characterize the metabolic clearance of compounds, namely: antibody inhibition, correlation analysis, chemical inhibitors and cDNA-expressed CYPs. As expected the science underlying these tools has developed over the past two decades reducing the need to use several approaches simultaneously to make unequivocal conclusions regarding the CYP isoform responsible for the metabolism of a drug of interest. For the purposes of the current chapter, only the latter two are discussed. The readers are referred to recent reviews that describe in detail the science behind antibody inhibition and correlation analysis [87–89].

8.5.1
Chemical Inhibition

Ideally an approach of this type should employ a pool of human liver microsomes, or several lots from individual donors, with the intent that all CYP activities are representative of an average in the population. The experimental approach used should follow well defined conditions to ensure the most reliable result. The substrate concentration used should be lower/equal to the K_M. In most cases a concentration of 1 µM should suffice. Since CYP enzymes are very versatile enzymes, they can bind and metabolize a wide range of substrates and inhibitors with diverse chemical structures. Thus, it is unlikely that "absolutely specific inhibitors" can be found. However, well characterized "highly selective inhibitors" with respect to individual human CYP isoforms have been identified (see Table 8.1). Kinetic data generated in these experiments should then be analyzed using a linear fit of the natural logarithm of the ratio of the compound peak area to the internal standard peak area against time and the disappearance rate constant (k) determined from the gradient of this line. These rate constants determined in the presence ($k_{(I)}$) and absence (k) of chemical inhibitor are then used to calculate the percentage of contribution of each CYP enzyme to the *in vitro* metabolism of test compound using Equation 8.2 and subsequently the $f_{CL\ CYP}$.

$$\text{\% contribution} = \frac{(-k)-(-k_{(I)})}{(-k)} \times 100\% \tag{8.2}$$

It is not always possible to identify a totally specific inhibitor. In such instances one of two approaches may be used. The inhibitor concentration is chosen such that it does not effect other activities, but may not inhibit the targeted enzyme 100%. For example, if a "specific" CYP inhibitor was only found to inhibit the target enzyme by 80%, then a correction factor of 1.25 need be applied to any percentage inhibitions observed. Alternately a higher concentration is used which maximally inhibits the targeted activity also has some cross-reactivity against other enzymes. In this instance the sum of percent contributions likely exceeds 100% and therefore all values are adjusted down.

The application of chemical inhibitors in studies of this type can provide sound scientific information to make early decisions during drug discovery. However, as the majority of high turnover compounds are screened out, a major proportion of compounds for which phenotyping information is required, are low to intermediate clearance compounds. As such care needs to be taken when interpreting data from more metabolically stable compounds. This is best illustrated for compounds metabolized by more than one CYP, where the inclusion of a specific inhibitor results in no turnover, precluding an exact measurement of a percent contribution.

8.5.2
Recombinant Human CYP Enzymes

The use of rCYPs has grown over recent years, due in part to the increased availability of materials provided by commercial vendors (e.g., Gentest Corp., Invitrogen Corp., Oxford Biomedical Research Inc.) and in part because the results from studies utilizing these systems can be unambiguously assigned to a particular CYP. However, when choosing a system, it is important to use well characterized sources that report important information such as the CYP protein:reductase:cytochrome b_5 ratio. Differences in this ratio between the recombinant systems can lead to in appropriate study designs [92]. Experiments using rCYPs follow a similar approach to that of chemical inhibitors. Parent loss ($[S] < = K_M$) is followed in the presence of the rCYPs of choice. An ideal starting concentration for each of the rCYPs should be high enough to observe metabolism, but not too high to introduce artifacts associated with non-specific binding. In early screening as with the use of chemical inhibitors, only the major CYPs need be investigated (CYPs 1A2, 2B6, 2C8, 2C9, 2C19, 2D6, 3A4). The individual Cl_{int} values ($\mu L/min/pmol$ CYP; calculated for each rCYP) require subsequent scaling to the corresponding Cl_{int} values for that CYP in human liver microsomes [93]. The sum of the individual Cl_{int} values should approach that measured in liver microsomes. In brief a correction factor is needed to account for the difference between the Cl_{int} per unit amount of CYP (intrinsic activity or turnover number) in liver microsomes and rCYP enzymes. Such differences have been reported to be attributed to differences in the concentrations of accessory proteins and the lipid microenvironment of the enzyme [94–96]. This discrepancy is overcome by using relative activity factors (RAF), which define the amount of rCYP required to give an equivalent reaction velocity to that of the particular liver microsome sample used (Equation 8.3) [97, 98].

$$\text{RAF}(\text{pmol rhCYP/mg HLM}) = \frac{V_{max}\text{HLM (nmol/min/mg HLM)}}{V_{max}\text{rhCYP (nmol/min/pmol rhCYP)}} \quad (8.3)$$

However this approach does not address inter-individual variability in CYP expression nor the apparent substrate specificity of RAFs. This may be overcome through the use of intersystem extrapolation factors (ISEFs) which compare the intrinsic activities of rCYP versus liver microsomes and provide CYP abundance scaling by mathematical means. This employs the RAF approach and adjusts for the actual amount of liver microsomes CYP present (measured by immunochemistry) rather than a theoretical amount (Equation 8.4). Such corrections can be made using nominal specific contents of individual CYP proteins in liver microsomes or more appropriately employ modeling and simulation software (e.g., SIMCYP; www.simcyp.com) which takes into account population-based variability in CYP content.

$$\text{VISEF} = \frac{V_{max}\text{HLM (nmol/min/mg HLM)}}{V_{max}\text{rhCYP (nmol/min/pmol rhCYP)} \cdot \text{HLM CYP abundance (pmol/mg HLM)}} \quad (8.4)$$

Although corrections for RAFs in Equation 8.4 are based upon V_{max} values (VISEF), Cl_{int} ISEF value can also be used. Such approaches have successfully been used to extrapolate *in vitro* data to predict the *in vivo* DDI risk [93], although there still remains some uncertainty around the most appropriate index reaction conditions (i.e., HLM source, rCYP source, use of single or multiple probe substrate(s)) that should be used to generate the RAF value [93]. The $f_{CL\,CYP}$ for any contributing CYP is then determined from the sum of the individual contributing rCYP Cl_{int} values (µL/min/mg protein).

8.6
Predictions of Drug–Drug Interactions

In recent years, the utility of *in vitro* inhibition data to predict *in vivo* DDI was demonstrated. The underlying principles for this approach had been known for many years [99], but demonstration that these early concepts could be used practically in the prediction of clinical DDI was only obtained over the past few years. The principles can be applied for new compounds as the potential perpetrator of an interaction as well as the potential victim. The equation described by Rowland and Matin [99] forms the basis of this approach:

$$\text{magnitude of DDI} = \frac{\text{AUC}_{inhibited}}{\text{AUC}_{control}} = \frac{1}{\frac{f_{CL}}{1+\left(\frac{[I]_{in\,vivo}}{K_i}\right)} + (1-f_{CL})} \quad (8.5)$$

The terms $AUC_{inhibited}$ and $AUC_{control}$ refer to the exposures when co-administered and not co-administered with a second drug, respectively. The term f_{CL} refers to the fraction of clearance that is mediated by the enzyme that is affected. K_i is the reversible inhibition constant and $[I]_{in\ vivo}$ is the concentration of the inhibitor available to bind to the affected enzyme *in vivo*. When dealing with an irreversible inactivator, the structure of the relationship remains the same but the $[I]_{in\ vivo}/K_i$ term is replaced with $([I]_{in\ vivo} \cdot k_{inact})/(k_{deg} \cdot ([I]_{in\ vivo} + K_I))$, in which k_{inact} is the maximum inactivation rate constant, K_I is the concentration of inactivator at which the observed inactivation rate is half of the maximum, and k_{deg} is the *in vivo* first order rate of degradation of the affected enzyme.

8.6.1
New Compounds as Potential DDI Perpetrators

For predicting whether the new compound will be a perpetrator of DDI, defining $[I]_{in\ vivo}$ and K_i is what is required. As discussed above, in hit to lead screening, abbreviated methodologies (*in vitro* and *in silico*) are applied to provide an indication of the potential to inhibit. Use of such data for predictions of DDI is done with greater risk, since the input value will not be as accurate as if measured with a standard approach. For reversible inhibition, a general rule of thumb says that compounds with inhibition potencies less than 1 µM tend to more frequently cause DDI [100]. However, it is not just the intrinsic potency but also the concentration of inhibitor *in vivo* that will impact on the magnitude of a DDI. But in an examination of over 100 CYP-based DDI, if the *in vitro* inhibition potency was at 1 µM or below, there was a greater than 80% chance that there would be a DDI with a magnitude of greater than twofold [37]. It is therefore not unreasonable to use early CYP inhibition screens (which are run using a test compound concentration of 1–5 µM) to flag those compounds that could cause DDI.

Prediction of DDI from *in vitro* inactivation data has also been accomplished. However, unlike the aforementioned simple cutoff that can be applied to inhibition data, no such simple cutoff criterion has been well established for mechanism-based inactivation kinetic parameters. Ratios of k_{inact}/k_{deg} and $[I]_{in\ vivo}/K_I$ have been shown to be related to the magnitude of DDI [50]. The early screens previously discussed rely upon abbreviated approaches to identify mechanism-based inactivation as an issue rather than provide quantitative data for predictions of DDI.

To make quantitative predictions of DDI for the new compound as perpetrator, a reliable estimate of a relevant *in vivo* concentration is needed. What is truly needed is knowledge of the concentration of the inhibitor available to bind to the enzyme. For liver, if the well accepted free-drug hypothesis (which underwrites fundamental drug action principles in pharmacology) is applied for DDI, then the use of a free intracellular liver concentration is needed. For inhibitors that are permeable through membranes, the free concentration in the portal vein should serve as the closest proxy for free intracellular concentration in the liver. Diminished permeability as well as active uptake and efflux from liver cells can confound this relationship. Nevertheless, use of estimates of unbound portal vein concentrations (which can be estimated from

Table 8.2 Comparison of pharmacological target and CYP inhibition potencies for selected oral drugs, in order of DDI magnitude. Data compiled from [104–106].

Drug	CYP	Pharmacological target	CYP potency (μM)	Target potency (μM)	Potency ratio	DDI magnitude
Ketoconazole	CYP2D6	Lanosterol 14α-demethylase	14	0.064	220	1.0
Ketoconazole	CYP1A2	Lanosterol 14α-demethylase	12	0.064	190	1.1
Terbinafine	CYP1A2	Squalene epoxidase	6.0	0.005	1200	1.2
Ketoconazole	CYP2C19	Lanosterol 14α-demethylase	4.7	0.064	73	1.4
Sertraline	CYP2D6	5HT reuptake transporter	0.9	0.0003	3000	1.5
Citalopram	CYP2D6	5HT reuptake transporter	15	0.0016	9400	1.5
Ketoconazole	CYP2C9	Lanosterol 14α-demethylase	3.0	0.064	47	1.8
Fluconazole	CYP2C9	Lanosterol 14α-demethylase	5.5	0.051	110	4.3
Terbinafine	CYP2D6	Squalene epoxidase	0.02	0.005	4	4.9
Fluconazole	CYP2C19	Lanosterol 14α-demethylase	2.9	0.051	59	6.3
Fluoxetine	CYP2D6	5HT reuptake transporter	0.13	0.0008	160	10
Ketoconazole	CYP3A	Lanosterol 14α-demethylase	0.01	0.064	0.16	17

dose) serve as reasonably reliable values for $[I]_{in\ vivo}$ in predicting DDI for reversible inhibitors [101, 102]. For inactivation, unbound systemic concentrations appear to be more reliable for DDI predictions [61]. The difference may be an indication of the fundamentally different PK/PD relationships that would be expected for reversible and irreversible "antagonists of a receptor." In early drug research, the knowledge needed to make an estimate of any *in vivo* inhibitor concentration (irrespective of the controversy around which to use) may not be present. The only information available may be the intrinsic potency for the pharmacological target of interest. In the absence of any other information, comparing the potency for the CYP enzyme and the target receptor can be of some use. If these two values are comparable, the likelihood of a DDI issue is greater. If the compound is to be administered orally, a cushion between the target potency and CYP inhibition potency must be included to account for the greater concentrations that are in the intestine and liver during absorption. A list of examples for this comparison is in Table 8.2.

8.6.2
New Compounds as Potential DDI Victims

For the new compound as victim, *in vitro* data to predict f_{CL} by the enzyme that is affected is what is critical to determine an accurate prediction. *Bona fide* values for f_{CL} are hard to obtain, even for well established drugs. At best, values are estimates and intersubject variability in the term probably overwhelms any investment in attempts to gain highly precise values. However, it is important to note that the sensitivity of the prediction of DDI increases markedly as the value of the f_{CL} exceeds 0.9 (Figure 8.4).

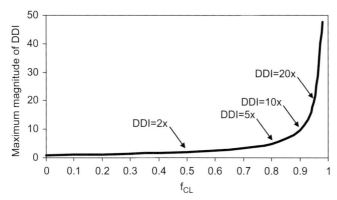

Figure 8.4 Sensitivity of DDI magnitude as a function of f_{CL}.

Values for f_{CL} can be obtained by one of three methods [102]:

1. If the enzyme is subject to genetic polymorphism with an allele coding for a nonfunctional enzyme, the comparison of the pharmacokinetics of a drug in subjects homozygous for the null allele to control subjects can yield a value for f_{CL}.

2. If one assumes that an inhibitor or inactivator, selective for an enzyme in question, can be dosed in such a manner so as to completely abolish the activity of an enzyme *in vivo*, then a clinical DDI study using that inhibitor can be used to estimate f_{CL} for that enzyme for the victim drug.

3. Using data from a human radiolabel ADME study in which metabolic pathways are fully delineated, in combination with *in vitro* data that identifies which enzymes are responsible for which metabolic pathways, values of f_{CL} can be estimated.

However, in early drug research, such data are not available. Thus, even more crude estimates must be used for f_{CL}. Since most of the important DDI are mediated by effects on the CYP enzymes, a three-tiered approach can be used to gain an assessment for f_{CL} for prediction of DDI for the new compound as a victim of DDI:

1. What fraction of clearance will occur via excretion of unchanged drug (i.e., renal or biliary) versus metabolism?
2. What fraction of metabolic clearance will be mediated by CYP enzymes versus other drug-metabolizing enzymes?
3. What fraction of CYP mediated metabolic clearance will be mediated by specific CYP enzymes?

The first question can be addressed by examining the amount of unchanged drug that is excreted in urine and bile of laboratory animals. It is generally accepted that, while there can be differences in metabolite profiles of drugs in animals and humans, overall clearance mechanisms will generally be consistent across species. For example, if a drug has a high f_{CL} by renal secretion in animals, then this will also

Table 8.3 Predicting the impact of CYP inhibitors on new compounds: values for $[I]_{in\ vivo}/K_i$ that can be inserted into the Rowland–Matin equation[a].

Perpetrator drug	Daily dose (mg)	CYP enzyme	$\dfrac{[I]_{in\ vivo}}{K_i}$
Fluconazole	300 (QD)	CYP2C9	5.5
Fluvoxamine	100 (QD)	CYP1A2	7.0
Fluvoxamine	87.9 (QD)	CYP2C19	8.9
Ketoconazole	400 (QD)	CYP3A	30 and 7500[b]
Quinidine	200 (QD)	CYP2D6	17

[a]Values were back calculated from actual in vivo DDI data for fluconazole and S-warfarin ($f_{CL,CYP2C9} = 0.91$), fluvoxamine and theophylline ($f_{CL,CYP1A2} = 0.8$), fluvoxamine and S-mephenytoin ($f_{CL,CYP2C9} = 1$), ketoconazole and midazolam ($f_{CL,CYP3A,hepatic} = 0.93$), and quinidine and desipramine ($f_{CL,CYP2D6} = 0.9$).
[b]Values for hepatic and intestinal terms, respectively.

be the case in humans, especially if this is observed in more than one animal species.

The fraction that is cleared by metabolism can be CYP- or non-CYP-mediated. In almost all cases, metabolic clearance is mediated by the liver and (for orally administered agents) by the gut as well. To gain an estimate of the fraction of metabolic clearance that is mediated by CYP, an experiment wherein the consumption of the new compound is studied in human hepatocytes in the presence and absence of 1-aminobenotrazole (ABT), is a chemical tool that can serve as a pan-CYP inactivator [90]. Also, visual inspection of the structure of the compound can lead to precluding some types of enzymes from being involved in clearance. (For example, if there is no substituent that can be subject to conjugative metabolism, then enzymes that catalyze these reactions can be eliminated from consideration.) After the f_{CL} for total CYP mediated metabolism is established, the experiments that were described earlier (Section 8.5, Reaction Phenotyping) can be done to address which specific CYP enzymes can be employed to define the values for f_{CL} for individual enzymes. When an estimate for f_{CL} is obtained, predictions of DDI can be made using standard perpetrators known to cause high inhibition/inactivation of the target enzyme. Values for $[I]_{in\ vivo}/K_i$ for some standard perpetrators that can be used in the Rowland–Matin equation are listed in Table 8.3.

The process is a bit more complicated for orally administered CYP3A-cleared compounds because a portion of the DDI can occur in the intestine during the first pass. The principles described above are the same, except that: (i) the value of f_{CL} term for the intestine can essentially be assumed as unity; and (ii) the value of $[I]_{in\ vivo}$ for the perpetrator is higher than that used for liver. Importantly, the extent to which the new compound is extracted by the intestine, which is a function of the intrinsic clearance (CL_{int}) of the new compound by CYP3A4, plays a major role in the potential magnitude of the DDI. High CL_{int} compounds can be subject to greater DDI [103].

8.7
Summary

DDI can have serious consequences in terms of product labeling and safety. It is therefore important to evaluate DDI potential at an early stage in drug discovery where changes to the molecule are still possible. In hit to lead profiling, there is still sufficient time to design out DDI, assuming the structural features required for pharmacological activity are not the perpetrators of the inhibition. In the first instance this may be achieved through *in silico* predictions to triage compound libraries. This can be followed up with appropriate *in vitro* assays. In a screening environment, all the principles of the definitive "gold standard" assay must be applied whilst increasing assay throughput. Reducing time at the bench is achieved through assay automation, abbreviated assays (e.g., single point determinations) and cocktail assays. Reducing analytical time may be accomplished through judicious choice of substrate (e.g., fluorescent plate-based assays) or assay protocol (e.g., ligand binding assay vs activity assay), however the caveats of these assays should be weighed up against the time savings incurred. Predicting *in vivo* DDI from *in vitro* data is a complex task. In hit to lead profiling it is unlikely that all the information needed to make a DDI prediction is available. DDI perpetrators are, therefore, most often ranked in terms of their own intrinsic potency or relative to the potency of the pharmacological target. In the case of a DDI victim drug, where f_{CL} is so important, compounds can again be ranked in terms of the balance of clearance mechanisms. And finally, whilst this chapter focuses on CYP enzymes, the same principles can be applied to any enzyme or transporter providing the tools to do the job are available (e.g., *in silico* models, specific substrates/inhibitors, recombinant systems).

List of Abbreviations

ADME	Absorption, distribution, metabolism and excretion
AhR	Aryl hydrocarbon receptor
CAR	Constitutive androstane receptor
Cl_{int}	Intrinsic clearance
CYP	Cytochrome P450
DDI	Drug–drug interactions
DMSO	Dimethyl sulfoxide
EC_{50}	Half maximal effective concentration
FMO	Flavin-containing monooxygenase
GST	Glutathione-S-transferase
HIV	Human immunodeficiency virus
HLM	Human liver microsomes
HPLC	High-performance liquid chromatography
IC_{50}	Inhibitor concentration to achieve half maximal activity
ISEF	Intersystem extrapolation factor
LC/MS/MS	Liquid chromatography/mass spectrometry/mass spectrometry

LC/UV	Liquid chromatography/ultraviolet detection
MAO	Monoamine oxidase
MBI	Mechanism-based inhibition
MIC	Metabolic intermediate complex
Mo-CO	Molybdenum-containing oxidase
MPO	Multi parameter optimization
NADPH	Nicotinamide adenine dinucleotide phosphate, reduced
NCE	New chemical entity
OC	Oral contraceptive
pK_a	Negative logarithm of ionization constant Ka
PSA	Polar surface area
PXR	Pregnane X receptor
QSAR	Quantitative structure–activity relationship
RAF	Relative activity factor
RPM	Revolutions per minute
SBDD	Structure-based drug design
SPA	Scintillation proximity assay
UGT	Uridine 5′-diphospho-glucuronosyltransferase (or UDP-glucuronosyltransferase)
AUC	Total area under plasma concentration time curve
F_{CL}	Fraction of clearance
[I]	Inhibitor concentration
k	Rate constant
k_{deg}	Degradation rate constantt
$k_{(I)}$	Rate constant in presence of inhibitor
K_i	Reversible inhibition constant
K_I	Enzyme inactivation constant
k_{inact}	Maximum rate of inactivation
K_M	Michaelis constant (concentration at 50% V_{max})
[S]	Substrate concentration
V_{max}	Maximum rate of reaction

References

1 Smith, C.C., Bennett, P.M., Pearce, H.M., Harrison, P.I., Reynolds, D.J., Aronson, J.K. and Grahame-Smith, D.G. (1996) Adverse drug reactions in a hospital general medical unit meriting notification to the Committee on Safety of Medicines. *British Journal of Clinical Pharmacology,* **42**, 423–429.

2 Issa, A.M., Phillips, K.A., Van Bebber, S., Nidmarthy, H.G., LAsser, K.E., Haas, J.S., Alldredge, B.K., Wachter, R.M. and Bates, D.W. (2007) Drug Withdrawals in the United States: A systematic review of the evidence and analysis of trends. *Current Drug Safety,* **2**, 177–185.

3 Huang, S.M. and Lesko, L.J. (2004) Drug–drug, drug-dietary supplement, and drug-citrus fruit and other food interactions: what have we learned? *Journal of Clinical Pharmacology,* **44**, 559–569.

4 Spina, E. and Perucca, E. (1994) Newer and older antidepressants: a comparative review of drug interactions. *CNS Drugs*, **2**, 479–497.

5 Isbister, G.K. and Buckley, N.A. (2005) The pathophysiology of serotonin toxicity in animals and humans: implications for diagnosis and treatment. *Clinical Neuropharmacology*, **28**, 205–214.

6 de Groot, M.J., Kirton, S.B. and Sutcliffe, M.J. (2004) In silico methods for predicting ligand binding determinants of cytochromes P450. *Current Topics in Medicinal Chemistry*, **4**, 1803–1824.

7 Refsgaard, H.H.F., Jensen, B.F., Christensen, I.T., Hagen, N. and Brockhoff, P.B. (2006) In silico prediction of cytochrome P450 inhibitors. *Drug Development Research*, **67**, 419–429.

8 Stoner, C.L., Gifford, E., Stankovic, C., Lepsy, C.S., Brodfuehrer, J., Prasad, J.V. and Surendran, N. (2004) Implementation of an ADME enabling selection and visualization tool for drug discovery. *Journal of Pharmaceutical Sciences*, **93**, 1131–1141.

9 Stoner, C.L., Advances in data reporting, visualization and decision making in the drug discovery process. www.touchbriefings.com/pdf/2911/stoner.pdf (19th June).

10 Wester, M.R., Yano, J.K., Schoch, G.A., Yang, C., Griffin, K.J., Stout, C.D. and Johnson, E.F. (2004) The structure of human cytochrome P450 2C9 complexed with flurbiprofen at 2.0-A resolution. *Journal of Biological Chemistry*, **279**, 35630–35637.

11 Yano, J.K., Wester, M.R., Schoch, G.A., Griffin, K.J., Stout, C.D. and Johnson, E.F. (2004) The structure of human microsomal cytochrome P450 3A4 determined by X-ray crystallography to 2.05 A resolution. *Journal of Biological Chemistry*, **279**, 38091–38094.

12 Williams, P.A., Cosme, J., Vinkovic, D.M., Ward, A., Angove, H.C., Day, P.J., Vonrhein, C., Tickle, I.J. and Jhoti, H. (2004) Crystal structures of human cytochrome P450 3A4 bound to metyrapone and progesterone. *Science*, **305**, 683–686.

13 Williams, P.A., Cosme, J., Ward, A., Angove, H.C., Matak Vinkovic, D. and Jhoti, H. (2003) Crystal structure of human cytochrome P450 2C9 with bound warfarin. *Nature*, **424**, 464–468.

14 Jefcoate, C.R. (1978) Measurement of substrate and inhibitor binding to microsomal cytochrome P-450 by optical-difference spectroscopy. *Methods in Enzymology*, **52**, 258–279.

15 Wester, M.R., Johnson, E.F., Marques-Soares, C., Dijols, S., Dansette, P.M., Mansuy, D. and Stout, C.D. (2003) Structure of mammalian cytochrome P450 2C5 complexed with diclofenac at 2.1 A resolution: evidence for an induced fit model of substrate binding. *Biochemistry*, **42**, 9335–9345.

16 Kalgutkar, A.S., Gardner, I., Obach, R.S., Shaffer, C.L., Callegari, E., Henne, K.R., Mutlib, A.E., Dalvie, D.K., Lee, J.S., Nakai, Y., O'Donnell, J.P., Boer, J. and Harriman, S.P. (2005) A comprehensive listing of bioactivation pathways of organic functional groups. *Current Drug Metabolism*, **6**, 161–225.

17 Jones, D.R., Ekins, S., Li, L. and Hall, S.D. (2007) Computational approaches that predict metabolic intermediate complex formation with CYP3A4 (+b5). *Drug Metabolism and Disposition: The Biological Fate of Chemicals*, **35**, 1466–1475.

18 Lightning, L.K., Jones, J.P., Friedberg, T., Pritchard, M.P., Shou, M., Rushmore, T.H. and Trager, W.F. (2000) Mechanism-based inactivation of cytochrome P450 3A4 by L-754,394. *Biochemistry*, **39**, 4276–4287.

19 Kumar, S., Kassahun, K., Tschirret-Guth, R.A., Mitra, K. and Baillie, T.A. (2008) Minimizing metabolic activation during pharmaceutical lead optimization: progress, knowledge gaps and future directions. *Current Opinion in Drug Discovery & Development*, **11**, 43–52.

20 Shimada, T., Yamazaki, H., Mimura, M., Inui, Y. and Guengerich, F.P. (1994) Interindividual variations in human liver cytochrome P-450 enzymes involved in the oxidation of drugs, carcinogens and toxic chemicals: studies with liver microsomes of 30 Japanese and 30 Caucasians. *Journal of Pharmacology and Experimental Therapeutics*, **270**, 414–423.

21 Yuan, R., Madani, S., Wei, X.X., Reynolds, K. and Huang, S.M. (2002) Evaluation of cytochrome P450 probe substrates commonly used by the pharmaceutical industry to study in vitro drug interactions. *Drug Metabolism and Disposition: The Biological Fate of Chemicals*, **30**, 1311–1319.

22 Williams, J.A., Hyland, R., Jones, B.C., Smith, D.A., Hurst, S., Goosen, T.C., Peterkin, V., Koup, J.R. and Ball, S.E. (2004) Drug–drug interactions for UDP-glucuronosyltransferase substrates: a pharmacokinetic explanation for typically observed low exposure (AUCi/AUC) ratios. *Drug Metabolism and Disposition: The Biological Fate of Chemicals*, **32**, 1201–1208.

23 Chauret, N., Gauthier, A. and Nicoll-Griffith, D.A. (1998) Effect of common organic solvents on in vitro cytochrome P450-mediated metabolic activities in human liver microsomes. *Drug Metabolism and Disposition: The Biological Fate of Chemicals*, **26**, 1–4.

24 Uchaipichat, V., Mackenzie, P.I., Guo, X.H., Gardner-Stephen, D., Galetin, A., Houston, J.B. and Miners, J.O. (2004) Human udp-glucuronosyltransferases: isoform selectivity and kinetics of 4-methylumbelliferone and 1-naphthol glucuronidation, effects of organic solvents, and inhibition by diclofenac and probenecid. *Drug Metabolism and Disposition: The Biological Fate of Chemicals*, **32**, 413–423.

25 Zientek, M., Miller, H., Smith, D., Dunklee, M., Heinle, L., Thurston, A., Lee, C., Hyland, R., Fahmi, O. and Burdette, D. (2009) Development of an in vitro drug–drug interaction assay to simultaneously monitor five cytochrome P450 isoforms and performance assessment using drug library compounds. *Journal of Pharmacological and Toxicological Methods*, in press.

26 Cohen, L.H., Remley, M.J., Raunig, D. and Vaz, A.D. (2003) In vitro drug interactions of cytochrome p450: an evaluation of fluorogenic to conventional substrates. *Drug Metabolism and Disposition: The Biological Fate of Chemicals*, **31**, 1005–1015.

27 Jenkins, K.M., Angeles, R., Quintos, M.T., Xu, R., Kassel, D.B. and Rourick, R.A. (2004) Automated high throughput ADME assays for metabolic stability and cytochrome P450 inhibition profiling of combinatorial libraries. *Journal of Pharmaceutical and Biomedical Analysis*, **34**, 989–1004.

28 Gao, F., Johnson, D.L., Ekins, S., Janiszewski, J., Kelly, K.G., Meyer, R.D. and West, M. (2002) Optimizing higher throughput methods to assess drug–drug interactions for CYP1A2, CYP2C9, CYP2C19, CYP2D6, rCYP2D6, and CYP3A4 in vitro using a single point IC (50). *Journal of Biomolecular Screening*, **7**, 373–382.

29 Moody, G.C., Griffin, S.J., Mather, A.N., McGinnity, D.F. and Riley, R.J. (1999) Fully automated analysis of activities catalysed by the major human liver cytochrome P450 (CYP) enzymes: assessment of human CYP inhibition potential. *Xenobiotica*, **29**, 53–75.

30 Venkatakrishnan, K., von Moltke, L.L., Obach, R.S. and Greenblatt, D.J. (2003) Drug metabolism and drug interactions: application and clinical value of in vitro models. *Current Drug Metabolism*, **4**, 423–459.

31 Bu, H.Z., Knuth, K., Magis, L. and Teitelbaum, P. (2000) High-throughput cytochrome P450 inhibition screening via cassette probe-dosing strategy. IV. Validation of a direct injection on-line

guard cartridge extraction/tandem mass spectrometry method for simultaneous CYP3A4, 2D6 and 2E1 inhibition assessment. *Rapid Communications in Mass Spectrometry,* **14**, 1943–1948.

32 Bu, H.Z., Knuth, K., Magis, L. and Teitelbaum, P. (2001) High-throughput cytochrome P450 (CYP) inhibition screening via cassette probe-dosing strategy: III. Validation of a direct injection/on-line guard cartridge extraction-tandem mass spectrometry method for CYP2C19 inhibition evaluation. *Journal of Pharmaceutical and Biomedical Analysis,* **25**, 437–442.

33 Bu, H.Z., Knuth, K., Magis, L. and Teitelbaum, P. (2001) High-throughput cytochrome P450 (CYP) inhibition screening via a cassette probe-dosing strategy. V. Validation of a direct injection/on-line guard cartridge extraction--tandem mass spectrometry method for CYP1A2 inhibition assessment. *European Journal of Pharmaceutical Sciences,* **12**, 447–452.

34 Bu, H.Z., Magis, L., Knuth, K. and Teitelbaum, P. (2000) High-throughput cytochrome P450 (CYP) inhibition screening via cassette probe-dosing strategy. I. Development of direct injection/on-line guard cartridge extraction/tandem mass spectrometry for the simultaneous detection of CYP probe substrates and their metabolites. *Rapid Communications in Mass Spectrometry,* **14**, 1619–1624.

35 Bu, H.Z., Magis, L., Knuth, K. and Teitelbaum, P. (2001) High-throughput cytochrome P450 (CYP) inhibition screening via a cassette probe-dosing strategy. VI. Simultaneous evaluation of inhibition potential of drugs on human hepatic isozymes CYP2A6, 3A4, 2C9, 2D6 and 2E1. *Rapid Communications in Mass Spectrometry,* **15**, 741–748.

36 Bu, H.Z., Magis, L., Knuth, K. and Teitelbaum, P. (2001) High-throughput cytochrome P450 (CYP) inhibition screening via cassette probe-dosing strategy. II. Validation of a direct injection/on-line guard cartridge extraction-tandem mass spectrometry method for CYP2D6 inhibition assessment. *Journal of Chromatography. B, Biomedical Sciences and Applications,* **753**, 321–326.

37 Obach, R.S., Walsky, R.L., Venkatakrishnan, K., Houston, J.B. and Tremaine, L.M. (2005) *In vitro* cytochrome P450 inhibition data and the prediction of drug–drug interactions: qualitative relationships, quantitative predictions, and the rank-order approach. *Clinical Pharmacology and Therapeutics,* **78**, 582–592.

38 Smith, D., Sadagopan, N., Zientek, M., Reddy, A. and Cohen, L. (2007) Analytical approaches to determine cytochrome P450 inhibitory potential of new chemical entities in drug discovery. *Journal of Chromatography. B, Analytical Technologies in the Biomedical and Life Sciences,* **850**, 455–463.

39 Walsky, R.L. and Obach, R.S. (2004) Validated assays for human cytochrome P450 activities. *Drug Metabolism and Disposition: The Biological Fate of Chemicals,* **32**, 647–660.

40 Youdim, K.A., Lyons, R., Payne, L., Jones, B.C. and Saunders, K. (2009) An automated, high-throughput, 384 well Cytochrome P450 cocktail IC50 assay using a rapid resolution LC–MS/MS endpoint. *Journal of Pharmaceutical and Biomedical Analysis,* in press.

41 Di, L., Kerns, E.H., Li, S.Q. and Carter, G.T. (2007) Comparison of cytochrome P450 inhibition assays for drug discovery using human liver microsomes with LC-MS, rhCYP450 isozymes with fluorescence, and double cocktail with LC-MS. *International Journal of Pharmaceutics,* **335**, 1–11.

42 Tucker, G., Houston, B. and Huang, S. (2001) Optimizing drug development: strategies to assess drug metabolism/transporter interaction potential – toward a consensus. *Pharmaceutical Research,* V18, 1071–1080.

43 Walsky, R.L., Obach, R.S., Gaman, E.A., Gleeson, J.P. and Proctor, W.R. (2005) Selective inhibition of human cytochrome P4502C8 by montelukast. *Drug Metabolism and Disposition: The Biological Fate of Chemicals*, **33**, 413–418.

44 Cawley, G.F., Batie, C.J. and Backes, W.L. (1995) Substrate-dependent competition of different P450 isozymes for limiting NADPH-cytochrome P450 reductase. *Biochemistry*, **34**, 1244–1247.

45 West, S.B. and Lu, A.Y. (1972) Reconstituted liver microsomal enzyme system that hydroxylates drugs, other foreign compounds and endogenous substrates. V. Competition between cytochromes P-450 and P-448 for reductase in 3,4-benzpyrene hydroxylation. *Archives of Biochemistry and Biophysics*, **153**, 298–303.

46 Weaver, R., Graham, K.S., Beattie, I.G. and Riley, R.J. (2003) Cytochrome P450 inhibition using recombinant proteins and mass spectrometry/multiple reaction monitoring technology in a cassette incubation. *Drug Metabolism and Disposition: The Biological Fate of Chemicals*, **31**, 955–966.

47 Fontana, E., Dansette, P.M. and Poli, S.M. (2005) Cytochrome p450 enzymes mechanism based inhibitors: common sub-structures and reactivity. *Current Drug Metabolism*, **6**, 413–454.

48 Hollenberg, P.F., Kent, U.M. and Bumpus, N.N. (2008) Mechanism-based inactivation of human cytochromes p450s: experimental characterization, reactive intermediates, and clinical implications. *Chemical Research in Toxicology*, **21**, 189–205, Epub 2007 Dec 4.

49 Kalgutkar, A.S., Obach, R.S. and Maurer, T.S. (2007) Mechanism-based inactivation of cytochrome P450 enzymes: chemical mechanisms, structure-activity relationships and relationship to clinical drug–drug interactions and idiosyncratic adverse drug reactions. *Current Drug Metabolism*, **8**, 407–447.

50 Venkatakrishnan, K., Obach, R.S. and Rostami-Hodjegan, A. (2007) Mechanism-based inactivation of human cytochrome P450 enzymes: strategies for diagnosis and drug–drug interaction risk assessment. *Xenobiotica*, **37**, 1225–1256.

51 Polasek, T.M. and Miners, J.O. (2007) In vitro approaches to investigate mechanism-based inactivation of CYP enzymes. *Expert Opinion on Drug Metabolism and Toxicology*, **3**, 321–329.

52 Ghanbari, F., Rowland-Yeo, K., Bloomer, J.C., Clarke, S.E., Lennard, M.S., Tucker, G.T. and Rostami-Hodjegan, A. (2006) A critical evaluation of the experimental design of studies of mechanism based enzyme inhibition, with implications for in vitro-in vivo extrapolation. *Current Drug Metabolism*, **7**, 315–334.

53 Van, L.M., Heydari, A., Yang, J., Hargreaves, J., Rowland-Yeo, K., Lennard, M.S., Tucker, G.T. and Rostami-Hodjegan, A. (2006) The impact of experimental design on assessing mechanism-based inactivation of CYP2D6 by MDMA (Ecstasy). *Journal of Psychopharmacology* (Oxford, England), **20**, 834–841. Epub 2006 Feb 14.

54 Riley, R.J., Grime, K. and Weaver, R. (2007) Time-dependent CYP inhibition. *Expert Opinion on Drug Metabolism and Toxicology*, **3**, 51–66.

55 Kent, U.M., Juschyshyn, M.I. and Hollenberg, P.F. (2001) Mechanism-based inactivators as probes of cytochrome P450 structure and function. *Current Drug Metabolism*, **2**, 215–243.

56 Polasek, T.M., Elliot, D.J., Somogyi, A.A., Gillam, E.M., Lewis, B.C. and Miners, J.O. (2006) An evaluation of potential mechanism-based inactivation of human drug metabolizing cytochromes P450 by monoamine oxidase inhibitors, including isoniazid. *British Journal of Clinical Pharmacology*, **61**, 570–584.

57 Yamamoto, T., Suzuki, A. and Kohno, Y. (2004) High-throughput screening for the assessment of time-dependent inhibitions of new drug candidates on

recombinant CYP2D6 and CYP3A4 using a single concentration method. *Xenobiotica*, **34**, 87–101.

58 Atkinson, A., Kenny, J.R. and Grime, K. (2005) Automated assessment of time-dependent inhibition of human cytochrome P450 enzymes using liquid chromatography-tandem mass spectrometry analysis. *Drug Metabolism and Disposition: The Biological Fate of Chemicals*, **33**, 1637–1647.

59 Fairman, D.A., Collins, C. and Chapple, S. (2007) Progress curve analysis of CYP1A2 inhibition: a more informative approach to the assessment of mechanism-based inactivation? *Drug Metabolism and Disposition: The Biological Fate of Chemicals*, **35**, 2159–2165, Epub 2007 Sep 6.

60 Bertelsen, K.M., Venkatakrishnan, K., Von Moltke, L.L., Obach, R.S. and Greenblatt, D.J. (2003) Apparent mechanism-based inhibition of human CYP2D6 *in vitro* by paroxetine: comparison with fluoxetine and quinidine. *Drug Metabolism and Disposition: The Biological Fate of Chemicals*, **31**, 289–293.

61 Obach, R.S., Walsky, R.L. and Venkatakrishnan, K. (2007) Mechanism-based inactivation of human cytochrome p450 enzymes and the prediction of drug–drug interactions. *Drug Metabolism and Disposition: The Biological Fate of Chemicals*, **35**, 246–255, Epub 2006 Nov 8.

62 Yasuda, K., Ranade, A., Venkataramanan, R., Strom, S., Chupka, J., Ekins, S., Schuetz, E. and Bachmann, K. (2008) A comprehensive *in vitro* and in silico analysis of antibiotics that activate PXR and Induce CYP3A4 in liver and intestine. *Drug Metabolism and Disposition: the Biological Fate of Chemicals*.

63 Smith, D.A. (2000) Induction and drug development. *European Journal of Pharmaceutical Sciences*, **11**, 185–189.

64 Strong, J. and Huang, S. (2008) U.S. regulatory perspective: drug–drug interactions, in *Drug–drug Interactions in Pharmaceutical Development* (ed. A.P. Li), John Wiley and Sons Inc., pp. 201–226.

65 Benedetti, M.S. (2000) Enzyme induction and inhibition by new antiepileptic drugs: a review of human studies. *Fundamental & Clinical Pharmacology*, **14**, 301–319.

66 Stanley, L.A., Horsburgh, B.C., Ross, J., Scheer, N. and Wolf, C.R. (2006) PXR and CAR: nuclear receptors which play a pivotal role in drug disposition and chemical toxicity. *Drug Metabolism Reviews*, **38**, 515–597.

67 Tirona, R.G. and Kim, R.B. (2005) Nuclear receptors and drug disposition gene regulation. *Journal of Pharmaceutical Sciences*, **94**, 1169–1186.

68 Novak, R.F. and Woodcroft, K.J. (2000) The alcohol-inducible form of cytochrome P450 (CYP 2E1): role in toxicology and regulation of expression. *Arch. Pharmaceutical Research*, **23**, 267–282.

69 Kliewer, S.A. and Willson, T.M. (2002) Regulation of xenobiotic and bile acid metabolism by the nuclear pregnane X receptor. *Journal of Lipid Research*, **43**, 359–364.

70 Jones, S.A., Moore, L.B., Wisely, G.B. and Kliewer, S.A. (2002) Use of *in vitro* pregnane X receptor assays to assess CYP3A4 induction potential of drug candidates. *Methods in Enzymology*, **357**, 161–170.

71 Zhu, Z., Kim, S., Chen, T., Lin, J.H., Bell, A., Bryson, J., Dubaquie, Y., Yan, N., Yanchunas, J., Xie, D., Stoffel, R., Sinz, M. and Dickinson, K. (2004) Correlation of high-throughput pregnane X receptor (PXR) transactivation and binding assays. *Journal of Biomolecular Screening*, **9**, 533–540.

72 Cui, X., Palamanda, J., Norton, L., Thomas, A., Lau, Y.Y., White, R.E. and Cheng, K.C. (2002) A high-throughput cell-based reporter gene system for measurement of CYP1A1 induction. *Journal of Pharmacological and Toxicological Methods*, **47**, 143–151.

73 Luo, G., Cunningham, M., Kim, S., Burn, T., Lin, J., Sinz, M., Hamilton, G., Rizzo, C., Jolley, S., Gilbert, D., Downey, A., Mudra, D., Graham, R., Carroll, K., Xie, J., Madan, A., Parkinson, A., Christ, D., Selling, B., LeCluyse, E. and Gan, L.S. (2002) CYP3A4 induction by drugs: correlation between a pregnane X receptor reporter gene assay and CYP3A4 expression in human hepatocytes. *Drug Metabolism and Disposition: The Biological Fate of Chemicals*, **30**, 795–804.

74 El-Sankary, W., Gibson, G.G., Ayrton, A. and Plant, N. (2001) Use of a reporter gene assay to predict and rank the potency and efficacy of CYP3A4 inducers. *Drug Metabolism and Disposition: The Biological Fate of Chemicals*, **29**, 1499–1504.

75 Lemaire, G., de Sousa, G. and Rahmani, R. (2004) A PXR reporter gene assay in a stable cell culture system: CYP3A4 and CYP2B6 induction by pesticides. *Biochemical Pharmacology*, **68**, 2347–2358.

76 Raucy, J., Warfe, L., Yueh, M.F. and Allen, S.W. (2002) A cell-based reporter gene assay for determining induction of CYP3A4 in a high-volume system. *Journal of Pharmacology and Experimental Therapeutics*, **303**, 412–423.

77 Noracharttiyapot, W., Nagai, Y., Matsubara, T., Miyata, M., Shimada, M., Nagata, K. and Yamazoe, Y. (2006) Construction of several human-derived stable cell lines displaying distinct profiles of CYP3A4 induction. *Drug Metab. Pharmacokinet.*, **21**, 99–108.

78 Persson, K.P., Ekehed, S., Otter, C., Lutz, E.S., McPheat, J., Masimirembwa, C.M. and Andersson, T.B. (2006) Evaluation of human liver slices and reporter gene assays as systems for predicting the cytochrome p450 induction potential of drugs *in vivo* in humans. *Pharmaceutical Research*, **23**, 56–69.

79 Sinz, M., Kim, S., Zhu, Z., Chen, T., Anthony, M., Dickinson, K. and Rodrigues, A.D. (2006) Evaluation of 170 xenobiotics as transactivators of human pregnane X receptor (hPXR) and correlation to known CYP3A4 drug interactions. *Current Drug Metabolism*, **7**, 375–388.

80 Swales, K. and Negishi, M. (2004) CAR, driving into the future. *Molecular Endocrinology* (Baltimore, MD), **18**, 1589–1598.

81 Harmsen, S., Koster, A.S., Beijnen, J.H., Schellens, J.H. and Meijerman, I. (2008) Comparison of two immortalized human cell lines to study nuclear receptor-mediated CYP3A4 induction. *Drug Metabolism and Disposition: The Biological Fate of Chemicals*, **36**, 1166–1171.

82 Hariparsad, N., Carr, B.A., Evers, R. and Chu, X. (2008) Comparison of immortalized Fa2N-4 cells and human hepatocytes as *in vitro* models for cytochrome P450 induction. *Drug Metabolism and Disposition: The Biological Fate of Chemicals*, **36**, 1046–1055.

83 Mills, J.B., Rose, K.A., Sadagopan, N., Sahi, J. and de Morais, S.M. (2004) Induction of drug metabolism enzymes and MDR1 using a novel human hepatocyte cell line. *Journal of Pharmacology and Experimental Therapeutics*, **309**, 303–309.

84 Ripp, S.L., Mills, J.B., Fahmi, O.A., Trevena, K.A., Liras, J.L., Maurer, T.S. and de Morais, S.M. (2006) Use of immortalized human hepatocytes to predict the magnitude of clinical drug–drug interactions caused by CYP3A4 induction. *Drug Metabolism and Disposition: The Biological Fate of Chemicals*, **34**, 1742–1748.

85 Lamb, D.C., Waterman, M.R., Kelly, S.L. and Guengerich, F.P. (2007) Cytochromes P450 and drug discovery. *Current Opinion in Biotechnology*, **18**, 504–512, Epub 2007 Nov 19.

86 Miners, J.O., Knights, K.M., Houston, J.B. and Mackenzie, P.I. (2006) *In vitro-in vivo* correlation for drugs and other compounds eliminated by glucuronidation in humans: pitfalls and promises. *Biochemical Pharmacology*, **71**, 1531–1539, Epub 2006 Feb 7.

87 Bachmann, K.A. (2002) Genotyping and phenotyping the cytochrome p-450 enzymes. *American Journal of Therapy*, 9, 309–316.

88 Venkatakrishnan, K., Von Moltke, L.L. and Greenblatt, D.J. (2001) Human drug metabolism and the cytochromes P450: application and relevance of *in vitro* models. *Journal of Clinical Pharmacology*, 41, 1149–1179.

89 Zhang, H., Davis, C.D., Sinz, M.W. and Rodrigues, A.D. (2007) Cytochrome P450 reaction-phenotyping: an industrial perspective. *Expert Opinion on Drug Metabolism and Toxicology*, 3, 667–687.

90 Williams, J.A., Hurst, S.I., Bauman, J., Jones, B.C., Hyland, R., Gibbs, J.P., Obach, R.S. and Ball, S.E. (2003) Reaction phenotyping in drug discovery: moving forward with confidence? *Current Drug Metabolism*, 4, 527–534.

91 Huang, S.M., Temple, R., Throckmorton, D.C. and Lesko, L.J. (2007) Drug interaction studies: study design, data analysis, and implications for dosing and labeling. *Clinical Pharmacology and Therapeutics*, 81, 298–304.

92 Kumar, V., Rock, D.A., Warren, C.J., Tracy, T.S. and Wahlstrom, J.L. (2006) Enzyme source effects on CYP2C9 kinetics and inhibition. *Drug Metabolism and Disposition: The Biological Fate of Chemicals*, 34, 1903–1908, Epub 2006 Aug 23.

93 Dickins, M., Galetin, A. and Proctor, N. (2007) Modelling and simulation of pharmacokinetic aspects of cytochrome P450-based metabolic drud-drug interactions, in *Comprehensive Medicinal Chemistry II*, vol. 5 (eds J.B. Taylor and D.J. Triggle), Elsevier Ltd, Oxford, pp. 827–846.

94 Tang, W. and Stearns, R.A. (2001) Heterotropic cooperativity of cytochrome P450 3A4 and potential drug–drug interactions. *Current Drug Metabolism*, 2, 185–198.

95 Nakajima, M., Tane, K., Nakamura, S., Shimada, N., Yamazaki, H. and Yokoi, T. (2002) Evaluation of approach to predict the contribution of multiple cytochrome P450s in drug metabolism using relative activity factor: effects of the differences in expression levels of NADPH-cytochrome P450 reductase and cytochrome b(5) in the expression system and the differences in the marker activities. *Journal of Pharmaceutical Sciences*, 91, 952–963.

96 Venkatakrishnan, K. and Obach, R.S. (2005) *In vitro-in vivo* extrapolation of CYP2D6 inactivation by paroxetine: prediction of nonstationary pharmacokinetics and drug interaction magnitude. *Drug Metabolism and Disposition: The Biological Fate of Chemicals*, 33, 845–852.

97 Crespi, C.L. (1995) Xenobiotic-metabolizing human cells as tools for pharmacological and toxicological research, in *Advances in Drug Research* (eds U.A. Meyer and B. Testa), Academic Press, New York, pp. 179–235.

98 Proctor, N.J., Tucker, G.T. and Rostami-Hodjegan, A. (2004) Predicting drug clearance from recombinantly expressed CYPs: intersystem extrapolation factors. *Xenobiotica*, 34, 151–178.

99 Rowland, M. and Matin, S.B. (1973) Kinetics of drug–drug interactions. *Journal of Pharmacokinetics and Biopharmaceutics*, 1, 553–567.

100 Wrighton, S.A., Schuetz, E.G., Thummel, K.E., Shen, D.D., Korzekwa, K.R. and Watkins, P.B. (2000) The human CYP3A subfamily: practical considerations. *Drug Metabolism Reviews*, 32, 339–361.

101 Kanamitsu, S., Ito, K. and Sugiyama, Y. (2000) Quantitative prediction of *in vivo* drug–drug interactions from *in vitro* data based on physiological pharmacokinetics: use of maximum unbound concentration of inhibitor at the inlet to the liver. *Pharmaceutical Research*, 17, 336–343.

102 Obach, R.S., Walsky, R.L., Venkatakrishnan, K., Gaman, E.A.,

Houston, J.B. and Tremaine, L.M. (2006) The utility of *in vitro* cytochrome P450 inhibition data in the prediction of drug–drug interactions. *Journal of Pharmacology and Experimental Therapeutics*, **316**, 336–348.
103 Galetin, A., Hinton, L.K., Burt, H., Obach, R.S. and Houston, J.B. (2007) Maximal inhibition of intestinal first-pass metabolism as a pragmatic indicator of intestinal contribution to the drug–drug interactions for CYP3A4 cleared drugs. *Current Drug Metabolism*, **8**, 685–693.
104 Baldessarini, R.J. (2001) Drugs and the treatment of psychiatric disorders. Depression and anxiety disorders, *Goodman and Gilman's The Pharmacological Basis of Therapeutics*, 10th edn (eds J.G. Hardman and L.E. Limbird), McGraw Hill, pp. 447–483.
105 Georgopapadakou, N.H. and Bertasso, A. (1992) Effects of squalene epoxidase inhibitors on Candida albicans. *Antimicrobial Agents and Chemotherapy*, **36**, 1779–1781.
106 Trosken, E.R., Adamska, M., Arand, M., Zarn, J.A., Patten, C., Volkel, W. and Lutz, W.K. (2006) Comparison of lanosterol-14 alpha-demethylase (CYP51) of human and Candida albicans for inhibition by different antifungal azoles. *Toxicology*, **228**, 24–32.

9
Plasma Protein Binding and Volume of Distribution: Determination, Prediction and Use in Early Drug Discovery

Franco Lombardo, R. Scott Obach, and Nigel J. Waters

9.1
Introduction: Importance of Plasma Protein Binding

The importance of plasma protein binding primarily resides in its impact on pharmacokinetic properties such as clearance and volume of distribution, as well as potency and CNS penetration. However plasma protein binding is generally not, in itself, a deciding factor when consideration is given to the advancement of a compound to further studies and development, nor does a change in plasma protein binding mean much from a clinical relevance perspective [1]. Plasma protein binding is rather a "modulator" or a "buffer" of the free drug concentration; and a nice treatment of this aspect is offered by Trainor [2]. Also, as explained in the following sections, the values are generally reported as equilibrium values and they are determined in plasma with little or no consideration toward possible physiological variability of plasma protein content and the on/off rate. Thus, they represent "bulk" values and relevant examples of apparent exceptions are presented in the following section, with caveats mentioned in the section on the determination of plasma protein binding values. One more word of caution in interpreting the results can be offered when dealing with highly protein-bound compounds. A small percent difference, for example, 3% difference between 99% bound and 96% bound represents a fourfold difference in free fraction, while a 3% difference between say 76% bound and 73% bound represents only a 1.1-fold difference in free fraction. And, of course, a value of 99.9% bound versus a value of 99% bound represents a 10-fold difference, but measuring a value of >99% with confidence is generally problematic.

9.2
Impact of Plasma Protein Binding on PK, Exposure, Safety Margins, Potency Screens and Drug–Drug Interaction

According to the free drug hypothesis only the unbound drug is available to act at physiological sites of action, whether it is the intended pharmacological target, or action at an undesired site with potential toxicological consequences and a schematic

Hit and Lead Profiling. Edited by Bernard Faller and Laszlo Urban
Copyright © 2009 WILEY-VCH Verlag GmbH & Co. KGaA, Weinheim
ISBN: 978-3-527-32331-9

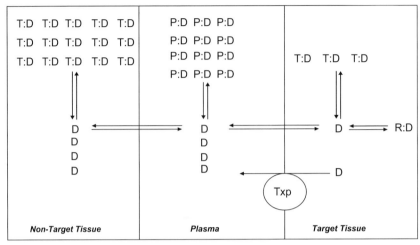

Figure 9.1 In this scheme, there are three compartments represented, the central (plasma) compartment, the target compartment, and all other tissues compartment. The letters represent the following: D = drug, P = plasma protein, T = non-specific tissue binding sites, R = target receptor, Txp = drug transporter. All binding interactions are reversible and the drug can readily traverse the membranes that divide the various compartments. In the plasma, the scheme shows 12 drug molecules bound and four free, indicating a value for fu of 0.25. The drug can readily penetrate the non-target tissues and there is binding capacity for the drug in these tissues. The fu(tissue) value is 0.16, which is lower than the plasma free fraction, but the free concentration is still the same (4D). In the target tissue, there is also non-specific binding capacity as well binding to the target receptor. The fu(target tissue) is 0.33, but the free drug concentration is lower (2D) due to active transport from the tissue. If both target and non-target tissues are included together, the fu(tissue) value would be 0.20 (6/30).

representation of the partition phenomena between plasma and target as well as non-target tissues is shown in Figure 9.1. In either case, assessing drug exposure as the area under the plasma concentration–time curve (AUC) or maximal plasma concentration (C_{max}), expressed in their free forms (i.e., unbound AUC, unbound C_{max}) can be paramount. In pharmacodynamic studies of the azole antifungals, Andes et al. [3] using a mouse model of disseminated candidiasis, showed that the free AUC-to-MIC (minimum inhibitory concentration) ratio was the pharmacokinetic–pharmacodynamic (PK-PD) parameter most predictive of efficacy for voriconazole. This correlated well with large clinical studies on voriconazole, where free drug AUC was considered rather than total drug AUC [4]. Similar work on the fluoroquinolone antibiotics has shown free AUC/MIC ratio to be a successful predictor of efficacy in a rat model of pneumococcal pneumonia, and in the case of moxifloxacin, the free AUC/MIC was similar to that reported in human [5]. In clinical studies of the bcr-abl/c-kit inhibitor, imatinib, in patients with advanced gastrointestinal stromal tumors, hematotoxicity was assessed as percent absolute neutrophil count and percent platelets. These parameters were correlated to the estimated AUC at steady state, with correlations using unbound AUC being stronger than those to total AUC [6]. In addition to assessing and understanding PK-PD and exposure–toxicity relationships, expressing AUC and C_{max} in their free forms allows direct compound comparisons to be made at the lead and candidate selection phases of drug discovery.

There are cases where differences in plasma protein binding arising as a result of inter-species variation or in numerous disease states, can affect the pharmacokinetics and pharmacodynamics of a drug. In Phase I clinical studies on the antitumor agent, UCN-01, the clearance and steady state distribution volume were markedly lower than that expected from studies in preclinical species. The percent unbound in human plasma at 1 μg/mL was <0.02% compared to 0.42, 1.75 and 1.17% in dog, rat and mouse respectively. Further studies illustrated UCN-01 binds to a single, saturable high-affinity binding site on human α1-acid glycoprotein (AAG), with an association constant (K_a) of 803×10^6 L/mol [7]. This K_a is >10-fold higher than for typical ligands such as dipyridamol, disopyramide and thioridazine (K_a 15.5×10^6, 1×10^6 and 63×10^6 L/mol, respectively). As well as a cause of species variation, plasma proteins can lead to variation in clinical response. Albumin concentrations (physiologically around 40 g/L in humans) are known to vary in a number of diseases and altered physiological states, including liver and renal disease, surgery, trauma, pneumonia and sepsis. In many cases, patients with burns, cirrhosis or nephrotic syndrome, may have plasma albumin concentrations as low as 20–30% of normal, down at ~10 g/L. Hypoalbuminemia leads to an increase in free fraction and has been observed with the NSAIDs, diflunisal, naproxen, phenylbutazone and salicylate [8]. As an acute phase protein, plasma concentrations of AAG are known to be increased in a number of pathologies, including trauma, inflammation, bacterial infection and cancer, while the generally accepted physiological value is around 0.75 g/L. It is thought to serve a protective function by binding toxic entities such as lectins, endotoxins and bacterial lipopolysaccharide, but in doing so also acts to lower free therapeutic drug levels. The clinical pharmacokinetics of imatinib in cancer patients has been shown to be dependent on the levels of circulating AAG. The inter-individual variability in imatinib clearance was significantly reduced when normalized for the plasma AAG concentration [6]. Comparable clinical findings have been presented on the anti-arrhythmic agent, pilsicainide, where patients with increased levels of C-reactive protein and AAG exhibited lower clearance and increased total plasma concentrations of pilsicainide [9].

The impact of plasma protein binding on the extent of renal drug clearance has been investigated *in vitro* and *in vivo*, although not in parallel with the plethora of work in the area of drug transporters. The organic anion, p-aminohippurate, binds with low affinity to serum albumin ($K_a \sim 2.3 \times 10^3$ L/mol) and its renal clearance of ~10 mL/min/kg greatly exceeds that of the glomerular filtration rate (GFR, ~1.8 mL/min/kg) indicating efficient active tubular secretion. In contrast, ochratoxin A (OTA), a naturally occurring mycotoxin, binds with high affinity to serum albumin (K_a 5×10^6 L/mol, more than 1000 times that of p-aminohippurate) leading to a renal clearance of only 0.002 mL/min/kg. This occurs despite the fact OTA is a high affinity substrate of the organic anion transporters (OATs) expressed on the proximal tubular membrane [10]. The importance of free drug concentrations in transporter-mediated clearance has been investigated *in vitro* using ochratoxin A, estrone sulfate and methotrexate. In both oocyte expression systems and the MDCK cell line transfected with human OAT1, the presence of albumin (0.5% w/v, eightfold lower than *in vivo* concentrations) essentially eliminated the uptake of OTA. This was confirmed using OAT1 substrates, estrone-3-sulfate (ES) and methotrexate (MTX), that bind to albumin with lower affinity (OTA > ES > MTX). Increasing albumin concentrations to physiological levels did not inhibit the accumulation of MTX in hOAT1-expressing oocytes, and is in agreement with *in vivo* data where the renal CL ($\sim$2.8 mL/min/kg) exceeds GFR (human GFR$\sim$1.8 mL/min/kg). Accumulation of ES in hOAT1-expressing oocytes was significantly inhibited by albumin concentrations >0.5% (w/v), correlating well with ES renal CL *in vivo* ($\sim$0.04 mL/min/kg) indicating no active secretion. The understanding of active drug transport in drug disposition has expanded greatly in recent years and the role of plasma protein binding may need to be carefully considered in extrapolation to the *in vivo* situation.

The prediction of clinical CYP-mediated drug–drug interactions (DDI) from *in vitro* data using models based on the ratio of inhibitor concentration [I] to the inhibition constant, K_i, also relies on assessment of fraction unbound in plasma and there are many reports discussing the relative merits of total and unbound inhibitor concentration [11–13]. With respect to reversible CYP inhibition, the use of unbound hepatic inlet inhibitor concentration is considered most predictive whilst for time-dependent CYP inhibition the unbound systemic C_{max} appears to be more relevant [14]. Although the use of different inhibitor concentrations depending on the inhibitory mechanism requires further investigation, it is clear the free, as opposed to total, drug concentration is crucial.

The consensus with respect to plasma protein binding displacement interactions is that they are of minor clinical significance ([15]; [1]). For two highly bound drugs proposed to cause a plasma protein binding displacement interaction, the pharmacokinetic implications can be thought of as follows: (i) the displacer causes the volume of distribution of the displaced drug to increase, as less displaced drug is in the plasma compared with tissues, as the tissue:plasma equilibrium is re-established; (ii) any increase in free levels of the displaced drug is also available for drug elimination. Hence, any increase in pharmacological effect of the displaced drug is transient and cannot be sustained. Thus, the overall result of displacement is that it may cause a minor transient increase in free drug concentration and effect, but the mean steady-state free drug concentration will be unaltered. It is the interpretation of total drug concentrations when using therapeutic drug monitoring that can be affected. An example of this type of interaction is seen when valproic acid and phenytoin are co-administered and the interpretation of total phenytoin concentration is confounded by the increase in free fraction [16].

Although PPB displacement has little clinical significance as a mechanism of DDI itself, it can confound the *in vitro* prediction of metabolic DDI such that an increase in free fraction of a drug by a displacer increases its hepatic clearance based on total plasma drug concentration that, in turn, may mask a concomitant effect of the displacer as an enzyme inhibitor in decreasing drug clearance. One such example is that of warfarin and gemfibrozil, where the expected increase in total warfarin AUC, as a result of gemfibrozil-mediated CYP2C9 inhibition, is not observed. Interestingly, this may be the case for many 2C9 interactions given the overlapping SAR with serum albumin affinity. Hence, equations describing human serum albumin displacement are incorporated into quantitative DDI models like SimCyp [17]. Although PPB displacement for serum albumin is a rare event, it may be key for AAG, which is easier to saturate and as an acute phase protein, exhibits variable expression dependent on disease state, genetics and so on.

The impact of plasma or serum drug binding on *in vitro* potency is a common observation in drug discovery programs where addition of the plasma or serum fraction to the *in vitro* system expressing the target receptor/enzyme, renders a drop-off in activity. The presence of serum albumin (typically bovine or human) or whole serum (e.g., fetal calf) lowers the free drug concentrations resulting in a rightward shift in the IC_{50} or EC_{50} potency curve. This was recently demonstrated using cocaine-induced sodium channel blockade in cardiac myocytes, where the presence of α1-acid glycoprotein (AAG) reversed the action of cocaine in a dose-dependent manner [18]. Similarly, the intracellular accumulation of the HIV protease inhibitors, saquinavir, ritonavir and indinavir, was shown to be reduced by the presence of increasing concentrations of AAG *in vitro*, impacting on antiviral activity *in vitro* [19]. An important consideration with *in vitro* cell culture assays is the usual requirement for 10% fetal calf serum in order to maintain cell viability, with cultures typically not being able to tolerate growth media containing >50% human serum. This leads to two incorrect assumptions that: (i) the absence of human serum represents a protein- or serum-free potency measure (despite 10% fetal calf serum being a component); (ii) the presence of 50% human serum (and 10% FCS) representing the full effect of serum binding [16].

9.3
Methodologies for Measuring Plasma Protein Binding

There are a multitude of approaches applied to the measurement of plasma protein binding and several of them are presented in Table 9.1. They typically fall into three categories: *in vitro*, *in vivo* and higher-throughput surrogate methods. In addition, a number of analytical technologies are employed including, but not limited to, UV and fluorescence [20], nuclear magnetic resonance [21], circular dichroism [22] and surface plasmon resonance [23] spectroscopy; but the focus here is on methods currently in widespread use throughout pharmaceutical R&D.

In vitro assessment of plasma protein binding requires a technique capable of separating free and bound drug for subsequent analysis and usually involves some form of ultrafiltration, ultracentrifugation or equilibrium dialysis. Ultrafiltration forces the aqueous plasma component containing the free drug through a selective, semipermeable membrane aided by vacuum, positive pressure or centrifugation. It is a simple, relatively rapid (15–45 min) procedure that has been formatted into 96-well plates [24–26]. This approach can suffer from compound adsorption issues to both the device and filter, and protein leakage across the filter can lead to erroneous determinations of free fraction for highly bound compounds. Efforts have been made to overcome some of the drawbacks associated with the ultrafiltration technique.

Table 9.1 Summary of approaches to PPB determination in vitro.

Methodology		Advantages	Disadvantages	Reference
Ultrafiltration		Simple, rapid, 96-well format.	Adsorption issues, protein leakage.	[24–27]
Ultracentrifugation		Minimal non-specific binding and osmotic volume shifts.	Large plasma volumes required, long assay time, issues such as sedimentation, back diffusion and viscosity. Potential for lipoprotein contamination of plasma water layer.	[28, 29]
Equilibrium Dialysis	Standard ED	High-throughput, 96-well format.	Long incubation time – compound instability and plasma degradation. Issues of pH drift and osmotic volume shifts (can be corrected for). Membrane adsorption/non-specific binding[a].	[30–32]
	Rapid ED	Incubation times can be shorter – minimizing volume shifts. Amenable to automation. High throughput.	Membrane adsorption/non-specific binding[a].	[36, 37]
	Comparative ED	Relative binding useful for highly bound compounds.	Mixing plasma types can influence binding properties. Time to reach equilibrium can exceed 24 h.	[38, 39]

Table 9.1 (*Continued*)

Methodology	Advantages	Disadvantages	Reference
Erythrocyte distribution in plasma and buffer	No need for mechanism to separate bound and free drug – adsorption issues minimized. For highly bound compounds, analytical precision no longer a prerequisite.	Low throughput, more complex assay format.	[40]
PAMPA	Binding constants obtained for protein in solution. No requirement for mass balance or equilibrium.	Binding measurement made on protein of interest rather than whole plasma.	[41]
HPLC	Rapid, simple, high-throughput.	Binding specificity of immobilized protein assumed to be same as in solution. Non-specific binding and adsorption issues. Binding measurement made on protein of interest rather than whole plasma.	[42–45]

[a]Impacts on mass balance but should not affect concentration ratio if system is at equilibrium.

By utilizing two centrifugations and using the proteinaceous retentate from a control plasma sample, it is possible to aid compound solubility and perturb non-specific binding, as demonstrated for a series of corticosteroids [27]. Ultracentrifugation uses centrifugal forces in excess of 10^5 g in order to separate the aqueous phase from proteinaceous material [28]. There is no membrane and so non-specific binding is minimized, with negligible potential for osmotic volume shifts. However, ultracentrifugation uses large plasma volumes (~2 mL/sample), can take 12–16 h and introduces issues such as sedimentation, back-diffusion and viscosity. Another major concern is the potential for lipoprotein contamination of the plasma water layer that is generated [29].

Equilibrium dialysis has tended to be the "gold standard" in most drug metabolism laboratories with a number of high throughput approaches being reported recently [30–32]. In all cases, equilibrium dialysis comprises two chambers divided by a selective, semi-permeable membrane with a plasma "retentate" on one side and a buffer "dialysate" on the other. This system is then incubated over the course of hours (6–24 h) usually at a physiologically relevant temperature (37 °C) before the retentate and dialysate chambers are sampled and analyzed for drug concentrations. Long incubation times can confound the determination of fraction unbound values as a result of compound instability or degradation of plasma components as reported, for example, for quinidine [33]. The observation and impact of pH drift on protein binding over long incubation times has also been reported [34, 35]. Membrane adsorption and non-specific binding can impact on mass balance, but as long as the system is in equilibrium this does not affect the concentration ratio. With long equilibration times, the osmotic pressure of the plasma proteins can induce volume shifts, driving the flow of fluid from the buffer chamber to the plasma side. The dilution of the plasma by the net flow of buffer can alter binding properties in an unpredictable way by influencing factors such as ionic strength and pH. If retentate and dialysate volumes are measured post-incubation, the volume shift itself can be easily corrected for using the Boudinot equation shown below.

$$fu_p = 1 - \frac{(C_{plasma} - C_{buffer}) \cdot (V_{plasma}^{final} / V_{plasma}^{initial})}{(C_{plasma} - C_{buffer}) \cdot (V_{plasma}^{final} / V_{plasma}^{initial}) + C_{buffer}}$$

As part of this, an important phenomenon is the Gibbs–Donnan effect where charged proteins held on the retentate side draw low molecular weight ions across the membrane to achieve electroneutrality, leading to an uneven distribution of small ions. This can be overcome by using isotonic phosphate buffers. Attempts to improve the throughput and laborious nature of ED assays has included development of rapid equilibrium dialysis (RED) offering shorter experiment times and being amenable to automation. The dialysis cell format with an increased surface area to volume ratio enables potentially shorter equilibration times with minimal volume shift [36]. A comparative analysis of the RED and standard ED approaches using a diverse subset of compounds showed the value of this assay to increase throughput and reduce experiment time without compromising data accuracy or robustness [37].

A variant on the equilibrium dialysis protocol was recently reported. Comparative equilibrium dialysis places plasma from two different sources (e.g., species, individuals, etc.) on either side of the dialysis membrane. The total concentration at equilibrium on each side represents the ratio between the respective fu values, and as such is a measure of the relative binding. This has been proposed for species comparisons and for highly bound compounds where determining the actual fu can be complicated by analytical precision and sensitivity [38]. However, other groups have shown it is likely that mixing plasma types changes the binding properties by mixing of low MW fractions. This was confirmed using dialyzed blank plasma in a subsequent ultrafiltration experiment. Due to this inherent problem and the time to reach equilibrium exceeding 24 h, the authors did not recommend this approach [39]. For highly bound compounds with high lipophilicity and potential apparatus adsorption problems, Schuhmacher *et al.* [40] proposed measuring a plasma-free fraction based on distribution between erythrocytes and aqueous, proteinaceous solutions. By performing incubations containing resuspended erythrocytes and diluted plasma or buffer in glass tubes and without the need for a mechanism to separate plasma-free drug from plasma-bound drug, adsorption issues were minimized. With this approach, plasma fu was calculated as the ratio of the partition coefficients of erythrocytes:plasma and erythrocytes:buffer, accounting for the hematocrit in both cases. This type of "biological dialysis" precludes the accurate measurement of low drug concentrations which are prone to error.

A novel application of the parallel artificial membrane permeability assay (PAMPA) system to measuring protein binding constants was demonstrated recently [41]. The apparent permeability of 11 test compounds was measured in the presence and absence of human serum albumin in the donor compartment, and by solving the differential equations describing the kinetics of membrane permeability, membrane retention and protein binding, the authors were able to obtain the Kd. With the protein in solution rather than immobilized and without the need for mass balance or equilibrium conditions, this approach provides an attractive alternative to existing methods with the potential to be applied to an array of other soluble proteins.

Much work has been reported on the development and application of surrogate systems to assess plasma protein binding. Chromatographic methodologies whereby HSA or AAG is chemically bonded to silica-based stationary phases were first reported by Wainer and colleagues about 15–20 years ago [42, 43]. This approach measures a chromatographic retention factor (k') which is directly related to the proportion of molecules in the stationary phase and in the mobile phase, and so from this a percent bound value can be obtained describing the interaction between the immobilized protein and test compound of interest. Although, typically a UV endpoint is employed making it a rapid and straightforward method, the underlying assumption is that the chemically bonded protein retains the binding specificity and conformational mobility of the native protein. In addition, there is potential for non-specific binding and adsorption issues with the silica support and long retention times. Reasonable correlations have been reported between HSA binding and literature values, although this has not been the case in studies using immobilized AAG [44, 45]. This is possibly a reflection of the fact this type of method is not truly representative of whole blood plasma, lacking the full complement of plasma proteins and using high concentrations of organic solvent (up to 30% organic, depending on chemistry). The speed and simplicity offered by this approach has been somewhat superseded by the increased throughput of standardized *in vitro* methods utilizing whole plasma as detailed above. A variation on the HPLC methodology, TRANSIL technology, involves immobilization of HSA onto the inert surface of silica beads suspended in PBS buffer [46]. After compound addition and mixing, the beads are separated by low speed centrifugation and the resultant supernatant is analyzed by UV or MS. Validation has been performed on a range of compounds but there are few reported applications in the literature. Other similar approaches include gel filtration which was applied historically to investigate a number of protein–ligand interactions [47], and more recently solid phase microextraction (SPME) which measures the partitioning of drug between plasma proteins and a SPME fiber [48]. In a similar manner, charcoal has been used as a binding "sink", so PPB can be measured as the time course of decline of the percent bound drug remaining in plasma while the free drug is removed by charcoal adsorption. This can prove useful in alleviating some of the issues of non-specific binding observed with highly lipophilic compounds [49].

Accurate determination of drug-free fraction *in vivo* is a complex undertaking but has been achieved with some success using microdialysis. Based on the dialysis principle, microdialysis comprises a probe inserted into the tissue of interest through which fluid is delivered. The probe is made up of a hollow fiber that is permeable to water and low MW molecules, and during the perfusion, molecular exchange by diffusion occurs in both directions. Dialysate samples are then analyzed online by standard techniques, such as LC–MS, with appropriate analyte separation by LC or CE. In pharmacokinetic studies, the major advantage over conventional blood sampling is the collection of protein-free samples allowing measurement of unbound drug concentrations. Microdialysis coupled with simultaneous blood sampling then enables the *in vivo* determination of plasma protein binding, with each sampling technique giving a measure of free and total drug concentration, respectively. Microdialysis has been used to investigate the temporal profile and saturation of protein binding of irbesartan [50] as well as obtaining binding parameters for drugs such as flurbiprofen [51], methotrexate [52] and valproate [53]. The use of this approach in pharmacokinetic and pharmacodynamic studies was nicely reviewed by Höcht *et al.* [54], although due to issues of complexity and the availability of *in vitro* alternatives, the method has not been reported to be applied to PPB determination in drug discovery.

9.4
Physicochemical Determinants and *In Silico* Prediction of Plasma Protein Binding

The physicochemical determinants of plasma protein binding and the *in silico* prediction of the latter have been examined by several authors [55–57] and generally found to coincide with lipophilicity (generally expressed by $\log P_{oct}$ or $\log D_{oct}$) and, for acidic compounds, charge was also found to be important, considering the presence of basic ionized residues in the binding sites of albumin. It is a common observation that the vast majority of acidic compounds tend to be largely bound to albumin, in particular, and to yield a correspondingly higher bound fraction relative to basic and neutral compounds although there are exceptions to this "rule".

Plasma protein binding typically shows a sigmoidal relationship when the data are plotted against lipophilicity, as shown by van de Waterbeemd et al. [55] on a data set of approximately 150 compounds, comprising neutral, acidic and basic molecules. In a more recent analysis reported by Obach et al. [57] the sigmoidal trend was linearized by transforming the fu data into the logarithm of the apparent affinity constant logK calculated as log bound/free. The set of 554 compounds used shows that an increase in lipophilicity, expressed as calculated logP, correlates with an increase in logK for all charge classes (neutral, basic, acidic and zwitterionic molecules) and this parameter, together with charge, is essentially the only parameter for which a relationship with logK exists. Charge is important as well, even for basic compounds, because the latter tend to bind to α1-acid glycoprotein due to electrostatic interactions with acidic residues on the protein.

Many attempts have been made at predicting plasma protein binding from structures only, with a variety of statistical approaches and sizes of data set; and the recent work of Gleeson [56] as well as the review recently published by Egan [58], both citing several examples of prior work, are mentioned here as leading references. It should be noted, when considering in silico approaches and their performance that, while plasma protein binding is generally determined as an equilibrium property, the binding process is not controlled by bulk properties alone, such as lipophilicity, and that, for example, structural differences may be important determinants of binding, especially when considering the diverse binding sites present on albumin.

The review article by Egan examines several predictive approaches, from fairly simple ones, using only one variable and showing a sigmoidal relationship [55], to increasingly more complex approaches where non-linear equations were successfully used to predict percent protein binding for neutral, basic and zwitterionic compounds across a set of 302 compounds, but where a similar attempt was used for acidic compounds the result was a poor fitting model [59].

Gleeson [56] used plasma protein binding data in human and rat, encompassing approximately 900 compounds for the human set and approximately 1500 compounds in rat, which were both split 75% (training set) to 25% (test set), yielding a training set in human of 686 compounds. Like Obach et al. [57], he used the logK value (with K being a pseudo-equilibrium constant calculated as the ratio bound/free). Several parameters, including polar surface area, hydrogen-bond donor and acceptor indicators and estimation of their strength, as well as logD and logP and the extent of ionization, were calculated and a PLS approach used. Extensive statistical validation and comparative work were presented together with model limitations and we mention two of the conclusions reported by the author. One is that the model can be used to rank compounds according to the criteria of whether they will be bound greater than 99%. If a compound is predicted to be 95% bound, the author commented, it is highly likely that the actual value is <99% given the r^2 and RMSE of the model, 0.56 and 0.55, respectively, with a 70% confidence that its range would be 86.0–98.4% and a corresponding interval of the experimental value of 92.3–96.8% bound. Thus, the author concludes that, while the model may not be predictive enough to predict subtle changes during lead optimization, it could be used to rank virtual possibilities. We submit, however, that plasma protein binding is probably not amenable to use as a ranking tool and in a predictive fashion but, rather, it is an eminently experimental parameter that aids in rationalizing differences in total versus intrinsic clearance and differences between *in vitro* versus *in vivo* potency. Or, in other words, it aids in understanding the composite nature of PK rather than offering basis to prioritize synthesis and choice of compounds. Second, the analysis of the model descriptors confirms that lipophilicity, size (molecular weight) and charge type/extent of ionization are the key descriptor types, and the addition of an acidic group (or a decrease in its pK_a) was found to increase binding while the addition (or the increase in basic pK_a) of a basic group was generally found to lead to decreased binding in line with other work and generally observed "rules" which were also recently discussed by the same author [60].

9.5
Volume of Distribution: General Considerations and Applications to Experimental Pharmacokinetics and Drug Design

The volume of distribution is a parameter that can be calculated from plasma drug concentration versus time data (expressed as area under the curve or AUC), according to the two equations shown below, for terminal or steady-state volume of distribution, respectively.

$$VD_\beta = \frac{\text{Dose}}{\text{AUC} \cdot k_{el}}$$

$$VD_{ss} = \frac{\text{Dose} \cdot \text{AUMC}}{\text{AUC}^2}$$

In these equations k_{el} is the elimination rate constant and AUMC is the area under the first moment curve. A treatment of the statistical moment analysis is of course beyond the scope of this chapter and those concepts may not be very intuitive, but AUMC could be thought of, in a simplified way, as a measure of the "concentration–time" average of the time–concentration profile and AUC as a measure of the "concentration" average of the profile. Their ratio would yield MRT, a measure of the "time average" of the profile termed in fact mean residence time. Or, in other words, the time–concentration profile can be considered a statistical distribution curve and the AUC and MRT represent the "zero" and "first" moment with the latter being calculated from the ratio of AUMC and AUC.

By itself, volume of distribution does not provide any insight into mechanisms of drug distribution, however it is a useful descriptive index of how well the drug partitions away from the central plasma compartment. Volume of distribution is dependent on the extent of plasma binding and peripheral tissue binding, which are dependent on the binding capacity of each of these compartments and the affinity of the drug for specific plasma and tissue macromolecules and structures:

$$VD \propto \frac{f_{b(tissues)}}{f_{b(plasma)}} = \frac{f_{u(plasma)}}{f_{u(tissues)}}$$

Clearly, the mechanistic contributors to the extent of plasma and tissue binding are numerous, and the VD term represents a simplistic picture of potentially hundreds, maybe thousands, of individual tissue binding interactions. Despite this possible complexity, there may be a few individual types of tissue binding that are mostly responsible for tissue partitioning, and as described elsewhere in this chapter, this phenomena may be more related to non-specific interactions that are a function of gross physicochemical properties of the drug than specific binding interactions.

The larger the VD, the longer the $t_{1/2}$, since the time it will take for the drug to reemerge from the tissues can drive the $t_{1/2}$ (or mean residence time if it is the steady-state VD that is being considered). Thus, in medicinal chemistry drug design efforts, when faced with a predicted short half-life, there is temptation to drive towards higher VD to gain a longer $t_{1/2}$ (in essence, leveraging tissue binding as an internal reservoir of drug that slowly re-enters the systemic circulation and becomes available to the pharmacological target). However, while there has been description of some limited successes using this approach (e.g., amlodipine vs felodipine [61]), this is generally not a good strategy because:

1. Structural modifications needed to alter VD generally need to alter physicochemical properties (e.g., lipophilicity, charge, etc.) which in turn alter other pharmacokinetic characteristics of the molecule and may not be tolerated by the pharmacophore of the target.

2. If intrinsic potency remains the same, the dose must be greater in order to "fill the tissue reservoirs" and attain the same unbound efficacious concentration. Non-specific tissue capacity will take up a greater proportion of the dosed drug.

3. Many of the structural modifications that can lead to increased VD also lead to increased rates of metabolism, hence clearance, and results in a zero-sum effect on half-life.

4. Very large VD values can be frequently associated with drugs that can exhibit phospholipidosis. It is important to note that this is not a cause and effect relationship, but a general trend. Furthermore, drugs that exhibit high tissue binding are difficult to remove by hemodialysis, in the event that a deleterious event, such as overdose, must be treated.

In order to increase the predicted human $t_{1/2}$, it is a generally more successful strategy to design new molecules with the intent to decrease the free clearance. However, while designing new molecules to attain specific VD values may not be a fruitful endeavor, the prediction of VD is still an important activity in drug design because it is an important component of predicting $t_{1/2}$ and mean residence time (MRT):

$$t_{1/2} = \frac{0.693 \cdot VD_\beta}{CL} \quad \text{and} \quad MRT = \frac{VD_{ss}}{CL}$$

in which VD_β and VD_{ss} refer to terminal phase and steady-state VD values, respectively. (For drugs that exhibit multiphasic concentration vs time profiles, the MRT will be a better indicator than $t_{1/2}$ of the potential dosing frequency needed and expected accumulation ratio that will occur with repeated administration.)

9.5.1
Prediction of Human Volume of Distribution

Over the years, several types of methods were developed to predict human VD. Because VD is thought to be more dependent of overall physicochemical properties of drugs contributing to non-specific binding rather than specific structural attributes responsible for specific protein–ligand interactions, prediction of VD is more successful than prediction of clearance. The methods vary in their accuracy and labor needed to gather the needed input data; generally with an inverse relationship between the accuracy and labor. Different approaches are applicable at various stages during drug design. In early efforts, when there are hundreds of compounds being considered for a given therapeutic target receptor/enzyme, approaches must be simple and high throughput. Applications of *in silico* methods are probably best in most cases at this stage, since compounds would not even need to be synthesized to accomplish these predictions. As the number of compounds being considered for further development decreases, there is a greater need for increased confidence in the VD prediction. Reliance on laboratory data increases at this later stage and may include approaches that use *in vitro* data and/or pharmacokinetic data from laboratory animal species. These three types of VD prediction approaches are described below and the reader is referred to a recent detailed discussion of these methods [62].

9.5.1.1 Prediction of Human Volume of Distribution from Animal Pharmacokinetic Data

If VD is truly more dependent on non-specific interactions between drug and tissues, then the differences that could be observed across the species for the VD of a drug is more a function of differences in body tissue compositions among animals versus humans than specific structural attributes of the drug. Drugs that exhibit high VD in animals also exhibit high VD in humans; drugs that exhibit low VD in animals also exhibit low VD in humans. This logic, taken to an extreme, would suggest that the VD for a set of drugs in humans should correlate to VD values for these same drugs in a laboratory animal species, such as rat. This is exactly the approach described by Caldwell et al. [63] in which a linear correlation was derived between human and rat VD values for a set of 144 drugs such that the VD measured in rat, uncorrected for body weight, could merely be multiplied by 188 to obtain the human VD prediction.

Other investigators suggested the same approach but used the monkey as the laboratory species [64].

VD is a function of both tissue binding and plasma protein binding, and while the former may be comprised of a multiplicity of non-specific interactions dependent on gross physicochemical characteristics, the latter is generally a function of just a few interactions (i.e., binding to albumin, α_1-acid glycoprotein, lipoproteins), albeit this is also more driven by physicochemical characteristics rather than specific ligand–receptor type interactions (see Section 9.4). Thus, it is possible to observe differences in plasma protein binding across species, although these differences are not usually large. Nevertheless, *in vitro* measurements of plasma protein binding are fairly easy to make and can be used to correct human VD predictions made from animal VD data. Such a correction is employed in two methods, one which only uses pharmacokinetic data from dogs and one in which pharmacokinetic data from multiple animal species are required [65]. In the dog–human VD proportionality approach, dog VD (per body weight) is measured and corrected to free VD by dividing by the unbound fraction in dog plasma. The free VD in dog is assumed to be equal to that in human, and the human VD is obtained by multiplying this value by the free fraction in human plasma. Thus, differences in plasma protein binding can be considered in the prediction. In the other method, VD and plasma protein binding are measured in multiple species, and used to make estimates of the fraction unbound in tissues ($f_{u(tissue)}$) for each species using the Oie–Tozer equation which relates $f_{u(plasma)}$, $f_{u(tissue)}$, VD_{ss} and several physiological volumes [66]:

$$VD_{ss} = V_P(1 + R_{E/I}) + f_u V_P(V_E/V_P - R_{E/I}) + \frac{V_R f_u}{f_{ut}}$$

The parameters V_P, V_E and $R_{E/I}$ are the plasma and extracellular fluid volumes and the extravascular to intravascular protein (albumin) ratio, respectively. Their values in human, as an example, are 0.0436 and 0.151 L/kg, respectively, with a $R_{E/I}$ ratio of 1.4. V_R is defined as the physical space into which the drug distributes minus the extracellular space and its value, in human, is taken as 0.380 L/kg. f_u and f_{ut} are defined as above.

The $f_{u(tissue)}$ values are averaged for the species, this average is assumed to be the value for human, inserted back into the Oie–Tozer equation and combined with the measured value of $f_{u(plasma)}$ in human to obtain a predicted value for human VD. However, despite its increased complexity it does not offer additional accuracy over the above mentioned dog–human proportionality method and may only be most appropriate when plasma protein binding shows considerable inter-species variability.

Finally, no discussion of human pharmacokinetic predictions is complete without a consideration of allometric scaling [67–69]. In general, allometry is the examination of relationships between size and function and it has been applied to the prediction of human pharmacokinetic parameters from animal pharmacokinetic parameters for decades [70]. Allometry has been shown to work reasonably well for predicting human VD from animal VD data, probably because volumes of plasma and various tissue across species are allometrically scaleable to body weight, a notion reinforced by the frequent observation that the allometric exponent ("b" in the equation below) is typically unity for scaling VD:

$$VD = a \cdot W^b$$

in which a is the allometric coefficient and W is body weight for each species. The VD values measured in various species are plotted against their body weights (on a logarithmic scale), and the VD value for human is extrapolated from 70 kg. The method suffers from a need to generate VD values in potentially multiple species, and if the single species methods described above can work, the impetus for using allometry may be diminished in the spirit of decreasing unneeded animal experimentation.

9.5.1.2 Prediction of Human Volume of Distribution from *In Vitro* Data

Since VD is a function of relative tissue and plasma binding, it follows that if these measurements could be made *in vitro*, then the data could be used to predict VD. Furthermore, if tissue binding is driven by physicochemical properties, such as lipophilicity, then it also follows that physicochemical measurements could serve as surrogates for tissue binding propensity. *In vitro* tissue binding and physicochemical measurements form the basis of *in vitro* approaches to predict human VD.

In considering tissue binding and its role in VD, the identities of the most important tissues must be known. Some tissues have a high binding affinity but lack a high capacity (e.g., binding of cationic drugs in melanin-containing structures of the eye), while others have a high capacity because of their mass but affinity may not be great (e.g., muscle, bone, skin, adipose). Thus, selection of which tissues to include in an *in vitro* tissue binding experiment and whether to combine tissues is not well established. Furthermore, there are practical limitations to conducting tissue binding experiments: the tissues must be diluted in order to make homogenates and most investigators use animal tissues as surrogates for human tissues. Finally, these methods mostly rely upon developing correlations between tissue binding and VD [71, 72] and with one exception [73] do not mathematically scale the binding data using physiologically based pharmacokinetic modeling.

Since tissue binding is likely related to physicochemical properties, other investigators derived methods to predict human VD from such data [74–77]. Poulin and Thiel categorize tissues into two types: adipose and non-adipose. For the latter value, octanol:water partitioning is used as a surrogate while for adipose, olive oil:water partitioning is used. These values are combined with physiological constants for these tissue volumes, along with plasma and blood volumes, to predict human VD. In the methods described by Lombardo et al. [75], Lombardo et al. [76] and Hollosy et al. [77], HPLC methods are used as surrogates for physicochemical measurements, and these are used in correlations to tissue binding. In the former method, the ElogD parameter (i.e., $logD^{7.4}$ obtained by reverse phase HPLC) is measured, and together with the fraction unbound in plasma (f_u) and fraction ionized (f_i) based on pK_a, it is used to predict the fraction unbound in tissue (f_{ut}) via a multiple linear regression equation. The correlation derived between ElogD, f_u, f_i and f_{ut} from known drugs is used to predict tissue binding, and combined with measured plasma binding to predict VD in human, for the compound of interest. In the latter method, albumin and phospholipid HPLC columns are used as surrogates for plasma and tissue binding, respectively under the assumption that these two entities are what give the greatest drive to plasma and tissue binding. The data are correlated to human VD to show that these measurements can be made to predict VD for new compounds.

9.5.1.3 Prediction of Human Volume of Distribution from *In Silico* Methods

The types of physicochemical parameters used in the *in vitro* prediction approaches can also be derived computationally, suggesting that purely *in silico* approaches are possible for predicting VD. In an early method, compounds were separated by charge type before deriving a relationship between a single computed physicochemical parameter and human VD [78], however the method accuracy was not high enough to merit its use in drug design efforts.

Additional efforts at developing computational models for predicting human VD were more successful and used more computed descriptors as well as several statistical approaches (e.g., partial least squares, neural networks, stepwise regression, classification and regression trees, and random forest [79–82]). As expected, lipophilicity and charge type play an important role in these models. The general approach for model building has been to use large datasets of human VD data to develop the models and then to test them using subsets of the data that were not used in model building. It is important to note that the predictive accuracy of test sets from these models has now approached the accuracy of aforementioned methods that use animal or *in vitro* data. The advantage is that no laboratory experimentation is needed, no compound needs to be synthesized and the VD prediction can be made from a proposed structure alone. In this way, medicinal chemists can query proposed compounds and understand how various substituents can influence VD.

9.6
Relationship Between Clearance, VDss and Plasma Protein Binding

As already alluded, VD and plasma protein binding are intrinsically linked, as VDss is a weighted mean ratio of tissue and plasma binding affinity, with VD corrected for species/individual differences in PPB (unbound VD) in many cases remaining constant for a given compound. In addition, free fraction in plasma is a key determinant of clearance *in vivo*, together with intrinsic clearance (CL_{int}); a measure of the efficiency of drug turnover or elimination not restricted by organ blood flow. A number of physiological models are applied to drug clearance, with the well stirred model being the most commonly used.

$$CL_H = \frac{Q_H \cdot f_u \cdot CL_{int}}{Q_H + f_u \cdot CL_{int}}$$

From this model it is clear that, for example, highly bound drugs with high CL_{int} can exhibit low clearance. A common medicinal chemistry strategy to increase $t_{1/2}$ is to lower CL by modulating PPB towards higher binding. Although this tends to reduce CL, it also lowers VD to a similar extent, as plasma binding is increased, thus having negligible effect on the $t_{1/2}$.

9.7
Summary and Conclusions

Throughout this chapter we discuss the importance of plasma protein binding and its relationship with clearance and volume of distribution. We also illustrate experimental and computational methods for the determination of both plasma protein binding and volume of distribution, ranging from *in vitro* to *in vivo* to *in silico* approaches, and we close this chapter with some considerations along those lines. On the subject of physicochemical determinants and *in silico* or *in vitro* prediction we point out that there is a correlation between plasma protein binding and lipophilicity and that a correlation can be found between volume of distribution and lipophilicity as well. Charge, in contrast, modulates those relationships in a somewhat opposite way, since negatively charged compounds tend to be more tightly bound to plasma protein (albumin) and tend to have lower volume of distribution as well as lower clearance values, while the opposite is generally true for positively charged compounds. These are of course broad generalizations; and exceptions are known and have been discussed.

The prediction of volume of distribution, based on largely although not exclusively passive diffusion phenomena, can be achieved with reasonable accuracy with *in silico* methods, over and above available *in vivo* and *in vitro* methods, with obvious advantages in terms of time, cost of synthesis and animal use. However, an accurate prediction of plasma protein binding, in the high range (e.g., $\geq$98% bound) is still difficult to achieve, and a small error in prediction (or determination) in the high range yields a large error in terms of fold difference in free fraction, which is ultimately what matters when evaluating the concentration of drug free to interact with a receptor or enzyme. These errors in prediction are also rooted in the difficulty in obtaining very high accuracy measurements, at least routinely. However, it may be possible to confidently explore trends and classify molecules, depending on the predicted value, on the basis of the likelihood that they have a very large ($\geq$98% bound) percent bound or not, as reported by Gleeson [56].

We discuss, largely on the basis of the commentary by Benet and Hoener [1], the fact that changes in plasma protein binding are seldom of clinical relevance since most drugs (whether high or low extraction ratio compounds) are administered orally and mostly cleared by the liver. We also illustrate caveats regarding the use of volume of distribution in trying to increase $t_{1/2}$ citing, among other factors, the likelihood that structural modification leading to an increase in VD also leads to an increase in clearance and thus to a zero-sum effect, making this an "indirect" link between the two otherwise independent parameters.

Finally, we note that plasma protein binding is generally determined on a "retrospective" or "interpretation" basis, and it is seldom determined routinely, as a primary parameter and/or in a screening mode, while several other characterization studies are instead conducted on a given compound. The advent of faster experimental methods, and of course experience with the application of *in silico* methods, may change this approach but it is doubtful that it will greatly impact the decision-making process on the selection of a compound, as we alluded to in Section 9.4.

References

1. Benet, L.Z. and Hoener, B. (2002) Changes in plasma protein binding have little clinical relevance. *Clinical Pharmacology and Therapeutics*, **71**, 115–121.
2. Trainor, G. (2007) The importance of plasma protein binding in drug discovery. *Expert Opinion on Drug Discovery*, **2**, 51–64.
3. Andes, D., Marchillo, K., Stamstad, T. and Conklin, R. (2003) *In vivo* pharmacokinetics and pharmacodynamics of a new triazole, voriconazole, in a murine candidiasis model. *Antimicrobial Agents and Chemotherapy*, **47**, 3165–3169.
4. Pfaller, M.A., Diekema, D.J., Rex, J.H., Espinel-Ingroff, A., Johnson, E.M., Andes, D., Chaturvedi, V., Ghannoum, M.A., Odds, F.C., Rinaldi, M.G., Sheehan, D.J., Troke, P., Walsh, T.J. and Warnock, D.W. (2006) Correlation of MIC with outcome for Candida species tested against voriconazole: analysis and proposal for interpretive breakpoints. *Journal of Clinical Microbiology*, **44**, 819–826.
5. Olsen, K.M., Gentry-Nielsen, M., Yue, M., Snitily, M.U. and Preheim, L.C. (2006) Effect of ethanol on fluoroquinolone efficacy in a rat model of pneumococcal pneumonia. *Antimicrobial Agents and Chemotherapy*, **50**, 210–219.
6. Delbaldo, C., Chatelut, E., Re, M., Deroussent, A., Seronie-Vivien, S., Jambu, A., Berthaud, P., Le Cesne, A., Blay, J.-Y. and Vassal, G. (2006) Pharmacokinetic-pharmacodynamic relationships of imatinib and its main metabolite in patients with advanced gastrointestinal stromal tumors. *Clinical Cancer Research*, **12**, 6073–6078.
7. Fuse, E., Tanii, H., Kurata, N., Kobayashi, H., Shimada, Y., Tannini, T., Sasaki, Y., Tanigawara, Y., Lush, R.D., Headlee, D., Figg, W.D., Arbuck, S.G., Senderowicz, A.M., Sausville, E.A., Akinaga, S., Kuwabara, T. and Kobayashi, S. (1998) Unpredicted clinical pharmacology of UCN-01 caused by specific binding to human α1-acid glycoprotein. *Cancer Research*, **58**, 3248–3253.
8. Lin, J.H., Cocchetto, D.M. and Duggan, D.E. (1987) Protein binding as a primary determinant of the clinical pharmacokinetic properties of non-steroidal anti-inflammatory drugs. *Clinical Pharmacokinetics*, **12**, 402–432.
9. Fukumoto, K., Tanemura, M., Tsuchishita, Y., Kusumoto, M., Matsumoto, K., Kamakura, S. and Ueno, K. (2005) Effect of protein binding of pilsicainide on the pharmacokinetics. *Drug Metabolism and Pharmacokinetics*, **20**, 183–186.
10. Bow, D.A.J., Perry, J.L., Simon, J.D. and Pritchard, J.B. (2006) The impact of plasma protein binding on the renal transport of organic anions. *Journal of Pharmacology and Experimental Therapeutics*, **316**, 349–355.
11. Ito, K., Chiba, K., Horikawa, M., Ishigami, M., Mizuno, N., Aoki, J., Gotoh, Y., Iwatsubo, T., Kanamitsu, S. and Kato, M. (2002) Which concentration of the inhibitor should be used to predict *in vivo* drug interactions from *in vitro* data? *AAPS Pharmsci*, **4**, E25.
12. McGinnity, D.F., Tucker, J., Trigg, S. and Riley, R.J. (2005) Prediction of CYP2C9-mediated drug-drug interactions: a

13 Obach, R.S., Walsky, R.L., Venkatakrishnan, K., Gaman, E.A., Houston, J.B. and Tremaine, L.M. (2006) The utility of *in vitro* cytochrome P450 inhibition data in the prediction of drug-drug interactions. *Journal of Pharmacology and Experimental Therapeutics*, **316**, 336–348.

comparison using data from recombinant enzymes and human hepatocytes. *Drug Metabolism and Disposition: The Biological Fate of Chemicals*, **33**, 1700–1707.

14 Venkatakrishnan, K. and Obach, R.S. (2007) Drug-drug interactions via mechanism-based cytochrome P450 inactivation: points to consider for risk assessment from *in vitro* data and clinical pharmacologic evaluation. *Current Drug Metabolism*, **8**, 449–462.

15 Rolan, P.E. (1994) Plasma protein binding displacement interactions–why are they still regarded as clinically important? *British Journal of Clinical Pharmacology*, **37**, 125–128.

16 Boffito, M., Back, D.J., Blaschke, T.F., Rowland, M., Bertz, R.J., Gerber, J.G. and Miller, V. (2003) Protein binding in antiretroviral therapies. *AIDS Research and Human Retroviruses*, **19**, 825–835.

17 Christensen, H., Baker, M., Tucker, G.T. and Rostami-Hodjegan, A. (2006) Prediction of plasma protein binding displacement and its implications for quantitative assessment of metabolic drug-drug interactions from *in vitro* data. *Journal of Pharmaceutical Sciences*, **95**, 2778–2787.

18 Ma, Y., Peters, N.S. and Henry, J.A. (2006) α1-Acid glycoprotein reverses cocaine-induced sodium channel blockade in cardiac myocytes. *Toxicology*, **220**, 46–50.

19 Jones, K., Hoggard, P.G., Khoo, S., Maher, B. and Back, D.J. (2001) Effect of α1-acid glycoprotein on the intracellular accumulation of the HIV protease inhibitors saquinavir, ritonavir and indinavir *in vitro*. *British Journal of Clinical Pharmacology*, **51**, 99–102.

20 Chignell, C.F. (1969) Optical studies of drug-protein complexes II. Interaction of phenylbutazone and its analogues with human serum albumin. *Molecular Pharmacology*, **5**, 244–252.

21 Liu, M., Nicholson, J.K., Parkinson, J.A. and Lindon, J.C. (1997) Measurement of biomolecular diffusion coefficients in blood plasma using two-dimensional ^{1}H-^{1}H diffusion-edited total-correlation NMR spectroscopy. *Analytical Chemistry*, **69**, 1504–1509.

22 Bertucci, C., Salvadori, P. and Domenici, E. (1997) *The Impact of Stereochemistry on Drug Development and Use*, Wiley, New York, pp. 521–543.

23 Frostell-Karlsson, A., Remaeus, A., Roos, H., Andersson, K., Borg, P., Hämäläinen, M. and Karlsson, R. (2000) Biosensor analysis of the interaction between immobilized human serum albumin and drug compounds for prediction of human serum albumin binding levels. *Journal of Medicinal Chemistry*, **43**, 1986–1992.

24 Bowers, W.F., Fulton, S. and Thompson, J. (1984) Ultrafiltration vs equilibrium dialysis for determination of free fraction. *Clinical Pharmacokinetics*, **9** (S1), 49–60.

25 Fung, E.N., Chen, Y.H. and Lau, Y.Y. (2003) Semi-automatic high-throughput determination of plasma protein binding using a 96-well plate filtrate assembly and fast liquid chromatography-tandem mass spectrometry. *Journal of Chromatography B*, **795**, 187–194.

26 Zhang, J. and Musson, D.G. (2006) Investigation of high-throughput ultrafiltration for the determination of an unbound compound in human plasma using liquid chromatography and tandem mass spectrometry with electrospray ionization. *Journal of Chromatography B*, **843**, 47–55.

27 Taylor, S. and Harker, A. (2006) Modification of the ultrafiltration technique to overcome solubility and non-specific binding challenges associated with the measurement of plasma protein binding of corticosteroids. *Journal of Pharmaceutical and Biomedical Analysis*, **41**, 299–303.

28. Richards, E.G. and Schachman, H.K. (1957) A differential ultracentrifuge technique for measuring small changes in sedimentation coefficients. *Journal of the American Chemical Society*, **79**, 5324–5325.

29. Simon, N., Dailly, E., Combes, O., Malaurie, E., Lemaire, M., Tillement, J.P. and Urien, S. (1998) Role of lipoproteins in the plasma binding of SDZ PSC 833 a novel multidrug resistance-reversing cyclosporin. *British Journal of Clinical Pharmacology*, **45**, 173–175.

30. Banker, M.J., Clark, T.H. and Williams, J.A. (2003) Development and validation of a 96-well equilibrium dialysis apparatus for measuring plasma protein binding. *Journal of Pharmaceutical Sciences*, **92**, 967–974.

31. Kariv, I., Cao, H. and Oldenburg, K.R. (2001) Development of a high throughput equilibrium dialysis method. *Journal of Pharmaceutical Sciences*, **90**, 580–587.

32. Wan, H. and Rehngren, M. (2006) High-throughput screening of protein binding by equilibrium dialysis combined with liquid chromatography and mass spectrometry. *Journal of Chromatography. A*, **1102**, 125–134.

33. Guentert, T.W. and Øie, S. (1982) Factors influencing the apparent protein binding of quinidine. *Journal of Pharmaceutical Sciences*, **71**, 325–328.

34. Hinderling, P.H. and Hartmann, D. (2005) The pH dependency of the binding of drugs to plasma proteins in man. *Therapeutic Drug Monitoring*, **2005**, **27**, 71–85.

35. Kochansky, C.J., McMasters, D.R., Lu, P., Koeplinger, K.A., Kerr, H.H., Shou, M. and Korzekwa, K.R. (2008) Impact of pH on plasma protein binding in equilibrium dialysis. *Molecular Pharmacology*, **5**, 438–448.

36. Huang, T.-N. (2006) Dialysis device for equilibrium dialysis U.S. Pat. Appl. Publ. 13 pp. US 2006102547.

37. Waters, N.J., Jones, R., Williams, G. and Sohal, B. (2008) Validation of a rapid equilibrium dialysis approach for the measurement of plasma protein binding. *Journal of Pharmaceutical Sciences*, **97**, 4586–4595.

38. Collins, J.M. and Klecker, R.W. (2002) Evaluation of highly bound drugs: Interspecies, inter-subject and related comparisons. *Journal of Clinical Pharmacology*, **42**, 971–975.

39. Eriksson, M.A.L., Gabrielsson, J. and Nilsson, L.B. (2005) Studies of drug binding to plasma proteins using a variant of equilibrium dialysis. *Journal of Pharmaceutical and Biomedical Analysis*, **38**, 381–389.

40. Schuhmacher, J., Bühner, K. and Witt-Laido, A. (2000) Determination of the free fraction and relative free fraction of drugs strongly bound to plasma proteins. *Journal of Pharmaceutical Sciences*, **89**, 1008–1021.

41. Lázaro, E., Lowe, P.J., Briand, X. and Faller, B. (2008) New approach to measure protein binding based on a parallel artificial membrane assay and human serum albumin. *Journal of Medicinal Chemistry*, **51**, 2009–2017.

42. Domenici, E., Bertucci, C., Salvadori, P., Motellier, S. and Wainer, I.W. (1990) Immobilized serum albumin: Rapid HPLC probe of stereoselective protein-binding interactions. *Chirality*, **2**, 263–268.

43. Aubry, A.F., Markoglou, N., Descorps, V., Wainer, I.W. and Félix, G. (1994) Evaluation of a chiral stationary phase based on mixed immobilized proteins. *Journal of Chromatography. A*, **685**, 1–6.

44. Valko, K., Nunhuck, S., Bevan, C., Abraham, M.H. and Reynolds, D.P. (2003) Fast gradient HPLC method to determine compounds binding to human serum albumin Relationships with octanol/water and immobilized artificial membrane lipophilicity. *Journal of Pharmaceutical Sciences*, **92**, 2236–2248.

45. Singh, S.S. and Mehta, J. (2006) Measurement of drug-protein binding by immobilized human serum albumin-HPLC and comparison with ultra-filtration. *Journal of Chromatography B*, **834**, 108–116.

46 Hartmann, T., Schmitt, J., Rohring, C., Nimptsch, D., Noller, J. and Mohr, C. (2006) ADME related profiling in 96 and 384 well plate format – a novel and robust HT-assay for the determination of lipophilicity and serum albumin binding. *Current Drug Delivery*, **3**, 181–192.

47 Cooper, P.F. and Wood, G.C. (1968) Protein binding of small molecules: new gel filtration method. *Journal of Pharmacy and Pharmacology*, **20**, 150S–156.

48 Musteata, F.M., Pawliszyn, J., Qian, M.G., Wu, J.-T. and Miwa, G.T. (2006) Determination of drug plasma protein binding by solid phase microextraction. *Journal of Pharmaceutical Sciences*, **95**, 1712–1722.

49 Yuan, J., Yang, D.C., Birkmeier, J. and Stolzenbach, J. (1995) Determination of protein binding by *in vitro* charcoal adsorption. *Journal of Pharmacokinetics and Biopharmaceutics*, **23**, 41–55.

50 Höcht, C., Opezzo, J.W. and Taira, C. (2003) Validation of a new intra-arterial microdialysis shunt probe for the estimation of pharmacokinetic parameters. *Journal of Pharmaceutical and Biomedical Analysis*, **31**, 1109–1117.

51 Evrard, P.A., Cumps, J. and Verbeeck, R.K. (1996) Concentration-dependent plasma protein binding of flurbiprofen in the rat: an *in vivo* microdialysis study. *Pharmaceutical Research*, **13**, 18–22.

52 Maia, M.B., Saivin, S., Chatelut, E., Malmary, M.F. and Houin, G. (1996) *In vitro* and *in vivo* protein binding of methotrexate assessed by microdialysis. *International Journal of Clinical Pharmacology and Therapeutics*, **34**, 335–341.

53 Nakashima, M., Takeuchi, N., Hamada, M., Matsuyama, K., Ichikawa, M. and Goto, S. (1994) *In vivo* microdialysis for pharmacokinetic investigations: a plasma protein binding study of valproate in rabbits. *Biological & Pharmaceutical Bulletin*, **17**, 1630–1634.

54 Höcht, C., Opezzo, J.A.W. and Taira, C.A. (2004) Microdialysis in drug discovery. *Current Drug Discovery and Technology*, **1**, 269–285.

55 van de Waterbeemd, H., Smith, D.A. and Jones, B.C. (2001) Lipophilicity in PK design: methyl, ethyl, futile. *Journal of Computer-Aided Molecular Design*, **15**, 273–286.

56 Gleeson, M.P. (2007) Plasma protein binding affinity and its relationship to molecular structure: an in-silico analysis. *Journal of Medicinal Chemistry*, **50**, 101–112.

57 Obach, R.S., Lombardo, F. and Waters, N.J. (2008) Trend analysis of a database of intravenous pharmacokinetic parameters in humans for 670 compounds. *Drug Metabolism and Disposition: The Biological Fate of Chemicals*, **36**, 1385–1405.

58 Egan, W.J. (2007) Computational models for ADME. *Annual Reports in Medicinal Chemistry*, **42**, 449–467.

59 Yamazaki, K. and Kanaoka, M. (2004) Computational prediction of plasma protein binding precent of diverse pharmaceutical compounds. *Journal of Pharmaceutical Sciences*, **93**, 1480–1494.

60 Gleeson, M.P. (2008) Generation of a set of simple, interpretable ADMET rules of thumb. *Journal of Medicinal Chemistry*, **51**, 817–834.

61 Smith, D.A., Jones, B.C. and Walker, D.K. (1996) Design of drugs involving the concepts and theories of drug metabolism and pharmacokinetics. *Medicinal Research Reviews*, **16**, 243–266.

62 Obach, R.S. (2007) Prediction of human volume of distribution using *in vitro*, *in vivo* and in silico approaches. *Annual Reports in Medicinal Chemistry*, **42**, 469–488.

63 Caldwell, G.W., Masucci, J.A., Yan, Z. and Hageman, W. (2004) Allometric scaling of pharmacokinetic parameters in drug discovery: Can human CL Vss and t1/2 be predicted from in-vivo rat data? *European Journal of Drug Metabolism and Pharmacokinetics*, **29**, 133–143.

64 Ward, K.W. and Smith, B.R. (2004) A comprehensive quantitative and qualitative evaluation of extrapolation of

intravenous pharmacokinetic parameters from rat, dog, and monkey to humans II. Volume of distribution and mean residence time. *Drug Metabolism and Disposition: The Biological Fate of Chemicals*, **32**, 612–619.

65 Obach, R.S., Baxter, J.G., Liston, T.E., Silber, B.M., Jones, B.C., MacIntyre, F., Rance, D.J. and Wastall, P. (1997) The prediction of human pharmacokinetic parameters from preclinical and *in vitro* metabolism data. *Journal of Pharmacology and Experimental Therapeutics*, **283**, 46–58.

66 Øie, S. and Tozer, T.N. (1979) Effect of altered plasma protein binding on apparent volume of distribution. *Journal of Pharmaceutical Sciences*, **68**, 1203–1205.

67 Mahmood, I. and Balian, J.D. (1996) Interspecies scaling: a comprehensive study for the prediction of clearance and volume using two or more than two species. *Life Sciences*, **59**, 579–585.

68 Mahmood, I. (1999) Prediction of clearance, volume of distribution and half-life by allometric scaling and by use of plasma concentrations predicted from pharmacokinetic constants: a comparative study. *Journal of Pharmacy and Pharmacology*, **51**, 905–910.

69 Karalis, V. and Macheras, P. (2002) Drug disposition viewed in terms of the fractal volume of distribution. *Pharmaceutical Research*, **19**, 697–704.

70 Boxenbaum, H. (1984) Interspecies pharmacokinetic scaling and the evolutionary-comparative paradigm. *Drug Metabolism Reviews*, **15**, 1071–1121.

71 Schuhmann, G., Fichtl, B. and Kurz, H. (1987) Prediction of drug distribution *in vivo* on the basis of *in vitro* binding data. *Biopharmaceutics & Drug Disposition*, **8**, 73–86.

72 Bjorkman, S. (2002) Prediction of the volume of distribution of a drug: which tissue-plasma partition coefficients are needed? *Journal of Pharmacy and Pharmacology*, **54**, 1237–1245.

73 Jones, H.M., Parrott, N., Jorga, K. and Lave, T. (2006) A novel strategy for physiologically based predictions of human pharmacokinetics. *Clinical Pharmacokinetics*, **45**, 511–542.

74 Poulin, P. and Thiel, F.P. (2002) Prediction of pharmacokinetics prior to *in vivo* studies. 1. Mechanism-based prediction of volume of distribution. *Journal of Pharmaceutical Sciences*, **91**, 129–156.

75 Lombardo, F., Obach, R.S., Shalaeva, M.Y. and Gao, F. (2002) Prediction of volume of distribution values in humans for neutral and basic drugs using physicochemical measurements and plasma protein binding data. *Journal of Medicinal Chemistry*, **45**, 2867–2876.

76 Lombardo, F., Obach, R.S., Shalaeva, M.Y. and Gao, F. (2004) Prediction of human volume of distribution values for neutral and basic compounds 2. Extended data set and leave-class-out statistics. *Journal of Medicinal Chemistry*, **47**, 1242–1250.

77 Hollosy, F., Valko, K., Hersey, A., Nunhuck, S., Keri, G. and Bevan, C. (2006) Estimation of volume of distribution in humans from high throughput HPLC-based measurements of human serum albumin binding and immobilized artificial membrane partitioning. *Journal of Medicinal Chemistry*, **49**, 6958–6971.

78 Lobell, M. and Sivarajah, V. (2003) In silico prediction of aqueous solubility, human plasma protein binding, and volume of distribution of compounds from calculated pKa and AlogP98 values. *Molecular Diversity*, **7**, 69–87.

79 Ghafourian, T., Barzegar-Jalali, M., Hakimiha, N. and Cronin, M.T.D. (2004) Quantitative structure-pharmacokinetic relationship modeling: apparent volume of distribution. *Journal of Pharmacy and Pharmacology*, **56**, 339–350.

80 Ghafourian, T., Barzegar-Jalali, M., Dastmalchi, S., Khavari-Khorasani, T., Hakimiha, N. and Nokhodchi, A. (2006) QSPR models for the prediction of apparent volume of distribution. *International Journal of Pharmaceutics*, **319**, 82–97.

81 Gleeson, M.P., Waters, N.J., Paine, S.W. and Davis, A.M. (2006) In silico human and rat Vss quantitative structure-activity relationship models. *Journal of Medicinal Chemistry*, **49**, 1953–1963.

82 Lombardo, F., Obach, R.S., DiCapua, F.M., Bakken, G., Lu, J., Potter, D.M., Gao, F., Miller, M.D. and Zhang, Y. (2006) A hybrid mixture discriminant analysis-random forest computational model for the prediction of volume of distribution in human. *Journal of Medicinal Chemistry*, **49**, 2262–2267.

10
Putting It All Together
Pamela Berry, Neil Parrott, Micaela Reddy, Pascale David-Pierson, and Thierry Lavé

10.1
Challenges in Drug Discovery

The integration of discovery data is the key to selecting good compounds for development. Drug discovery is increasingly "data rich" with high-throughput chemistry generating numerous compounds which are rapidly screened for pharmacological and pharmacokinetic properties. This vast amount of data is used to drive the decision-making process for compounds to be moved into development. The most common method for selecting compounds is to eliminate compounds that fail to meet criteria for DMPK, safety and pharmacological screens, and then pick the best candidate from the remaining compounds based on efficacy and other concerns. But consider, for example, a choice between the following compounds: compound A has excellent efficacy in a rat pharmacology bioassay, good permeability but low solubility, and much higher plasma protein binding in humans than in rats, while compound B has good efficacy, permeability and solubility, but has protein binding in humans similar to that of rats. Which compound should be chosen to move forward? We suggest integrating all available preclinical data using physiologically based pharmacokinetic (PBPK) modeling and, whenever feasible, incorporating pharmacology data to develop the PK/PD (PK/pharmacodynamic) relationship, to come up with the most accurate, quantitative interpretation of the dataset and, therefore, the most science-driven selection of the clinical candidate [1].

The need for integration of data from diverse sources leads to an increased use of mechanism-based models during drug discovery and the early phases of drug development. Biological mechanism-based models allow separation of biological and compound-specific components and are thus, by design, capable of integrating information about various processes.

Furthermore biological mechanism-based models which are built on the basis of human physiological parameters provide the opportunity to translate *in vitro* and/or *in silico* data into knowledge which is relevant for the situation in man. This approach allows optimization and selection of compounds based on the expected human profile rather than mice or rat data which might be irrelevant for human [2].

Hit and Lead Profiling. Edited by Bernard Faller and Laszlo Urban
Copyright © 2009 WILEY-VCH Verlag GmbH & Co. KGaA, Weinheim
ISBN: 978-3-527-32331-9

A key aspect during drug discovery is the need to understand the concentration–effect relationship. This understanding is crucial as the optimal pharmacokinetic properties of compounds need to be defined in the context of their relationship to the efficacy profile. Because mechanism based PK/PD models explicitly distinguish drug-specific properties and biological system specific properties, these PK/PD models offer the properties needed for integrating *in vitro* preclinical data and extrapolating to man [3, 4]. These models allow prediction of *in vivo* drug effects based on *in vitro* data (such as receptor affinity) generated during drug discovery.

Another challenge is uncertainty in the data and knowledge gaps in the processes driving the pharmacokinetic and efficacy profiles of drug candidates. Models offer the possibility to translate such uncertainty into a measure of confidence in the simulation and/or prediction. Quantifying key uncertainties and providing a range of possible outcomes that could be reasonable based on current knowledge contributes to more informed decision making [1, 2].

This chapter describes the utility of PBPK and PK/PD modeling for integrating available information in support of early drug discovery. The ability to gain better insight into compound properties and simulate the expected outcome of our compounds in man will enable improved decision making. Some methodological aspects are presented in this chapter. The potential and the limitations of the proposed approaches at various stages of the discovery process are discussed and illustrated with a number of examples.

10.2
Methodological Aspects

10.2.1
PBPK

As with classic compartment pharmacokinetic models, PBPK models can be used to simulate drug plasma concentration versus time profiles. However, PBPK models differ from classic PK models in that they include separate compartments for tissues involved in absorption, distribution, metabolism and elimination connected by physiologically based descriptions of blood flow (Figure 10.1).

Volumes and flows are based on actual measured tissue volumes and blood flows to various organs, which have been tabulated for many species [5]. The basic approach for the development of a PBPK model, including model formulation, parameterization and validation, was described in detail by Clewell *et al.* [1]. These authors also included discussions on technical topics ranging from numerical solutions of PBPK models to sensitivity analysis.

PBPK models require physicochemical and biochemical parameters along with physiological parameters. Historically, PBPK models were developed using a combination of *in vitro* data and/or *in vivo* PK data for a specific compound, and the amount of data necessary for model development was seen as prohibitive for application in the pharmaceutical industry. However, recent PBPK modeling papers

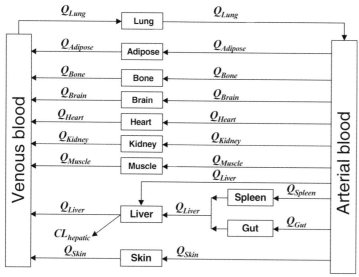

Figure 10.1 Schematic diagram of a PBPK model.

demonstrated the parameterization of generic models using *in silico*, *in vitro* and *in vivo* data typically generated in preclinical development [6–12]. PBPK models can incorporate *in silico* and/or *in vitro* data for solubility, permeability, lipophilicity (logP) and pKa, as well as plasma protein binding data. Also, metabolic stability data (e.g., microsomes or hepatocytes), when scaled appropriately, can be used to estimate clearance for compounds with metabolism as the primary mechanism of elimination.

One important advance making PBPK modeling accessible was a mechanistic approach for predicting tissue:blood partition coefficients (Pt:p) drugs [13]. For this approach, it was assumed that drug distributes homogenously into tissue and plasma by passive diffusion. Non-specific binding to lipids is estimated from drug lipophilicity (logP, logD). Specific, reversible binding to common plasma and tissue proteins is approximated based on plasma protein binding (f_{up}). Improved methods have been developed for calculating Pt:p for moderate-to-strong bases [14] and for acids, very weak bases, neutrals and zwitterions [15, 16]. Another method, reported to be equally applicable to neutral, acidic, basic, or multiply charged compounds, predicts Pt:p values based on the binding to phospholipid membranes, pKa and binding in blood [17].

Another important advance adding to the value of PBPK modeling in the pharmaceutical industry are physiological, mechanistic models developed to describe oral absorption in humans and preclinical species. Oral absorption is a complex process determined by the interplay of physiological and biochemical processes, physicochemical properties of the compound and formulation factors. Physiologically based models to predict oral absorption in animals and humans have recently been reviewed [18, 19] and several models are now commercially available. The commercial models have not been published in detail because of proprietary reasons but in essence they are transit models segmenting the gastrointestinal tract

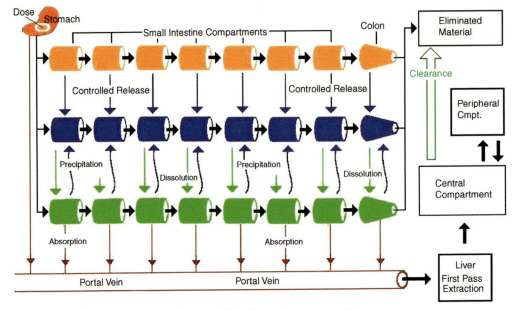

Figure 10.2 Schematic diagram of the advanced compartmental absorption and transit (ACAT) model [18].

into different compartments with the kinetics of transit, dissolution and uptake described by differential equations. For example, the model underlying GastroPlus is known as the advanced compartmental absorption and transit (ACAT) model [18] (Figure 10.2) and is a semi-physiologically based transit model, consisting of nine compartments corresponding to different segments of the digestive tract. Oral absorption simulations take *in vitro* and *in silico* input data such as solubility, permeability, particle size, logP, pKa (ionization constant) and dose. A similar mechanistic physiologically based model (advanced dissolution, absorption and metabolism; ADAM) was also recently implemented in the Simcyp population-based ADME simulator. A different physiological approach was been proposed [20, 21] that describes the GI tract not as a series of compartments but as a tube with spatially varying properties, with transport through this tube modeled as continuous plug flow with dispersion.

These powerful oral absorption models are a key feature of PBPK modeling software packages made available to scientists whose specialty is not mathematic modeling. Multiple software packages using physiology-based whole-body models for the simulation of the PK behavior, including absorption, distribution, metabolism and elimination. Cloe PK (Cyprotex; www.cyprotex.com) can be a powerful tool for early-stage PK predictions and compound prioritization. Software packages such as GastroPlus (Simulations Plus Inc.; www.simulations-plus.com), Simcyp (Simcyp; www.simcyp.com) and PK-Sim (Bayer Technology Services; www.pksim.com) make PBPK/mechanistic modeling accessible to pharmaceutical scientists.

Although PBPK modeling software packages can save time and require no programming effort, PBPK models can be developed using platforms such as MATLAB, Berkeley Madonna and acslXtreme. For example, Peters [22] reported using MATLAB to implement a PBPK model including a description of oral pharmacokinetics to assess any "lineshape" mismatch between simulated and observed oral profiles to gain mechanistic insights into pharmacokinetic processes affecting the lineshape of oral pharmacokinetics time-course data. The author proposed a strategy for identifying mechanisms impacting PK, such as saturation of clearance, enterohepatic recirculation, extrahepatic elimination, and processes impacting oral absorption, such as drug-induced delays in gastric emptying and regional variation in gut absorption. A custom-designed PBPK model takes significant resource to develop (both in terms of developing the model and the expertise to use the model effectively); however, a custom-designed PBPK modeling platform would be powerful and flexible, allowing integration of PBPK with PK/PD and/or disease modeling.

10.2.2
PK/PD

PK/PD evaluations provide crucial information on the potency and tolerability of the drug *in vivo*. PK/PD analysis is a multilayered process which starts with plotting the right data in the right way (including/excluding protein binding, assuming minimal/maximal effect, assuming direct effect/hysteresis, etc.) and becomes more elaborate by incorporating simple empirical (data-driven) models (direct effect/indirect effect etc.), comparisons with calculated receptor occupancy based on exposure and *in vitro* binding measurements, to more mechanistically or physiologically based models typically combining data from very heterogeneous sources (e.g., in house concentration time course, *in vitro* parameters, literature data from competitors).

The time course of drug effects is the result of many factors, including formulation, pharmacokinetic and pharmacodynamic properties, as well as physiological factors such as circadian rhythms, homeostatic mechanisms and disease progression. Given this complexity, the analysis of the time course of drug response using PK/PD models represents a much more efficient way to deal with pharmacological effects than the use of simple methods based upon single parameters such as onset time and peak effects, or integrated effects such as the area under time–effect curves. Potential complexities during the time course of drug action include: delayed distribution from plasma to the effect site, indirect mechanisms of action, irreversible binding to receptor, development of tolerance, rebound, metabolite interactions, changes in protein binding and irreversible effects. However, different models have been developed to describe each of these situations. Current methods of integrating various system complexities into these models were reviewed recently [3, 4, 23].

Mechanism-based PK/PD models contain specific expressions to characterize the different stages between drug administration and clinical effects, namely: target site distribution, target binding and activation, pharmacodynamic interactions, transduction, homeostatic feedback mechanisms and effects on disease progression [3, 4, 23]. Such models are parameterized to describe: (i) drug-specific properties; (ii) biological system specific properties. This mechanistic basis is crucial for improved prediction of *in vivo* drug effects; for example, *in vitro* information on receptor affinity can be used to predict target effects as well as potentially downstream effects at an early discovery stage.

Often PK/PD models are developed using classic PK models to describe plasma concentrations, which is often appropriate when PK samples are obtained during the PD assay so that plasma concentrations are most accurately simulated. A PBPK/PD model may be particularly useful when PK data are not available for a given PD assay, when a PD effect is not related to free plasma concentrations but instead is related to the free concentration in a target tissue, or when a PK/PD model must be extrapolated to humans.

10.3
Strategic Use of PBPK During Drug Discovery

PBPK modeling can be a powerful tool for integrating available *in silico* and *in vitro* data to gain mechanistic insight. In the paradigm of PBPK modeling introduced by the pharmaceutical industry, data generated throughout the drug development process can be integrated and updated efficiently. The results of PBPK modeling can be used to determine the most critical assays to include in the screening cascade to provide more informative data to chemists. However, to ensure that modeling can be used to best advantage, a modeling strategy should be considered when making data generation choices. At early stages, while characterizing a series of compounds, enough data must be generated to assess the accuracy of the *in silico* properties and the ability of predictive PBPK/PD to make predictions of sufficient quality for making decisions.

The data integration process can begin even before compounds are generated, that is, with virtual compounds. For example, compound structures and *in silico* properties can be entered from a company database into an sdf file and then imported into a PBPK model such as the one available in GastroPlus, which can interface with ADMET Predictor for the generation of additional *in silico* parameters. Of course, the *in silico* predictions for a series of compounds should be verified appropriately before being used to make decisions. These batch files can be run in a high-throughput manner, providing some idea of the compounds' PK properties even before synthesis.

The preliminary models can be used to select compounds for synthesis and to determine which data is most important to generate to understand the PK properties of a particular compound or series. As compounds are generated and at first low-throughput and then high-throughput data become available, the model can be updated and when possible validated against *in vivo* PK data in animals. Mismatches between model predictions and data indicate missing mechanisms or inadequate data. If the model prediction does not match the data, the model can be used to develop hypotheses for additional experimentation. Thus, PBPK modeling allows integration of *in silico* and *in vitro* data, and the model itself becomes a repository of information for what is known for a series of compounds or a specific compound.

The model is only as good as the data used as input. Therefore, it is important to use a model in ways appropriate for the level of data that was available for its development. At early stages, when only *in silico* and high-throughput screening data are available, model applications such as sensitivity analysis to determine key factors impacting absorption, distribution and elimination would be most appropriate. At later stages, when high-throughput screening data and perhaps some more definitive *in vitro* data and/or limited *in vivo* PK data are available, the model could be used to determine if the compound could achieve efficacy with BID or QD dosing. When definitive data (*in vivo* and *in vitro*) are generated and the model is verified to the extent possible, it can be used to make estimates such as the human PK at the efficacious dose.

10.4
Strategic Use of PK/PD During Drug Discovery

PK/PD modeling provides a scientific basis for understanding the relationship between the time course of the plasma concentration and the drug effect and for the prediction of drug effect in humans with regard to efficacy and safety. During lead identification, PK/PD modeling can be used to support the definition of the target profile, to understand the balance needed between PK and PD properties and to guide lead optimization efforts. Furthermore, with the integration of *in vitro* (PK and PD) data relevant for human, PK/PD modeling provides the opportunity to base decisions on expected human PK/PD profiles rather than observed profiles in the animals. The quantitative information on functional effects might be very limited at the early stages of the drug discovery processes. At this stage however, the use of *in vitro* target-related binding information together with knowledge of the target distribution in the body may be very valuable to obtain initial estimate of the therapeutic dosing regimen in man at an early stage.

Target effect considerations represent the initial steps of PK/PD model building which can then be extended to include downstream effects such as molecular target activation, physiological measures, pathophysiological measures and clinical ratings [3, 4] as our drug candidates move through the discovery and development process.

10.5
Application During Lead Identification

Recent publications discuss the utility of physiologically based pharmacokinetic models to predict the pharmacokinetics of discovery compounds in the rat [7, 9]. The following examples show the utility of applying these methods at an even earlier stage.

During lead identification, multiple series are evaluated for the potential to yield drug-like compounds, that is, the appropriate combination of potency, physicochemical and ADMET properties expected to meet the target product profile. Typically, one or more representative compounds from each series are characterized to uncover any inherent liabilities. Data generated during this evaluation may include *in vitro* determinations of metabolic stability, permeability, solubility, lipophilicity and protein binding, as well as rat pharmacokinetic data. Previously, modeling activities in lead identification typically focused on *in silico* predictions of individual physicochemical and ADMET properties. Employing the PBPK approach at this stage allows integration of all the available data into a composite picture of compound behavior.

PBPK simulations using GastroPlus software equipped with the PBPK Plus module (Simulations Plus; Lancaster, Calif., USA) have been used to guide some Roche lead identification programs. Typically, a structure data file containing one or more compounds is imported into GastroPlus so that *in silico* properties can be calculated using the ADMET Predictor software. The calculation of *in silico* parameters allows the prediction of complete intravenous and oral profiles from the structure and an estimate of clearance; however, minimal data requirements needed for adequate predictions must be established for each series. Care should be taken when using *in silico* values for sensitive parameters. For example, using *in silico* values for pKa- and pH-dependent solubility factors should be adequate for many compounds that are unionized or are completely ionized at physiologically relevant pH (e.g., from pH 1 in the GI tract to ca. pH 7.4 in the ileum), but the appropriateness of the *in silico* predictions should be carefully examined for compounds that are only partially ionized at physiological pH. The PBPK approach may not be useful for all series in early discovery. Failure of the approach usually indicates a deficiency in the dataset or the occurrence of a process impacting the pharmacokinetics of the compounds that was not incorporated into the model.

The extension of PBPK simulation to include pharmacodynamic endpoints is very powerful at this stage to guide the project team with respect to the key properties to consider for optimization, as demonstrated in the example below.

Example 10.1

In an anticoagulant project at Roche, guidance was provided with modeling and simulation in order to estimate the required potency and bioavailability to cover the patient in terms of anticoagulation over the dosing interval with more than 1.5-fold but less than fivefold prolongation of prothrombin time. Another question addressed with modeling and simulation was related to the impact of the different pharmacokinetic and efficacy parameters to be optimized on the coagulation profile *in vivo*.

The analysis was completed for 12 compounds for which protein binding, renal and hepatic clearances and microsomal data were available. Plasma concentration versus time profiles in the rat were also available for these compounds. The approach taken was to simulate the individual processes (metabolic clearance, renal clearance, distribution, pharmacological activity). The ability of the PBPK model to simulate the *in vivo* behavior of the compound was verified in the rat. Thus, the metabolic clearance of the compounds could be reasonably well simulated, based on microsomal data and assuming no binding to microsomes: less than twofold deviation between the observed and predicted clearance was achieved for about eight of the

12 compounds. Renal clearance was predicted using a model based on artificial neural networks using the structural descriptors hydrophobic surface, hydrophilic volume and molecular weight. For all compounds, the volume of distribution was remarkably similar and corresponded approximately to extracellular space (i.e., 0.3 L/kg). These parameters (renal clearance, metabolic clearance, extracellular distribution) allowed reasonable simulations of the intravenous plasma versus time concentrations profiles in the rat.

Using human physiology and *in vitro* data and clinically relevant input parameters (i.e., metabolic stability in human hepatocytes and microsomes as well as prothrombin time measured in various batches of human plasma) the model was extended to human. This human PK/PD model was then used to investigate the impact of the various physicochemical, pharmacokinetic and pharmacodynamic properties on the anticoagulant profile (i.e., prothrombin time) expected in man.

Example 10.2
In a virology program at Roche, modeling and simulation was included in the early profiling of potential lead series. For these early compounds, *in silico* estimates were used for most of the physicochemical parameters; measured values were substituted when available. Simulations of pharmacokinetics in the rat were compared against measured *in vivo* PK data for several compounds in a series before performing human projections. Since oral exposure for compounds with low aqueous solubility tends to be underestimated if solubility in a physiologically relevant medium is not used in the model [7], measured solubility in simulated human intestinal fluid was obtained for compounds with aqueous solubility <10 µg/mL. Human jejunal permeability was converted from 21-day Caco-2 assay data, using a previously established inhouse correlation. For fairly soluble compounds exhibiting an efflux in the Caco-2 assay, the permeability measured in the presence of the Pgp inhibitor elacridar may provide a better estimate of permeability at saturating conditions. Clearance was predicted from microsome or hepatocyte data using the well stirred model, assuming equivalent binding to plasma and liver microsomes. The tissue distribution was predicted using the tissue composition models [14–16]. Simulations of pharmacokinetics in the rat were compared against measured profiles for several compounds of a series before performing human projections using the corresponding dataset shown to be predictive for the rat.

In this project, compound A from a potential lead series was a neutral compound of MW 314 with low aqueous solubility (<1 µg/mL) and moderate permeability (5.6×10^{-6} cm/s in the presence of 2 µM elacridar). Systemic clearance, volume and AUC following a 0.5 mg/kg intravenous dose to rats were well predicted (within twofold) from scaled microsomal clearance and *in silico* prediction of pKa, logP and unbound fraction in plasma. Figure 10.3a shows the predicted oral profile compared to the observed data from two rats dosed orally at 2 mg/kg. The additional inputs for the oral prediction were the Caco-2 permeability and measured human fed-state simulated intestinal fluid (FeSSIF, 92 µg/mL). The oral pharmacokinetic parameters T_{max}, C_{max}, AUC and bioavailability were well predicted. Simulation of higher doses of compound A predicted absorption-limited

230 | *10 Putting It All Together*

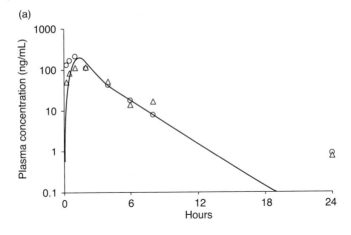

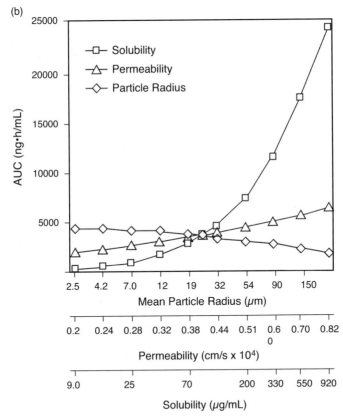

Figure 10.3 (a) Predicted oral profile compared to the observed data from two rats dosed orally at 2 mg/kg. (b) Parameter sensitivity analysis.

exposure in the rat, indicating potential difficulty in achieving sufficient exposures in toxicity studies. This conclusion was not intuitive given compound A's favorable oral pharmacokinetics at the dose tested in rats; bioavailability was estimated to be approx. 36% at 2 mg/kg, but the maximum absorbable dose (MAD) was projected to be achieved by 10 mg/kg. Parameter sensitivity analysis indicated that solubility is the key parameter limiting absorption of compound A. Modest gains would be expected from increasing permeability, but reducing particle size would have little effect on the absorption of this compound (Figure 10.3b). Thus, using minimal investment of resources, modeling and simulation approaches were able to highlight potential development hurdles and suggest solutions at a very early stage. In addition, these approaches have the potential of saving Pharmaceutics resources by reducing unnecessary investigations into micronized formulations.

Similar approaches were used to predict the pharmacokinetics of three representative compounds of a another potential lead series from this program. All were neutral compounds with a mean MW of 470, low aqueous solubility ($\leq 1\,\mu g/mL$), moderate lipophilicity, and low to moderate Caco-2 permeability (0.4–1.5×10^{-6} cm/s). Measured FeSSIF solubility (9–72 µg/mL) and unbound fraction in rat plasma (<1.0 to 6.4%) were used in the predictions. PBPK predictions for the rat (0.5 mg/kg IV, 2 mg/kg PO) were made for all three compounds and compared with the observed data. All intravenous and oral pharmacokinetic parameters were reasonably well predicted within twofold of the observed values. Following verification of the PBPK approach in the rat, human oral projections could be made with confidence for this series. Human PBPK projections for compound B, which exhibited the highest exposure of the three compounds in the rat, were made to evaluated the series potential for achieving the target product profile. The predicted human MAD for this compound was 700 mg. The projected maximum exposures at this dose were barely within the range of efficacious trough concentrations required by the target product profile. Clearly, substantial improvements in the pharmacokinetics of this series would be needed to achieve sufficient exposures to assess efficacy and tolerability in the clinic. Parameter sensitivity analysis performed around the 10 mg/kg human dose (Figure 10.4) indicated that improvements in solubility would have the maximum effect on the absorption of these compounds. Improvements in permeability would also result in increased absorption, but little benefit would be expected from reducing particle size. However, increases in particle size would result in decreased absorption. Validation of the PBPK approach in rats and projection to the human model for a series at the lead identification stage should guide the development of screening paradigms as the program transitions to the lead optimization phase, defining the key parameters affecting human PK and providing a quantitative assessment of their desired ranges.

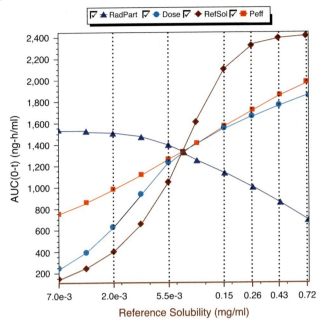

Figure 10.4 Parameter sensitivity analysis performed around the 700 mg dose. RadPart: particle radius; RefSol: reference solubility.

10.6
Application During Lead Optimization

Determination of *in vivo* PK is considerably more costly than *in vitro* screening, and thus there is interest in optimizing resources by using simulation to prioritize compounds for *in vivo* testing. Furthermore, the *in vivo* PK evaluation is restricted to rat or mice at this stage, therefore approaches that provide the possibility to simulate the expected outcome in man are of great value. However, acceptance of this approach requires extensive validation. The practical value of generic physiologically based models of pharmacokinetics at the early stage of drug discovery was recently evaluated [7, 9].

In the study by Parrott *et al.* [7], a generic PBPK model was applied to predict plasma profiles after intravenous and oral dosing to the rat for a set of 68 compounds from six different chemical classes. The compounds were selected without particular bias and so are considered representative of current Roche discovery compounds. The physicochemical properties of the compounds are rather different from those of marketed compounds; in particular they have higher lipophilicity (mean logP = 4) and lower aqueous solubility as well as a tendency to be neutral at physiological pH. The more extreme property values can present experimental determination challenges and so for consistency all predictions were made on the basis of calculated lipophilicity and protein binding while *in vitro* measurements of intrinsic clearance in hepatocytes, ionization, solubility and permeability were used for all compounds.

In a first stage, distribution was predicted with tissue composition-based equations and the estimated tissue partition coefficients were combined with clearance estimated by direct scaling of hepatocyte intrinsic clearance in a PBPK model as described earlier.

In a second stage GastroPlus was used to simulate oral absorption, and oral profiles were produced by feeding this predicted input into a compartmental disposition model fitted to the mean observed intravenous data.

For intravenous dosing simulations 60% of the clearance and volume predictions were within twofold of the observed values and the ranking of compounds by predicted versus observed parameters showed correlation coefficients of 0.8 and 0.6 for clearance and volume respectively. For oral dosing simulations, 40% of the predicted AUC values were within twofold of observed values and the mean fold error was 4.1. For compounds with measured solubility less than 0.012 mg/mL only 10% of predictions were within twofold, while for compounds with higher solubility 70% were within twofold [7] (see Figure 10.5).

Overall, this study indicated that generic simulation of pharmacokinetics at the lead optimization stage could be useful to predict differences in pharmacokinetic parameters of threefold or more based upon minimal measured input data. Fine discrimination of pharmacokinetics (less than twofold) should not be expected due to the uncertainty in the input data at the early stages. It is also apparent that verification of simulations with *in vivo* data for a few compounds of each new compound class was required to allow an assessment of the error in prediction and to identify invalid model assumptions.

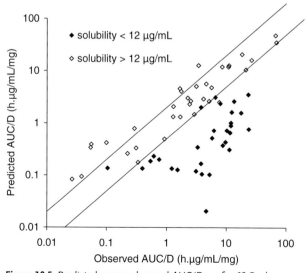

Figure 10.5 Predicted versus observed AUC/Dose for 68 Roche compounds [6].

The value of PBPK for simulating the *first time in animal* study was illustrated also by Germani *et al.* [9]. In this study, the model was used to predict the plasma pharmacokinetics obtained in 24 rat and two mouse pharmacokinetic studies. This study was restricted to the prediction of disposition profiles (i.e., profiles observed after intravenous administration of the compounds). The administered compounds were synthesized as part of a number of different discovery programs. The simulated profiles were generally in agreement with the observed ones. Plasma clearance and mean residence times were well predicted: average fold errors were 2.7 and 2.5, respectively, with approximately one-half of the cases predicted within a twofold of observed. Some over prediction of plasma clearance was observed in the range of low clearance values, in case of compounds with logP = 5 and protein binding of 99%. In contrast, slight underestimations were observed for molecules with logP near zero and protein binding of 99.9%. The error in the volume of distribution at steady state (Vss) was higher, but still acceptable (average fold error was 3.7).

As discussed earlier, PBPK simulations can be extended to include target effects, that is, receptor binding. In a recent Roche antiobesity project, PBPK/PD simulations including target effects were performed in order to get a better understanding of the efficacy or lack of efficacy of compounds tested in a subchronic food intake model. PK/PD simulated brain receptor occupancy for all compounds tested in a 3-day *in vivo* food intake model in the rat. Such simulations were performed based on *in vitro* parameters for DMPK and efficacy (*in vitro* K_i, *in vitro* microsomal clearance, buffer solubility, logD, pKa, unbound fraction in plasma) and using a PBPK model to predict *in vivo* concentration–time profiles in the rat. The simulations of receptor occupancy were performed under the assumption that unbound concentration in plasma is close to unbound concentration in the brain. Interestingly these PK/PD simulations indicated that *in vivo* active compounds exhibited high (>60%) and sustained (>8 h) receptor occupancy while lower sustained receptor occupancies were predicted for inactive compounds (Figure 10.6). A cross-validation of predicted receptor occupancy with observed ex vivo receptor occupancy was also performed proving the validity of the simulations and of the assumptions used.

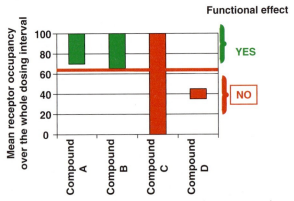

Figure 10.6 Simulations of receptor occupancy for active (green bars) and inactive compounds (red bars).

Such examples extend PBPK simulations to prediction of target effect and appear very powerful for generation of insights into the efficacy/lack of efficacy *in vivo* in relation to receptor occupancy. Consequently, such PBPK/PD simulations can be used as a filter between high-throughput screening and *in vivo* efficacy in order to prioritize compounds expected to be active *in vivo*.

10.7
Application During Clinical Lead Selection

An example showing the utility of such an approach was provided recently [6]. In this example, *in vitro* and *in vivo* data for five potential clinical candidates were combined in PK/PD models to estimate the effective human dose and associated exposure and to aid in the selection of the most promising compound. To ensure that the decision was based on significant differences between the compounds, estimates of variability and/or uncertainty were carried through in the modeling of the PK and PD. The five compounds were from the same structural class and had similar physicochemical properties. Molecular weights were in the range 406–472 and all compounds were largely unionized at physiological pH. LogP values ranged from 2.1 to 2.9 and permeability was good for all compounds, while solubility ranged from 0.009 to 2.2 mg/mL. *In vitro* receptor binding and plasma protein binding in rat and human and *in vivo* PK and PD data in rat were also available for all compounds.

In a first step the scaling of intrinsic clearances determined in rat hepatocytes was compared to *in vivo* clearance. When taking account of non-linearity, the estimated hepatic metabolic clearance values were in reasonable agreement with observed total clearances, which ranged from 7 to 35 mL/min/kg, and it was considered reasonable to estimate the expected clearances in human by a similar scaling of human hepatocyte data. The error around the mean predicted human clearance was based on the variability seen in different batches of human hepatocytes.

Volume of distribution predicted from tissue composition-based equations showed an average fold error of 2.2 and the correlation of predicted versus observed volume for the five compounds was poor. For the prediction of volume of distribution it was assumed that the volume in human (L/kg) was the same as the observed volume in the rat (ranging from 0.9 to 2.8 L/kg for the five compounds). Due to the uncertainty in the prediction of volume, the error range associated with this parameter was set as a uniform distribution over a twofold range.

There was a direct relationship between the effect and the plasma concentration in the rat pharmacodynamic data and it was well described by a simple E_{max} model. Based on preclinical models for efficacy, a 90% effect was considered as the target for therapeutic effect. Finally the human C_{90} (human concentration corresponding to 90% effect, C90_man) was estimated by accounting for the different affinities and unbound fractions of each compound for the rat and human receptors as follows:

$$C90\_man = C90\_rat.(Ki\_man/Ki\_rat).(fu\_rat/fu\_man) \quad (10.1)$$

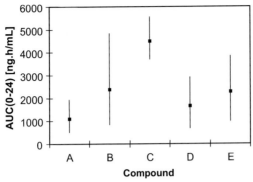

Figure 10.7 Simulated AUC at steady state for five potential clinical candidate compounds. Symbols give the mean prediction while lines indicate a 95% confidence range [6].

where Ki_man and Ki_rat are the affinities in man and rat, and fu_man and fu_rat are the unbound fraction in plasma in man and rat, respectively.

Finally, absorption in the rat was shown to be well predicted by GastroPlus, since good agreement was seen between simulated and observed oral profiles, and so the predicted human pharmacokinetics and pharmacodynamics were combined in a GastroPlus model of human to allow for estimation of the effective steady-state doses and exposures after repeated oral dosing. Incorporation of variability and uncertainty was achieved using some stochastic simulations. The predicted effective doses and associated exposures including error ranges on the predictions were then provided for the various potential clinical candidates (see Figure 10.7).

This example showed that the PBPK approach assists a sound decision on the selection of the optimal molecule to be progressed by integrating the available information and focusing the attention onto the expected properties in human. The predicted efficacious AUC values shown in Figure 10.7 were combined with early toxicological data to estimate safety margins, while the associated dose estimates for the five molecules were combined with chemical supply and formulation data to assess compound developability. After weighing these considerations compound D was selected for progression. Importantly, the method aided the decision by effectively summarizing a variety of *in vitro* and *in vivo* preclinical data including estimation of variability and uncertainty in the predictions (Figure 10.8).

10.8
Limitations with Current Methodology and Approaches

Physiologically based models show improved performance over more empirical methods. The PBPK approach is based upon solid physiological principles and can be extended to include additional relevant processes. Also, besides satisfactory

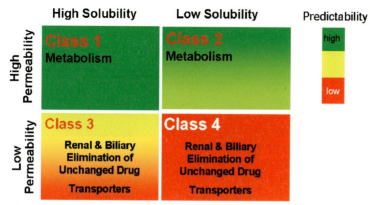

Figure 10.8 Predictability of systemic exposure profile using a PBPK approach and Biopharmaceutics Drug Disposition Classification System (adapted from Wu and Benet [24]).

prediction capabilities, an approach based on a mechanistic framework can lead to greater insights into the behavior of compounds and offers more potential in the early stages of drug development since it does not require *in vivo* data in several species as is needed for allometric scaling.

Some caution is required with some chemical classes and compound properties related to low solubility, high lipophilicity, major impact of active transport processes on elimination and distribution. It is therefore recommended that PBPK models should only be applied after verification of the simulations with *in vivo* pharmacokinetics for a few compounds of a given chemical class. Such verification will help to identify invalid model assumptions or missing processes where additional data is needed.

The applicability of PBPK models can be described in the context of the BDDCS classification [24]. PBPK models are very predictive for class 1 and class 2 compounds. However for poorly soluble compounds, the use of aqueous solubility is shown to be inadequate for reliable prediction of oral absorption in physiologically based models [7]. In such cases, it is recommended to use solubility measured in simulated intestinal fluids (FeSSIF, FaSSIF). Such data proved to be very relevant to simulate the oral absorption of BCS 2 (low solubility, high permeability) compounds [25].

Important limitations of the PBPK approach are realized for class 3 and 4 compounds with significant active distribution/absorption processes, where biliary elimination is a major component of the elimination process or where the assumptions of flow-limited distribution and well mixed compartments are not valid and permeability-limited distribution is apparent. These drawbacks could be addressed by the addition of permeability barriers for some tissues and by the incorporation of a more complex liver model which addresses active uptake into the liver, active efflux into the bile, biliary elimination and enterohepatic recirculation. However, this improvement to current methodologies requires the availability of the appropriate input data for quantification of the various processes involved as well as validation of the corresponding *in vitro* to *in vivo* scaling approaches.

A number of limitations related to PK/PD modeling are also a reality in situations where predictability of the animal model to man is questionable, where the time course of the pharmacodynamic effect cannot be assessed for drug candidates and when, for example, no accessible/"valid" pharmacodynamic endpoint for PK/PD is available. The relevance of the animal model for human could be addressed to some extent at least by measuring relative potency in animal versus man *in vitro*. In situations where no relevant PD endpoint is available (e.g., for CNS efficacy models), effects at target level (i.e., enzyme inhibition, receptor occupancy) might represent a valuable alternative. In this context however the level and duration of target effect required for clinical efficacy requires careful considerations.

10.9
Conclusions

The physiological and mechanistic basis of PBPK and PK/PD models provides several benefits for data integration during early discovery. Recent reports and examples demonstrate the utility of PBPK models using the data typically generated during preclinical development at early stages for guiding projects and prioritizing *in vivo* experimentation and predicting human PK. The powerful capability of extending these models to PD at the early stage are also illustrated with a few examples, but this has definitely not yet been fully exploited by the pharmaceutical industry.

References

1 Clewell, H.J., Reddy, M.B., Lave, T. and Andersen, M.E. (2008) Physiologically based pharmacokinetic modeling, in *Preclinical Development Handbook: ADME and Biopharmaceutical Properties* (ed. S.C. Grad), John Wiley and Sons, Hoboken, New Jersey.

2 Lavé, T., Parrott, N., Grimm, H.P., Fleury, A. and Reddy, M. (2007) Challenges and opportunities with modelling and simulation in drug discovery and drug development. *Xenobiotica*, 37, 1295–1310.

3 Danhof, M., de, J., Joost De, L., Elizabeth, C.M., Della, P., Oscar Ploeger, B.A. and Voskuyl, R.A. (2007) Mechanism-based pharmacokinetic-pharmacodynamic modeling: biophase distribution, receptor theory, and dynamical systems analysis. *Annual Review of Pharmacology and Toxicology*, 47, 357–400.

4 Danhof, M., de, L., Elizabeth, C.M., Della, P., Oscar, E., Ploeger, B.A. and Voskuyl, R.A. (2008) Mechanism-based pharmacokinetic-pharmacodynamic PK-PD modeling in translational drug research. *Trends in Pharmacological Sciences*, 29, 186–191.

5 Brown, R.P., Delp, M.D., Lindstedt, S.L., Rhomberg, L.R. and Beliles, R.P. (1997) Physiological parameter values for physiologically based pharmacokinetic models. *Toxicology and Industrial Health*, 13, 407–484.

6 Parrott, N., Jones, H., Paquereau, N. and Lavé, T. (2005) Application of full physiological models for pharmaceutical drug candidate selection and extrapolation of pharmacokinetics to man. *Basic Clinical Pharmacology and Toxicology*, 96, 193–199.

7 Parrott, N., Paquereau, N., Coassolo, P. and Lavé, T. (2005) An evaluation of the utility of physiologically based models of pharmacokinetics in early drug discovery. *Journal of Pharmaceutical Sciences*, **94**, 2327–2343.

8 Jones, H., Parrott, N., Jorga, K. and Lavé, T. (2006) A novel strategy for physiologically based predictions of human pharmacokinetics. *Clinical Pharmacokinetics*, **45**, 511–542.

9 Germani, M., Crivori, P., Rocchetti, M., Burton, P.S., Wilson, A.G.E., Smith, M.E. and Poggesi, I. (2005) Evaluation of a physiologically-based pharmacokinetic approach for simulating the first-time-in-animal study. *Basic Clinical Pharmacology and Toxicology*, **96**, 254–256.

10 Leahy, D.E. (2004) Drug discovery information integration: virtual humans for pharmacokinetics. *Drug Discovery Today: Biosilico*, **2**, 78–84.

11 De Buck, S.S., Sinha, V.K., Fenu, L.A., Gilissen, R.A.H.J., Mackie, C.E. and Nijsen, M.J. (2007) The prediction of drug metabolism, tissue distribution, and bioavailability of 50 structurally diverse compounds in rat using mechanism-based absorption, distribution, and metabolism prediction tools. *Drug Metabolism and Disposition: The Biological Fate of Chemicals*, **35**, 649–659.

12 De Buck, S.S., Sinha, V.K., Fenu, L.A., Nijsen, M.J., Mackie, C.E. and Gilissen, R.A.H.J. (2007) Prediction of human pharmacokinetics using physiologically based modeling: a retrospective analysis of 26 clinically tested drugs. *Drug Metabolism and Disposition: The Biological Fate of Chemicals*, **35**, 1766–1780.

13 Poulin, P. and Theil, F.P. (2000) A priori prediction of tissue: plasma partition coefficients of drugs to facilitate the use of physiologically-based pharmacokinetic models in drug discovery. *Journal of Pharmaceutical Sciences*, **89**, 16–35.

14 Rodgers, T., Leahy, D. and Rowland, M. (2005) Physiologically based pharmacokinetic modeling 1: predicting the tissue distribution of moderate-to-strong bases. *Journal of Pharmaceutical Sciences*, **94**, 1259–1276.

15 Rodgers, T. and Rowland, M. (2006) Physiologically based pharmacokinetic modeling 2: predicting the tissue distribution of acids, very weak bases, neutrals and zwitterions. *Journal of Pharmaceutical Sciences*, **95**, 1238–1257.

16 Rodgers, T. and Rowland, M. (2007) Mechanistic approaches to volume of distribution predictions: understanding the processes. *Pharmaceutical Research*, **24**, 918–933.

17 Schmitt, W. (2008) General approach for the calculation of tissue to plasma partition coefficients. *Toxicology In Vitro: An International Journal Published in Association with BIBRA*, **22**, 457–467.

18 Agoram, B., Woltosz, W.S. and Bolger, M.B. (2001) Predicting the impact of physiological and biochemical processes on oral drug bioavailability. *Advanced Drug Delivery Reviews*, **50** (Suppl 1), S41–S67.

19 Parrott, N.J. and Lavé, T. (2002) Prediction of intestinal absorption: comparative assessment of commercially available software. *European Journal of Pharmaceutical Sciences*, **17**, 51–61.

20 Willmann, S., Schmitt, W., Keldenich, J. and Dressman, J.B. (2003) A physiologic model for simulating gastrointestinal flow and drug absorption in rats. *Pharmaceutical Research*, **20**, 1766–1771.

21 Willmann, S., Schmitt, W., Keldenich, J., Lippert, J. and Dressman, J.B. (2004) A physiological model for the estimation of the fraction dose absorbed in humans. *Journal of Medicinal Chemistry*, **47**, 4022–4031.

22 Peters, S.A. (2008) Evaluation of a generic physiologically based pharmacokinetic model for lineshape analysis. *Clinical Pharmacokinetics*, **47**, 261–275.

23 Mager, D.E. and Jusko, W.J. (2008) Development of translational pharmacokinetic-pharmacodynamic models. *Clinical Pharmacology and Therapeutics*, **83**, 909–912.

24 Wu, C.Z. and Benet, L.Z. (2005) Predicting drug disposition via application of BCS: transport/absorption/elimination interplay and development of a biopharmaceutics drug disposition classification system. *Pharmaceutical Research*, **22**, 11–23.

25 Jones, H.M., Parrott, N., Ohlenbusch, G. and Lavé, T. (2006) Predicting pharmacokinetic food effects using biorelevant solubility media and physiologically based modelling. *Clinical Pharmacokinetics*, **45**, 1213–1226.

Part III

11
Genetic Toxicity: *In Vitro* Approaches for Hit and Lead Profiling
Richard M Walmsley and Nicholas Billinton

11.1
Introduction

As the flow of new drugs to market continues to reduce, there is ever greater interest in the causes of compound attrition in drug discovery. Whilst aspects of ADME/Tox profiling were considered in the preceding chapters, this chapter focuses on a specific type of toxicity, namely genetic toxicity (or genotoxicity). Some 12–15% of candidate attrition is due to adverse genotoxicity safety assessment [1]. Reducing this to perhaps 3–5% would be a significant reduction in late-stage attrition and its associated costs, and is probably achievable by early profiling.

Genotoxicity assessment has traditionally been the domain of the late-preclinical safety assessment departments, in which GLP testing for regulatory submission is preceded by relatively small-scale screening exercises. Perhaps a couple of dozen compounds from a discovery program representing several chemistries are reduced to a main candidate, with a backup in the same chemistry and an example from a different chemistry. Some of these assays are simply cutdown regulatory assays and others were more specifically developed for the screening of perhaps hundreds of compounds in a year. This chapter reviews these current late screening tools and considers which might be appropriate for hit and lead profiling, which requires the capability to test thousands or tens of thousands of compounds per year.

Currently failures resulting from genotoxic liability occur late and with significant expense, arising from mechanistic studies in animals, delay in first time in human (FTIH) phase zero/one clinical trials and going to market, or even late abandonment and loss of all investment in the program. It is therefore a valuable exercise to gain this information earlier in discovery. This chapter investigates the possibilities of genotoxicity screening as part of compound profiling.

The ultimate aim of early genotoxicity profiling is to reduce the number of candidate drugs that carry an unforeseen genotoxic hazard. This is because exposure to genotoxins can increase the risk of developing cancers and/or germ line mutations in mammals. In discussing the utility of genotoxicity assessment in the context of profiling, it is important to distinguish between hazard assessment and safety

Hit and Lead Profiling. Edited by Bernard Faller and Laszlo Urban
Copyright © 2009 WILEY-VCH Verlag GmbH & Co. KGaA, Weinheim
ISBN: 978-3-527-32331-9

assessment because the data are used differently at these extremes of the drug discovery process. When there are still perhaps thousands of hits to choose from, a reliable positive result (hazard) can either contribute to a low ranking for development, or be used as an attrition tool. From this it is clear that a profiler needs the genotoxicity "screening" input to exhibit high specificity: wrongly classifying noncarcinogens as carcinogens could lead to the loss of potentially valuable drugs. Much later, in candidate selection, when there may be fewer than 20 compounds left, reliable negative results (safety) are required to carry the drug forward into development and FTIH studies. Thus safety assessment groups require high sensitivity: wrongly classifying carcinogens as noncarcinogens allows compounds to continue their ever more expensive progress to the clinic via animal studies before the liability is identified. An additional difference in approach to data is that whilst the profiler is only interested in hazard, the safety expert is more interested in the human relevance of the underlying mechanism causing hazard.

The ideal genotoxicity test should have high specificity and high sensitivity; it should generate negative results for noncarcinogens and positive results for genotoxic carcinogens. In reality there is a trade-off between specificity and sensitivity, which is clear from the predictive properties of the commonly used genotoxicity tests (Figure 11.1; graph derived from data in [2]). This compromise needs to be understood and recognized when developing testing strategies at different stages in discovery and development. Whilst high specificity often comes at the expense of sensitivity, for screening this is less of a concern, as genotoxins "missed" in a

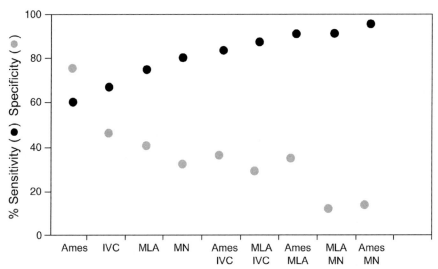

Figure 11.1 The sensitivity and specificity of the *in vitro* regulatory tests in the prediction of rodent carcinogenicity.
IVC, *in vitro* chromosome aberration; MLA, mouse lymphoma assay; MN, micronucleus test. Upper dark circles, sensitivity; lower light circles, specificity.

screening exercise will be picked up in later GLP studies – though in much lower numbers than is achieved in a strategy without the early screen.

Genetic toxicity testing generates quantitative data and genetic toxicologists recognize that genotoxins are not all equal. Compounds that are genotoxic in any particular *in vitro* assay may or may not have no-effect levels (NOELS). There are potent genotoxins, active at low concentrations, and weak genotoxins, active at high concentrations. Genotoxins might produce large or small increases in the measured outputs. In making a safety assessment, exposure and dose are both considered, so a weak genotoxin might be an acceptable drug if the therapeutic dose is not high. Exceptions are allowed in the case of life-threatening diseases, and in the special case of antivirals and antineoplastic agents, genotoxicity can also provide the mechanism of action. The practical aim of screening for genotoxic potential much earlier than safety assessment should probably be to identify potent genotoxins, as these would be the most challenging to carry forward in safety assessment. The result should be that fewer problem compounds are needlessly carried forward as candidates, or that safety assessment laboratories are provided with an early warning of the arrival of compounds requiring mechanistic investigation.

The traditional paradigm positions genotoxicity assessment in the hands of experts in safety assessment departments, who perform labor-intensive assays on very small numbers of compounds. However, it is now possible to envisage a situation in which the potent genotoxins are identified by robots and computer programs, in the same way as other liabilities in ADME/Tox. The increasing appearance of publications that discuss genotoxicity in an earlier screening context reflects a growing willingness to consider genotoxicity hazard assessment as a welcome extension to the utility of genotoxicity data. Here we introduce the philosophical, scientific and practical aspects of genotoxicity which are relevant to those intending to introduce screening programs.

11.2
Definitions

For the purposes of this chapter, genotoxins are defined as agents that cause genome damage. This damage includes all quantifiable changes in DNA base sequence (mutagenesis), chromosome number (aneugenesis), chromosome rearrangements (translocation) as well as single- and double-strand breaks (clastogenesis). Direct damage to DNA may be caused by a compound or its metabolic product reacting or interacting with DNA, for example, either to form adducts or, through subsequent processing, to alter a DNA base. Indirect damage is a consequence of interference with either the enzymes associated with DNA replication and repair, or with the ordered segregation of chromosomes during mitosis. Some authors use the term "indirect acting agents", to describe promutagens/progenotoxins – compounds which become genotoxins following metabolism – but here we use the former. To detect these many different types of DNA/genome damage, a variety of methods has evolved. In this chapter, many of these are considered in terms of their utility as early screening methods.

Aside from the sensitivity and specificity parameters used in the prediction of genotoxic carcinogenicity, there are several other terms commonly used in the assessment of genotoxicity tests. For example, the sensitivity and specificity terms are often combined to give an overall figure for "concordance". This is of value only if approximately equal numbers of carcinogens and noncarcinogens were assessed in generating the dataset, but can be very misleading if the numbers are not equal [3]. It is valuable to compare new screening versions of an existing test with their regulatory counterparts and in this case it is appropriate to calculate the predictivity of the new test format with respect to the existing test as percentage agreement with positive or negative results, though in these cases the terms sensitivity and specificity should be avoided.

11.3
Major Challenges for Early, Predictive Genotoxicity Testing

DNA is a constant regardless of the kingdom of life in which it resides, so both bacterial cells and mammalian cells can produce viable models for the identification of direct-acting genotoxins. However, bacteria provide a less complete model for the detection of indirect agents and aneugens. In prokaryotes, less complex packaging of DNA and single circular chromosome topology led to the evolution of structurally different enzymes that interact with DNA compared with those in eukaryotes that evolved with the more complex chromatin in multiple linear chromosomes. Thus agents that affect replication, recombination and repair of DNA in bacteria might not have similar effects in mammals. Bacteria also lack mitosis and meiosis and are therefore deficient in the detection of important events in the development of cancer, including karyotype instability and aneugenesis. Finally, the mechanisms for chemical defense also followed evolutionarily different pressures between the free-living bacteria and the often more-protected metazoan cells and this is, in part, reflected by differences in xenobiotic metabolism, which again can impact on the relevance of genotoxicity results from different species.

It is clear that individual targets for particular genotoxic compounds are not all present in all cell types, or even in all mammals. The corollary of this is that no single test is effective in the identification of all genotoxins. It is also necessary to recognize that not all carcinogens act through genotoxic mechanisms, so that even very effective genotoxicity screening strategies allow compounds to progress that give positive results in rodent carcinogenicity assays. The identification of nongenotoxic carcinogens is beyond the scope of this chapter. Finally, *Homo sapiens* is the species of interest, but genetic toxicologists are ultimately constrained by the use of different animal models which do not always reproduce human patterns of tumor development and chemical sensitivity. This reflects the unfortunate truth that different mammalian species and to a lesser extent individuals within a species have differences in drug absorption, distribution through the tissues, metabolism, excretion and receptor distribution. Those issues are covered in other chapters: metabolism is only considered here in the context of progenotoxin metabolism.

The assessment of metabolites often requires complex preclinical studies and there are currently no cell-based assays that fully reproduce the *in vivo* metabolism of the human liver, or other tissues. The rodent S9 liver extracts used as an exogenous source of metabolism are incomplete metabolic surrogates, and perhaps more relevantly here, their properties are inappropriate for handling on an automated HTS platform.

Most of the current *in vitro* mammalian assays were developed for late-stage safety assessment, with full appreciation of the limitations in non-animal systems. However, for many years there was an emphasis on developing high sensitivity without corresponding attention to specificity. The result has been the poor prediction of *in vivo* hazard. It is clear from the Physicians Desk Reference that the regulatory agencies were expedient in their assessment of drug submissions, as about 25% of pharmaceuticals registered for use with clinical indication, excluding antineoplastic and antiviral drugs, have positive data from *in vitro* mammalian genotoxicity tests: the positive results were concluded not to be relevant to humans [4]. Subsequent studies of data from both drug submissions [5] and other chemicals in the public domain [2] reveal the same pattern. It is clear that, whilst the Ames test and *in vivo* chromosome aberration assessments have high specificity, the *in vitro* mammalian tests for mutation and chromosome aberration have poor specificity (see Figure 11.1). At the regulatory level, this was recognized in proposed revisions to the ICH S2 guidance [6] which provide a new option for the registration of new pharmaceuticals, whereby the Ames test is the only required *in vitro* assay (see Table 11.1). The implications for this are discussed in a later section.

Table 11.1 Comparison of current and proposed revised ICH guidelines.

ICH S2B	ICH S2 (R1)	
	Option 1	Option 2
Ames and repeat 5 mg/plate	Ames one complete assay; tested to first precipitating dose	Ames one complete assay; tested to first precipitating dose
In vitro mammalian cell assay: chromosome aberrations; or *tk* mutations in mouse lymphoma cells 10 mM	*In vitro* mammalian cell assay: chromosome aberrations; or *tk* mutations in mouse lymphoma cells; or *in vitro* micronucleus assay 1 mM or 0.5 mg/ml top concentration	No *in vitro* mammalian assay
In vivo cytogenetic assay	*In vivo* cytogenetic assay integrated into 28 d rodent toxicity study, provided it is adequate to support clinical trials and sampling within a day of last day of dosing	*In vivo* cytogenetic assay and a 2nd *in vivo* endpoint, integrated with 28 d rodent assay and 1st *in vivo* endpoint if possible

Screening and profiling is not subject to regulatory approval not least because initial hits are not the chemicals that become drugs. This is reflected in the observations of Teague and co-workers [7], that lead optimization generally increases molecular weight of hits by one-third or more before reaching one of Lipinski's fives (m.w. 500 for lead-likeness [8]). Some of the more recently developed genotoxicity screening tests reflect a departure from the traditional focus on sensitivity and mechanism, to reflect the reliance on specificity to drive confident attrition – mechanism is unimportant if a compound is to be rejected early.

Since the advent of *in vitro* genotoxicity testing, the completion of the human genome project has lead to new disciplines within genetic toxicology – the "omics". The study of global gene expression from transcription and translation to a protein's various posttranslational states and intracellular location(s) increasingly provide tools for novel drug target identification, as well as tools that are beginning to give clues about the more common toxicological response patterns. These technologies and the interpretation of their data are not yet sufficiently developed for screening at the throughput required for profiling, so they are not considered further in this chapter. However in an integrated approach to safety assessment, genetic toxicologists will increasingly have access to data from broader toxicogenomic approaches; and such data are already becoming useful in confirming mechanism of drug action and adverse reaction.

A final challenge for early screening is the detection of genotoxic impurities and synthetic intermediates which can create occupational/manufacturing as well as patient safety issues. This again is a complex issue because the material screened from a library might be synthesized and purified by different routes to a drug that enters the clinic. These issues are addressed in a later section.

11.4
Practical Issues for Genotoxicity Profiling: Vehicle, Dose, Dilution Range and Impurity

11.4.1
Vehicle and Dose

The *in vitro* tests described in this chapter exploit living cells. Most libraries are held in DMSO which, like other undiluted organic solvents such as ethanol and acetone, is lethal to living cells. For this reason, DMSO has to be diluted in aqueous buffers to about 1% (v/v). This in turn sets the maximum compound concentration that can be tested, along with compound solubility. Generally, a pharmaceutical library will be held at between 10 and 50 mM in >98% DMSO, so dilution sets the upper limit for testing between 100 and 500 µM. This is of course rather lower than the current (10 mM) and proposed (1 mM) regulatory test limits set by the ICH. This implies that a screen cannot be expected to give an accurate prediction of regulatory testing. However, the regulatory levels are generally far in excess of the level that might be achieved or tolerated in subsequent *in vivo* tests; they are certainly higher than the concentration at which most biological, enzyme-catalyzed reactions would reach half their maximum velocity. In the more recent history of pharmacological development, molecules are generally active in the submicromolar range. Thus it is probably both more biologically and more pharmacologically relevant to screen at even lower concentrations than those imposed by the need for dilution.

11.4.2
Dilution Range

In contrast to the true high-throughput screening paradigm of single-point data, genotoxicity data should be derived from a range of compound concentrations for the information to be of value to the compound profiler. Genotoxins pose a particular problem because they kill cells at high concentrations where genome damage becomes overwhelming. In eukaryotic cells they trigger cell cycle delay and ultimately apoptosis. As a consequence, testing at a single concentration might only allow the conclusion that a compound causes growth inhibition or death. The lowest effect doses for different genotoxins in an individual assay can vary enormously. Taking data from the *GADD45a*-GFP assay [9] as an example, amongst the aneugens, vincristine sulfate exhibits $25\,000\times$ the potency of colchine; and, amongst the nucleoside/nucleotide analogs, 5-azacytidine shows a potency $24\,000\times$ that of didanosine. If these compounds were only tested at $100\,\mu M$, the more potent genotoxins, vincristine and 5-azacytidine would simply kill the test cells, without an indication of genotoxicity. In the regulatory tests there is a requirement to limit toxicity, but in screening there is not the luxury of range finding. A range of concentrations increases the opportunity to generate useful data. In a lead optimization program a range of exposures allows the selection of modifications that progressively reduce genotoxicity or segregate genotoxic effects from pharmacological efficacy.

The NIH set up a Chemical Genomics Center (NCGC) in 2007 to reproduce the facilities found in the best of the pharmaceutical company screening programs. NCGC runs a variety of tests at 15 dilutions from a highest concentration of about $92\,\mu M$ and, in the examples above, this would detect the genotoxicity of the most potent compounds, but not the least potent – and most likely irrelevant positive results.

11.4.3
Purity

Purity, or potential impurity, can be a confounding factor for any *in vitro* screens and can arise as a theoretical risk from *in silico* predictions, as well as an actual risk from synthesis. The quality of a compound in a library is relevant to any screening exercise, but there are particular issues relevant to genotoxicity screening. Whilst most useful drugs are nonreactive by design, the synthesis of novel small molecules is almost inevitably achieved through the use of reactive chemicals; and these might persist as contaminants in the library samples. Amongst these, many, including alkylators, aromatic nitro and aromatic amines, commonly are active in mutagenicity assays.

A potent genotoxic impurity might falsely identify a compound as hazardous. A related challenge is the presence of intermediates in synthesis, some of which might be readily anticipated, such as structural isomers, and others which might not be anticipated and might pose a genotoxic hazard. The increased scale in production that is required once a compound reaches development might actually follow a different synthetic route and/or allow for greater investment in purity. In such cases, a positive result for a discovery compound that arose because of an intermediate is not at all relevant. This topic has been the subject of industry wide discussion, leading to proposals for the determination, testing and control of specific impurities in pharmaceuticals [10] as well as some investigation of how structure based assessment can support safety assessment of impurities [11] (see below). The actual risk posed by an impurity/intermediate will depend on whether or not it is actually present, and how much of it is present. In theory, this requires the development of new analytical methods to detect and measure the compound, and if the *in silico* prediction is to be followed up, the purification or *de novo* synthesis of the intermediate for *in vitro* or *in vivo* testing. A similar scenario arises from the consideration of genotoxic metabolites that might either be predicted, or detected during *in vitro* studies with S9, or inferred/detected in animals.

Detailed reiteration of other issues raised in the consideration of impurities is beyond the scope of the present discussion, though it is relevant to consider the concept of a "threshold of toxicological concern" (TTC) as it relates to genotoxicity. Essentially, a TTC defines a level of acceptable exposure to known carcinogens and is expressed as a level of daily dose that would increase the number of cancers in the populations by only a negligible level. The European Medicines Agency have proposed that "a TTC value of 1.5 µg/day intake of a genotoxic impurity is considered to be associated with an acceptable risk (excess cancer risk of <1 in 100 000 over a lifetime) for most pharmaceuticals. From this threshold value, a permitted level in the active substance can be calculated based on the expected daily dose. Higher limits may be justified under certain conditions such as short-term exposure periods" [12]. Delaney [13] summarized a variety of reasons to see this as an over-cautious limit, including inappropriate linear extrapolation from TD_{50} values and reliance on carcinogenicity data from rodent studies that substantially overestimates human risk. Perhaps a more direct way to focus on the absurdity of this virtually zero risk approach is to remember that the actual lifetime risk of all cancers in human is 30–40 000 per 100 000 and that humans consume gram quantities of known rodent carcinogens every day [14]. A risk of 1 in 100 000 in fact approximates to a lifetime risk of death by lightning strike.

11.5
Computational Approaches to Genotoxicity Assessment: "*In Silico*" Assessment

The prediction of genotoxicity based on chemical structure began in earnest after Ashby and Tennant [15, 16] established that there are correlations between chemical structure, *Salmonella* mutagenicity and carcinogenicity – and that genotoxic and nongenotoxic carcinogens do not follow the same rules. In the subsequent early development of *in silico* methods there was an inevitable reliance on the Ames and rodent carcinogenicity data contained in those papers, not least because these provided the only readily available datasets. This is still a rapidly evolving field and before considering the current tools and their application, it is worth exploring in a little more detail the challenges that are now being addressed in the development of ever more sophisticated models. These challenges fall into two groups: (i) the biological relevance of the carcinogenicity and genotoxicity test data; (ii) the breadth of chemistry in the molecular structures included.

Much of the historical carcinogenicity data was derived from animals exposed to chronic sublethal doses of a test chemical. This can lead to cell damage and cell death, which in turn requires cell division to replace lost cells. DNA replication is intrinsically very accurate, but mutations occur in every cell at every division and this itself can increase the risk of cancer independently of the cause of increased cell division. Thus, building a rule around a molecule which will never reach such concentrations in man is likely to overestimate hazard ([14] and references therein). As discussed elsewhere in this chapter, the Ames test itself has high specificity, so Ames-positive compounds are very likely to be genotoxic carcinogens and hence their structures are of value in modeling. However, its relatively low sensitivity means that there are many Ames-negative compounds which are both *in vitro* and *in vivo* genotoxins and carcinogens. Without data from these Ames-negative genotoxic compounds, the predictive model is deficient. This gap is increasingly filled by the inclusion of data from the current regulatory *in vitro* mammalian genotoxicity tests though, as discussed elsewhere, this generates its own problems: their poor specificity sometimes produces positive results for compounds which are not *in vivo* genotoxins or carcinogens. This contributes to the risk of the model generating false predictions of hazard.

Reactive molecules are not generally good drug candidates and the original Ashby and Tennant rules were not derived from drug-like molecules. Instead they were largely derived from "industrial" chemicals, including pesticides, herbicides and others chemicals of environmental concern. These are often highly electrophilic and reactive. Of course reactive molecules are important in the synthesis of drugs as reactants or intermediates, because they may remain as impurities. They may also be generated by the metabolism of drugs. These various putative reactive derivatives might not exist, they might not be detectable and they can certainly be challenging and costly to synthesize. A study of the potential value of *in silico* methods in risk assessment for impurities found that *in silico* methods are already very effective in this application [11].

Snyder and co-authors [17] analyzed the extent to which the limitations above might influence the accuracy of three different *in silico* methods (DEREK for Windows, TOPKAT, MCASE) by using them to predict the genotoxicity of 394 marketed pharmaceuticals. Their general conclusions were that the *in silico* methods had poor sensitivity in the prediction of genotoxicity in pharmaceuticals. Since then there have been concerted efforts to improve the models by populating the chemical structure databases with more drug-like molecules and collecting data from chemical classes that have alerting structures within them but are not all genotoxic or carcinogenic.

Two branches of genotoxicity assessment based on molecular structure have emerged. The first branch is based on mathematical algorithms which generate a statistical assessment of risk by the definition of quantitative structure–activity relationships (QSAR), based on correlations between molecular structure and genotoxicity endpoints. Examples of these are MC4PC (MultiCASE), MDL-QSAR (MDL), BioEpisteme (Prous Science), Predictive Data Miner (LeadScope) [18]. In general these methods have high specificity and low sensitivity. The second branch adds research information gathered by human experts to the structure, such as molecular context of the alert, as well as mechanisms of genotoxicity, activities and reactivities to build knowledge-based expert system rules for correlation with genotoxicity endpoints (DEREK for Windows, LHASA). These methods have a lower specificity but higher sensitivity. It is likely therefore that, as with the *in vitro* tests, the best strategy is to consider a combination of *in silico* approaches: a preliminary study has shown this to be the case [18]. This would not be so compound-hungry as combining *in vitro* tests, so perhaps an easier decision to justify. The final section of this chapter considers the combination of both *in silico* and *in vitro* approaches. Here we look at the *in silico* information in isolation.

Yang and co-authors [19] undertook a comprehensive effort to integrate genotoxicity data from multiple databases, incorporating private databases from four private industrial sources, including pharma. The latter considerably increase coverage of pharma space despite only using general structure feature statistics rather than actual chemical structures. Principal component analysis was applied to reveal multiple domain correlations between chemical structures/features with semimechanistic data from the genotoxicity test battery: Bacterial (Ames) and mammalian (MLA) mutation, *in vitro* chromosome aberration and *in vivo* (rodent) micronucleus formation. The broader collection of chemicals and genotoxicity endpoints should allow the generation of a weight of evidence approach to the generation of an *in silico* genotoxicity hazard profile that also contains advice on follow up testing – if the compound is to progress.

11.5.1
How Should *In Silico* Methods be Applied in Hit and Lead Profiling?

It makes sense to use data mining of structural features and molecular properties to assist in the building of alerts for more precise structural features. Various *in vitro* testing results can be used to describe structures at the compound and feature levels. These profiles can be used either to build weight of evidence strategies or as predictors for prediction models.

Computational methods allow speedy "virtual" research. Thus genotoxicity profiling can start before a compound has been synthesized so that chemists can avoid the synthesis of compounds with readily predictable liabilities. However because the current predictive power of computational methods derives from genotoxicity data, which as a whole tend to overpredict *in vivo* hazard, *in silico* methods should perhaps be seen as more of a trigger for *in vitro* follow-up where alerts arise in a compound series that is otherwise proving drug-like and effective. An effective knowledge based expert system can also give insight into mode of action and suggest an appropriate *in vitro* follow-up test to discover whether the prediction is borne out. The results of such tests can then feed back into the development of ever more sophisticated tools.

11.6
Genotoxicity Assays for Screening

In this section, regulatory genotoxicity is briefly introduced to give context to the use of early profiling. Next, the various regulatory and screening tests are considered in three basic classes, according to the endpoint of the assay: gene mutation, chromosome damage, including single- and double-strand breaks and aneugenesis and genotoxin-induced gene expression. The regulatory assays are well described elsewhere and the reader is referred to other sources for current regulatory guidelines and references therein. Screening assays derived from regulatory assays are described, noting protocol differences from the parent assays, as well as the strengths and weaknesses of all the assays which might be considered for use in the profiling context (see Table 11.2).

The current ICH harmonized tripartite guideline for genotoxicity testing of pharmaceuticals (S2B) defines a standard battery of tests, including both *in vitro*

Table 11.2 Properties of tests suitable for profiling.

Test endpoint	Category	Validation: transfer	Application	Throughput
Bacterial mutation	Ames II	Yes : Yes	Candidates and leads	50/wk; 2500/yr
Bacterial mutation	Biolum	Yes : No	Candidates	20/wk; 1000/yr
Bacterial reporter	*Escherichia* SOS	Yes : Yes	Candidates and leads	180/wk; 9000/yr
Yeast deletion	DEL	Yes : No	Candidates	Unknown
Yeast reporter	RAD54-GFP	Yes : Yes	Candidates and leads	160/wk; 8000/yr
Mammalian DNA damage	MNT imaging	Yes : Yes	Candidates	55/wk; 2750/yr
Mammalian DNA damage	MNT flow	Yes : Yes	Candidates	40/wk; 2000/yr
Mammalian DNA damage	Comet	Yes : Yes	Candidates	30/wk; 1500/yr
Mammalian reporter	GADD45a-GFP	Yes : Yes	Candidates and leads	200/wk; 10 000/yr

and *in vivo* tests and intending that the constituent tests should be complementary. The three-test battery consists of the bacterial gene mutation test, the *in vitro* mammalian cell test (cytogenetic evaluation of chromosomal damage or mouse lymphoma forward mutation tk assay) and *in vivo* test for genetic damage that allows additional relevant factors, such as ADME, to be incorporated. The *in vivo* assays suggested to be most capable of meeting these ends are based in rodent haematopoietic cells and comprise either assessment of chromosomal damage in bone marrow cells or micronuclei in bone marrow or peripheral blood erythrocytes. If all the tests in the battery give negative results then this is usually considered sufficient to demonstrate the lack of genotoxic activity. However, according to the current guideline, compounds yielding positive results in this standard battery may require more extensive testing.

Follow-up testing guidance is also provided in the form of the ICH S2A "Guidance on specific aspects of regulatory genotoxicity tests for pharmaceuticals". This current guidance suggests that for a compound producing biologically relevant positive results in one or more *in vitro* tests, further useful information may be obtained by performing another *in vivo* test in an alternative tissue. The target tissue for the compound and the endpoint measured in the *in vitro* test both impact on the choice of the additional *in vivo* test.

In 2008, the ICH proposed revisions to the ICH S2 battery guideline and guidance on specific aspects documents (Table 11.1). In the combined revision, S2(R1), there is a new option for regulatory submissions in which the bacterial mutation assay is the only required *in vitro* test, but two *in vivo* endpoints are required [6]. Further advice is offered on the choice of *in vivo* test and top concentration for testing. ICH guidelines do not affect the development of an effective early screening strategy – indeed the new guidance offers a little more flexibility. It is not anticipated that early profiling and screening will replace the regulatory battery in the near future.

11.6.1
Gene Mutation Assays

The bacterial and mammalian cell assays for gene mutation were developed to measure statistically significant increases in the numbers of mutant colonies derived from rare events: many millions of exposed cells must be plated out to allow the assessment of mutation frequency. The *Salmonella typhimurium* reverse mutation assay ("Ames" test) is carried out in a variety of different mutant strains selected to identify the various classes of mutation. The test generates many hundreds of Petri dishes for counting and is not practical for profiling.

The "mouse lymphoma assay" is in fact just one of several mammalian cell assays designed to determine increases in mutation rate. It focuses on the thymidine kinase (tk) assay in murine lymphoma cells (L5178Y), though tk data have also been produced from the human lymphoblastoid cell line TK6, and at the hgprt (hypoxanthine–guanine phosphoribosyl-transferase) locus in Chinese Hamster ovary or lung (V79) cells and mouse lymphoma cells. Since Ames mutation data and often mammalian cell mutation data may cause the abandonment of a drug, efforts are being made to increase throughput of the tests for candidate selection. Few are suited to hit and lead profiling in their present form.

11.6.2
The Ames Test and Variants

Many laboratories use "cutdown" versions of the regulatory *Salmonella* reverse mutation assay in which a reduced set of strains is used, and a smaller number of colonies may be counted to estimate mutation rate [20]. Whilst practical for candidate selection this is still not suitable for profiling factories. The most recent development in the bacterial mutation assays has been the incorporation, into the *Salmonella* tester strains, of a gene encoding a light-emitting protein under the control of the constitutively expressed kanamycin resistance gene to create the "BioLum" Ames test. Cells that can form colonies (and in the Ames test this means revertant colonies selected for histidine prototrophy) emit light and as a consequence they are readily counted using electronic imaging systems. The resolution of these devices means that very much smaller colonies can be counted. This in turn allows for higher cell densities to be plated, in microplate format – with the concomitant reduction in use of plastic ware and test article [1]. Initial validation work was performed in 24-well microplates with a throughput of around 20 compounds/week, though the authors felt that the simple protocol and amenability to automation should mean that significantly higher throughputs are possible. At present this assay version is not widely available.

An alternative to counting colonies is to use fluctuation tests (cited in OECD 471) in which wells containing a specified number of cells are scored, and the mutation rates derived statistically. A further improvement in the efficiency of these methods is the use of "mixes" of tester strains in addition to single strains. After a series of handling and treatment steps in larger volumes, cells are transferred to 384-well microplates for incubation and the fluctuation test assessment. This means that much of the assay preparation can be efficiently handled robotically. Wells are scored positive when cell proliferation can be detected with colorimetric indicators of cell growth (e.g., purple to yellow change), permitting the use of spectrophotometric plate readers for data collection. The method can be established by the end-user laboratory and is also available commercially as either "Ames MPF" or "Ames II" (Xenometrix by Endotell GmbH). The difference between the two commercially available assays lies in the *Salmonella* strains employed: Ames MPF uses up to four of the classic TA strains (98, 100, 1535, 1537) whilst Ames II uses TA98 and then a TA mix, consisting of the TA700X series of strains.

The Ames II test is reported to use at least threefold less test compound and sixfold less plasticware than the traditional Ames test (Xenometrix), and whilst it is still rather plastic-hungry for profiling purposes, one study reported screening 2698 compounds in a little more than a year [21]. An interlaboratory "ring trial" with 19 coded compounds concluded that the method provides an effective screening alternative to the standard Ames test [22].

11.6.3
Mammalian Cell Mutation Assays

The "mouse lymphoma assay" detects gene mutations as well as chromosomal mutations, with the difference inferred from colony size and confirmed by secondary assays. Both colony-counting and well-counting methods are used in microplate format for the calculation of mutant frequency. Cells are first exposed to the test chemical, then after a wash step they are allowed an expression/recovery phase before an estimate of cell growth, another wash step, then plating for growth and finally assessment: the assay length runs into weeks rather than hours or days. Small and large colony types are identified by inspection. The slower growth of mammalian cells, coupled with the complex handling protocols, make these the least tractable assays to adapt for use in hit and lead profiling. At present there are no reports of these assays being used routinely earlier than candidate selection.

11.6.4
Saccharomyces cerevisiae ("Yeast") Mutation Assays

The use of yeast cells as a eukaryotic complement to the Ames test led to the development of several protocols for the detection of mutation, gene conversion and recombination. The formal introduction of methods [23] followed by much development work from Zimmermann's laboratory led to large systematic studies [24, 25] and OECD guidelines for the test battery (OECD 480, 481). However the assays are now rarely used, at least in part because of concerns over low sensitivity, thought to reflect limited permeability of the cell wall.

An intrachromosomal recombination assay ("DEL") based on a genetically engineered *HIS3* locus in *Saccharomyces cerevisiae* [26] was developed as both a colony-counting and a well-counting assay. Nine chemicals were used in a proof of principle for higher-throughput screening in a 96- or 384-well format modified into a colorimetric assay [27]. The assay is reported to detect carcinogenic compounds, including those for which a genotoxicity mechanism has not previously been reported. At present, the assay is not widely available and throughput is not known, so it is too early to realize whether this method will become widespread or to understand its value.

11.7
Chromosome Damage and Aberration Assays

11.7.1
Aberrations

Gross rearrangements of chromosomes fall into several categories including translocations, large insertions/deletions, the loss or gain of whole chromosomes and double- or single-stranded DNA breakage. Since chromosomes only condense and become visible during mitosis, most test protocols require treatment with a mitotic poison (such cytochalasin B), such that all cells in the exposed population can be scored rather than the subpopulation that happen to be in mitosis at the analytical time point (OECD 473). Some tools and systems are appearing on the market for aiding mitotic index and chromosome aberration scoring, for example, the Pathfinder technology from IMSTAR (Paris, France). Metasystems GmbH (Altlussheim, Germany) also provides a metaphase locating software called Metafer MSearch. Such systems have the potential to speed up the identification of metaphase cells, and use chromosome "painting" to help identify the type of aberration. At present, automated high-throughput scoring of translocations, insertions and deletions has not replaced microscopic examination and it remains to be seen how widespread such systems will become. In a recent review of methods focusing on human cells, the authors commented that: "even the best automated system may never replace a skilled observer" [28]. These methods are not yet sufficiently mature for profiling.

11.7.2
Micronuclei

There has been rather more progress in the automated detection of clastogens and aneugens. Nuclear membrane forms around chromosomes and chromosome fragments that fail to segregate into nuclei during anaphase. This might be a consequence of failures in the mitotic machinery or chromosome breakage, which generates fragments without centromeres. These smaller "micronuclei" can be identified and counted using two quite different approaches: high resolution imaging and flow cytometry. In both cases, DNA-specific dyes are crucial in resolving nuclei and micronuclei and imaging is reliant on careful optimization of the parameters used to distinguish DNA-containing bodies.

Diaz and co-workers [29] published an evaluation of an automated MNT assay using fluorescent microscopy coupled with image analysis software from Cellomics (Pitsburg, USA). The results showed high concordance with data collected by manual scoring. The speed of scoring limited throughput to 11 compounds/day (at multiple dilutions, with and without S9). This throughput approaches the minimum levels required for screening and the ever-increasing processing power and data storage available to assay developers will doubtless increase this, though the sample preparation protocols remain relatively complex. Alternative imaging systems and analysis software are also available from, for example, IMSTAR and Metasystems, with reductions in analysis time down to 4–5 min/slide rather than the 25 min/slide for scoring manually. The Metasystems Metafer system allows up to 80 slides to be loaded into an automatic slide feeder.

Flow cytometric assessment generates results that reproduce microscopic methods for the *in vivo* assessment of micronucleus frequency in peripheral blood micronucleated reticulocytes [30] and the method is increasingly applied in *in vitro* assessments. Litron Laboratories (Rochester, N.Y., USA) recently launched their "MicroFlow *In Vitro*" kit for the *in vitro* micronucleus test, following a six-compound interlaboratory evaluation [31]. This method permits 50 samples to be analyzed over the course of 3.5 h, including incubation times, leading to a possible throughput of 40 compounds/week or perhaps 2000 compounds/year.

11.7.3
"Comet" Assay

The electrophoresis of the nuclear content of individual cells, followed by DNA staining, gives rise to microscopic images reminiscent of comets hurtling across the night sky – giving the name to the comet assay. It is a relatively simple assay, though has several handling steps. The comet "head" contains giant (75 μm) supercoiled loops of DNA, liberated from higher order chromatin packaging by high salt treatment. The "tail" contains loops in which there has been at least one single-stranded break, leading to a more extended relaxed supercoil. The more single-strand breaks there are, the more relaxed loops are formed and the greater proportion of staining migrates into the tail. Double-strand breaks, and under alkaline conditions where there are two single-strand breaks in the same loop, lead to fragmentation of the loops and altered tail structure. Smaller fragments of DNA including the mitochondrial (5.6 μm), or apoptotic fragments are beyond the resolution of the gels, and do not contribute to the head or tail staining. Thus the comet assay, in alkaline or neutral conditions, should detect single- and double-stranded breaks, but not "pure" aneugens. In alkaline conditions however, breakage can occur at alkaline labile sites, including sites where the base has been lost from the sugar/phosphate backbone. Modified assays, in which lesion-specific nuclease treatment is included, can be used to reveal oxidative damage. Readers are referred to the excellent review by Collins and co-workers [32] for more detail on data generation and interpretation.

In the routine comet assay, a user can operate at a maximum throughput of 8–12 compounds/week, limited by sample and cell preparation, and also by the imaging and scoring. There are a number of imaging and software analysis solutions currently available from companies such as IMSTAR, Metasystems and Perceptive Instruments Ltd (Haverhill, UK). The assay has also been developed into a higher throughput format that accommodates four compounds each tested at ten dilutions in a 96-well microplate. In this method, cells are still transferred to slides for scoring [33], and with robotic handling, data from six compounds/day can be analyzed. A new protocol in development utilizes a multichamber plate which can be used for both cell treatment and electrophoresis [34]. The throughput is therefore potentially 1500 compounds/year, approaching the minimum requirements for late profiling.

11.7.4
DNA Adduct Assessment

Analysis of DNA adducts is used in mechanistic analysis but it is not suited to profiling at present because of the complexities in sample preparation and analysis. There are no formal guidelines for testing.

11.7.5
Gene Expression Assays

Microbes and metazoans are exposed to a variety of toxic stresses and have evolved appropriate defenses and repair mechanisms. Some of these systems are regulated at the protein level, but others are regulated at the transcriptional level, allowing the development of reporter assays. These transcriptional responses can be used to provide an earlier marker for genotoxin exposure in a whole population of cells, rather than the detection of the endpoints discussed above, in which genotoxic stress leads to fixation of mutations or chromosomal aberrations/damage in a small subpopulation.

11.7.5.1 Prokaryotic

Early progress in bacterial recombinant DNA technology lead to the first generation of reporters, which exploited the DNA damage inducible genes of the "SOS" operon [35]. These genes variously encode proteins involved in excision repair, recombinational repair and DNA polymerase. Reporters for both the *sfiA* gene (SOS chromotest: [36]) and *umuC* [37] have been used to drive β-galactosidase synthesis, which can be assessed using a colorimetric assay. A review of SOS chromotest data from 751 compounds [38] revealed that for the 452 compounds which also had Ames data, there was agreement between the tests for 82% of compounds. A number of alternative SOS reporters have been developed to drive expression of the *lux* operon which allows luminometric data collection. These include the commercially available Vitotox assay (Gentaur Molecular Products BVBA, Brussels, Belgium) which exploits the *recN* gene [39] as well as reporters for *recA*, *uvrA*, *alkA* [40] and *umuC* [41]. In a limited comparison of data from seven genotoxins and six environmental samples generated using *recA*-lux, *umuC* and *sfi* reporter assays, the umuC test performed the best [42]. The simplicity of these systems and low compound requirement recommends their use, though they are less accurate in prediction of Ames data than the more cumbersome fluctuation tests.

The SOS-*umuC* assay allows three compounds to be assessed over seven dilutions on a 96-well microplate. A user can prepare up to 15 assay microplates/day, meaning that a user can profile around 180 compounds/week or around 10 000 compounds/year.

11.7.5.2 Eukaryotic

The first eukaryotic gene regulation assay used green fluorescent protein (GFP) as a reporter for induction of the yeast *RAD54* gene – a member of the recombinational repair family of genes (GreenScreen GC; Gentronix Ltd, UK). A screening validation study [43] demonstrated that the assay detected a different spectrum of compounds to bacterial genotoxicity assays; and it was suggested that, together with a high throughput bacterial screen, the two would provide an effective preview of the regulatory battery of genotoxicity tests. This proposal was subsequently justified in a study of 2698 proprietary compounds from the Johnson & Johnson compound library [21].

With a format in which four compounds are tested per 96-well microplate, with robust host cells and rapid assay time, it is possible to assess up to 160 compounds/week, even without automation. Beyond this throughput, compound supply and data collection become the rate-limiting factors.

Broader reservation about yeast tests led the same group to develop a human cell assay in which GFP was used as a reporter for induction of the *GADD45a* gene [9]. Significantly, the TK6 cell line was chosen not only because of its human origins, but also due to its wild-type p53 status: other mammalian cell lines in common use are insufficient or deficient in p53 and this compromises the success of the DNA damage response. The resultant *GADD45a*-GFP assay (GreenScreen HC; Gentronix Ltd) responds to all classes of genotoxin including S9-generated metabolites [44], and in contrast to the regulatory *in vitro* mammalian assays, demonstrates high specificity without compromising sensitivity. This 96-well microplate assay is becoming widely used and its transfer to other laboratories has been systematically evaluated [45].

The format of the *GADD45a*-GFP assay is very similar to the *RAD54*-GFP yeast assay in that four compounds are tested on a 96-well microplate, though the assay incubation time is longer (48 h instead of 16 h) due to the nature of the assay host cells. An operator can achieve a throughput of 80–100 compounds/week, though this can be significantly improved with a reformatted version of the assay in which the number of compounds tested per 96-well plate is increased. In a recent study using this higher-throughput assay format, a library of 1266 pharmacologically active compounds (LOPAC; Sigma-Aldrich Co. Ltd.) was screened [46]. The potential throughput from this assay format could be as high as 36 000 compounds/year.

A second p53 responsive reporter has been described which exploits elements of the p53R2 gene which encodes a subunit of ribonucleotide reductase, linked to a luciferase gene [47, 48]. It has been validated against diverse mechanistic classes of genotoxin. To perform this assay, the p53 wild-type cell line MCF-7 is transiently transfected with two plasmids: one with the p53R2 reporter and the second with constitutively expressed control (driven by elements of CMV promoter). Between 4 and 6 h after transfection, cells are exposed to test materials (five dilutions) for 24 h, then washed three times, lysed and assayed. It is not yet known how well the assay transfers to other laboratories and the protocol is quite complex for adaptation to high throughput.

11.8
Using Data from *In Vitro* Profiling: Confirmatory Tests, Follow-Up Tests, and the Link to Safety Assessment and *In Vivo* Models

A theme throughout this chapter is the difference between genotoxicity assessment in hazard profiling and safety assessment applications. This comes more acutely into focus in this section where the follow-up to positive profiling tests is considered. The default expectation is that the follow-up for a positive early profiling test would be removal of the compound from the collection going forward: the aim of a screening program is to reduce the proportion of compounds that give positive results in GLP submissions. Under current safety assessment practice, positive genotoxicity test results are more likely to be followed-up to investigate mechanism and risk, as regulatory tests are carried out on candidate pharmaceuticals very close to their human phase 0 (microdosing) and phase I clinical trials. As noted earlier, this is likely to culminate in expensive delays in the early clinical trials, and is associated with the disruption and increased costs related to urgent animal testing. These can in turn contribute to go/no go decisions on the development program. This is not the case with results derived from early profiling.

Profiling can occur when the properties of compounds identified in other screening tests are already informing lead optimization chemists. Compound choice is still wide and the investment per compound is still low, such that a positive result can be used to drive early-stage attrition. If the choice of compounds is not wide, which might reflect either the therapeutic indication of the drug or the nature of the target, then there are two avenues for immediate follow-up. First, lead optimization chemists can be alerted to the need to focus on the segregation of useful pharmacology from unwanted genotoxicity. Second, the compound file/profile/cv should be annotated to indicate the possible need for follow-up by safety assessment teams to consider mechanism of action. A positive result need not be the end of a program, but would immediately reduce the ranking of the compound: only in very particular cases would a potent genotoxin be carried forward.

In the following paragraphs the links between *in vitro* and *in vivo* models are explored in the context of providing information to be included in a compound file at the hit profiling stage. The different follow-up strategies for results from particular profiling assays are considered. The longer term prospects for *in vivo* screening are briefly reviewed.

11.8.1
Annotations from Screening Data

All annotations/alerts should carry basic information, including the assay type, the result, the top dose tested, the solvent and any additional information generated, such as control, lowest effective concentration, level of effect, or associated toxicity data. Annotations and appropriate alerts should be included, even where the result is negative, and they should be specific to the screening strategy. For a strategy based solely on mutation endpoints a negative result should generate an alert that genotoxicity assessment is incomplete and an *in vitro* aneugenicity or clastogenicity assay is still required. For a strategy based solely on aneugenicity or clastogenicity, a negative result should generate an alert that assessment is incomplete and an *in vitro* mutation assay should be prioritized at a later next stage. For a strategy using a reporter assay that is not endpoint-specific, a negative result should generate an alert for a complementary assay: for example a bacterial assay after a eukaryotic screen or a eukaryotic assay after a bacterial screen.

Most of the *in vitro* assays are described with an additional protocol for the assessment of metabolites; however, it is unclear whether genuine high-throughput screening assays would be performed routinely with a source of exogenous metabolism such as S9. This seems unlikely because of S9 handling difficulties in a "factory" situation, for example, S9 is heat-labile and frozen samples create problems associated with frost. If there are no data from assays incorporating S9, then an alert should be generated to reflect that metabolites have not been investigated, and this alert might be strengthened by linkage to data from metabolic liability assays or *in silico* approaches (see above and see Chapter 7).

11.8.2
Annotations from Positive Screening Data

11.8.2.1 Gene Mutation Assays

For the majority of cases a positive result from the relatively high specificity Ames test would be sufficient to prevent a compound proceeding to *in vivo* testing and on into development. It follows that a positive result in a screening test with high predictivity of the Ames test would constitute a major hazard in the compound profile, and lead to considerably reduced ranking of the compound for development. In the regulatory safety assessment framework, it is generally only Ames negative compounds, with ("unique") positive results from the low specificity mammalian cell assays which trigger further tests. It follows that a positive result from a profiling test that exhibits high predictivity of positive MLA test results would represent a lower hazard than an Ames screening positive and would hence have a higher ranking for development. In either case, the compound file should be annotated with an alert for a confirmatory *in vitro* test for mutation (if the compound remains live) at a later stage. The confirmatory assay might be a simple repeat assay, as the high compound requirement for full GLP testing would inevitably delay the retest. A second alert would notify the need for a lead optimization program that replaces the compound with a nongenotoxic derivative. A third alert should notify the genotoxicity safety assessment team that the compound is a priority for mechanistic investigation if the series continues and this in turn should trigger the potential need for coordination of testing with a 28 day toxicity study, which might then be scheduled earlier.

11.8.2.2 Chromosome Damage Assays

A positive result from an MNT profiling assay would lower the ranking of the compound for development to a lesser extent than an Ames profiling assay. Again the compound file should be annotated with an alert for a confirmatory *in vitro* test (if the compound remains live), along with a second alert to the lead optimization chemists. Whilst a third alert should still notify the genotoxicity safety assessment team that the compound is a priority for mechanistic investigation if the series continues, with the associated need for coordination of *in vivo* studies, this would be a lower priority than an Ames profiling positive. Given the lower specificity of these screens, a secondary high specificity screen, for example the *GADD45a*-GFP assay, might be advised prior to candidate selection.

11.8.2.3 Reporter Assays

A positive result from a bacterial reporter assay would lower the ranking of the compound for development. The compound file should be annotated with an alert for a confirmatory *in vitro* test (if the compound remains live), in this case it might be a screening Ames at a later stage. There should also be a second alert to the lead optimization chemists. A third alert should still notify the genotoxicity safety assessment team that the compound is a priority for mechanistic investigation if the series continues, with the associated need for coordination of *in vivo* studies, this would be a lower priority than an Ames profiling positive.

A positive result from a eukaryotic reporter assay would lower the ranking of a compound for development, alert lead optimization chemists and similarly trigger a confirmatory assay and alert safety assessment.

11.9
Can a Genetic Toxicity Profile Inform *In Vivo* Testing Strategies?

The first regulatory *in vivo* assay is routinely the micronucleus test using either bone marrow or peripheral blood cells from only one sex of a rodent. It remains the most sensitive, though not perfect, predictor of rodent and human genotoxic carcinogenesis [49]. The second *in vivo* test is more focused on which regulatory *in vitro* test(s) gave the positive result(s). With appropriate planning it is generally possible to use different tissues from the same animals that are used for the initial haematopoietic MNT test. There is not yet consensus on the second *in vivo* test, though the comet assay is gaining support.

A positive result from a mutation assay (Ames, large colonies in MLA/tk or HGPRT mutation) suggests the use of an *in vivo* test for DNA damage such as unscheduled DNA synthesis (UDS OECD 486), or P32-postlabelling to detect DNA adduct formation (no OECD guideline). A recent review identified 120 rodent carcinogens where the *in vivo* MNT gave negative or equivocal results and there were other *in vivo* data to consider: UDS has very poor sensitivity [49] and adduct assessment is generally reserved for compounds where reactive metabolites are suggested. The alkaline comet assay is now considered appropriate. The other alterative is to use one of the genetically engineered rodent mutation assays (MutaMouse, Big Blue), though these are expensive and time-consuming, so unlikely to be used routinely for both tissues/endpoints. Advice regarding choice of tissue will be dependent on other factors such as the target tissue of the drug, though this may not be available when screening alerts are recorded; and as such a discussion is beyond the scope of this chapter.

A positive result from a chromosome aberration assay (MNT, cytogenetic analysis or small colonies in MLA) suggests a second *in vivo* assay for clastogenesis or aneugenesis. Centromere staining of mitotic cells allows the distinction of aneugens and clastogens.

Follow-up for positive results in reporter assays specifically developed for profiling screening would by default be *in vivo* MNT, though additional information might be generated during the regulatory *in vitro* testing. Kirkland and Speit [49] recommend the comet assay as a second *in vivo* test of choice, since the limited data available suggests it identifies more of the carcinogens missed by MNT. However, more recently attention was drawn to the assessment of Pig-a mutations [50, 51]. This X-linked gene provides a readily scored mutant phenotype as a consequence of its essential role in the anchoring of GPI proteins in the membrane. Mutant cells are distinguished by their inability to bind GPI-linked proteins such as CD59, CD55, CD24. Furthermore, wild-type cells are killed by aerolysin, a bacterial toxin that uses the GPI anchor to mediate lysis. Thus aerolysin resistance is a direct selection for Pig-a mutants, which can then be cloned and sequenced to determine the nature of the mutation.

11.9.1
Prospects for *In Vivo* Profiling of Hits and Leads for Genotoxicity

It might seem unimaginable to have an *in vivo* hit and lead profiling tool, but between cultured cells and various mammalian models there are numerous other animal models that might be considered. It is clearly desirable to have an early insight into the additional ADME properties that are only detectable in living animals. There will always be the caveat from rodent, canine and even primate studies that metabolism can vary a great deal, though this is not in itself a reason not to search for readily collectable and useful data from nonmammalian animals. This section simply notes the better known examples of fish (Vertebrata), fly (Insecta) and worm (Nematoda). None is yet developed to a stage where profiling is really feasible, but all have sequenced genomes and sufficient biochemical and genomic information to confirm conservation of the main DNA damage response and repair pathways. All have some published data demonstrating successful extraction of genotoxicity data.

Zebrafish (*Brachydanio/Danio rerio*) embryos can be produced in large numbers and carry sufficient nutrients within the egg sack to allow development within microplate volumes [52, 53]. Mutation frequency has been estimated indirectly using transgenic fish [54] and UDS, comet, MNT and alkaline filter elution methods have been used effectively [55]. At present, there has been insufficient study of the model to understand predictivity of mammalian genotoxicity, and none of the methods has been demonstrated at throughputs sufficient for hit and lead screening.

For the sex-linked recessive lethal test in *Drosophila melanogaster*, fruit flies can be bred in large numbers and are cheaper to maintain than mammals. This led to early interest in their potential use in mutagen detection. Mutations in sex-linked (chromosome X-linked) genes are phenotypically evident in males, so mutations in essential genes lead to reduced numbers of male progeny in controlled matings. This provides a measure of mutation frequency [56]. An OECD guideline has been produced (OECD 477) and a coded compound study carried out [57]. Publication numbers suggest that the test is only rarely used in safety assessment. Its use in screening presents interesting automation and image analysis challenges for the controlled mating, phenotypic scoring and counting of flies.

The nematode *Caenorhabditis elegans* is extraordinarily well described. It was the first animal genome to be sequenced [58] and its entire development has been described, right down to individual cell lineages from the zygote [59]. Its role in biomedical science was recently reviewed by Leung and co-authors [60] who note the conservation of all the major DNA damage response and repair pathways. The worm is small and readily cultured in microplates, though at present there have been no validation studies for genotoxicity assessment.

11.10
What to Test, When and How?

Genotoxicity data should become an important part of a compound's profile and can provide value in decision making at all stages in discovery from libraries containing millions of compounds to leads progressing to candidate selection. Each is here considered in turn.

11.10.1
Profiling Entire Libraries: >100 000 Compounds/Year

At the outset, *in silico* methods can assist in compound design to avoid the most hazardous structures and in the design of safest synthetic routes to avoid hazardous synthetic intermediates. The *in vitro* screening methods could allow segregation of genotoxins into a sublibrary. If a new therapeutic campaign is initiated where genotoxicity is allowable or expected, for example antineoplastics or antivirals, then those compounds are included, but if genotoxicity is unacceptable they are excluded. A whole library screen does not mean that genotoxicity ceases to be a problem. As discussed earlier in this chapter, no screen picks up all genotoxins, so appropriate alerts will remain for unassessed hazards. Furthermore, the chemical differences that evolve during the move from hit-likeness to lead-likeness and drug-likeness introduce new structures.

None of the genotoxicity assays described here have been used for whole large libraries, as none have sufficient throughput. This is not least because most assay developers do not have access to the instrumentation required for developing HTS or ultra-HTS methods. The only feasible approach would be to adopt a progressive longer-term strategy, and collect the data over a period of a year or more.

11.10.2
Profiling Hits: 10 000–100 000 Compounds/Year

The first level of genotoxicity testing likely to be used in the near future is hit profiling. For numerical reasons, hits from a discovery campaign can be considered alongside smaller complete libraries of natural products and specialist collections enriched for particular target types (inhibitors of kinases, proteases, HDACs, etc.). All would benefit from the early inclusion of genotoxicity data in the profile. Of the assays considered here only the four that were developed as screening assays might be scalable to hit profiling: the bacterial Ames II and SOS reporters, the yeast *RAD54*-GFP reporter and the human *GADD45a*-GFP reporter. Of these the first two provide an early warning for Ames-positives, and the second two also preview aneugens and clastogens and so on missed by Ames. The most effective screen would combine two tests. As early as 2004, Kitching et al. [61] compiled validation data for 71 compounds from the GreenScreen GC (yeast) test with published SOS/*umu* data. Of the 71 compounds, 54 (76%) had positive data in cancer studies, so the selection is not typical of broader pharmacological space. Also, 32 (45%) were positive in Green-Screen GC and 32 compounds were positive with SOS/*umu*. Finally, 22 (31%) were positive for both tests and each test had ten unique positives. In a second more recent study, data were generated from 2351 potential drug candidates during preregulatory screening using both Ames II and the GreenScreen GC (yeast) assay [21]. This is a more "open" pharmacological space; and 164 (7%) were positive in Ames II, with and/or without S9 metabolic activation and 176 (7.5%) were positive in the Green-Screen GC assay without S9. Just 12 (7%) of the 176 GreenScreen GC positives were also positive in Ames II. This study further confirms that the bacterial Ames II and yeast assays each detect a different but overlapping spectrum of genotoxins. Overall, 14% had a positive result in either or both tests and this is within the known range of attrition rate of candidates due to genotoxic hazard. In a third study of a further 1684 compounds, using GreenScreen HC (human cell) and Ames II, there was a similarly small overlap (12.5% = 31 compounds) between the two assays. Aside from again confirming the different endpoints covered by bacterial and mammalian cell tests, this collection had only about half the prevalence of positive results in both assays, revealing how markedly genotoxicity results can vary with the chemistry.

A combination of two tests is clearly better than one, but at this early stage, when there is still more chemical development likely, one is probably enough. Given that *in silico* methods are most effective in the identification or designing out of Ames positive compounds, a single eukaryotic screening test would probably be optimum.

11.10.3
Profiling in Lead Optimization: 2000–10 000 Compounds/Year

At this level of throughput genetic toxicity screening is already happening in some of the larger pharmaceutical companies; and examples of screening data are described above. More assays are available at the lower end of this range and it is appropriate to consider which option will be selected for subsequent regulatory submissions. Using the current ICH S2B guidelines or ICH S2(R1) option one, where both Ames and *in vitro* mammalian test data are required, many would follow the conservative approach and use a bacterial screen with one of the "screening" micronucleus tests, such as flow cytometry or imaging. These mammalian tests will most likely lead to a high prevalence of positive data (35% or more), corresponding to the level seen in marketed pharmaceuticals for these tests, though of course many of these positives will not give positive *in vivo* data. The consequence of this is that many potentially valuable nonhazardous leads might be discarded before the selection of candidates is complete, or a great deal of follow-up will be required. To reduce this risk, a secondary screen of MNT positives with the higher specificity *GADD45a*-GFP test would identify the subset of compounds liable to give positive results in later *in vivo* tests. Many of the remaining MNT positives could become useful drugs once mechanistic studies establish the nonrelevance of the positive data. Others might prefer to follow the more radical ICH S2(R1) option two, where only Ames *in vitro* data is required for submissions. In these cases there is a broader selection of assays from which to choose a tool to identify the compounds inevitably missed by Ames, and so avoid frequent *in vivo* failures. In the absence of informative *in silico* data, a high specificity eukaryotic test would obviously be preferred.

11.11
Summary

There is a growing list of genotoxicity assays that could provide data at the throughput required for hit and lead profiling. Several of these have a high enough specificity to provide reliable hazard warnings, and they each suggest a positive prevalence of around 7% in pharmaceutical space. Because individual tests cover different but overlapping classes of genotoxins, the overall level of genotoxicity in a library that can be detected by combining approaches seems close to the level of candidate attrition due to genotoxicity. This suggests that early profiling offers excellent prospects for a significant reduction in late stage failure. It also offers an overall increase in efficiency for later regulatory genotoxicity safety assessment, by providing an early alert for projects likely to require mechanistic investigation.

Acknowledgments

The authors would like to thank Chihae Yang for advice on *in silico* methods, Andy Scott for Figure 11.1, David Tweats for Table 11.1 and Jacky van Gompel for providing unpublished screening data.

References

1 Aubrecht, J., Osowski, J.J., Persaud, P., Cheung, J.R., Ackerman, J., Lopes, S.H. and Ku, W.W. (2007) Bioluminescent *Salmonella* reverse mutation assay: a screen for detecting mutagenicity with high throughput attributes. *Mutagenesis*, 22, 335–342.

2 Kirkland, D., Aardema, M., Henderson, L. and Muller, L. (2005) Evaluation of the ability of a battery of three *in vitro* genotoxicity tests to discriminate rodent carcinogens and non-carcinogens I. Sensitivity, specificity and relative predictivity. *Mutation Research*, 584, 1–256.

3 Bruner, L.H., Carr, G.J. and Curren, R.D. (2002) An investigation of new toxicity test method performance in validation studies: 3. sensitivity and specificity are not independent of prevalence or distribution

of toxicity. *Human & Experimental Toxicology*, **21**, 325–334.

4 Snyder, R.D. and Green, J.W. (2001) A review of the genotoxicity of marketed pharmaceuticals. *Mutation Research*, **488**, 151–169.

5 Matthews, E.J., Kruhlak, N.L., Cimino, M.C., Benz, R.D. and Contrera, J.F. (2006) An analysis of genetic toxicity, reproductive and developmental toxicity, and carcinogenicity data: I. Identification of carcinogens using surrogate endpoints. *Regulatory Toxicology and Pharmacology*, **44**, 83–96.

6 US Federal Register (2008) International Conference on Harmonisation: draft guidance on S2(R1) genotoxicity testing and data interpretation for pharmaceuticals intended for human use, availability, 73, p. 59.

7 Teague, S.J., Davis, A.M., Leeson, P.D. and Prea, T. (1999) The design of leadlike combinatorial libraries. *Angewandte Chemie-International Edition*, **38**, 3743–3748.

8 Lipinski, C.A., Lombardo, F., Dominy, B.W. and Feeney, P.J. (1997) Experimental and computational approaches to estimate solubility and permeability in drug discovery. *Advanced Drug Delivery Reviews*, **23**, 3–25.

9 Hastwell, P.W., Chai, L.-L., Roberts, K.J., Webster, T.W., Harvey, J.S., Rees, R.W. and Walmsley, R.M. (2006) High-specificity and high-sensitivity genotoxicity assessment in a human cell line: Validation of the GreenScreen HC GADD45a-GFP genotoxicity assay. *Mutation Research*, **607**, 160–175.

10 Müller, L., Mauthe, R.J., Riley, C.M., Andino, M., De Antonis, D., Beels, C., DeGeorge, J. De Knaep, F. et al. (2006) A rationale for determination, testing and control of genotoxic impurities. *Regulatory Toxicology and Pharmacology*, **44**, 198–211.

11 Dobo, K.L., Greene, N., Cyr, M.O., Caron, S. and Ku, W.W. (2006) The application of structure-based assessment to support safety and chemistry diligence to manage genotoxic impurities in active pharmaceutical ingredients during drug development. *Regulatory Toxicology and Pharmacology*, **44**, 282–293.

12 EMEA Guideline on the limits of genotoxic impurities. http://www.emea.europa.eu/pdfs/human/swp/519902en.pdf.

13 Delaney, E.J. (2007) An impact analysis of the application of the threshold of toxicological concern concept to pharmaceuticals. *Regulatory Toxicology and Pharmacology*, **49**, 107–124.

14 Ames, B.N. and Gold, L.S. (2000) Paracelsus to parascience: the environmental cancer distraction. *Mutation Research*, **447**, 3–13.

15 Ashby, J. (1985) Fundamental structural alerts to potential carcinogenicity or non-carcinogenicity. *Environmental Mutagenesis*, **7**, 919–921.

16 Ashby, J. and Tennant, R.W. (1991) Definitive relationships among chemical structure, carcinogenicity and mutagenicity for 301 chemicals tested by the U.S. NTP. *Mutation Research*, **257**, 229–306.

17 Snyder, R.D., Pearl, G.S., Mandakas, G., Choy, W.N., Goodsaid, F. and Rosenblum, I.Y. (2004) Assessment of the sensitivity of the computational programs DEREK, TOPKAT, and MCASE in the prediction of the genotoxicity of pharmaceutical molecules. *Environmental and Molecular Mutagenesis*, **43**, 143–158.

18 Matthews, E.J., Kruhlak, N.L., Benz, R.D., Contrera, J.F., Marchant, C.A. and Yang, C. (2008) Combined use of MC4PC, MDL-QSAR, BioEpisteme, Leadscope PDM, and Derek for Windows software to achieve high-performance, high-confidence, mode of action-based predictions of chemical carcinogenesis in rodents. *Toxicol Mech Methods*, **18**, 189–206.

19 Yang, C., Hasselgren, C.H., Boyer, S., Arvidson, K., Aveston, S., Dierkes, P., Benigni, R., Benz, R.D. et al. (2008) Understanding genetic toxicity through data mining: the process of building knowledge by integrating multiple genetic

toxicity databases. *Toxicol Mech Methods*, **18**, 277–295.
20 Burke, D.A., Wedd, D.J. and Burlinson, B. (1996) Use of the Miniscreen assay to screen novel compounds for bacterial mutagenicity in the pharmaceutical industry. *Mutagenesis*, **11**, 201–205.
21 van Gompel, J., Woestenborghs, F., Beerens, D., Mackie, C., Cahill, P.A., Knight, A.W., Billinton, N., Tweats, D.J. et al. (2005) An assessment of the utility of the yeast GreenScreen assay in pharmaceutical screening. *Mutagenesis*, **20**, 449–454.
22 Flückiger-Isler, S., Baumeister, M., Braun, K., Gervais, V., Hasler-Nguyen, N., Reimann, R., Van Gompel, J., Wunderlich, H. et al. (2004) Assessment of the performance of the Ames II™ assay: a collaborative study with 19 coded compounds. *Mutation Research*, **558**, 181–197.
23 Mortimer, R.K. and Manney, T.R. (1971) Mutation induction in yeast, in *Chemical Mutagens: Principles and Methods for their Detection*, Vol. 1 (ed. A. Hollaender), Plenum Press, New York.
24 Zimmermann, F.K., von Borstel, R.C., von Halle, E.S., Parry, J.M., Siebert, D., Zetterberg, G., Barale, R. and Loprieno, N. (1984) Testing of chemicals for genetic activity with *Saccharomyces cerevisiae*, in Report to the US Environmental Protection Agency Gene-Tox Program. *Mutation Research*, **133**, 199–244.
25 Parry, E.M. and Parry, J.M. (1985) The assay of genotoxicity of chemicals using the budding yeast Saccharomyces cerevisiae, in *Mutagenicity Testing, A Practical Approach* (eds S. Venitt and J.M. Parry), IRL Press, Oxford.
26 Schiestl, R.H., Gietz, R.D., Mehta, R.D. and Hasting, P.J. (1989) Carcinogens induce intrachromosomal recombination in yeast. *Carcinogenesis*, **10**, 1445–1455.
27 Hontzeas, N., Hafer, K. and Schiestl, R.H. (2007) Development of a microtiter plate version of the yeast DEL assay amenable to high-throughput toxicity screening of chemical libraries. *Mutation Research*, **634**, 228–234.
28 Mateuca, R., Lombaert, N., Aka, P.V., Decordier, I. and Kirsch-Volders, M. (2006) Chromosomal changes: induction, detection methods and applicability in human biomonitoring. *Biochimie*, **88**, 1515–1531.
29 Diaz, D., Scott, A., Carmichael, P., Shi, W. and Costales, C. (2007) An assessment of the performance of an automated scoring system (Cellomics) for the *in vitro* micronucleus assay in CHO-K1 cells. *Mutation Research*, **630**, 1–13.
30 Witt, K.L., Livanos, E., Kissling, G.E., Torous, D.K., Caspary, W., Tice, R.R. and Recio, L. (2008) Comparison of flow cytometry- and microscopy-based methods for measuring micronucleated reticulocyte frequencies in rodents treated with nongenotoxic and genotoxic chemicals. *Mutation Research*, **649**, 101–113.
31 Bryce, S.M., Avlasevich, S.L., Bemis, J.C., Lukamowicz, M., Elhajouji, A., Van Goethem, F., De Boeck, M., Beerens, D. et al. (2008) Interlaboratory evaluation of a flow cytometric, high content *in vitro* micronucleus assay. *Mutation Research*, **650**, 181–195.
32 Collins, A.R., Oscoz, A.A., Brunborg, G., Gaivão, I., Giovannelli, L., Kruszewski, M., Smith, C.C. and Stetina, R. (2008) The comet assay: topical issues. *Mutagenesis*, **23**, 143–151.
33 Kiskinis, E., Suter, W. and Hartmann, A. (2002) High throughput Comet assay using 96-well plates. *Mutagenesis*, **17**, 37–43.
34 Witte, I., Plappert, U., de Wall, H. and Hartmann, A. (2007) Genetic toxicity assessment: Employing the best science for human safety evaluation part III: The comet assay as an alternative to *in vitro* clastogenicity tests for early drug candidate selection. *Toxicological Sciences*, **97**, 21–26.
35 Radman, M. (1975) SOS repair hypothesis: Phenomenology of an inducible DNA repair which is accompanied by

mutagenesis. *Basic Life Sciences*, **5**, 355–367.

36 Quillardet, P., Huisman, O., D'Ari, R. and Hofnung, M. (1982) SOS Chromotest, a direct assay for induction of an SOS function in *Escherichia coli* K-12 to measure genotoxicity. *Proceedings of the National Academy of Sciences of the United States of America*, **79**, 5971–5975.

37 Reifferscheid, G. and Heil, J. (1996) Validation of the SOS/*umu* test using test results of 486 chemicals and comparison with the Ames test and carcinogenicity data. *Mutation Research*, **369**, 129–145.

38 Quillardet, P. and Hofnung, M. (1993) The SOS chromotest: a review. *Mutation Research*, **297**, 235–279.

39 Verschaeve, L., Van Gompel, J., Thilemans, L., Regniers, L., Vanparys, P. and van der Lelie, D. (1999) VITOTOX bacterial genotoxicity and toxicity test for the rapid screening of chemicals. *Environmental and Molecular Mutagenesis*, **33**, 240–248.

40 Vollmer, A.C., Belkin, S., Smulski, D.R., Van Dyk, T.K. and LaRossa, R.A. (1997) Detection of DNA damage by use of *Escherichia coli* carrying *recA'::lux*, *uvrA'::lux*, or *alkA'::lux* reporter plasmids. *Applied and Environmental Microbiology*, **63**, 2566–2571.

41 Schmid, C., Reifferscheid, G., Zahn, R.K. and Backmann, M. (1997) Increase in sensitivity and validity of the SOS/umu-test after replacement of the beta-galactosidase reporter gene with luciferase. *Mutation Research*, **394**, 9–16.

42 Flegrova, Z., Skarek, M., Bartos, T., Cupr, P. and Holoubek, I. (2007) Usefulness of three SOS-response tests for genotoxicity detection. *Fresenius Environmental Bulletin*, **16**, 1369–1376.

43 Cahill, P.A., Knight, A.W., Billinton, N., Barker, M.G., Walsh, L., Keenan, P.O., Williams, C.V. Tweats, D.J. et al. (2004) The GreenScreen genotoxicity assay: a screening validation programme. *Mutagenesis*, **19**, 105–119.

44 Jagger, C., Tate, M., Cahill, P.A., Hughes, C., Knight, A.W., Billinton, N. and Walmsley, R.M. (2008) Assessment of the genotoxicity of S9-generated metabolites using the GreenScreen HC GADD45a–GFP assay. *Mutagenesis*, doi: 10.1093/mutage/gen050.

45 Billinton, N., Hastwell, P.W., Beerens, D., Birrell, L., Ellis, P., Maskell, S., Webster, T.W., Windebank, W., *et al.* (2008) Interlaboratory assessment of the GreenScreen HC GADD45a-GFP genotoxicity screening assay: An enabling study for independent validation as an alternative method. *Mutation Research*, **653**, 23–33.

46 Knight, A.W., Birrell, L. and Walmsley, R.M. (2009) Development and validation of a higher throughput screening approach to genotoxicity testing using the *GADD45a-GFP* GreenScreen HC assay. *Journal of Biomolecular Screening*, in press.

47 Ohno, K., Taaka-Azuma, Y., Yoneda, Y. and Yamada, T. (2005) Genotoxicity test system based on p53R2 gene expression in human cells: Examination with 80 chemicals. *Mutation Research*, **588**, 45–57.

48 Ohno, K., Ishihata, K., Tanaka-Azuma, Y. and Yamada, T. (2008) A genotoxicity test system based on p53R2 gene expression in human cells: Assessment of its reactivity to various classes of genotoxic chemicals. *Mutation Research*, doi: 10.1016/j.mrgentox.2008.07.002.

49 Kirkland, D. and Speit, G. (2008) Evaluation of the ability of a battery of three *in vitro* genotoxicity tests to discriminate rodent carcinogens and non-carcinogens III. Appropriate follow-up testing *in vivo*. *Mutation Research*, **654**, 114–132.

50 Miura, D., Dobrovolsky, V.N., Kasahara, Y., Katsuura, Y. and Heflich, R.H. (2008) Development of an *in vivo* gene mutation assay using the endogenous Pig-A gene: I. Flow cytometric detection of CD59-negative peripheral red blood cells and CD48-negative spleen T-cells from the rat.

Environmental and Molecular Mutagenesis, **49**, 614–621.

51 Phonethepswath, S., Bryce, S.M., Bemis, J.C. and Dertinger, S.D. (2008) Erythrocyte-based Pig-a gene mutation assay: Demonstration of cross-species potential. *Mutation Research*, **657**, 122–126.

52 Spitsbergen, J.M. and Kent, M.L. (2003) The state of the art of the zebrafish model for toxicology and toxicologic pathology research-advantages and current limitations. *Toxicologic Pathology*, **31**, 62–87.

53 Rubinstein, A.L. (2006) Zebrafish assays for drug toxicity screening. *Expert Opinion on Drug Metabolism and Toxicology*, **2**, 231–240.

54 Amanuma, K., Takeda, H., Amanuma, H. and Aoki, Y. (2000) Transgenic zebrafish for detecting mutations caused by compounds in aquatic environments. *Nature Biotechnology*, **18**, 62–65.

55 Diekmann, M., Waldmann, P., Schnurstein, A., Grummt, T., Braunbeck, T. and Nagel, R. (2004) On the relevance of genotoxicity for fish populations II: genotoxic effects in zebrafish (*Danio rerio*) exposed to 4-nitroquinoline-1-oxide in a complete life-cycle test. *Aquatic Toxicology*, **68**, 27–37.

56 Sobels, F.H. and Vogel, E. (1976) The capacity of Drosophila for detecting relevant genetic damage. *Mutation Research*, **41**, 95–106.

57 Vogel, E., Blijleven, W.G.H., Kortselius, M.J.H. and Zijlstra, J.A. (1981) Mutagenic activity of 17 coded compounds in the sex-linked recessive lethal test in Drosophila melanogaster, in *Progress in Mutation Research, Volume 1: Evaluation of Short-Term Tests Carcinogens* (eds F.J. de Serres and J. Ashby), Elsevier, Amsterdam.

58 The C. elegans Sequencing Consortium (1998) The *C. elegans* sequencing consortium. *Science*, **282**, 2012–2018.

59 Sulston, J.E., Schierenberg, E., White, J.G. and Thomson, J.N. (1983) The embryonic cell lineage of the nematode *Caenorhabditis elegans*. *Developmental Biology*, **100**, 64–119.

60 Leung, M.C.K., Williams, P.L., Benedetto, A., Au, C., Helmcke, K.J., Aschner, M. and Meyer, J.N. (2008) *Caenorhabditis elegans*: an emerging model in biomedical and environmental toxicology. *Toxicological Sciences*, doi: 10.1093/toxsci/kfn121.

61 Kitching, J., Burlinson, B., Wing, M.G. and Walmsley, R.M. (2004) Finding the optimum approach for genetic toxicology screening. *The Toxicologist*, **78**, 132.

12
In Vitro Safety Pharmacology Profiling: an Important Tool to Decrease Attrition

Jacques Hamon and Steven Whitebread

12.1
What is "*In Vitro* Safety Pharmacology Profiling?"

"Safety pharmacology" is a term which started to be used in the early 1990s, specifically for the *in vivo* pharmacology assays designed to detect adverse effects of drugs in preclinical development. At that time, *in vitro* pharmacology was included under the term "general pharmacology", which encompassed all *in vivo* and *in vitro* assays designed to characterize the pharmacology of a clinical candidate, including both desired and undesired effects [1–3]. The concept of using general pharmacology to profile drugs for safety or "pharmacological toxicity" was already well understood [4]. In 2001, some guidance for the industry was published (ICH S7A) defining safety pharmacology studies as those studies that investigate the potential undesirable pharmacodynamic effects of a substance on physiological functions in relation to exposure within the therapeutic range and above [5]. While the S7A guidance largely deals with *in vivo* safety pharmacology studies, it states that *in vitro* studies on receptors, enzymes, transporters and ion channels can also be used as test systems and data from ligand binding and enzyme assays, suggesting that a potential for adverse effects should be taken into consideration when designing safety pharmacology studies. We classify these studies as "*in vitro* safety pharmacology" and the routine testing of compounds during early drug discovery we call "*in vitro* safety pharmacology profiling" [6].

In vitro safety pharmacology assays have been around for more than 35 years – ever since the first *in vitro* pharmacology assays were developed to measure binding or activity at a specific protein. Initially of course, they were used to discover new medicines acting through such targets. However, it quickly became clear, especially for those working in the cardiovascular and neuroscience fields, that many of these targets were also responsible for unwanted side effects seen in animal experiments and humans, and testing (profiling) of new drug candidates against a number of these safety-related targets (also called "antitargets" [7]) was performed.

Hit and Lead Profiling. Edited by Bernard Faller and Laszlo Urban
Copyright © 2009 WILEY-VCH Verlag GmbH & Co. KGaA, Weinheim
ISBN: 978-3-527-32331-9

The best example of a safety-related target is probably the hERG (human ether-a-go-go-related gene) potassium channel. This target is strongly implicated in QT prolongation and can result in the potentially fatal type of arrhythmia, torsades de pointes (TdP), which has been one of the main causes of drug withdrawals in recent years (see Chapter 16). We review more specifically a number of other important targets for early *in vitro* safety pharmacology assessment in the next sections of this chapter.

The main aim of *in vitro* safety pharmacology profiling is to characterize the secondary pharmacology profile of compounds in discovery, using a core battery of human *in vitro* assays designed to predict potential adverse drug reactions, the ultimate goal being to reduce late stage attrition [8, 9]. *In vitro* safety pharmacology profiling is "nothing new", but thanks to faster throughput assay technologies, cloned human proteins, miniaturization, robotics and a rapidly expanding knowledge base, it can be put to more efficient use much earlier in the drug discovery process to guide medicinal chemists in the lead selection and optimization phases.

We do not address early toxicology profiling in this section, that is, those phenotypic assays for which molecular targets are hardly known and which attempt to be predictive of the standard later stage assays, such as those covering genotoxicity, hepatotoxicity or phototoxicity. These are all covered elsewhere in this book.

12.2
Examples of Drug Failures Due to Secondary Pharmacology

Of the 16 drugs withdrawn from the market between 1992 and 2002, 15 (94%) were withdrawn due to toxic events and adverse drug reactions and eight compounds were withdrawn due to a well defined mechanism of action [10]. As examples, fenfluramine (Pondimin) and dexfenfluramine (Redux), two appetite-suppressant agents, were withdrawn due to cases of valvular heart disease linked to a secondary activity at the serotonin 5HT2B receptor. Pergolide (Permax), a drug used for the treatment of Parkinson's disease, was removed from the market in 2007 for the same adverse reaction and was also shown to display secondary 5HT2B agonist activity. Rapacuronium (Raplon), a rapidly acting, nondepolarizing neuromuscular blocker used in modern anaesthesia, to aid and enable endotracheal intubations, was withdrawn from the United States market by the manufacturer in 2001 [11]. This was due to a risk of fatal bronchospasm linked to a muscarinic M2 antagonist activity. Amineptine (Survector), an atypical tricyclic antidepressant, was withdrawn from the market for multiple adverse effects including acneiform eruptions, hepatotoxicty and addiction. The latter effect was attributed to its dopaminergic properties. An older example is the case of PCP (Sernyl), introduced as a dissociative anaesthetic agent in 1963, but withdrawn two years later due to hallucinations experienced by about 30% of the patients. This adverse effect was the reason for the use of PCP as a drug on the street in the 1970s under the names "angel dust" or "peace pill". This effect is linked to its NMDA antagonist property, but also to its complex pharmacological profile affecting monoamine transporters, the cholinergic system, the sigma and opioid receptors and some ion channels [12].

A number of mechanism of actions are known to be linked with serious adverse effects which prevent some compounds from reaching the market. One example is PDE4 inhibition. Despite the efforts of most major pharmaceutical companies to develop safe PDE4 inhibitors for the treatment of asthma or COPD, none have so far been marketed, due in particular to emetic side effects most probably linked with their primary pharmacology. In other cases, drugs were not withdrawn from the market, but their prescription decreased dramatically following the late characterization of adverse effects. Such is the case with MAO inhibitors. The use of the first generation of nonselective monoamine oxidase inhibitors as neuropsychiatric drugs was seriously limited, mainly because of what became known as the "cheese reaction". This reaction is due to the presence of tyramine in many fermented foodstuffs including cheese that are not deaminated by MAO in the intestine of the patients treated with MAO inhibitors. The consequence can be a severe hypertensive reaction induced by the absorbed tyramine [13].

A different example concerns fialuridine, a uridine analog that was being developed for the treatment of hepatitis B before it was stopped in Phase II trials, due to fatal mitochondrial hepatotoxicity [14]. This hepatotoxicity was found to be enhanced by filuridine being actively transported into the mitochondria by the human equilibrative nucleoside transporter (hENT1, adenosine transporter). It was then shown that, unlike in humans, the mouse ENT1 is not incorporated into the mitochondrial membrane [15]. This explains why the toxicity was not picked up in animal experiments. Although not a true secondary pharmacology, screening of compounds in a hENT1 assay might prevent such deaths in future. Species differences are common and this example demonstrates that human *in vitro* assays could be more predictive of human ADRs than animal experiments.

It is important to keep in mind that about 30% of the late failures during drug development occur due to toxicity and safety issues [16]. Also, once a drug reaches the market, the chance of receiving a black box warning is rather high [17], sometimes dramatically impacting the sales. Furthermore, ADRs are believed to be a leading cause of death in the United States [18]. All of these facts show the need for an early characterization of the potential adverse effect profiles of new chemical entities (NCE), starting early in the discovery stage. This need is even reinforced by an apparent increase in regulatory caution by the FDA, which possibly led to a decrease of drug approvals and an increase in the late drug discovery stage attrition rate [19].

12.2.1
Components

12.2.1.1 Target Selection
A key point for the success of a good *in vitro* safety profile is the selection of the targets or pathways to include in such a profile in order to cover both a large spectrum of

adverse effects and the pharmacological space. Each target has to be linked to a known adverse or unwanted effect. It should be noted that a pharmacological effect may be the "wanted" or primary therapeutic effect in some cases, but in most other cases it would be "unwanted". The hypnotic or sedative agent zolpidem (a benzodiazepine receptor agonist) for instance is useful for its intended clinical use, but such a property is not wanted for most medications. So, a first strategy is to start from the known failures due to safety issues: Serotonin 5HT2B agonism as an example to avoid "fen-phen"-type disasters or PDE4 inhibition to avoid emetic side effects. However, the different types of adverse effects need to be considered.

Adverse drug reactions (ADRs) are classified into five main types: A–E [20, 21]. The main type, A, which accounts for about 75% of all ADRs, is caused by dose-dependent primary or secondary pharmacology. If the molecular target which mediates the ADR is known, then this type can be predicted by *in vitro* safety pharmacology profiling. By definition, the idiosyncratic toxicities, or type B, which account for most of the remaining ADRs, cannot be predicted (although this may change as they become better understood). However, some teratogenic effects which are included in type D can be predicted, for example, those which are mediated through the endothelin or retinoic acid receptors [22, 23].

Table 12.1 shows the most commonly occurring type A ADRs associated with the clinical use of drugs, sorted by therapeutic areas. These would be the main ADRs which *in vitro* safety pharmacology assays should aim to detect. It is clear that, especially at an early stage, an oncology program must consider mainly life-threatening adverse effects while a program on a chronic treatment for hypertension or the treatment of nasal congestion as examples must consider a wider range of potential adverse effects.

Each of these adverse effects is often related to different targets or pathways. For instance, sedation could be linked to an interaction with the histaminergic, alpha2 adrenergic or opioid receptors, but also with GABAergic transmission and many other targets. The list of potential targets is extensive when considering effects in various organs.

12.2.1.2 Target Annotation

Critical to any safety prediction based on *in vitro* safety pharmacology profiling is an accurate and comprehensive knowledge base to enable links to be made between activities at individual targets and side effects seen in the clinic. Traditionally, this is done by searching the primary literature for hints from *in vitro* and *in vivo* animal pharmacology experiments. This is of course still an essential source and can be the only way for those targets where no known ligand has yet been tested in humans. Ideally, however, the annotation should be based on known human clinical evidence, such as the primary and secondary pharmacologies of known drugs and phenotypic information from human genetic mutations. The challenge is to link data on known side effects to the targets through which they are mediated. This requires an overall assessment of all the available *in vitro* and *in vivo* data from animals and humans. One way to do this is to apply *in silico* prediction models (see Chapter 13).

Table 12.1 Major type A adverse effects associated with the clinical use of drugs.

GI tract	Hematology	Dermatology	Cardiovascular
Hepatitis/hepato-cellular damage	Agranulocytosis	Erythemas	Arrhythmias
Constipation	Hemolytic anemia	Hyperpigmentation	Hypotension
Diarrhea	Pancytopenia	Photodermatitis	Hypertension
Nausea/vomiting	Thrombocytopenia	Eczema	Congestive heart failure
Ulceration	Megaloblastic anemia	Urticaria	Angina/chest pain
Pancreatitis	Clotting/bleeding	Acne	Pericarditis
Dry mouth	Eosinophilia	Alopecia	Cardiomyopathy
Endocrine	Respiratory	Psychiatric	Musculoskeletal
Thyroid dysfunction	Airway obstruction	Delirium, confusion	Myalgia/myopathy
Sexual dysfunction	Pulmonary infiltrates	Depression	Rhabdomyolysis
Gynecomastia	Pulmonary edema	Hallucination	Osteoporosis
Addison syndrome	Respiratory depression	Schizophrenia/paranoia	
Galactorrhea	Nasal congestion		
Metabolic	Renal	Neurological	Ophthalmic/Otological
Hyperglycemia	Nephritis	Seizures	Disturbed color vision
Hypoglycemia	Nephrosis	Tremor	Cataract
Hyperkalemia	Tubular necrosis	Sleep disorders	Optic neuritis
Hypokalemia	Renal dysfunction	Peripheral neuropathy	Retinopathy
Metabolic acidosis	Bladder dysfunction	Headache	Glaucoma
Hyponatremia	Nephrolythiasis	Extrapyramidal effects	Corneal opacity
Hyperuricemia	Drowsiness		Deafness
			Vestibular disorders

Literature searching has been made much easier and faster with the current generation of search engines, but much of the drug side effect and related data has not been published in the primary literature and is only to be found in sources such as unpublished regulatory reports and drug labels. Information on drugs which failed during development is particularly difficult to find. However, much of this information has been collated and made available through web-based databases, some of which are freely available, although others are commercial. A list of some of the freely available databases is given in Table 12.2. Some restrictions may apply to their use. Some commercial databases are listed in Table 12.3.

12.2.1.3 Examples of *In Vitro* Safety Pharmacology Profiling Panels

Different panels of assays are most generally used at different stages of the drug discovery process covering only the most critical targets for safety (targets linked with life-threatening adverse effects or safety targets known to display a high hit rate) or a broad range of targets potentially involved in many different diseases. Some examples can be found among the *in vitro* safety profiles offered by different contract

Table 12.2 Some freely available web-based databases providing drug annotation.

Name and URL	Comment
FDA Center for Drug Evaluation and Research http://www.fda.gov/cder/site/default.htm http://www.fda.gov/cder/aers/default.htm	Includes drug information and regulatory guidance. Useful pages within this site include the Adverse Event Reporting System (AERS, a web-based reporting system for adverse events; this also gives drug safety and ADR information, including FDA safety alerts), the FDA Orange Book and Drugs@FDA (listed separately).
FDA Electronic Orange Book http://www.fda.gov/cder/ob/default.htm	Up-to-date information on all drug approvals and withdrawals in the US. Includes applicant, dosage form, proprietary name, date approved, patent information. Does not include drug label information or safety information.
Drugs@FDA http://www.accessdata.fda.gov/scripts/cder/drugsatfda/index.cfm	Similar to the Orange Book, but drugs listed alphabetically, therefore easier to browse.
RxList The Internet Drug Index http://www.rxlist.com/script/main/hp.asp	Alphabetically index of drugs (trade name only), giving detailed information, including structure, indications, safety. Provides a ranked list of the top 200 most prescribed drugs.
MedlinePlus drug information http://www.nlm.nih.gov/medlineplus/druginformation.html	Alphabetical index of drugs, herbs and supplements listed separately. Indications, ADRs, but no structure. For herbs and supplements grades are given according to whether the claimed activities are scientifically proven or not.
DailyMed (current medication information) http://www.dailymed.nlm.nih.gov/dailymed/about.cfm	Alphabetical listing of drugs. Provides FDA approved drug labels.
DrugDigest http://www.drugdigest.org/DD/Home	Similar to DailyMed, but search only, no browsing.
Common terminology criteria for adverse events (cancer therapy evaluation program) http://resadm.uchc.edu/hspo/ investigators/files/Common%20Toxicity%20Criteria_version%203.0.pdf	Categorizes ADRs according to MedDRA terminology, including severity grades.
PharmGKB (the pharmacogenetics and pharmacogenomics knowledge base) http://www.pharmgkb.org/index.jsp	Free database, but registration requested. Genes, pathways, drugs and diseases database. No structures.

Table 12.2 (Continued)

Name and URL	Comment
BIDD (BioInformatics and Drug Design group) http://xin.cz3.nus.edu.sg/group/sitemap.htm	Various databases, including: drug adverse reaction target (DART) database.
Drug Withdrawals http://www.ganfyd.org/index.php?title=Drug_withdrawals	List of UK drug withdrawals and changes in indication for use.
Fact and Comparisons http://online.factsandcomparisons.com/index.aspx?	Comprehensive monographs on individual drugs and drug classes. ADRs given with levels of incidence. Also available on CD-ROM.
List of bestselling drugs http://en.wikipedia.org/wiki/List_of_bestselling_drugs	Ranked list of the 200 best selling drugs.
Online Mendelian Inheritance in Man (OMIM) http://www.ncbi.nlm.nih.gov/sites/entrez?db=OMIM	Catalog of human genes and genetic disorders. Can provide genetic evidence for linking ADRs to interactions with specific targets.
Gene Cards http://www.genecards.org/	Comprehensive genomic and proteomic information.
NIMH Psychoactive Drug Screening Program: Receptor Affinity Database http://kidb.bioc.cwru.edu/pdsp.php	Receptor affinities of drugs and reference compounds.
DrugBank [24] http://www.drugbank.ca/	Extensive chemical and pharmacological annotation of 4800 compounds, including >1480 FDA-approved small molecule drugs and >3200 experimental drugs. Annotation includes drug target and indication information, but not ADRs.
Matador http://matador.embl.de	A manually annotated database linking drugs to targets.
UN list of banned, withdrawn, severely restricted or not approved pharmaceuticals [25] http://www.un.org/esa/coordination/CL12.pdf	Comprehensive world list of withdrawn drugs giving the reasons for withdrawal.

research organizations (CROs), which are heavily used by most of the small and major pharmaceutical companies:

- The "general safety profile" from CEREP including 155 *in vitro* assays specifically designed to identify potential side effects of drug candidates (not in a specific pathology).

Table 12.3 Some commercial web-based databases providing drug annotation.

Name and URL	Comment
GVK Biosciences	http://www.gvkbio.com/informatics.html
Prous Science Integrity	http://integrity.prous.com
PharmaPendium	http://www.pharmapendium.com
GeneGo	http://www.genego.com/
Biovista	http://www.biovista.com/
MedicinesComplete	http://www.medicinescomplete.com/mc/
Facts and Comparisons	http://www.factsandcomparisons.com/

- The "adverse reaction enzymes" profile from MDS Pharma including 41 enzymatic assays to predict moderate to serious adverse effects.
- The "LeadProfilingScreen" from MDS Pharma dedicated also to the adverse effect prediction.
- The "general side effect profile" from Caliper with 65 different targets.
- The "broad safety" and "focused safety" panels of functional GPCR assays offered by Millipore.

As opposed to selectivity profiling panels which generally include only related targets from the same family, the *in vitro* safety pharmacology panels are composed of a high diversity of targets, including representatives from GPCRs, ion channels, different families of enzymes, transporters and nuclear receptors, the main criteria being their link with ADRs. The GPCRs are often the most important target family represented in these panels. It reflects the fact that more than 30% of the marketed drugs are GPCR modulators and that most diseases can be impacted by some GPCRs [26]. With the increase in kinase drug discovery targets, broad kinase selectivity profiling has become very important. However, much less is known about the safety relevance of individual kinases than, for instance, for GPCRs. This is in part due to the fact that there are relatively few drugs for kinase targets in the clinic which could provide the necessary ADR annotation. This is certainly a field which needs expanding in future. Table 12.4 gives some examples of "safety targets" with the potential consequences of target interaction.

12.3
Processes

12.3.1
Assay Requirements and Technologies

The first requirement of an *in vitro* safety profiling assay is to be as predictive as possible of an adverse event, given all the limitations of *in vitro* assays and the other important parameters to consider in combination, such as physicochemical

Table 12.4 List of targets often included in *in vitro* safety pharmacology panels and the potential major consequences of receptor interaction.

Targets		Possible consequences of target interaction
Serotonin 5-HT 1A receptor	HTR1A	*Agonism*: Induces a behavioural syndrome characterized by flat body posture and head weaving in rats – In humans, 5-HT1A agonists, such as Buspirone, induce light-headedness, miosis, nervousness or agitation. They may also induce hypothermia, decrease blood pressure and heart rate. *Antagonism*: No side effects clearly defined – May have cognition enhancing effects useful for Alzheimer disease's (see Lecozotan).
Serotonin 5-HT 2B receptor	HTR2B	*Agonism*: Cardiac valvulopathy, fibroblast mitogenesis, hypertension. *Antagonism*: No side effects clearly defined, but cardiac effects cannot be excluded, especially at embryonic stage.
Adenosine 2a receptor	ADORA2A	*Agonism*: Inhibition of platelet aggregation, anti-inflammation and neuroprotective effects, coronary vasodilation, decreased blood pressure, increased plasma renin activity and sleep induction. *Antagonism*: Increased platelet aggregation, hypertension, nervousness (tremor, agitation), arousal, insomnia, cerebral and coronary vasodilation (in microvessels only).
Adenosine 3 receptor	ADORA3	*Agonism*: Immunosuppression, hypotension, anti-ischaemic (cardioprotective), pro-ischaemic (cerebral), cell necrosis, cell proliferation and angiogenesis. *Antagonism*: might cause myocardial ischaemia, proinflammatory effects, hypertension and interfere with the regulation of cell growth.
Adrenergic Alpha 1A receptor	ADRA1A	*Agonism*: Smooth muscle contraction (prostate in particular, effects on the lower urinary tract) and cardiac positive ionotropy, arrhythmia. *Antagonism*: Orthostatic hypotension and other blood pressure related adverse effects and impact on various aspects of sexual function.
Adrenergic Alpha 2A receptor	ADRA2A	*Agonism*: Sedation – anesthetic-sparing effect – central hypotensive and hypothermic actions, hyperglycemia. *Antagonism*: May induce gastrointestinal prokinetic effects.

Table 12.4 (Continued)

Targets		Possible consequences of target interaction
Adrenergic Beta 1 receptor	ADRB1	*Agonism*: May stimulate cardiac muscle (increase heart rate and force of contraction) and contributes to the relaxation of blood vessels. *Antagonism*: May stress cardiovascular performance.
Dopamine D1 receptor	DRD1	*Agonism*: May induce dyskinesia, extreme arousal, locomotor activation, vasodilatation and hypotension. *Antagonism*: Tremor.
Dopamine Transporter	SLC6A3	*Inhibitors* will prevent dopamine uptake (cocaine-like drugs). Important effects on locomotor activity, motivation, reward and cognition, dopaminergic hyperactivity, ADHD, depression, Parkinsonism, psychotic disorders, seizure, dystonia, dyskinesia.
Histamine H1 receptor	HRH1	*Agonism*: Allergic reaction. *Antagonism*: Sedation.
Muscarinic M1 receptor	CHRM1	*Agonism*: May increase blood pressure, heart rate and sympathetic outflow – May be involved in the regulation of circadian rhythm. *Antagonism*: Disruption of cognitive functions such as learning and memory.
Muscarinic M2 receptor	CHRM2	*Agonism*: Vagal effects (key role in the control of heart rate and smooth muscle activity); Bradycardia. *Antagonism*: May induce cardiac side effects (palpitations, dysrhythmia) or peripheral edema. bronchoconstriction can result from presynaptic M2 receptor antagonism if postsynaptic M3 receptors are not also blocked.
Opiate mu receptor	OPRM1	*Agonism*: Analgesia, Sedation, Physical dependence, Bowel dysfunction, Respiratory depression, Modulation of cough reflex.
Thromboxane A2 receptor	TBXA2R	*Agonism*: Vaso-, bronchoconstriction, platelet aggregation, myocardial ischemia, heart failure. *Antagonism*: could cause bleeding by inhibiting platelet aggregation.

Table 12.4 (Continued)

Targets		Possible consequences of target interaction
Progesterone receptor	PGR	*Agonism*: May cause loss of bone mineral density, bleeding disorders and promote breast cancer in females, and gestagenic effects in males. *Antagonism*: can cause excessive menstrual bleeding, uterine cramping, endometrial hyperplasia; contraindicated in young females.
Nicotinic receptor central	CHRNA2	*Agonism*: May play a role in the modulation of a number of neurotransmitters (e.g., dopaminergic, serotoninergic, glutamatergic) with effects on cognitive and motor function. They exhibit analgesic activity and may stimulate autonomic cardiovascular, respiratory and gastrointestinal function (palpitation/nausea). *Antagonism*: Muscle relaxants and anti-hypertensive agents. A number of neurotoxins (e.g., bungarotoxin, conotoxins) display also an antagonist action on different nicotinic acetylcholine receptor subtypes.
PCP receptor (NMDA channel)	GRIN1	*Agonism*: Anesthetic properties, may induce psychosis (schizophrenia like), hallucination, delirium and disoriented behavior, may cause seizures, neurotoxicity.
Epidermal growth factor receptor (HER1)	EGFR	*Activation*: Increased cell proliferation, angiogenesis, metastasis and decreased apoptosis. *Inhibition*: Skin rash, cancer metastasis.
Cathepsin D	CTSD	*Inhibition*: Neurodegeneration.
Phosphodiesterase 3A	PDE3A	*Inhibition*: May induce positive cardiac ionotropic effects.
Phosphodiesterase 4D	PDE4D	*Inhibition*: Emesis, Arteritis.
Monoamine Oxidase A	MAOA	*Inhibition*: May induce severe hypertensive crisis (known as "the Cheese reaction") – Centrally mediated side effects such as the serotonin syndrome, dizziness, blurred vision and weakness.
Cyclooxygenase-1	PTGS1	*Inhibition*: May disrupt normal cellular homeostasis and disrupt the production of prostaglandins, causing elevated levels of gastrointestinal toxicity, gastric bleeding, pulmonary bleeding.

and ADME properties of the compounds. The assay has to be robust, reproducible, cost-effective, medium-throughput and use a small amount of compound. The revolution in this field came with the development of high-throughput screening (HTS) technologies. These HTS assays are the starting point of most therapeutic projects in all major pharmaceutical companies and, despite their limitations, allowed the identification of a number of NCEs [27]. The same assay technologies can be used for the early assessment of ADRs. Initially, profiling assays were largely based on radioligand-binding filtration assays, often nonhuman. For the low number of compounds that were typically tested in the past for safety, these were perfectly adequate. However, the newer screening technologies for binding or enzymatic inhibition assays, for example, scintillation proximity assay (SPA), fluorescent polarization (FP) and fluorescence resonance transfer (FRET) and for functional cell-based assays (e.g., measuring cAMP, IP, calcium or GTP) allowed safety profiling to be moved earlier in the drug discovery process where many more compounds can be tested. The required throughput is not so much "high", but "medium" and "fast". For this reason, other medium-throughput technologies, such as automated patch clamp systems for ion channels, high content imaging technologies and/or technologies described as more physiologically relevant such as those using impedance measurements, find their place in *in vitro* safety profiling. With the recent accent on cardiosafety profiling, the automated patch clamp systems in particular have become routine technologies to functionally test for ion channel blockers such as hERG, sodium (Nav1.5) and calcium (Cav1.2).

12.3.2
Binding and/or Functional Assays

Should a binding assay or a functional assay be used as the primary profiling assay for a given target; and which technology is most suitable? Both formats using various technologies are available for most targets from the various commercial providers. Depending on the target and mechanism of action(s) which need to be assessed, one assay may be better to use than another, that is, more predictive, more robust, or less expensive. Radioligand-binding studies were the first to be used on a large scale and demonstrated their usefulness in *in vitro* safety pharmacology profiling panels. These assays are generally very robust, easy to automate, high-throughput and cost-effective; and their predictivity can be good enough as a primary assay. Indeed, direct correlations between some ADRs and ligand-binding activities for some receptors can be demonstrated. Figure 12.1 shows some of these correlations, established first by CEREP [28], and which we confirmed at Novartis. Such correlations are very useful because they can give an indication as to how potent a compound has to be at the target before an ADR becomes a possibility (ADME data always have to be taken into account as well). It should however be pointed out that, even though a correlation can be demonstrated between certain target/ADR pairs, it does not necessarily mean that that particular target actually mediates the ADR. Due to similar pharmacophores between related and even unrelated targets, all might show such a correlation, while actually only one might mediate the effect. The latter might not even be included in the safety

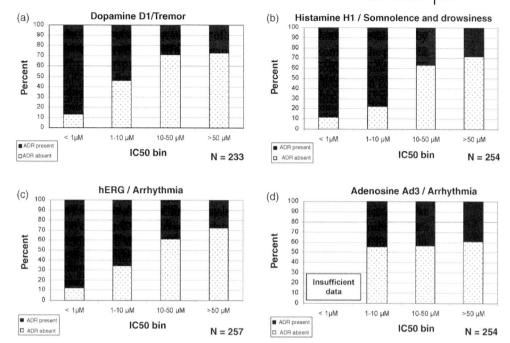

Figure 12.1 Examples of *in vitro* binding assays correlating with ADRs. Marketed drugs with known ADR profiles were tested in three different *in vitro* receptor binding assays and their IC$_{50}$s (concentration required to achieve 50% inhibition) were determined. The percentage of drugs having (black bars) and not having (dotted bars) the stated ADR is plotted for each IC$_{50}$ bin (X-axis). The receptor/ADR pairs dopamine D1 and tremor (a), histamine H1 and somnolence (b), and hERG and arrhythmia (c) all show a marked increase in the presence of the ADR in the lower IC$_{50}$ bins. As a control, the pair adenosine Ad3 and arrhythmia (d), shows no correlation, with the arrhythmia drugs evenly distributed across the IC$_{50}$ bins.

panel and might not even be known as the mediator of the effect. A typical example is the similarity between the different dopamine receptors. Many compounds show little selectivity between all five dopamine receptors; and the correlation between tremor and dopamine D1 receptor binding (shown in Figure 12.1) can also be found with all other dopamine receptors.

Binding assays generally require the availability of a high affinity ligand that can be chemically labeled (e.g., with a radioactive isotope or a fluorescent group) and often require overexpression of the target of interest in a given cellular system, which is not always easy to achieve. Another limitation is that a ligand-binding assay cannot usually provide any information on the mechanism of action (agonist/activator, antagonist/inhibitor) and cannot detect an indirect modulator of a given target. For GPCRs, when the ADR is clearly related to one particular mechanism of action, it may be of interest to consider the use of a functional assay as a primary assay rather than a follow-up to a binding assay. Especially when looking for GPCR agonism, a functional assay is often more sensitive than a binding assay and also detects compounds with allosteric effects. A cAMP quantification agonist assay on the histamine H2 receptor is much more valuable in an *in vitro* safety pharmacology profiling panel than a binding assay for the detection of a secondary histamine H2 agonist activity. This activity is known to induce positive inotropic effects on the human ventricle (amthamine is a cardiotonic agent) and potentially to stimulate gastric acid secretion, while H2 antagonists are known to be rather safe – ranitidine (Zantac) is among the most prescribed drugs without major adverse effects, although overdosing can cause muscular tremors, vomiting, dizziness and rapid respiration.

Likewise, functional agonist assays for the serotonin 5HT2 receptors (5HT2A, 5HT2B, 5HT2C) are more relevant for safety than binding assays. The latter tend to give a very high hit rate, but most of the binders are antagonists, for which no major ADRs have been reported.

Finally, and this could be the future of *in vitro* safety pharmacology profiling, new functional technologies, described to be more physiologically relevant, are being developed and may give an additional advantage to functional technologies over binding assays, especially when associated with the use of primary cells. However, there will always be a need for some binding experiments as primary profiling assays or follow-up assays in order to confirm the interaction with a given target.

12.3.3
Processes and Logistics

Even though profiling assay technologies are highly similar to screening assay technologies, the process and automation required are completely different and more complex. Instead of dealing with a very high number of compounds and plates to run in a given assay (as in high-throughput screening), one has to deal with a lower number of plates to test in a set of diverse assays. Fully automated systems need to be sufficiently flexible to handle assays using different reagents, conditions and technologies within the same run. They have to integrate different readers and require sophisticated scheduling software. Compound management can also be complex, as different sets of compounds often need to be tested in different panels or even individual assays.

A fast turn-around time has to be maintained, as it is part of the project flowchart and contributes to the optimization cycles of the different chemical scaffolds, together with the physichochemical properties and *in vitro* ADME data. At Novartis, rather than testing initially at a single concentration, we decided to perform direct full IC_{50} determinations in order to ensure not only a good turn-around time, but more importantly a good data quality. We thereby avoid the cherry picking and retesting of active compounds. The additional consumption of reagents when doing direct IC_{50} determination is largely compensated by the reduction of compound management tasks. Also, one can easily differentiate between inactive compounds and low-active compounds (micromolar range activities) and see the potential solubility issues (compounds showing activity at low concentrations, but not at the highest concentrations due to precipitation in the incubation medium). Each assay run includes at least one reference compound which is most generally included in each plate as an intra-plate control. A deviation of no more than threefold is generally accepted with the average value acquired during the assay validation step. Also, parameters such as the Z' value, the signal to background ratio, the percentage of nonspecific signal and other parameters linked with each technologies are systematically calculated for further validation.

Finally, all the data need to be registered in the company database together with all the details on how they were obtained. This is important, as it may contribute, sometimes several years later, to a drug data package to be used either inside the company for different decision points or externally as part of a regulatory dossier for health authorities. Although *in vitro* safety pharmacology profiling data are not officially requested by regulatory bodies, it is often one piece of data which helps to prove the good safety and selectivity profile of a drug. Data registration is also very important to get the full benefit of profiling activities, as it becomes a very rich source for data mining, allowing the development of *in silico* tools to drive drug discovery (see Chapter 13) or providing starting points for new therapeutic projects.

12.4
Application to Drug Discovery

12.4.1
How and When to Use *In Vitro* Safety Pharmacology Profiling

After the hit discovery process (often using high-throughput screening), early drug discovery is generally split into a "hit to lead" phase and a "lead optimization" phase, followed by the selection of development candidates (DCs) (Figure 12.2). *In vitro*

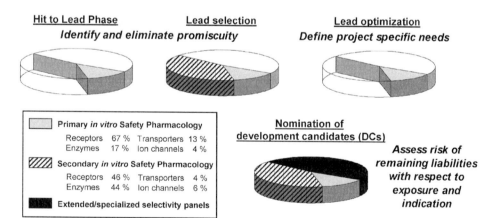

Figure 12.2 The use of *in vitro* safety pharmacology profiling during early drug discovery. A smaller (primary) panel of targets is usually sufficient during the hit to lead phase and lead optimization phases of a drug discovery program to detect promiscuous scaffolds and to pick up the most commonly occurring liabilities. At each phase transition, it is advisable to test the candidate compounds in a broader (secondary) panel, to detect the less commonly occurring liabilities. The broadest panel is used to test the final selection of development candidates.

safety pharmacology profiling can be applied to the first of these phases with the aim of identifying and avoiding chemical series which are inherently promiscuous. At this stage, the number of compounds that need to be tested can be relatively high, but it is usually sufficient to test them in a relatively small, but diverse (primary) panel of assays, thereby keeping the cost low. Most compounds at this stage have a rather low affinity for the primary target, often not very different from any off-target affinities. It is often believed that, as the primary target affinity is optimized, the off-target activities are lost. While this can happen, in most cases it does not succeed.

At lead selection, after which typically more chemistry effort is invested, the selected compounds can be profiled in a broader (secondary) panel of assays, hopefully confirming the selective nature of the leads. If this is the case, spot checking in the primary panel through the optimization phase may be sufficient to ensure selectivity is retained while the required potency at the primary target is achieved. If the selected leads are still rather promiscuous, or certain individual unwanted liabilities remain, these should be monitored by testing in the primary panel (or in additional individual assays) and improved upon during lead optimization. The broader panel can then be applied again to the selected development candidates for a final check and these may even be extended further to additional specialized panels for added security.

At this point in the program, key information from other *in vitro* and *in vivo* studies become available, such as efficacy, pharmacokinetics, potential drug–drug interactions, metabolites and some early toxicology. All of these factors combined enable a first integrated risk assessment to be made.

In vitro safety pharmacology profiling can also be applied to other stages of the drug discovery process. For instance, a broad profile may discover an unknown target for an orphan drug or during target feasibility studies, before starting a drug discovery program, any known reference or competitor compounds can be tested for an early assessment. Using profiling, salvinorin A was found to be the first naturally occurring non-nitrogenous opioid receptor subtype-selective agonist [29] and this result suggested that kappa opioid receptors may play a prominent role in the modulation of human perception. A study by Elphick *et al.* investigating the inhibition of human polyomavirus JCV infection by antipsychotics highlighted the importance of pharmacological profiling in discovering roles of receptors in diseases [30]. It is also by using the profiling of a number of antipsychotics that a link between muscarinic M3 receptor and type 2 diabetes was shown [31]. During later-stage development, new metabolites, especially human, may be discovered which should also be tested, plus competitor compounds as they become known. *In vitro* safety pharmacology profiling will also be very useful for back-up programs to improve on earlier compounds which suffer from unfavorable safety profiles.

12.4.2
Pharmacological Promiscuity and Its Clinical Interpretation

Most antipsychotic compounds are known to bind to many different receptors, especially those for serotonin, dopamine and histamine [32, 33]. Such pharmacological promiscuity is possibly required for certain central indications, such as psychosis, depression, Alzheimer's disease [34–37] and possibly also for cancer [38], but it is certainly also the source of the many known side effects of such drugs [39, 40]. Several authors use the term polypharmacology for this phenomenon [41–43], but this term was introduced for the broad pharmacology obtained by combination therapies, irrespective of the number of targets hit [44, 45]. Due to the higher risk of side effects occurring with pharmacologically promiscuous compounds, it makes sense to promote compounds during the research phase which are inherently selective.

The target hit rate (THR) was introduced to quantify the phenomenon of pharmacological promiscuity [46, 47]. THR is defined as the number of targets bound by a drug at a given concentration, expressed as a percentage of all targets tested, for instance in a panel of *in vitro* safety pharmacology assays. THR_{10} is the THR where a "hit" is defined as >50% inhibition at 10 µM. Compounds with a THR_{10} of <5% were defined as "selective", 5–20% as "medium promiscuous" and >20% as "promiscuous". A similar quantification was used by Leeson and Springthorpe [48], except that they used >30% inhibition at 10 µM. The THR is not a constant term, as it depends heavily on the number of targets tested and the degree of target diversity. It can however be used in a standardized profiling panel calibrated against known promiscuous compounds. The THR classification given above is used in the Novartis *in vitro* safety pharmacology profiling panel where >50 targets have been tested.

A THR analysis of 293 marketed drugs demonstrated that over 60% were selective (THR <5%; Figure 12.3). This group included 22 antipsychotics, which were all promiscuous. A subset of 132 of the most prescribed and best selling drugs, excluding any withdrawn drugs or antipsychotics, had only 5% "promiscuous" but 73%

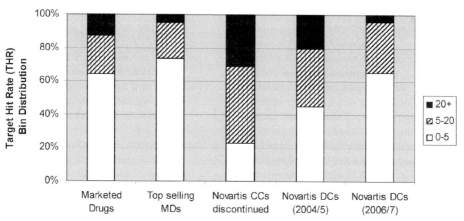

Figure 12.3 Target Hit Rates (THR) for marketed drugs and Novartis compounds. A THR of >20% is considered to be "promiscuous" (black), 5–20% "medium promiscuous" (hatched) and 0–5% "selective" (white). 65% of the "Marketed Drug" set of 293 compounds, including antipsychotics and withdrawn drugs, were selective, whereas only 13% were promiscuous. Promiscuity dropped to 5% in a subset of 132 most often prescribed and top selling drugs ("Top selling"). This contrasts with the 31% promiscuity found in the Novartis clinical candidates (CCs) which were discontinued. The most recent Novartis development candidates (DCs) on the other hand were very comparable to the best selling marketed drug set.

"selective". In contrast, of 26 Novartis clinical candidates (CCs) which failed to advance to human trials between 2001 and 2007, only six were selective. Novartis development candidates (DCs) from 2004 became more selective and can now be called "marketed drug-like", which suggests that compounds which might previously have failed during extensive animal toxicology studies are now being selected out during the research phase and should reduce the attrition rate in development.

It is important to point out that when a compound is pharmacologically promiscuous in a panel of 50 diverse targets, it is highly likely that the compound also hits several additional targets which are not included in the panel, thereby further increasing the liability risk. The reasons why certain compounds are more promiscuous than others and how promiscuity can be avoided is discussed in Chapter 13.

If pharmacological promiscuity is strongly reduced and only very few activities remain, a risk assessment has to be performed based on the therapeutic index.

12.4.3
Relevance of Potency and Therapeutic Index (TI)

In most drug discovery programs, the first goal is to achieve a high potency at the primary target and also a good selectivity against closely related targets. Optimally, *in vitro* potency correlates perfectly with activity *in vivo*, in both animals and humans, and the chosen compound is highly bioavailable, allowing a very low maximum free circulating concentration (C_{max}) at the therapeutic dose. Everything being equal, the fold selectivity against other targets *in vitro* can then be used to estimate the safety margin. Unfortunately there are so many factors working against this ideal situation that the fold selectivity *in vitro* is rarely equivalent to the actual therapeutic index (TI) in humans. A micromolar off-target activity may still be important, even if the affinity for the primary target is in the nanomolar range or lower.

Factors which can affect the TI include:
- Poor translation of *in vitro* to *in vivo* activity (e.g., due to poor accessibility of the target, up-/downregulation of target or endogenous ligand or compensatory effects).
- Poor translation of *in vivo* activity in animals to humans (e.g., due to species selectivity, different pharmacodynamics).
- Gender and age.
- General health of the patient.
- Circadian variations.
- Active human metabolites with lower TI.
- Drug–drug interactions.
- Accumulation in tissues.
- Low bioavailability.
- High protein binding.

If any of these factors influence the unwanted effects more favorably, then the TI will drop. This could occur in just a subset of patients, for instance those with genetic risk factors, and the side effect may therefore be seen only after a drug has been in the clinic for some while [49]. If it is a serious side effect, it could cause the drug to be withdrawn, or it may receive a black box warning [17]. If there is a potential for the recommended dose being exceeded, a higher therapeutic index may have to be applied.

Redfern et al. studied the occurrence of QT prolongation and the lethal arrhythmia torsades de pointes (see Chapter 16) in marketed drugs from the perspective of the therapeutic index [50]. This group proposed a therapeutic index of 30-fold, calculated from the free C_{max} at the therapeutic dose and the *in vitro* potency in the manual hERG patch clamp assay. This level, or even higher, seems to be generally followed by the industry.

Unfortunately such a precise estimation of the minimum TI is not available for most other targets, and each target is different. However, hERG may be considered to represent the extreme, and acceptable TIs for other targets could be 10-fold or less. For some targets, the area under the curve (AUC) may be more appropriate to use for the TI calculation than the C_{max}. For some indications, the medical need may outweigh the side effect potential, in which case a lower TI than usual may be acceptable. Considering that many drugs reach free C_{max} values in the micromolar range, off-target affinities in the micromolar range can, and do, result in side effects. As an example, grepafloxacin (withdrawn from the market in 1999 due to 13 hERG-related fatalities) had a hERG IC_{50} around 30 μM and free C_{max} values of around 20 μM [50].

12.4.4
Possible Benefits of Off-Target Effects

While *in vitro* safety pharmacology profiling is primarily designed to identify potential liabilities, the off-target data can be used to identify additional beneficial properties of the drug. These could enhance the efficacy of the drug, complement the intended indication, or allow a better positioning of it against competitor compounds. Activities at other targets could provide repositioning of the drug for new indications. This concept is actively being pursued by many companies for existing drugs [51, 52]. A newer generation of more selective compounds will however be more difficult to reposition and will probably require extensive additional optimization.

12.5
Conclusions and Outlook

In vitro safety pharmacology profiling is a very useful tool in the drug discovery process and contributes to the selection of the best chemical scaffolds for lead optimization. Promiscuous scaffolds and compounds with a high risk of failing can be avoided and potential development compounds with a lower risk pharmacological profile can be identified. As illustrated by the THR comparison of failed development compounds and the best selling drugs, we believe that this tool will help to reduce late drug attrition due to safety reasons. However, we need to improve the predictive value of existing assays, expand the number of *in vitro* assays which predict for ADRs and increase the number of ADRs which can be predicted.

Over the past two or three years, the industry has moved towards more functional cell-based profiling assays to complement the receptor-binding assays and to go deeper into the characterization of the mechanism of action. The use of imaging technologies or technologies described as being more physiological (e.g., cellular dielectric spectroscopy (CDS) [53], assays using primary cells [54, 55], emerging technologies for *in vivo* pharmacological assessment [56, 57]) may be among the next steps to explore in order to continue to improve our ability to provide an early safety assessment with simple, robust, inexpensive and medium-throughput assays.

Most importantly, our knowledge and understanding of the links between drug–protein interactions and adverse drug reactions has to extend into the whole pharmacological space [33]. The number and diversity of targets currently used during *in vitro* safety pharmacology profiling is not very great, considering the huge number of proteins which could potentially interact with a drug. These are variously estimated at between 3000 and 5000, of which about 800 are known to interact with small molecules and only about 300 which are targeted by approved drugs [33, 58, 59]. There is a tremendous push within the pharmaceutical industry to find novel drug targets and drugs to treat diseases with unmet medical needs. At the same time, the potential for each new drug target to also mediate side effects should be examined. New tools being developed which could help to address this problem include chemogenomics [33, 60] (see also Chapter 13) and gene-expression signatures [61].

References

1 Kinter, L.B., Gossett, K.A. and Kerns, W.D. (1993) Status of safety pharmacology in the pharmaceutical industry, 1993. *Drug Development Research*, **32** (4), 208–216.

2 Kinter, L.D. and Dixon, L.W. (1995) Safety pharmacology program for pharmaceuticals. *Drug Development Research*, **35** (3), 179–182.

3 Sullivan, A.T. and Kinter, L.B. (1995) Status of safety pharmacology in the pharmaceutical industry-1995. *Drug Development Research*, **35** (3), 166–172.

4 Williams, P.D. (1990) The role of pharmacology profiling in safety assessment. *Regulatory Toxicology and Pharmacology*, **12** (3), 238–252.

5 U.S. Food and Drug Administration (2001) International conference on harmonisation, S7A Safety pharmacology studies for human pharmaceuticals.

U.S. Food and Drug Administration, Washington.

6 Whitebread, S., Hamon, J., Bojanic, D. and Urban, L. (2005) *In vitro* safety pharmacology profiling: an essential tool for successful drug development. *Drug Discovery Today*, **10** (21), 1421–1433.

7 Vaz, R.J. and Klabunde, T. (eds) (2008) *Antitargets*, Wiley-VCH, Weinheim.

8 Wakefield, I.D., Pollard, C., Redfern, W.S., Hammond, T.G. and Valentin, J.P. (2002) The application of *in vitro* methods to safety pharmacology. *Fundamental and Clinical Pharmacology*, **16**, 209–218.

9 Kinter, L.B. and Valentin, J.-P. (2002) Safety pharmacology and risk assessment. *Fundamental and Clinical Pharmacology*, **16**, 175–182.

10 Schuster, D., Laggner, C. and Langer, T. (2005) Why drugs fail – A study on side

effects in new chemical entities. *Current Pharmaceutical Design*, **11**, 3545–3559.

11 Jooste, E., Klafter, F., Hirshman, C.A. and Emala, C.W. (2003) A mechanism for rapacuronium-induced bronchospasm: M2 muscarinic receptor antagonism. *Anesthesiology*, **98** (4), 906–911.

12 Morris, B.J., Cochran, S.M. and Pratt, J.A. (2005) PCP: from pharmacology to modelling schizophrenia. *Current Opinion in Pharmacology*, **5** (1), 101–106.

13 Gentili, F., Pizzinat, N., Ordener, C., Marchal-Victorion, S., Maurel, A., Hofmann, R., Renard, P., Delagrange, P. et al. (2006) 3-[5-(4,5-dihydro-1H-imidazol-2-yl)-furan-2-yl]phenylamine (Amifuraline), a promising reversible and selective peripheral MAO-A inhibitor. *Journal of Medicinal Chemistry*, **49**, 5578–5586.

14 McKenzie, R., Fried, M.W., Sallie, R., Conjeevaram, H., Di Bisceglie, A.M., Park, Y., Savarese, B., Kleiner, D. et al. (1995) Hepatic failure and lactic acidosis due to fialuridine (FIAU), an investigational nucleoside analogue for chronic hepatitis B. *New England Journal of Medicine*, **333**, 1099–1105.

15 Lee, E.-W., Lai, Y., Zhang, H. and Unadkat, J.D. (2006) Identification of the mitochondrial targeting signal of the human equilibrative nucleoside transporter 1 (hENT1): Implications for interspecies differences in mitochondrial toxicity of fialuridine. *The Journal of Biological Chemistry*, **281** (24), 16700–16706.

16 Kola, I. and Landis, J. (2004) Can the pharmaceutical industry reduce attrition rates? *Nature Reviews. Drug Discovery*, **3**, 711–715.

17 Lasser, K.E., Allen, P.D., Woolhandler, S.J., Himmelstein, D.U., Wolfe, S.M. and Bor, D.H. (2002) Timing of new black box warnings and withdrawals for prescription medications. *JAMA – Journal of the American Medical Association*, **287** (17), 2215–2220.

18 Lazarou, J., Pomeranz, B.H. and Corey, P.N. (1998) Incidence of adverse drug reactions in hospitalized patients. *JAMA – Journal of the American Medical Association*, **279**, 1200–1205.

19 Hughes, B. (2008) FDA drug approvals: a year of flux. *Nature Reviews. Drug Discovery*, **7** (2), 107–109, http://dx.doi.org/10.1038/nrd2514.

20 Redfern, W.S., Wakefield, I.D., Prior, H., Pollard, C.E., Hammond, T.G. and Valentin, J.-P. (2002) Safety pharmacology – a progressive approach. *Fundamental and Clinical Pharmacology*, **16**, 161–173.

21 Smith, D.A. and Schmid, E.F. (2006) Drug withdrawals and the lessons within. *Current Opinion in Drug Discovery and Development*, **9** (1), 38–46.

22 Spence, S., Anderson, C., Cukierski, M. and Patrick, D. (1999) Teratogenic effects of the endothelin receptor antagonist L-753,037 in the rat. *Reproductive Toxicology*, **13** (12), 15–29.

23 Niederreither, K. and Dollé, P. (2008) Retinoic acid in development: Towards an integrated view. *Nature Reviews. Genetics*, **9**, 541–553.

24 Wishart, D.S., Knox, C., Guo, A.C., Cheng, D., Shrivastava, S., Tzur, D., Gautam, B. and Hassanali, M. (2008) DrugBank: a knowledgebase for drugs, drug actions and drug targets. *Nucleic Acids Research*, **36**, D901–D906.

25 United Nations (2005) Consolidated list of products whose consumption and/or sale have been banned, withdrawn, severely restricted or not approved by governments. 12th issue. UN Office for Economic and Social Council Support and Coordination, pp. 595.

26 Wise, A., Gearing, K. and Rees, S. (2002) Target validation of G-protein coupled receptors. *Drug Discovery Today*, **7** (4), 235–246.

27 Fox, S., Farr-Jones, S., Sopchak, L., Boggs, A., Nicely, H.W., Khoury, R. and Biros, M. (2006) High-throughput screening: update on practices and success. *Journal of Biomolecular Screening*, **11** (7), 864–869.

28 Krejsa, C.M., Horvath, D., Rogalski, S.L., Penzotti, J.E., Mao, B., Barbosa, F. and Migeon, J.C. (2003) Predicting ADME properties and side effects: The BioPrint approach. *Current Opinion in Drug Discovery and Development*, **6** (4), 470–480.

29 Roth, B.L., Baner, K., Westkaemper, R., Siebert, D., Rice, K.C., Steinberg, S., Ernsberger, P. and Rothman, R.B. (2002) Salvinorin A: A potent naturally occurring nonnitrogenous κ opioid selective agonist. *Proceedings of the National Academy of Sciences of the United States of America*, **99**, 11934–11939.

30 Elphick, G.F., Querbes, W., Jordan, J.A., Gee, G.V., Eash, S., Manley, K., Dugan, A., Stanifer, M. et al. (2004) The Human Polyomavirus, JCV Uses Serotonin Receptors to Infect Cells. *Science*, **306**, 380–1383.

31 Silvestre, J.S. and Prous, J. (2005) Research on adverse drug events I. Muscarinic M3 receptor binding affinity could predict the risk of antipsychotics to induce type 2 diabetes. *Methods and Findings in Experimental and Clinical Pharmacology*, **27** (5), 289–304.

32 Yildirim, M.A., Goh, K.-I., Cusick, M.E., Barabasi, A.-L. and Vidal, M. (2007) Drug—target network. *Nature Biotechnology*, **25**, 1119–1126.

33 Paolini, G.V., Shapland, R.H.B., Van Hoorn, W.P., Mason, J.S. and Hopkins, A.L. (2006) Global mapping of pharmacological space. *Nature Biotechnology*, **24**, 805–815.

34 DeVane, C.L. and Nemeroff, C.B. (2001) An evaluation of risperidone drug interactions. *Journal of Clinical Psychopharmacology*, **21**, 408–416.

35 Roth, B.L., Sheffler, D.J. and Kroeze, W.K. (2004) Magic shotguns versus magic bullets: selectively non-selective drugs for mood disorders and schizophrenia. *Nature Reviews. Drug Discovery*, **3**, 353–359.

36 Youdim, M.B.H. (2006) The path from anti Parkinson drug selegiline and rasagiline to multifunctional neuroprotective anti Alzheimer drugs ladostigil and M30. *Current Alzheimer Research*, **3**, 541–550.

37 Stephenson, V.C., Heydingb, R.A. and Weaver, D.F. (2005) The "promiscuous drug concept" with applications to Alzheimer's disease. *FEBS letters*, **579** (6), 1338–1342.

38 Hampton, T. (2004) "Promiscuous" anticancer drugs that hit multiple targets may thwart resistance. *The Journal of the American Medical Association*, **292** (4), 419–422.

39 Rochon, P.A., Normand, S.-L., Gomes, T., Gill, S.S., Anderson, G.M., Melo, M., Sykora, K., Lipscombe, L., et al. (2008) Antipsychotic therapy and short-term serious events in older adults with dementia. *Archives of Internal Medicine*, **168** (10), 1090–1096.

40 Whitebread, S., Hamon, J., Scheiber, J., Fekete, A., Azzaoui, K., Mikhailov, D., Lu, Q. and Urban, L. (2008) Broad-scale *in vitro* pharmacology profiling to predict clinical adverse effects. *American Drug Discovery*, **3** (2), 32–38.

41 Hopkins, A.L., Mason, J.S. and Overington, J.P. (2006) Can we rationally design promiscuous drugs? *Current Opinion in Structural Biology*, **16** (1), 127–136.

42 Aronov, A.M., McClain, B., Moody, C.S. and Murcko, M.A. (2008) Kinase-likeness and Kinase-Privileged Fragments: Toward Virtual Polypharmacology. *Journal of Medicinal Chemistry*, **51**, 1214–1222.

43 Whitlock, G.A., Fish, P.V., Fray, M.J., Stobie, A. and Wakenhut, F. (2008) Pyridyl-phenyl ether monoamine reuptake inhibitors: Impact of lipophilicity on dual SNRI pharmacology and off-target promiscuity. *Bioorganic and Medicinal Chemistry Letters*, **18**, 2896–2899.

44 Abe, C., Kikukawa, T. and Komatsu, Y. (1995) Combination therapy on murine arthritis - Salazosulfapyridine, bucillamine, and methotrexate. *International Journal of Immunotherapy*, **11**, 129–132.

45 Burcoglu-O'Ral, A., Erkan, D. and Asherson, R. (2002) Treatment of

catastrophic antiphospholipid syndrome with defibrotide, a proposed vascular endothelial cell modulator. *Journal of Rheumatology*, **29**, 2006–2011.

46 Hamon, J., Azzaoui, K., Whitebread, S., Urban, L., Jacoby, E. and Faller, B. (2006) In vitro safety pharmacology profiling. *European Pharmaceutical Review*, **2006** (1), 60–63.

47 Azzaoui, K., Hamon, J., Faller, B., Whitebread, S., Jacoby, E., Bender, A., Jenkins, J.L. and Urban, L. (2007) Modeling promiscuity based on *in vitro* safety pharmacology profiling data. *ChemMedChem*, **2**, 874–880.

48 Leeson, P.D. and Springthorpe, B. (2007) The influence of drug-like concepts on decision-making in medicinal chemistry. *Nature Reviews. Drug Discovery*, **6**, 881–890.

49 Wilke, R.A., Lin, W., Roden, D.M., Watkins, P.B., Flockhart, D., Zineh, I., Giacomini, K.M. and Krauss, R.M. (2007) Identifying genetic risk factors for serious adverse drug reactions: current progress and challenges. *Nature Reviews. Drug Discovery*, **6**, 904–916.

50 Redfern, W.S., Carlsson, L., Davis, A.S., Lynch, W.G., MacKenzie, I., Palethorpe, S., Siegl, P.K.S., Strang, I. et al. (2003) Relationships between preclinical cardiac electrophysiology, clinical QT interval prolongation and torsade de pointes for a broad range of drugs: evidence for a provisional safety margin in drug development. *Cardiovascular Research*, **58**, 32–45.

51 Ashburn, T.T. and Thor, K.B. (2004) Drug repositioning: identifying and developing new uses for existing drugs. *Nature Reviews. Drug Discovery*, **3**, 673–683.

52 O'Connor, K.A. and Roth, B.L. (2005) Finding new tricks for old drugs: An efficient route for public-sector drug discovery. *Nature Reviews. Drug Discovery*, **4**, 1005–1014.

53 Verdonk, E., Johnson, K., McGuinness, R., Leung, G., Chen, Y.W., Tang, H.R., Michelotti, J.M. and Liu, V.F. (2006) Cellular dielectric spectroscopy: A label-free comprehensive platform for functional evaluation of endogenous receptors. *Assay and Drug Development Technologies*, **4** (5), 609–619.

54 Meyer, T., Sartipy, P., Blind, F., Leisgen, C. and Guenther, E. (2007) New cell models and assays in cardiac safety profiling. *Expert Opinion on Drug Metabolism and Toxicology*, **3** (4), 507–517.

55 Pouton, C.W. and Haynes, J.M. (2007) Embryonic stem cells as a source of models for drug discovery. *Nature Reviews. Drug Discovery*, **6** (8), 605–616.

56 Houck, K.A. and Kavlock, R.J. (2008) Understanding mechanisms of toxicity: insights from drug discovery research. *Toxicology and Applied Pharmacology*, **227** (2), 163–178.

57 Barros, T.P., Alderton, W.K., Reynolds, H.M., Roach, A.G. and Berghmans, S. (2008) Zebrafish: an emerging technology for *in vivo* pharmacological assessment to identify potential safety liabilities in early drug discovery. *British Journal of Pharmacology*, **154**, 1400–1413.

58 Imming, P., Sinning, C. and Meyer, A. (2006) Drugs, their targets and the nature and number of drug targets. *Nature Reviews. Drug Discovery*, **5**, 821–834.

59 Overington, J.P., Al-Lazikani, B. and Hopkins, A.L. (2006) How many drug targets are there? *Nature Reviews. Drug Discovery*, **5**, 993–996.

60 Bender, A., Scheiber, J., Glick, M., Davies, J.W., Azzaoui, K., Hamon, J., Urban, L., Whitebread, S. and Jenkins, J.L. (2007) Analysis of pharmacology data and the prediction of adverse drug reactions and off-target effects from chemical structure. *ChemMedChem*, **2**, 861–873.

61 Lamb, J., Crawford, E.D., Peck, D., Modell, J.W., Blat, I.C., Wrobel, M.J., Lerner, J., Brunet, J.-P. et al. (2006) The Connectivity Map: Using Gene-Expression Signatures to connect small molecules, genes, and disease. *Science*, **313**, 1929–1935.

13
Knowledge-Based and Computational Approaches to *In Vitro* Safety Pharmacology

Josef Scheiber, Andreas Bender, Kamal Azzaoui, and Jeremy Jenkins

13.1
Introduction

Legitimate estimates suggest that developing a novel chemical entity (NCE) as a drug can cost up to U.S.$ 2 billion [1, 2]. Still, about 10% of NCEs show serious adverse drug reactions (ADR) after market launch [3]. The majority of these ADRs can be avoided if possible undesired off-target effects of the compound are understood very early during the drug discovery process, that is, before clinical trials are started.

This contribution focuses on computational methods that are used to assist and to guide *in vitro* preclinical safety pharmacology (PSP), a technology commonly applied in the pharmaceutical industry to evaluate compound selectivity profiles [4–8]. To develop compounds highly selective for a therapeutically relevant target and to avoid side effects or adverse drug reactions are key goals for every small-molecule drug discovery project. To achieve this, preclinical safety pharmacology approaches are commonly employed to screen compounds routinely in comparatively inexpensive, yet predictive assays to generate knowledge about possible polypharmacology. Thereby a comprehensive identification of possible liabilities can be achieved.

We outline the currently available environment and approaches that can be applied for thorough computational analyses of *in vitro* safety pharmacology data. After discussing desirable and necessary prerequisites for the data input from a computational perspective, we address how this data is used to predict a general promiscuity score for a single compound. This approach aims to answer the general question of whether a compound will hit many targets or will be selective. Finally, we demonstrate how to computationally reveal possible single-target liabilities. This has the objective of understanding why a certain compound is active against a defined undesired target on a molecular level.

The above approaches are collectively used to triage compounds prior to being screened in an *in vitro* safety pharmacology panel in order to prioritize compounds for testing and identify those which have the highest likelihood of being selective.

Hit and Lead Profiling. Edited by Bernard Faller and Laszlo Urban
Copyright © 2009 WILEY-VCH Verlag GmbH & Co. KGaA, Weinheim
ISBN: 978-3-527-32331-9

13.1.1
The Value of Safety Pharmacology Data: the Value and Relevance of Complete, Standardized Data Matrices for *In Silico* Prediction of Adverse Events

Screening hundreds of compounds against 80–100 targets/year is an expensive research endeavor; However, it is one of the crucial parts of preclinical safety assessment and is also required by regulatory authorities [9]. Beside a better understanding of compound bioactivity profiles, which in some cases can be reliably linked to clinically observed side effects, there is also a particular aspect of the generated data which makes it worthwhile to be analyzed in more detail.

In an ideal case, one can make a comprehensive assessment of *all* chemicals that have been profiled against *all* targets that have been used in safety assays assuming the assays stay constant, which is not always the case in practice. This generates what computational modelers call a "complete data matrix", with each combination of ligand and target being assigned an activity data point. While this observation seems trivial to an experimentalist, it is of tremendous value to the computational modeler who attempts to find unbiased patterns in the preclinical profiling data.

So why precisely should this aspect of bioactivity data be important? If 1000 ligands are tested exhaustively against 100 targets, or 2000 ligands are tested sporadically against 50% of available targets, why is the former preferred over the latter?

The value of "complete bioactivity data matrices" can be illustrated by compounds involved in the blockage of the hERG ion channel in the heart. The hERG channel is linked to QT prolongation and as a rare consequence, torsades de pointes (TdP), followed in some cases by cardiac arrest and death [10, 11]. The public bioactivity repository PubChem [12] recently released a hERG activity dataset (assay identifier 376). Figure 13.1a is a sample from this database. A group of compounds correspond to the well established hERG pharmacophore [13] which contains a basic nitrogen and one of a maximum of three lipophilic, aromatic moieties which are involved in pi-stacking inside the channel [13–17].

One could, at a first pass, consider the prediction of hERG channel blockers a solved problem, based on this information. Indeed, early predictive models for hERG blocking did precisely establish the above pharmacophore, on the basis of smaller datasets than the PubChem dataset, and found the model to be predictive. However, a closer look into the PubChem database also reveals unexpected compounds (Figure 13.1b) as active hERG blockers – how do these compounds fit into the model? The chemical structures exhibit different features from the traditional hERG pharmacophore; namely a negative charge conferred *via* a carboxylic acid moiety, decorated either by a benzoquinone/naphthalene system (CID 222 760), a large aromatic ring system consisting of four fused rings (CID 82 011) or a substituted benzene as well as a cyclohexane ring (CID 22 792). These features are not explainable by the "conventional" hERG hypothesis, and accordingly, these molecules would never have been predicted to be blockers. (We do not rule out the possibility of false positives, but the observation that very different chemical classes of compounds can be active against a given biochemical target holds true as a general rule.)

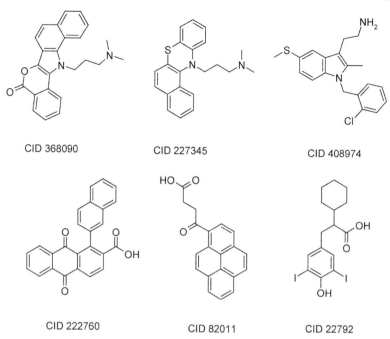

Figure 13.1 hERG compound data obtained from PubChem BioAssay AID 376. Upper line: "Conventional" hERG blockers. Lower line: "Atypical" hERG blockers which do not contain the conventional pharmacophore of a basic nitrogen, decorated by a set of lipophilic rings. (also see Chapter 16).

So what does this example illustrate when it comes to the exploitation of bioactivity data for *in silico* off-target prediction? The most crucial aspect is that a given area of chemical space can only be associated with bioactivity against a given target when chemically related compounds are experimentally found to be active. Even more fundamentally, compounds from a specific area of the chemical universe must be included in the assay run against that target. Bioactivity data points are often abstracted from literature or patent sources (see Table 13.2), thus, in practice they often contain different underlying chemistry in the assays that are compared. Since estimates of the size of chemical space of drug-like molecules are in the area of 10^{63} different entities [18], no experimental set of chemical ligands will ever explore this space exhaustively, and if different compound samples are used in each data source, a bias is introduced in each dataset. Still, it is possible that structures that are chemically very different can be similar in bioactivity in terms of their pharmacophores. However, conventional cheminformatics approaches can only incorporate knowledge that has already been generated and an expansion into a totally different chemistry from what is known is not readily predictable.

For the following scenario we assume that the same chemical descriptors are always used to describe the molecules under scrutiny – the case in every cheminformatics-based analysis. The situation of different areas of "chemical space" being associated with different biological datasets is illustrated in Figure 13.2. Let us take the hERG channel and histamine receptors as biological targets (arbitrarily chosen, but from the ligand-side related), and test random compounds in both assays. First it is evident that the areas of chemical space tested in each assay is much smaller than the total chemical space bioactive against that target – which matches the real situation that chemical space is difficult to sample, due to its sheer size. Again, if chemically different compounds are active against a target, computational approaches most often cannot describe this in perfect detail. But what is also apparent is that the areas of chemical space sampled for every activity class are different from each other – meaning, very different structural classes of compounds with very different substituents are being tested against both targets. Not surprisingly, the compounds found to be active against each target differ from one another, symbolized by the area of overlap between the two black circles and between the two gray circles. Although the total bioactive chemical space shared by both receptors is significant, this is not reflected in the models at all – since the sets of chemicals tested were so different to begin with.

However, when identical sets of compounds are tested against both (or all) targets of interest, this (while still not entirely addressing the problem of undersampling the huge chemical space) partly removes the *target-specific bias* of each individual activity set related to a particular receptor, as shown in Figure 13.3.

In this case, identical areas of chemical space are assayed against the whole target set and no additional "artificial" dataset bias is introduced into the final models. However, this still does not address the question of whether the bioactivity models employed to predict targets (or off-targets) is able to predict the bioactivity spectrum of a particular compound; this depends on whether the new compound is closer to the area covered by experiment, or further away from it.

While the coverage of similar chemical space in every assay is crucial for *in silico* analyses of bioactivity data, another factor that often hampers large-scale data analysis efforts is the consistency with which the data are generated – meaning, assay parameters can have a huge influence on the particular activity measured. Luckily, equivalent coverage of chemical space measured against every target in practice often (but not always) coincides with the presence of also comparable assay conditions: when a pharmaceutical company measures compound activity against a large set of GPCRs, then it is easier to keep assay conditions comparable than when abstracting bioactivity information from literature results measured in a multitude of different laboratories.

Apart from internal data generated from safety profiling in large pharmaceutical companies, very few service providers have generated activity matrices using the same ligands under consistent assay conditions. The largest example is the commercially available BioPrint database [19] generated by Cerep. In the year 2003 (when a comprehensive publication appeared on this dataset), the bioactivity matrix contained 1198 drugs marketed in the United States and other countries, 74 withdrawn drugs and compounds for which development has been halted, 50 prodrugs and metabolites, 47 herbal or nutritional actives, 36 veterinary drugs, 25 compounds in

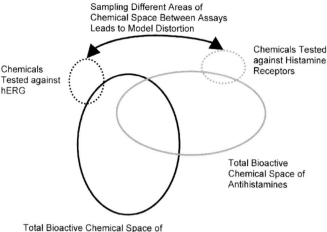

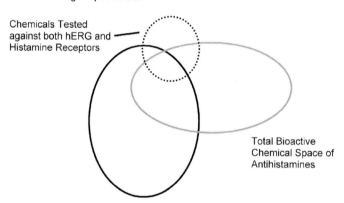

Figure 13.2 (a) Measuring substances for activity against two receptors (here the hERG channel and the histamine receptors) will give very different sets of active molecules, if the compounds tested against each receptor are very different in terms of chemical similarity. This is true even if a large area of bioactive chemical space is shared between activity classes – leading to models which are more likely to predict a given target over another, due to chemical bias in the underlying training set. (b) Investigating an identical area of chemical space for bioactivity against all interesting targets still under-samples chemical space considerably, but it diminishes target/dataset specific bias to a significant extent that would be introduced in the first case; thus it is preferred for modelling.

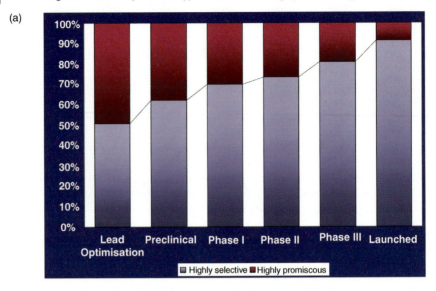

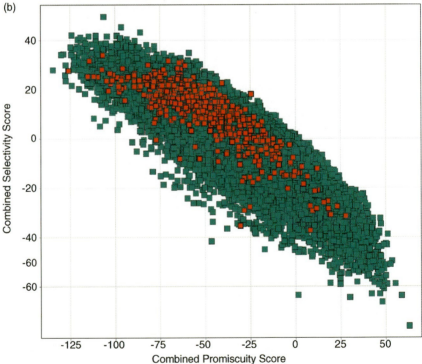

Figure 13.3 (a) Plot of selectivity score versus promiscuity score applied to MDDR. Red dots are marketed drugs. Marketed drugs clearly cluster when compared to other compounds in different drug discovery phases (green dots). (b) The predicted selectivity of compounds in different phases of the drug discovery process. This data is attributed to the dataset presented in the text.

development and 795 reference compounds selected for chemical diversity or biological activity [19], amounting to a total of 2225 compounds in the dataset. Each of those compounds were measured in 81 binding assays (out of which 54 were GPCRs), 39 enzyme assays, none ADME assays (for metabolic stability, permeability/efflux and chemical properties such as logD) and seven safety assays (e.g. cell viability assays). This dataset amounted to a total of more than 300 000 individual data points, which corresponds to the approximate size of preclinical safety pharmacology datasets available in a large pharmaceutical company.

There are two fundamentally distinct ways in which these bioactivity data matrices can be used. On the one hand, they can serve as the basis for "*in silico* safety profiling", namely the prediction of activities of novel compounds to individual targets by using the computational power provided by the large dataset. This approach is feasible where strong links between particular targets and undesired side effects are established or when many compounds have been screened in a repeated manner against the target. The hERG K^+ channel [11, 20–22], the 5-HT$_{2B}$ receptor [23] or the PXR nuclear hormone receptor [24] are typical examples which fall into this category. The goal of this type of analysis is to computationally predict the activity of compounds against the set of profiling panel targets; and for many compounds and depending on the modeling procedure used, a high confidence of activity against some targets can be achieved [25–27]. Ideally, and after extensive model validation, these "high-confidence" *in silico* predictions of compound activity or inactivity are useful for compound ranging and triaging and even would substitute for experimental testing, at least in the early stages of compound profiling. On the other hand, borderline actives (where the model is unable to provide predictions with a certain confidence) would be subject to experimental testing. Overall, activities for a given compound can thus be partly predicted (in the confident cases) and partly be measured experimentally (where the model is not able to make predictions with a given confidence), focusing efforts in safety profiling to understand key issues. These approaches are described in more details in the third part of this chapter.

A second computational use of preclinical profiling data is to predict *the number* of targets a compound is likely to be active against, which is also called the "promiscuity" of a compound. Promiscuous ligands are by their very nature more likely to show undesired and often ill-defined side effects. Ligand promiscuity should be distinguished from the phenomenon of promiscuous aggregation leading to "frequent hitters" due to the formation of micelles [28], which has also been the subject of *in silico* studies [20, 28]. The question of whether promiscuity is necessarily a disadvantage depends on its components and their relationship to the therapeutic indication because drugs hitting multiple desired targets (polypharmacology) also possess advantages for certain indications [29, 30]. However, the current consensus is that selective compounds, when all other things are equal, should be preferred over more promiscuous ones. The possibility of *in silico* promiscuity analysis crucially depends on the availability of a full bioactivity data matrix: Since training sets will be constructed for promiscuous compounds on the one hand (those which are active against a large fraction of the profiling targets, e.g., 10% or more of the complete set) and for selective compounds on the other hand (e.g., compounds which are active on

5% or less of all safety targets), datasets would be biased if compounds are only measured against a small number of targets. Such compounds would be assumed to be selective compounds, not due to experimental data, but due to the fact that "not measured" data points are usually assumed to be "inactive". Therefore, promiscuity prediction crucially depends on datasets where all compounds are measured against a large number of all targets.

In the remainder of this chapter, we discuss both approaches, for target and off-target prediction of compounds, as well as for the prediction of promiscuity, based in both cases on pharmaceutical safety profiling data.

13.2
"Meta Analysis" of Safety Pharmacology Data: Predicting Compound Promiscuity

13.2.1
Introduction

Promiscuous compounds carry various ADR liabilities and can severely restrict the use of the drug or prevent its entry into the clinic. Therefore, there is a clear interest to evaluate compound promiscuity or selectivity at the earliest possible phase of drug discovery – although there are exceptions when the design of compounds with multiple activities in a given pathway or cellular circuitry may be desirable. These include some well known examples in depression, schizophrenia [31], Alzheimer's disease [32], but also in oncology [33], showing that a weaker selectivity is key to the efficacy of a significant number of approved drugs. However, promiscuity in these cases is often limited to a particular subclass of targets (e.g., kinases). New paradigms to selectively modulate several molecular targets are also emerging, despite this multi-target approach being a challenge for medicinal chemists [34–36].

As mentioned earlier, a broad panel of *in vitro* safety pharmacology profiling assays have been implemented at Novartis to screen compounds for potential unwanted effects well before entering clinical trials [4, 5]. This *in vitro* safety pharmacology profile is essentially composed of noncellular binding assays, targeting a diverse set of receptors (GPCRs highly represented), nuclear receptors, transporters, enzymes and binding sites on ions channels with well documented associations to clinical ADRs [4, 5, 37, 38]. The central premise is that increasing selectivity for the desired primary target correlates with decreasing ADR frequencies arising from binding to off-targets or secondary targets identified in the safety profiling panel. Full IC_{50} determinations are systematically carried out and a large set of profiling data is now available. Previously, using a large set of safety pharmacology profiling data, we showed that the percentage of compounds which display promiscuous properties during the lead optimization stage is significant and in the range of 20–30% (according to the cut-off used) [4]. We also built models to predict promiscuity and selectivity for compounds using such matrix data. By mining the profiling data, we were able to define some general rules and structure activity relationships to distinguish between promiscuous and selective compounds. Consequently, we developed a simple scoring model based on a Naïve Bayesian (NB) classification for promiscuity and selectivity [39]. To improve the predictive power of the models, we further expanded the dataset to 5767 compounds tested on up to 79 targets – all selected for their known link with potential safety issues. For comparison, see recent articles that describe *in silico* approaches to discuss promiscuity and its linkage to side effects (using mainly the Cerep BioPrint dataset) [20, 40–42]. In our work, we compared the chemical properties of the compounds showing promiscuous properties to the selective compounds in this panel of assays in order to train a NB model [26, 27, 43, 44] that could predict compound promiscuity or selectivity. The following part of this chapter describes the set up and validation of the Bayesian model and its potential use in drug discovery.

13.2.2
Data Analysis

13.2.2.1 Hit Rate Parameter and Chemical Profiling

A set of 5767 compounds tested in at least 30 assays out of 79 was used. The full panel of targets can be found in previously published work [4]. The target hit-rate parameter (THR) was defined in order to assign each compound a measure for its selectivity or promiscuity across the whole assay panel. THR is defined as the ratio of the number of targets hit (i.e., >50% inhibition) by a compound to the number of targets tested at a given concentration. Both training and test set compounds are flagged according to their target hit-rate at $10\,\mu M$ (THR_{10}). Compounds with THR_{10} greater or equal to 20% were flagged as promiscuous (P); 1096 (19%) P compounds were found. Compounds with THR_{10} lower or equal to 5% were flagged as selective hits (S); 2910 (50%) S compounds were identified. Other compounds, having THR_{10} of 5–20%, were flagged as moderately promiscuous (MP); 1761 (31%) MP compounds were identified.

A considerable number of promiscuous compounds were found, although the vast majority of these compounds were submitted for profiling at the lead optimization stage. Some 21% showed activity lower than $5\,\mu M$ on at least eight different targets. However, this number is biased because projects that encounter pharmacological promiscuity submit more compounds than others. The origin of compounds and their promiscuity profile is reported in Table 13.1. Compounds originating from the neuroscience (NS) and respiratory disease areas (RDA) were less promiscuous. This is interesting as their target portfolio contains a significant number of GPCRs One explanation for this finding may be that their criteria to submit compounds to the safety panel are more stringent (compounds with a molecular weight (MW) <500 and low polar surface area). In fact, compounds from NS and RDA also have the lowest molecular weight average compared to compounds originated from other disease areas (Table 13.1). Another explanation could be that a crucial hit-to-lead criteria for NS compounds is GPCR selectivity. For other disease areas except oncology, the number of compounds submitted to the panel is lower and consequently the high number of promiscuous compounds could be explained by specific compounds encountering promiscuity problems during lead optimization.

Table 13.1 *Top section:* The mean value of molecular weight, calculated LogP and target hit rate for compounds originating from different disease areas. *Middle section:* Sensitivity and specificity of promiscuous models applied to the test set. Model FP uses fingerprint based descriptors. Model PC uses physicochemical based descriptors. *Bottom section:* Sensitivity and specificity of promiscuous models applied to the drugs set. Model FP uses fingerprint based descriptors. Model PC uses physicochemical based descriptors.

Disease area	Molecular weight mean	cLog P mean	THR mean
Bone and metabolism	492.8	3.68	21.3
Autoimmunity and transplantation	466.4	3.95	16.5
Cardiovascular	454.2	3.35	14.9
Oncology	461.9	3.46	12.1
Respiratory diseases	450.1	3.13	9.9
Nervous system	417.1	3.48	9.1
Others	458.5	3.47	8.1

Models	Bayesian score threshold	Sensitivity TH	Specificity	% of unclassified compounds
Model FP	0	0.97	0.89	41.6
Model FP	−10	0.94	0.86	27.5
Model PC	0	0.82	0.60	44.9
Model PC	−1	0.73	0.63	25.4
Combined score from model FP and PC	0	0.97	0.88	43.5
Combined score from model FP and PC	−10	0.93	0.85	28.9

Models	Bayesian score threshold	Sensitivity	Specificity	% of unclassified compounds
Model 1(FP)	0	0.97	0.89	40.1
Model 1(FP)	−10	0.84	0.87	21.2
Model 2 (PC)	0	0.34	0.88	35.8
Model 2 (PC)	−1	0.26	0.89	21.2
Combined score from model FP and PC	0	0.65	0.99	39.7
Combined score from model FP and PC	−10	0.40	0.99	23.8

To check the chemical diversity of the dataset, compounds were clustered in 843 singletons and 1836 chemical classes containing at least two molecules. The biggest cluster had 72 members. The singleton set contains only 10% of promiscuous compounds. Classes with more than 20 compounds contain a higher number of promiscuous compounds. In fact, classes with 20–30 members have 25% promiscuous members and classes with >30 members have 40% promiscuous members.

The explanation of this trend is that more compounds are submitted to the safety panel during the lead optimization when a series of compounds turns out to have off-target activities at safety targets.

As previously reported [39], the chemical profiles of all promiscuous compounds were compared to the selective compounds by using classic 2D molecular descriptors. Both calculated log P (AlogP) and MW were significantly higher for promiscuous compounds compared to selective compounds. The number of nitrogen atoms was also higher for promiscuous compounds, while the number of oxygen atoms was lower than for nonpromiscuous compounds. In contrast, the number of H-bond donor or acceptor atoms was not significantly different between the two groups of compounds.

To further investigate the influence of O and N atoms, functional groups were counted for each set of compounds. This analysis revealed that indole substructures are overrepresented in promiscuous compounds [45, 46]. Likewise, furan and piperazine rings are also more present in promiscuous compounds. Since the profiling panel contains a large number of GPCR targets, previously published findings suggested privileged substructures could be found in promiscuous compounds [30, 47, 48]. Others substructures were checked, but were not found to be represented higher in one group over the other. Carboxylic acids show a high selectivity probably due to the negative charge, which can lead to unfavorable interaction with many targets. For example, the benefits of carboxylic acids for avoiding hERG channel binding was recently shown as a magic SAR switch [49] (other acidic groups such as tetrazole or sulfonamide do not show such a large difference). In the new dataset, the 585 compounds with a carboxylic acid contain respectively 79% of selective, 19% of moderately promiscuous and only 2% of promiscuous compounds.

13.2.2.2 Computational Efforts: Generation of Hypotheses

One way to develop an *in silico* tool to predictive promiscuity is to apply a NB classifier for modeling, a technique that compares the frequencies of features between selective and promiscuous sets of compounds. Bayesian classification was applied in many studies and was recently compared to other machine-learning techniques [26, 27, 43, 51, 52].

In order to classify promiscuous and selective compounds, we used the NB modeling protocol available in Pipeline Pilot (Scitegic) [53]. The data was split randomly into 5193 compounds for modeling and 574 compounds for testing the models. In addition to the test set, 302 known drugs were also profiled and kept separate for testing the models. All sets were checked visually to ensure that no chemical classes were overrepresented in one set or the other.

The specificity and sensitivity of each model is reported in the middle and bottom of Table 13.1. In general, the models trained on only Scitegic fingerprints (Model FP) perform better than the other models. The combined score from Model FP and Model PC improve the prediction on the drug set which contains molecules chemically different that the test set and the training set. A relatively high enrichment was observed for both models although the selectivity model appears more accurate than the promiscuity model.

From the training set, four NB classifiers were built using Pipeline Pilot Software: two models for promiscuous and two models for selective compounds. The molecular descriptors used for the first two models (Models FP) were a combination of chemical fingerprints such as extended-connectivity fingerprints (ECFP_4) and functional-connectivity fingerprints (FCFP_4) [54–56]. The combination of both fingerprints gives the best sensitivity (SE) and specificity (SP; see definitions below). For the models (Models PC), we used mainly physicochemical descriptors, such as calculated log P, MW, number of H-bond donor/acceptor atoms and number of rotatable bonds. We also used the following descriptors that have a large difference on average between promiscuous and selective compounds: number of ring systems, number of nitrogen atoms, presence of carboxylic acids, presence of indole rings and number of terminal rotamers. In addition, we combined scores from models. The combined score is defined by the equation:

$$\text{Combined score} = (\text{score from Model PC}*10) + \text{score from Model FP}$$

To validate the classification models, the sensitivity SE and specificity SP of an individual model were evaluated by the equations:

$$SE_i = TP_i/(TP_i + FN_i)$$
$$SP_i = TN_i/(TN_i + FP_i)$$

where TP_i, TN_i, FP_i and FN_i represent, respectively, the number of true positives, true negatives, false positives and false negatives. TP_i, TN_i, FP_i and FN_i are the four different possible outcomes of a single prediction for a two-class case with classes "1" ("yes") and "0" ("no"). A false positive is when the outcome is incorrectly classified as "yes" (or "positive") when it is in fact "no" (or "negative"). A false negative is when the outcome is incorrectly classified as negative when it is in fact positive. True positives and true negatives are obviously correct classifications.

13.2.2.3 Promiscuity and Attrition Rate

The high attrition rate of new chemical entities (NCEs) in preclinical and clinical phases can be attributed to many factors. According to Kola and Landis [50], NCEs fail mainly to insufficient efficacy, bioavailability, safety, toxicological and economic reasons. All these factors are somehow interrelated – a less soluble drug might be less bioactive and thus less efficient. Additionally, the attrition rate can depend on the therapeutic area the drug comes from. For example, compounds tend to fail more for CNS and oncology indications than in other therapeutic areas [50].

Interestingly, but not surprisingly, attrition also correlates to the phase of the drug discovery process (i.e., discovery phase, clinical phase, marketed phase). To further investigate this further, we applied the models to compounds in different drug discovery phases from the MDL drug data report database (MDDR) [51]. The plot of selectivity score versus promiscuity score is reported in Figure 13.4. Marketed drugs were highlighted in the plot and clearly form a cluster when compared to other compounds in different drug discovery phases. For further study, we selected compounds in each phases and scored them. The top predicted promiscuous and selective for each phase are reported in Figure 13.4.

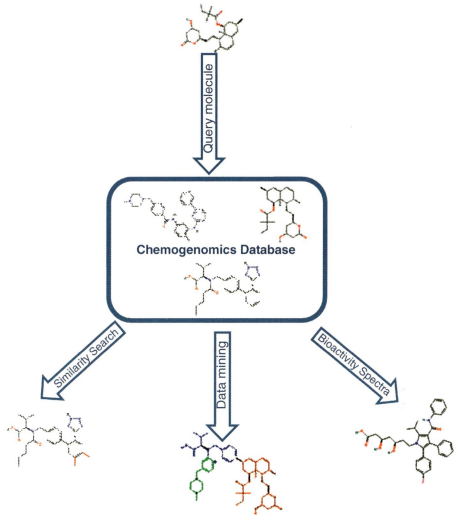

Figure 13.4 The outcome of the different target prediction methodologies: The targets associated to molecules exhibiting the degree of similarity shown in this figure are predicted for an input compound. Similarity searching finds targets that are hit by very similar molecules that share a common scaffold; data mining combines substructures from different molecules and thereby can come up with totally novel scaffolds that share substructures with the start database; Biospectra use existing biological profiles.

The combined score from the fingerprint and physicochemical models was the best to confirm a logical trend from lead optimization to launched drugs. Indeed, as shown in Figure 13.4, the best scored compounds were checked for the phase in which they belonged and the average scores suggested that, as a trend, compounds predicted as promiscuous are found more often in the lead optimization phase than in the launched phase. However, more compounds predicted as selective are in the launched phase than in the lead optimization phase.

13.2.2.4 Conclusion on Promiscuity Prediction

Compound activity against multiple biological targets is a property often observed at the lead selection phase of a drug discovery program. The introduction of high throughput screening of targets with compound libraries on the scale of millions will inevitably identify a significant number of promiscuous compounds. Selection of scaffolds at the early phase of drug discovery is now based on broad-scale profiling for drug-like characteristics, including minimal occurrence of ADRs. This can be done by introducing the *in vitro* safety pharmacology profile, as reported before by several groups [4, 5, 31].

By mining the more profiling data, we were able to improve the prediction of previously published models for promiscuous and selective compounds.

What is particularly interesting is that, when applied to a large database of compounds at different phases of the drug discovery process, the model shows a higher score (lower promiscuity) for marketed drugs than for compounds in early development or compounds which failed during clinical development. Although failure of drugs can arise from different factors, we found a clear correlation between promiscuity and attrition rate. This result demonstrates the usefulness of this predictive model of promiscuity and the importance of having a "clean profile" in the *in vitro* safety pharmacology panel (see also Chapter 12). Such a model can be used for virtual screening and lead optimization.

Going a step further, one can also try to predict single-target liabilities of compounds in Drug Discovery. These approaches are dealt with in the next section.

13.3
Prediction of Off-target Effects of Molecules Based on Chemical Structure

13.3.1
Introduction

Large-scale *in vitro* safety pharmacology profiling efforts (see Chapter 12) in combination with clinical databases laid the ground for the development of predictive *in silico* tools for clinical ADRs. These tools operate on chemical structure by leveraging information from increasingly available biologically annotated chemical databases. This part of the chapter provides an overview of recent studies in which ligand-based data-mining and similarity of chemical structures is used to elucidate target class or mechanism of action. These approaches reverse the paradigm of finding compounds for single targets, to finding targets for compounds by leveraging large-scale chemogenomics databases. For more detailed information see a recent review by Jenkins *et al.* [25].

The described applications rely heavily on the available information sources, which usually means small-molecule databases annotated with bioactivity data. Due to the lack of available GPCR crystal structures and the fact that safety pharmacology has currently a clear focus on GPCR targets (see the second part of this chapter), we focus only on ligand-based approaches for target prediction and leave out those methods that require a solved protein structure as an input for the analysis. For a seminal paper in this area the reader is referred to Xie et al. [57].

It is an exciting scientific challenge to develop predictive methods that capture off-target-related adverse drug reactions reliably with a comparatively small number of compounds and at a reduced number of targets to be screened. The perfect scenario of a full data matrix as a starting point was outlined in the first part of this chapter.

In general terms, there are compounds with two major preclinical profiles emerging from published studies: (i) compounds or structural classes which show high promiscuity and bind with various affinities to a large number of unrelated targets and (ii) compounds or structural classes which have high affinity to a specific class of targets or even only a single target. Approaches to find members of the first class are described in the second part of this contribution.

First, we deal with possible data sources and the requirements to enable target prediction exercises and then describe approaches that have been developed in recent years. The data sources go beyond the scope of safety profiling as literature knowledge about any targets with known ligands can also be used.

13.3.2
Available Databases and Desired Format

Minimum requirements for chemogenomics databases amenable to target fishing include high-quality machine-readable chemical structures that have been checked for chemical integrity. The targets or bioactivities reported for the compounds need to be consistent (i.e., using well established controlled vocabulary) and free of spelling or typing errors. Also, the target nomenclature has to follow agreed bioinformatics standards (e.g., Entrez Gene ID, Uniprot-Swissprot, Accession Number, NCBI RefSeq number) to enable more in-depth analysis and comparison of predictions. For target prediction protocols, well annotated data of compound–target pairings derived from secondary assays with activity values (e.g., IC_{50}, EC_{50}, K_d) calculated from multiple concentration points are most useful. Single data points from high-throughput screening are less desirable, although such data has been successfully used [58, 59]. Ideally, the database would have additional layers of annotation describing target family ontology (to truly be a chemogenomics database), normalized activity values, inactive as well as active compounds and data source (journal or patent citation). Each record of a compound–target pairing in fact describes a molecular event; thus the assay conditions and the type of cell, tissue or organism used are all influential on the activity measurement and should be included with the record. As mentioned above, assay results are only totally comparable when they are generated under the same conditions.

The following section outlines the more detailed requirements of databases used in target prediction for safety pharmacology. Also, Table 13.2 provides an overview of currently available databases and how far they reach the desired standard.

Table 13.2 An overview of databases amenable for target prediction.

Database	Description	Size	Target coverage	Standardization
Target and MedChem databases (GVK)	Large diverse collection of chemical series from medchem literature and patents	>2 Mio compounds	1.5 K from journals and patents	Most of the target names are standardized
AurSCOPE (Aureus)	Collection of target-focused knowledge-bases	500 K	Selected medicinal chemistry journals	Yes
stARLITe (BioFocus DPI)	Large diverse collection of chemical series from medchem literature	300 K	Selected medicinal chemistry journals	Yes, mostly RefSeq or ACCESSION
ChemBioBase Suite (Jubilant Biosys)	Target-centric ligand databases	1.4 Mio	Journals and patents	Yes
Bioprint (Cerep)	Drug-focused pharmacology/ADME profiling database, full matrix	2400	Experimentally determined data, full data matrix	Yes
WOMBAT (Sunset Molecular)	Large diverse collection of chemical series from medchem literature	178 K	Relevant medchem journals	Yes
PubChem BioAssay	Large diverse collection of compounds from various sources		Screening centers, vendors	Mostly yes, some gaps

The number of records in total, as well as the number of unique compounds and targets, is highly relevant. Both the diversity of target classes and the big target families need to be taken into account. This breadth and depth comes specifically from the scope and number of scientific journals and patents that are covered within the database. For these sources, the age of the annotation needs to be taken into account. It is also very important that especially human targets are covered.

Next, the process of generating the database needs to be evaluated. Pertinent questions are: is it generated with computational mining methods or by manual curation? If well done, the latter is preferable. How easy is it to merge external data into internal safety pharmacology data to get a broader picture of available chemogenomics space? Also, it is crucial to determine how amenable the data is for model building and should encompass the following factors:

1. Number of compounds with activity values per target;
2. Dynamic range of biological data per target;
3. Information provided showing that molecule is inactive;
4. Type and compatibility of biological data (IC_{50}, EC_{50}, K_i).

Next, the annotation depth of every entry has to be considered:

1. How are multiple activities provided for a compound or target?
2. Are activity values normalized to a standard unit? For example, how are percent inhibition values presented versus IC_{50} values?
3. Is update frequency and quality good enough that the database can be used in competitive intelligence assessment?
4. Is derivative work allowed, global access, price/molecules, price/target?
5. Has anyone claimed any IP on the database itself or attached licensing strings to data usage?

Once all these points have been considered and a decision has been made for the input database, different approaches can be used to actually predict possible targets for compounds undergoing a safety evaluation.

13.3.3
The Best Established Technologies for *In Silico* Target Fishing

The following summarizes three related computational approaches that enable the prediction of target or mechanism of action (MOA) from chemical structure: chemical similarity searching, data mining/machine learning and bioactivity spectra. Each of these technologies was developed to find new compounds for known targets but can also be used the other way round.

13.3.3.1 Similarity Searching in Databases

Chemical similarity searching for target prediction compares an orphan compound structure to a database of compounds with known targets. Any chemical descriptor or similarity metric can be used and more importantly similarity searching does not require a well curated database of normalized target names, although this would still be extremely helpful. Consequently, any database can be queried: the orphan compound is input and the similarity matches point to potential target classes. Similarity and substructure searching have been used for many years for target prediction to assess patent coverage around chemotypes – albeit unsystematically – with tools such as SciFinder. In more recent years, web-based search engines became available for finding chemically similar bioactive structures.

Although the searches themselves may take seconds to run, the amount of follow-up reading needed to align potential targets with compound phenotype can be time-intensive (imagine using SciFinder to predict targets for 10 000 hits from a cell-based screen). Further, how does one go about ranking the targets? Should only the target associated with the most similar compound be considered or also less similar compounds? Is target enrichment among similar compounds most important, given that some target classes are more represented than others? All these questions need to be addressed to establish a reliable target identification metric. Further, the technical disadvantage of similarity searching are clear: that prior knowledge of target class information is typically not incorporated in a way that focuses or improves the search. However, there are recent notable exceptions where search performance is improved by weighting molecular fingerprints with target class knowledge [60–63]. Similarity searching for target fishing can also be performed with 3D chemical descriptors. For example, Cleves and Jain demonstrated the predictive ability of 3D morphological descriptors [64]. While 2D descriptors are powerful for similarity searching in annotated databases, 3D descriptors may be more appropriate when the orphan compound has low 2D similarity to all database molecules [65]. In addition to chemical similarity searching for target fishing, target ontologies may be exploited to find new targets for compounds. In this case, compounds are not orphans, but rather a target is known; the goal then is to link new related targets to a compound on the basis of sequence similarity to the known target. For example, Schuffenhauer *et al.* demonstrated the relationship between similar compounds and similar targets in similarity searching [66] and Sheinerman *et al.* explored the relationship between kinase sequences and kinase inhibitor selectivity [67].

13.3.3.2 Data Mining in Annotated Chemical Databases

Given a large, diverse chemogenomics database as the starting point, data mining is the ideal approach for target prediction. Associations between target names and chemical substructures can be extracted automatically across target class sets with machine learning. Chemical features correlated with specific target binding are then stored as multiple-target models. Target prediction is therefore compound classification on a very large scale, involving thousands of individual target class models. By comparing orphan compound features with correlated features in each target class, target prediction can be achieved at very high speed. Models built from machine learning – in contrast to similarity searching – retain only the bits relevant for activity and ignore bits common to both actives and inactives. Table 13.2 provides a comparison of large, diverse databases on which target class model building is possible.

In the mid-1990s, V. Poroikov, D. Filimonov and others pioneered the *in silico* prediction of activity spectra for substances (PASS) by training models on the chemical features of activity classes [68, 69]. Recent successes were reported using the PASS technology to guide the design of novel cognition enhancers [70]. Niwa [71] later explored the use of probabilistic neural networks in combination with atom-type descriptors to predict targets for compounds. Bayesian modeling on chemogenomics database targets were carried out by Nidhi *et al.* [26] using extended connectivity fingerprints [72]. On a grander scale, several commercial and in-house databases containing 4.8 million compounds and 2876 targets were combined to create a global pharmacology map that was also explored by multiple-category Bayesian modeling [27]. One advantage of creating models on chemical fingerprints is the interpretability: substructures correlated with target binding can be backprojected onto orphan compound structure. In a recent review, Jenkins *et al.* describe the power of mining chemogenomics databases to link chemistry and biology [25].

13.3.3.3 Data Mining on Bioactivity Spectra

The activities of a compound across screening panels such as a preclinical profiling panel or other protein panels, cell line panels, HTS screening panels, or DNA microarrays can also be a type of signature, termed the "biological activity spectra", "bioactivity spectra" or just "biospectra". The biospectra of a compound is related to chemical structure [73] and therefore can be used predictively in either direction – predicting activities for compounds or predicting compounds for activities. The behavior of compounds across targets enables prediction of structure–property associations and provides probabilistic SAR. This needs to be distinguished from the promiscuity prediction that aims to answer the question: "is my compound promiscuous or not?" In contrast, the biospectra approach aims to link the immediate differences and similarities two compounds show over the *whole* panel to their physiological outcome.

Early work in this area by Kauvar et al. [74] showed that one can predict the binding of compounds to a new target when they are first screened against a reference panel of proteins and then a small, diverse subset of those compounds are screened against the new target. The binding signature of the diverse subset is an affinity fingerprint that can be compared to the panel binding of the whole compound set with stepwise linear regression to predict binding of the whole set to the new targets [74]. Similar compounds have similar affinity fingerprints although, interestingly, there are cases where structurally dissimilar compounds are not distant in affinity fingerprint space and vice versa [75]. Therefore, bioactivity spectra provide foresight that does not entirely overlap with structural predictions.

Bioactivity spectra also show great promise with respect to mining pharmacology data and predicting adverse drug reactions (ADRs) rather than primary targets, especially in the case of the BioPrint database (Cerep). For example, ADRs can be predicted for a compound on the basis of its "profile similarity" to other compounds with known ADRs [76], where the profile is determined in ligand-binding assays against a panel of targets [19, 40, 77].

Cytotoxicity data across multiple cell lines is another type of biospectra; extensive research has been carried out at the National Cancer Institute to deconvolute cytotoxicity and gene expression data to specific chemotypes, targets and modes of action using self-organizing maps [78, 79]. The question whether compound activities across multiple cell-based screens are the result of primary target binding or off-target binding was addressed by Klekota et al. by applying an entropy-based score to structurally clustered compounds to see whether their biospectra statistically reflected a single-target mechanism [80]. In the simplest scenario, compound activity refers to inhibition measurements or protein binding; however, the notion of compound activity can also be expanded to include its effect on gene expression patterns. The trend in linking chemical structure to mRNA profiles from microarray gene expression data recently emerged as a tool to drive postgenomics drug development [81].

For example, compound selection or design on the basis of similarity to other compounds with a desired global effect on cellular gene expression is now possible – a true clinical application of systems biology. In another intriguing study, Rosania showed that chemical substructures can be predictive of subcellular distribution, which could be highly relevant to the current topic of target prediction [82].

The main strength of the biospectra approach is also its main disadvantage: *in silico* predictions initially require experimental data collected across a matrix of targets or assays, which can be difficult to obtain, and is typically specialized in nature (e.g., kinase or pharmacology targets, cytotoxicity assays). This is described extensively in the first part of this chapter. In contrast to other described methods, biospectra do not work when there is no full data matrix available unless attempts are made to fill in missing activity values by modeling or statistical means.

Several studies have been conducted that combine large databases of molecules with machine-learning algorithms and these represent a proof of concept of what could be achieved to enrich our knowledge of potential toxicities. A network approach may assist in designing drugs with affinity for multiple targets [29] or avoiding off- or anti-targets. For example, an interaction network between 25 nuclear receptors was recently constructed on the basis of an annotated chemical library containing 2033 molecules [83], revealing potential cross-pharmacologies, with implications for the side effect prediction of small molecules. There have also been several attempts to establish relationships between molecular structure and broad biological activity and off-target effects (toxicity) [74]. For example, Fliri *et al.* presented biological spectra for a cross-section of the proteome [40]. Using hierachical clustering of the spectra similarities, they created a relationship between structure and bioactivity. This work was further extended to identify agonist and antagonist profiles at various receptors, correctly classifying similar functional activity in the absence of drug target information [40].

13.4
Future Directions

The public availability of data on drugs and drug-like molecules may make the types of analyses described above possible for scientists outside the private sector. For example, chemical repositories such as DrugBank [84], PubChem, PDSP (http://pdsp.med.unc.edu/pdsp.php), ChemSpider (www.chemspider.com) [31, 85] and others consist of target and small molecule data that could be used for extensive safety pharmacology analyses, as described above. These may also be linked to pathway analysis tools or gene expression databases like The Connectivity Map. In the future we envisage that the chemogenomics databases will need to be integrated with other informatics tools in order to fully leverage their content. Efforts to incorporate all available literature data from sources such as publications, databases and patents will be particularly valuable. We should caution that the curating of such data is not straightforward and is highly context-dependent.

A key issue will be the integration and federation of various data sources that are already available. One can imagine a data environment where all data from toxicogenomics to every biochemical assay around a compound is streamlined and easily accessible for every researcher. Having this kind of global molecule profile will also make it possible to describe the differences between compounds in detail and finally lead to novel ideas on how to improve lead compounds to ultimately make better drugs.

References

1 Adams, C.P. and Brantner, V.V. (2006) Estimating the cost of new drug development: is it really $802 million? *Health Affairs*, **25** (2), 420–428.
2 DiMasi, J.A., Hansen, R.W. and Grabowski, H.G. (2003) The price of innovation: new estimates of drug development costs. *Journal of Health Economics*, **22** (2), 151–185.
3 Schuster, D., Laggner, C. and Langer, T. (2008) Why drugs fail – a study on side effects in new chemical entities, in: *Antitargets: Prediction and Prevention of Drug Side Effects* (eds R.J. Vaz and T. Klabunde), Wiley-VCH Verlag GmbH 7 Co. KGaA, Weinheim, Germany.
4 Hamon, J., Azzaoui, K., Whitebread, S., Urban, L. and Faller, B. (2006) In vitro safety pharmacology profiling. *European Pharmaceutical Review*, **1**, 60–63.
5 Whitebread, S., Hamon, J., Bojanic, D. and Urban, L. (2005) Keynote review: in vitro safety pharmacology profiling: an essential tool for successful drug development. *Drug Discovery Today*, **10** (21), 1421–1433.
6 Wakefield, I.D., Pollard, C., Redfern, W.S., Hammond, T.G. and Valentin, J.P. (2002) The application of *in vitro* methods to safety pharmacology. *Fundamental & Clinical Pharmacology*, **16** (3), 209–218.
7 Williams, P.D. (1990) The role of pharmacological profiling in safety assessment. *Regulatory Toxicology and Pharmacology*, **12** (3 Pt 1), 238–252.
8 Bass, A., Kinter, L. and Williams, P. (2004) Origins, practices and future of safety pharmacology. *Journal of Pharmacological and Toxicological Methods*, **49** (3), 145–151.
9 Snodin, D.J. (2002) An EU perspective on the use of *in vitro* methods in regulatory pharmaceutical toxicology. *Toxicology Letters*, **127** (1–3), 161–168.
10 Curran, M.E., Splawski, I., Timothy, K.W., Vincent, G.M., Green, E.D. and Keating, M.T. (1995) A molecular basis for cardiac arrhythmia: HERG mutations cause long QT syndrome. *Cell*, **80** (5), 795–803.
11 Hoffmann, P. and Warner, B. (2006) Are hERG channel inhibition and QT interval prolongation all there is in drug-induced torsadogenesis? A review of emerging trends. *Journal of Pharmacological and Toxicological Methods*, **53** (2), 87–105.
12 PubChem, http://pubchem.ncbi.nlm.nih.gov/ (accessed June 2008).
13 Pearlstein, R.A., Vaz, R.J., Kang, J.S., Chen, X.L., Preobrazhenskaya, M., Shchekotikhin, A.E., Korolev, A.M., Lysenkova, L.N., Miroshnikova, O.V., Hendrix, J. and Rampe, D. (2003) Characterization of HERG potassium channel inhibition using CoMSiA 3D QSAR and homology modeling approaches. *Bioorganic & Medicinal Chemistry Letters*, **13** (10), 1829–1835.
14 Chen, J., Seebohm, G. and Sanguinetti, M.C. (2002) Position of aromatic residues in the S6 domain, not inactivation, dictates cisapride sensitivity of HERG and eag potassium channels. *Proceedings of the National Academy of Sciences of the United States of America*, **99** (19), 12461–12466.
15 Farid, R., Day, T., Friesner, R.A. and Pearlstein, R.A. (2006) New insights about HERG blockade obtained from protein modeling, potential energy mapping, and docking studies. *Bioorganic and Medicinal Chemistry*, **14** (9), 3160–3173.
16 Sanchez-Chapula, J.A., Navarro-Polanco, R.A., Culberson, C., Chen, J. and Sanguinetti, M.C. (2002) Molecular determinants of voltage-dependent human ether-a-go-go related gene (HERG) K+ channel block. *The Journal of Biological Chemistry*, **277** (26), 23587–23595.
17 Witchel, H.J., Dempsey, C.E., Sessions, R.B., Perry, M., Milnes, J.T., Hancox, J.C. and Mitcheson, J.S. (2004) The low-potency, voltage-dependent HERG blocker propafenone–molecular determinants and

drug trapping. *Molecular Pharmacology*, **66** (5), 1201–1212.

18 Bohacek, R.S., McMartin, C. and Guida, W.C. (1996) The art and practice of structure-based drug design: A molecular modeling perspective. *Medicinal Research Reviews*, **16** (1), 3–50.

19 Krejsa, C.M., Horvath, D., Rogalski, S.L., Penzotti, J.E., Mao, B., Barbosa, F. and Migeon, J.C. (2003) Predicting ADME properties and side effects: The BioPrint approach. *Current Opinion in Drug Discovery & Development*, **6** (4), 470–480.

20 Roche, O., Schneider, P., Zuegge, J., Guba, W., Kansy, M., Alanine, A., Bleicher, K., Danel, F., Gutknecht, E.-M., Rogers-Evans, M., Neidhart, W., Stalder, H., Dillon, M., Sjogren, E., Fotouhi, N., Gillespie, P., Goodnow, R., Harris, W., Jones, P., Taniguchi, M., Tsujii, S., von der Saal, W., Zimmermann, G. and Schneider, G. (2002) Development of a virtual screening method for identification of "frequent hitters" in compound libraries. *Journal of Medicinal Chemistry*, **45** (1), 137–142.

21 Sanguinetti, M.C. and Tristan-Firouzi, M. (2006) hERG potassium channels and cardiac arrhythmia. *Nature Chemical Biology*, **440**, 463–469.

22 Redfern, W.S., Carlsson, L., Davis, A.S., Lynch, W.G., MacKenzie, I., Palethorpe, S., Siegl, P.K., Strang, I., Sullivan, A.T., Wallis, R., Camm, A.J. and Hammond, T.G. (2003) Relationships between preclinical cardiac electrophysiology, clinical QT interval prolongation and torsade de pointes for a broad range of drugs: evidence for a provisional safety margin in drug development. *Cardiovascular Research*, **58** (1), 32–45.

23 Ekins, S. (2004) Predicting undesirable drug interactions with promiscuous proteins *in silico*. *Drug Discovery Today*, **9** (6), 276–285.

24 Ekins, S. and Erickson, J.A. (2002) A pharmacophore for human pregnane X receptor ligands. *Drug Metabolism and Disposition: The Biological Fate of Chemicals*, **30** (1), 96–99.

25 Jenkins, J.L., Bender, A. and Davies, J.W. (2006) *In silico* target fishing: Predicting biological targets from chemical structure. *Drug Discovery Today: Technologies*, **3** (4), 413–421.

26 Nidhi, G.M., Davies, J.W. and Jenkins, J.L. (2006) Prediction of biological targets for compounds using multiple-category bayesian models trained on chemogenomics databases. *Journal of Chemical Information and Modeling*, **46** (3), 1124–1133.

27 Paolini, G.V., Shapland, R.H.B., van Hoorn, W.P., Mason, J.S. and Hopkins, A.L. (2006) Global mapping of pharmacological space. *Nature Biotechnology*, **24** (7), 805–815.

28 McGovern, S.L., Caselli, E., Grigorieff, N. and Shoichet, B.K. (2002) A common mechanism underlying promiscuous inhibitors from virtual and high-throughput screening. *Journal of Medicinal Chemistry*, **45** (8), 1712–1722.

29 Csermely, P., Agoston, V. and Pongor, S. (2005) The efficiency of multi-target drugs: the network approach might help drug design. *Trends in Pharmacological Sciences*, **26** (4), 178–182.

30 Morphy, R. and Rankovic, Z. (2006) The physicochemical challenges of designing multiple ligands. *Journal of Medicinal Chemistry*, **49** (16), 4961–4970.

31 Roth, B.L., Sheffler, D.J. and Kroeze, W.K. (2004) Magic shotguns versus magic bullets: selectively non-selective drugs for mood disorders and schizophrenia. *Nature Reviews. Drug Discovery*, **3** (4), 353–359.

32 Stephenson, V.C., Heyding, R.A. and Weaver, D.F. (2005) The "promiscuous drug concept" with applications to Alzheimer's disease. *FEBS Letters*, **579** (6), 1338–1342.

33 Hampton, T. (2004) Panel reviews health effects data for assisted reproductive technologies. *The Journal of the American Medical Association*, **292** (24), 2961–2962.

34 Espinoza-Fonseca, L.M. (2006) The benefits of the multi-target approach in

drug design and discovery. *Bioorganic & Medicinal Chemistry*, **14** (4), 896–897.

35 Hopkins, A.L., Mason, J.S. and Overington, J.P. (2006) Can we rationally design promiscuous drugs? *Current Opinion in Structural Biology*, **16** (1), 127–136.

36 Mencher, S.K. and Wang, L.G. (2005) Promiscuous drugs compared to selective drugs (promiscuity can be a virtue). *BMC Clinical Pharmacology*, **5** (1), 3–13.

37 De Ponti, F., Poluzzi, E. and Montanaro, N. (2000) QT-interval prolongation by non-cardiac drugs: lessons to be learned from recent experience. *European Journal of Clinical Pharmacology*, **56** (1), 1–18.

38 Rothman, R.B., Baumann, M.H., Savage, J.E., Rauser, L., McBride, A., Hufeisen, S.J. and Roth, B.L. (2000) Evidence for possible involvement of 5-HT(2B) receptors in the cardiac valvulopathy associated with fenfluramine and other serotonergic medications. *Circulation*, **102** (23), 2836–2841.

39 Azzaoui, K., Hamon, J., Faller, B., Whitebread, S., Jacoby, E., Bender, A., Jenkins, J.L. and Urban, L. (2007) Modeling promiscuity based on *in vitro* safety pharmacology profiling data. *ChemMedChem*, **2** (6), 874–880.

40 Fliri, A.F., Loging, W.T., Thadeio, P.F. and Volkmann, R.A. (2005) Analysis of drug-induced effect patterns to link structure and side effects of medicines. *Nature Chemical Biology*, **1** (7), 389–397.

41 Keiser, M.J., Roth, B.L., Armbruster, B.N., Ernsberger, P., Irwin, J.J. and Shoichet, B.K. (2007) Relating protein pharmacology by ligand chemistry. *Nature Biotechnology*, **25** (2), 197–206.

42 Rolland, C., Gozalbes, R., Nicolai, E., Paugam, M.-F., Coussy, L., Barbosa, F., Horvath, D. and Revah, F. (2005) G-protein-coupled receptor affinity prediction based on the use of a profiling dataset: QSAR design, synthesis, and experimental validation. *Journal of Medicinal Chemistry*, **48** (21), 6563–6574.

43 Glick, M., Jenkins, J.L., Nettles, J.H., Hitchings, H. and Davies, J.W. (2006) Enrichment of high-throughput screening data with increasing levels of noise using support vector machines, recursive partitioning, and laplacian-modified naive bayesian classifiers. *Journal of Chemical Information and Modeling*, **46** (1), 193–200.

44 Xia, X., Maliski, E.G., Gallant, P. and Rogers, D. (2004) Classification of kinase inhibitors using a Bayesian model. *Journal of Medicinal Chemistry*, **47** (18), 4463–4470.

45 Rhee, M.H., Nevo, I., Bayewitch, M.L., Zagoory, O. and Vogel, Z. (2000) Functional role of tryptophan residues in the fourth transmembrane domain of the CB2 cannabinoid receptor. *Journal of Neurochemistry*, **75** (6), 2485–2491.

46 Wess, J., Nanavati, S., Vogel, Z. and Maggio, R. (1993) Functional-role of proline and tryptophan residues highly conserved among G-protein-coupled receptors studied by mutational analysis of the M3-muscarinic-receptor. *EMBO Journal*, **12** (1), 331–338.

47 Jacoby, E., Schuffenhauer, A., Popov, M., Azzaoui, K., Havill, B., Schopfer, U., Engeloch, C., Stanek, J., Acklin, P., Rigollier, P., Stoll, F., Koch, G., Meier, P., Orain, D., Giger, R., Hinrichs, J., Malagu, K., Zimmermann, J. and Roth, H.-J. (2005) Key aspects of the Novartis compound collection enhancement project for the compilation of a comprehensive chemogenomics drug discovery screening collection. *Current Topics in Medicinal Chemistry*, **5** (4), 397–411.

48 Schnur, D.M., Hermsmeier, M.A. and Tebben, A.J. (2006) Are target-family-privileged substructures truly privileged? *Journal of Medicinal Chemistry*, **49** (6), 2000–2009.

49 Zhu, B.-Y., Jia, Z.J., Zhang, P., Su, T., Huang, W., Goldman, E., Tumas, D., Kadambi, V., Eddy, P., Sinha, U., Scarborough, R.M. and Song, Y. (2006) Inhibitory effect of carboxylic acid group on hERG binding. *Bioorganic & Medicinal Chemistry Letters*, **16** (21), 5507–5512.

50 Kola, I. and Landis, J. (2004) Can the pharmaceutical industry reduce attrition rates? *Nature Reviews. Drug Discovery*, **3** (8), 711–715.

51 MDL (2006) MDL drug data report database (accessed December 2006).

52 Hann, M.M., Leach, A.R. and Harper, G. (2001) Molecular complexity and its impact on the probability of finding leads for drug discovery. *Journal of Chemical Information and Computer Sciences*, **41** (3), 856–864.

53 Scitegic *Pipeline Pilot 6.1*, Scitegic Inc., 9665 Chesapeake Drive, Suite 401, San Diego, CA 92123, USA: 2007.

54 Hert, J., Willett, P., Wilton, D.J., Acklin, P., Azzaoui, K., Jacoby, E. and Schuffenhauer, A. (2004) Comparison of topological descriptors for similarity-based virtual screening using multiple bioactive reference structures. *Organic and Biomolecular Chemistry*, **2** (22), 3256–3266.

55 Hert, J., Willett, P., Wilton, D.J., Acklin, P., Azzaoui, K., Jacoby, E. and Schuffenhauer, A. (2004) Comparison of fingerprint-based methods for virtual screening using multiple bioactive reference structures. *Journal of Chemical Information and Computer Sciences*, **44** (3), 1177–1185.

56 Morgan, H.L. (1965) The generation of a unique machine description for chemical structures-A technique developed at chemical abstracts service. *Journal of Chemical Documentation*, **5** (2), 107–113.

57 Xie, L., Wang, J. and Bourne, P.E. (2007) In silico elucidation of the molecular mechanism defining the adverse effect of selective estrogen receptor modulators. *PLoS Computational Biology*, **3** (11).

58 Spector, P.S., Curran, M.E., Keating, M.T. and Sanguinetti, M.C. (1996) Class III antiarrhythmic drugs block HERG, a human cardiac delayed rectifier K+ channel. Open-channel block by methanesulfonanilides. *Circulation Research*, **78** (3), 499–503.

59 Crisman, T.J., Parker, C.N., Jenkins, J.L., Scheiber, J., Thoma, M., Kang, Z.B., Kim, R., Bender, A., Nettles, J.H., Davies, J.W. and Glick, M. (2007) Understanding false positives in reporter gene assays: in silico chemogenomics approaches to prioritize cell-based HTS data. *Journal of Chemical Information and Modeling*, **47** (4), 1319–1327.

60 Bender, A., Jenkins, J.L., Glick, M., Deng, Z., Nettles, J.H. and Davies, J.W. (2006) "Bayes affinity fingerprints" improve retrieval rates in virtual screening and define orthogonal bioactivity space: when are multitarget drugs a feasible concept? *Journal of Chemical Information and Modeling*, **46** (6), 2445–2456.

61 Birchall, K., Gillet, V.J., Harper, G. and Pickett, S.D. (2006) Training similarity measures for specific activities: application to reduced graphs. *Journal of Chemical Information and Modeling*, **46** (2), 577–586.

62 Eckert, H., Vogt, I. and Bajorath, J. (2006) Mapping algorithms for molecular similarity analysis and ligand-based virtual screening: design of DynaMAD and comparison with MAD and DMC. *Journal of Chemical Information and Modeling*, **46** (4), 1623–1634.

63 Stiefl, N. and Zaliani, A. (2006) A knowledge-based weighting approach to ligand-based virtual screening. *Journal of Chemical Information and Modeling*, **46** (2), 587–596.

64 Cleves, A.E. and Jain, A.N. (2006) Robust ligand-based modeling of the biological targets of known drugs. *Journal of Medicinal Chemistry*, **49** (10), 2921–2938.

65 Nettles, J.H., Jenkins, J.L., Bender, A., Deng, Z., Davies, J.W. and Glick, M. (2006) Bridging chemical and biological space: "Target Fishing" using 2D and 3D molecular descriptors. *Journal of Medicinal Chemistry*, **49** (23), 6802–6810.

66 Schuffenhauer, A., Floersheim, P., Acklin, P. and Jacoby, E. (2003) Similarity metrics for ligands reflecting the similarity of the target proteins. *Journal of Chemical Information and Computer Sciences*, **43** (2), 391–405.

67 Sheinerman, F.B., Giraud, E. and Laoui, A. (2005) High affinity targets of protein kinase inhibitors have similar residues at

the positions energetically important for binding. *Journal of Molecular Biology*, **352** (5), 1134–1156.

68 Lagunin, A., Stepanchikova, A., Filimonov, D. and Poroikov, V. (2000) PASS: prediction of activity spectra for biologically active substances. *Bioinformatics (Oxford, England)*, **16** (8), 747–748.

69 Poroikov, V.V. and Filimonov, D.A. (2002) How to acquire new biological activities in old compounds by computer prediction. *Journal of Computer-Aided Molecular Design*, **16** (11), 819–824.

70 Geronikaki, A.A., Dearden, J.C., Filimonov, D., Galaeva, I., Garibova, T.L., Gloriozova, T., Krajneva, V., Lagunin, A., Macaev, F.Z., Molodavkin, G., Poroikov, V.V., Pogrebnoi, S.I., Shepeli, F., Voronina, T.A., Tsitlakidou, M. and Vlad, L. (2004) Design of new cognition enhancers: from computer prediction to synthesis and biological evaluation. *Journal of Medicinal Chemistry*, **47** (11), 2870–2876.

71 Niwa, T. (2004) Prediction of biological targets using probabilistic neural networks and atom-type descriptors. *Journal of Medicinal Chemistry*, **47** (10), 2645–2650.

72 Rogers, D., Brown, R.D. and Hahn, M. (2005) Using extended-connectivity fingerprints with laplacian-modified bayesian analysis in high-throughput screening follow-up. *Journal of Biomolecular Screening*, **10** (7), 682–686.

73 Young, D.W., Bender, A., Hoyt, J., McWhinnie, E., Chirn, G.-W., Tao, C.Y., Tallarico, J.A., Labow, M., Jenkins, J.L., Mitchison, T.J. and Feng, Y. (2008) Integrating high-content screening and ligand-target prediction to identify mechanism of action. *Nature Chemical Biology*, **4** (1), 59–68.

74 Kauvar, L.M., Higgins, D.L., Villar, H.O., Sportsman, J.R., Engqvist-Goldstein, A., Bukar, R., Bauer, K.E., Dilley, H. and Rocke, D.M. (1995) Predicting ligand binding to proteins by affinity finger-printing. *Chemistry & Biology*, **2** (2), 107–118.

75 Beroza, P., Villar, H.O., Wick, M.M. and Martin, G.R. (2002) Chemoproteomics as a basis for post-genomic drug discovery. *Drug Discovery Today*, **7** (15), 807–814.

76 Andreas, Bender, Davies, John W. and Jeremy, L.J. (2007) Analysis of pharmacology data and the prediction of adverse drug reactions and off-target effects from chemical structure. *ChemMedChem*, **2** (6), 861–873.

77 Fliri, A.F., Loging, W.T. and Volkmann, R.A. (2007) Analysis of system structure-function relationships. *ChemMedChem*, **2** (12), 1774–1782.

78 David, G. (2005) Covell Linking tumor cell cytotoxicity to mechanism of drug action: An integrated analysis of gene expression, small-molecule screening and structural databases. *Proteins: Structure, Function, and Bioinformatics*, **59** (3), 403–433.

79 Rabow, A.A., Shoemaker, R.H., Sausville, E.A. and Covell, D.G. (2002) Mining the national cancer institute's tumor-screening database: identification of compounds with similar cellular activities. *Journal of Medicinal Chemistry*, **45** (4), 818–840.

80 Klekota, J., Brauner, E., Roth, F.P. and Schreiber, S.L. (2006) Using high-throughput screening data to discriminate compounds with single-target effects from those with side effects. *Journal of Chemical Information and Modeling*, **46** (4), 1549–1562.

81 Fischer, H.P. and Heyse, S. (2005) From targets to leads: the importance of advanced data analysis for decision support in drug discovery. *Current Opinion in Drug Discovery & Development*, **8** (3), 334–346.

82 Rosania, G.R. (2003) Supertargeted chemistry: identifying relationships between molecular structures and their sub-cellular distribution. *Current Topics in Medicinal Chemistry*, **3** (6), 659–685.

83 Mestres, J., Couce-Martin, L., Gregori-Puigjane, E., Cases, M. and Boyer, S. (2006) Ligand-based approach to *in silico* pharmacology: nuclear receptor profiling.

Journal of Chemical Information and Modeling, **46**, 2725–2736.

84 Wishart, D.S., Knox, C., Guo, A.C., Shrivastava, S., Hassanali, M., Stothard, P., Chang, Z. and Woolsey, J. (2006) DrugBank: a comprehensive resource for *in silico* drug discovery and exploration. *Nucleic Acids Research*, **34** (Database issue), D668–D672.

85 Strachan, R.T., Ferrara, G. and Roth, B.L. (2006) Screening the receptorome: an efficient approach for drug discovery and target validation. *Drug Discovery Today*, **11** (15–16), 708–716.

Part IV

14
Discovery Toxicology Screening: Predictive, *In Vitro* Cytotoxicity
Peter J. O'Brien

14.1
Introduction

Safety considerations in drug discovery led to the introduction of several routine and well defined screens, for example, for genotoxicity, phototoxicity, and off-target pharmacology. More recently, there was also the introduction of *in vitro* cytotoxicity testing, especially using high-content analysis. This may be followed by short-term, *in vivo* toleration studies, especially with rats. The need for *in vitro* cytotoxicity assessment has long been recognized in discovery programs. However, they are used primarily to control interference during *in vitro* efficacy studies. Furthermore, their sensitivity is inadequate for revealing potential human toxicities that are chronic, low-grade, or occur with low frequency. Historically, toxicologists frequently rejected such screens for assessing toxicity potential because of their low sensitivity. Now, this sensitivity of cell-based models has been improved by an order of magnitude by incorporating several modifications, arising from: (i) identification of several critical features of cell-based safety models; (ii) demonstration of effective, cellular safety biomarkers; (iii) application of novel imaging and analysis technology and methodology; (iv) interpretation of cytotoxic concentrations relative to concentration associated with efficacy; (v) validation of *in vitro* biomarkers by correlation with well defined, clinical, human toxicity findings.

Screening effectiveness may be further enhanced by the inclusion of specific cell biomarkers for any past adverse effects of precedents or for any safety signals such that may have been flagged during theoretical assessment of potential for adverse target effects (e.g., immune suppression or stimulation), or by chemical class (e.g., phospholipidosis, vacuolation, mitochondrial DNA depletion). Lead optimization of efficacious compounds across and within chemical series can be substantially facilitated by effective cytotoxicity screens alongside *in vitro* assessments for bioavailability, off-target pharmacology, genotoxicity and (where relevant) phototoxicity. Following these *in vitro* assessments, short-term, *in vivo* toleration/toxicity studies may be effective for hit and lead screening for unexpected organ toxicities. These studies are typically conducted with repeat-dosing of rats over several days. They precede standard, regulatory safety pharmacology studies. At study termination, standard safety biomarkers are assessed, especially for hepato-, myelo-, nephro- and cardiac toxicities. *Ad hoc* safety biomarkers may also be assayed if indicated by any prior safety signals. Combined incorporation of *in vitro* cytotoxicity testing and *in vivo* toleration studies into a discovery safety assessment strategy is likely to substantially reduce the number of drug candidates making their way into drug development and failing due to unacceptable safety risk.

14.2
Basis of Need for Discovery Toxicology Screening

14.2.1
High Attrition at High Cost

A ten-year study of ten large pharmaceutical companies ended in 2000 and found only one in nine drugs survived from Phase I to registration, with success rate varying from 5 to 20% depending on therapeutic area. The financial impact of this attrition is high, given that costs of drug discovery and development were estimated at 800 million US dollars in 2001 and 900 million in 2004 [1]. At least half of this attrition was attributable to lack of efficacy and adverse safety [1].

14.2.2
High Proportion of Attrition Due to Adverse Safety

Analysis of safety attrition of approved drugs over a 25-year period ending in 1999 indicated that one approved drug was withdrawn and three drugs received black box warnings each year and a half [2]. Cardiotoxicity was responsible for most of any organ. Hepatotoxicity was responsible for more than a quarter of the toxicity. Of the 38 drugs withdrawn from the market by the US Food and Drug Agency between 1994 and 2006 because of toxicity, 17 were for cardiotoxicity and 14 for hepatotoxicity [3].

14.2.3
Discovery Screening Reduces Attrition by An Order of Magnitude

Lack of bioavailability and other adverse pharmacokinetic properties caused ~40% attrition in 1992. However, this attrition was reduced by an order of magnitude by 2000 to ~10%. This resulted in a substantial rise in the relative impact of adverse safety to one-third of attrition, whereas lack of efficacy had mildly less impact [1]. The basis of the decreased pharmacokinetic attrition may be reasonably attributable to the introduction of *in vitro* screening in drug discovery.

14.3
Obstacles to Discovery Toxicology Screening

Recognition of the importance of safety attrition and how it could be reduced by discover toxicology programs has only occurred recently. Thus, it is relatively new. It has been further limited by the lack of reliability of conventional *in vitro* models of target organ toxicity. In one study, these were demonstrated to have less than 25% predictivity for human toxicity potential [4]. However, as described below, high content analysis models improved this predictivity substantially. Application of *in vivo* studies is limited by their requirement for large amounts of compound as well as their poor predictivity. The latter is indicated, for example, by only half of compounds causing human hepatotoxicity generating hepatic safety signals in regulatory animal toxicity studies [5].

14.4
Need to Coordinate Cytotoxicity Screening with Other Discovery Safety Assessments

Cytotoxicity screening must be appropriately integrated into the safety assessment strategy that is now well established in drug discovery and encompasses multiple *in silico*, *in vitro* and *in vivo* approaches ([6], Table 14.1). It first begins with evaluation of the historical safety issues that are associated with precedents of the same chemical or pharmacologic class as the candidate compounds, or with their molecular target. Physicochemical properties known to be associated with adverse effects [7] and known toxicophores are screened for. These may be eliminated if they are separable from the desired pharmacologic and pharmacokinetic properties using structure–activity relationship (SAR) studies. Specific chemical structures historically associated with production of genotoxicity, phospholipidosis, phototoxicity and small numbers of target organ toxicities may be identified by screening through large databases [8].

Following *in silico* screens, there are numerous validated *in vitro* tests widely used in drug discovery. Candidate compounds are screened early for genetic toxicity related to both mutagenicity and chromosomal aberrations. Probably the next most well established *in vitro* safety screening is for off-target pharmacologic effects, in which a wide range of receptor, channel and enzyme interactions are screened for. Increased numbers of these is associated with increased safety risk. One such important test is for interaction with the hERG channel that is associated with prolongation of the QT interval detected in electrocardiograms. Phototoxicity potential, first indicated in the chemical structure, is identified by quantitative assessment of light absorption that has now become a regulatory requirement [9]. Compounds are also tested for their formation of reactive metabolites and reaction with glutathione [10].

After *in silico* and *in vitro* screening, short-term *in vivo* toleration (IVT) studies [7] are conducted to identify unexpected target organ toxicities, such as myelotoxicity and hepatotoxicity. The IVT is essentially an abbreviated version of regulatory, preclinical,

Table 14.1 Potential contributory role of HCA in discovery safety assessment (see genotoxicity and cytotoxicity).

Safety assessment approach	Comment
Scholarship	Evaluation of historical safety issues associated with chemical structure or molecular target
Physico-chemical properties	Toxicity potential has been demonstrated to be substantially decreased with compounds with low molecular weights and low polarity and lipophilicity
Toxicophore analysis	Evaluation of chemical moieties historically associated with safety issues, for example, genotoxicity, cationic amphiphilic drugs and phospholipidosis, tertiary amines that are charge neutral at physiologic pH and vacuolization
Ultraviolet and visible light absorption spectra	Phototoxicity potential assessed by 3T3 phototoxicity test if the molar extinction/absorption coefficient is less than 10 l/mol/cm
Molecular target distribution	Toxicity potential increases if the molecular target is found in tissues other than what are targeted therapeutically
Genotoxicity	Evaluation by toxicophore analysis and Ames type mutagencity test and chromosomal toxicity such as *in vitro* micronucleus test by HCA [21–23]
Off-target pharmacology	Evaluation of interaction of compound with a wide range of receptors and enzymes and proteins indicates that higher reactivity is associated with higher potential for toxicity
Cytotoxicity	Evaluated for confounding interpretation of *in vitro* efficacy assays, for predicting potential for human toxicity especially in liver but also if warranted by other safety assessments in bone marrow, kidney, neurons, immunocytes and so on. Also used for developing understanding of biochemical mechanisms of toxicity. HCA has been repeatedly demonstrated to be an effective tool in predictive toxicology. May also be used for certain translational safety biomarkers of toxicity [37]
Drug–drug interaction	Evaluation of potential for competition with other drugs for metabolism and clearance can affect the safety margin
Safety pharmacology	*In vitro* assays can test for hERG potassium channel interaction early in discovery, with *ex vivo* and *in vivo* assays being applied later in discovery. HCA assays are being developed for *in vitro* assessments of cardiac toxicity potential
Reactive metabolite screen	Reactive metabolites have been increasingly implicated in idiosyncratic toxicity
Short-term *in vivo* toleration (IVT) studies	Introduction into drug discovery, usually at late stage (earlier depending on safety signal generation) can bring attrition earlier than preclinical development. HCA may be used on blood cells to detect cytotoxicity [37]

animal toxicity studies used in drug development that has been brought into the later phase of drug discovery in order to take attrition earlier. However, where safety signals have been generated early and indicate increased potential for target organ toxicity, the IVT may be applied earlier to define SAR. To be effective, the IVT is customized to use low amounts of compound, has a rapid turnaround and is tailored to address the unexpected as well as the relevant safety signals previously generated.

14.5 Discovery Cytotoxicology

14.5.1 Biomarkers for Safety versus Efficacy for Screening

To identify effective safety biomarkers it is important to understand how they differ in their nature from an efficacy or even pharmacodynamic biomarker. First, it should be recognized that frequently drug toxicity is a side-effect and unrelated to the effect on the intended target or to the pharmacology of the drug. It more related to the drug's chemical properties or to a chemical moiety, which are unrelated to the therapeutic target (see examples below). This being said, it is also important to recognize that there are numerous drug toxicities that arise from an unintended interference with biochemical processes that have a component similar to, or are downstream of, the molecular target. Examples of these include certain antibiotic, antiretroviral and anticancer drugs, glitazones and statins. Mitochondrial function, calcium regulation, cell reproduction and oxidative stress are commonly the unintended targets of drug therapy. Since these are ubiquitous processes, and drug exposure is frequently systemic, blood cells with these processes may reveal early drug toxic effects. HCA has high potential as a clinical pathology tool for the detection of these effects.

Compared to efficacy, safety is typically more multifactorial, as it is dependent on homeostasis of virtually all cellular processes. A wider number and diversity of potential molecular and cellular effects of compound interactions may affect safety than may affect efficacy or bioavailability. Accordingly, cytotoxicity assessment is less specific, more multiparametric and extrapolatable with less certainty, unless there are specific safety signals indicated by the chemical structure or by its precedents. Extrapolation of safety biomarker data needs a greater foundation of mechanistic understanding of both *in vitro* and *in vivo* pathogenesis of toxicities, as well as rigorous, empirical validation of models.

14.5.2 Past Failure of Cytotoxicity Assessments

14.5.2.1 Insufficient Exposure

Historically, *in vitro* cytotoxicity tests have not been effective in predicting human toxicity potential [11]. This has been attributable largely to insufficiency of duration of exposure of cells and toxicant for cytotoxicity to be expressed. In one study of 23 drugs, 75% did not express their toxicity with only 24 h exposure, but only after several days [4]. Mitochondrial DNA and protein synthesis inhibitors, for example, take up to a week to show cytotoxic effects in many assays. Furthermore, dose–response curves are typically shifted to the left, toward increased sensitivity, with increasing duration of exposure from hours to days.

14.5.2.2 Measurement of Cell Death

The insensitivity of many assays is also due to their evaluation of events that are too late in the life cycle of cells, such as failure or death (Table 14.2) [11, 12]. At this point cells rupture and release cellular constituents or else allow penetration of extracellular substances. Causing cell death is not required for a compound in order for it to have significant toxicity. Also, the limited solubility of drugs might limit the ability to increase the drug concentration to a sufficient concentration for its adverse effect to be detected. For example, the assay of total ATP content of cell populations is frequently used for cytotoxicity assessment, but changes quite late in pathogenesis of cell failure. The lateness of this change reflects the tight regulation and buffering of

Table 14.2 Progressive response to sub-lethal cell stress.
The cellular responses in this table are listed in order of severity of stress [11, 36].

Cellular response	Example
Stress	For example, mitochondrial inhibitor, oxidant, substance accumulation (e.g., lipid, phospholipid, fluid)
Stress signal	For example, nrf-2, AP-1, NF-kB transcription factor translocation
Substrate consumption	Glutathione, ATP, glycogen
Induction	For example, antioxidant enzymes, mitochondrial, membrane hyperpolarization, mitochondrial biogenesis
Repair	Autophagocytosis of abnormal intracellular organelles
Stress susceptibility	Loss of functional reserve capacity
Dyshomeostasis	Mild impairment of energy and ionized calcium regulation
Dysfunction	Mild impairment of cell function, for example, proliferation
Degeneration	Mitochondrial permeability transition with membrane depolarization, cytochrome c release, and mitochondrial swelling and fragmentation; activation of caspases and cell death pathway, endonuclease fragmentation of DNA with chromatin and nuclear condensation; phosphatidyserine exposure on cell surface; cytoskeletal disruption with membrane blebbing
Failure	Marked impairment of energy homeostasis with volume contraction; impaired mitochondrial reductive activity with decreased ATP concentration (e.g., MTT, Alamar blue); organelle and cell swelling and distortion, cell lysis with intracellular enzyme release (e.g., LDH release)

ATP concentration by interconversions with other high-energy phosphates, such as creatine phosphate, and by replenishment by metabolic conversion of substrate stores, such as glycogen. This tight regulation is required because ATP in turn regulates activities of numerous metabolic pathways, cell functions and cell structure. Current assays for ATP are also significantly limited because there are no intracellular dyes for it and its concentration cannot be determined at the single-cell level.

Cytotoxicity measurement of events that are too early in the pathogenesis of cytotoxicity might also be ineffective for assessment of *in vivo* toxicity potential. For example, measurement of concentration of a noxious substance, byproduct or metabolite, or the activation of a signal transduction pathway is insufficient to conclude that a compound is toxic. This requires direct demonstration and measurement of the adverse effect, or of an adaptation to it.

14.5.3
Effective Cell-Based Assays for Marked and Acute Cytotoxicity

Assays are frequently needed to detect marked and acute cytotoxicity that may confound the interpretation of cell-based efficacy assays. Neutral red uptake is one of the most commonly used cytotoxicity assays and is used in the regulatory phototoxicity assay on NT3 fibroblasts [13]. It has been show to be more sensitive than assays for mitochondrial reductive capacity such as the tetrazolium reductase assays, ATP depletion assays, or for cell permeabilization or rupture such as dye uptake or lactate dehydrogenase leakage. Lysosomes take up, protonate and trap neutral red when cellular ATP production is sufficient to maintain pH gradients.

14.5.4
Characteristics of an Optimally Effective Cell Model of Toxicity

There are a number of key features essential for a cell-based model to be effectively predictive of toxicity (Table 14.3). First, as indicated above, it must be sensitive enough to reflect early, sublethal injury and not merely cell death.

Second, it must be able to detect chronic as well as acute toxicities, especially as it is the former that is the more common cause of safety attrition in the clinics. It is critical that cells be exposed to toxicants for sufficient time to allow expression of the cytotoxicity [6, 11, 14–16]. Three days of incubation of cells was effective for more than 95% human hepatotoxic drugs, whereas a single day of incubation was frequently ineffective [4] or produced cytotoxicity at a much higher concentration [4, 11, 14].

In order to screen effectively over a wide range of pathologies the screening assay needs to be a "catch all" measure of a ubiquitous process in cell injury. As there is no single measure yet described that will "catch all" toxicities sufficiently early, multiple parameters must be assessed. Live cell assays are the most sensitive indicators for detection of adverse effects.

There are also several important features of the cell type used that determine its effectiveness in predicting human toxicity. It should be of the same species as is

Table 14.3 Characteristics of an effective cell model for screening for sublethal cytotoxicity [4, 11, 33, 36].

Characteristic	Description
Sublethal	Measurement as opposed to measurement of cell death is required. Measurement of the noxious substance or a signal transduction event may be too early in the pathogenesis if cell injury as opposed to measurement of adaptive and adverse effects
Chronic	Most toxicities are expressed only after multiple days of exposure
"Catch all"	Includes measurements of adverse effect in common to all toxicities. There needs to be a "catch-all" measure of an activity that is affected in a final common pathway of cell injury
Mulitplex	Makes multiple measurements of different end points for different processes; a single end point assay will not identify most cytotoxicities
Morphometric and biochemical	Structural and functional measurement is complementary and additive
Mechanistic	Provides mechanistic information; signals generated in cytotoxicity assays need to indicate mechanisms to be followed up to derisk the compound
Single-cell resolution	Tracks individual live cells and discriminates them from dead cells and extracellular stain; allows identification of hormesis and separation of compensatory adaptation from degenerative change; allows more accurate identification of sequence of change in different cytotoxicity parameters as cells might not be synchronous or alike in their response
Live cell	Uses live cells under normophysiological conditions: cell function is substantially affected by temperature, humidity, and oxygenation, pH and osmolality, as well as media growth factors and attachment substrate
Predictive	High sensitivity and specificity and concordance with in vivo toxicity in species designed to be indicative of; inhibitor of DNA polymerize gamma for mitochondrial DNA synthesis by nucleoside reverse transcriptase inhibitors
Precise	High level of within-run, across-day, and across-laboratory precision; assay must be reproducible
Practical	Cells need to be widely commercially-available, standardized and quality managed, Assays need sufficient operational performance: throughput and cost-effectiveness; at least one to several hundred per week; assays are available that can be run at significantly less than U.S.$ 100 per compound, including materials, staff and instrumentation
Dose-responsive	Determines different response over range of concentrations
Cell features	Cells must have drug metabolism competence and be of the same species as predicting for. They must be well characterized and described in the literature

being modeled. Additionally it must have drug metabolic competency similar to that of the modeled species. If the assay is to be used widely, then practical considerations must be made, such as widespread availability of quality managed and standardized cells. The cell type should be well characterized and well understood, with extensive use reported in the scientific literature. HepG2 cells have been demonstrated to be one of the best cell models described for predicting human toxicity potential [4, 15, 16].

14.5.4.1 Need for Morphological and Functional Parameters

Assays that combine morphology and functional assessments are more predictive as they measure more parameters by using more and independent analytic approaches, such as dimensional image analysis and fluorescence intensity measurements. Morphological assessments provide information about the size and shape of cells and organelles, as well as the intracellular location, such as with transcription factor translocation or lysosomal sequestration. Thus assays measuring both morphology and function are making a more comprehensive evaluation over a wider spectrum of change.

14.5.4.2 Need for Multiple and Mechanistic Parameters

Cytotoxicity assessments are limited by their inability to measure multiple, mechanistic parameters that capture a wide spectrum of potential cytopathological changes [4, 11, 15–17]. The complexity of the biology behind a toxicological change requires several criteria for an effective cytotoxicity assay. First, there is no single parameter likely to be able to identify all toxicities, which immediately limits the utility of uniparametric assays. Assays with multiple parameters for key, multiple and different features are more predictive because they cover a wider spectrum of effects. Additionally, those assay parameters that represent fundamental, cellular mechanisms of pathogenesis rather than being purely descriptive are more potent.

14.5.4.3 Need for Single-Cell Monitoring

Assays that measure end points for cell populations rather than multiple individual cells might produce contradictory findings. These occur due to a failure to discriminate and correct for confounding effects of extracellular staining, dead cells, different cell types, or opposite effects in different cells.

For example, mitochondrial reductive capacity is decreased with decreased cell numbers but is increased with cells that are activated, such as lymphocytic immune activation, or if cells adapt to the stress associated with toxicity, such as during mitochondrial biogenesis. Thus, mitochondrial reductive capacity might be either increased or decreased with toxicity. Similar contradictory interpretations might occur with other cellular activities, for which there is a compensatory adaptive increase before their failure. This biphasic change is referred to as hormesis and occurs not only with reductive mitochondrial activity but also with mitochondrial number, cell number, mitochondrial membrane potential, antioxidant system activity and numerous other activities.

Finally, individual cell studies might be more accurate than cell population studies in which responses are variable over time or over different cells. Analysis of the sequence of changes in the different parameters might be important in elucidating the mechanisms and pathogenesis of toxicity.

14.5.4.4 Need for Effective Parameters

Critical for predictivity in a recent comprehensive study was the number and choice of parameters measured [4]. Early, sublethal effects on cell proliferation, cell morphology and mitochondria occurred consistently and ubiquitously with toxicity and when used collectively were most diagnostic. It is noteworthy that the toxicity of many drugs is attributable to various mitochondrial targets, including oxidative phosphorylation, fatty acid oxidation, Krebs cycling, membrane transport, permeability transition pore, proliferation and oxidative stress (Table 14.4).

Table 14.4 Mitochondrial targets for drug-induced inhibition [3, 4, 33, 36].

Target	Example
Oxidative phosphorylation	Inhibition of complexes (e.g., I by rotenone, fenofibrate and thiazolidinediones, IV by cyanide, V by oligomycin; depleters of coenzyme Q such as amitryptyline); redox cyclers (diverting electrons to form reactive oxygen and nitrogen species, e.g., quinones, bipyridyls); uncouplers of electron transport from ATP synthesis (e.g., protonophores, tolcapone, flutamide, cocaine, furosemide, fatty acids, non-steroidal anti-inflammatory drugs)
Fatty acid beta-oxidation	Inhibition by valproate, tetracyclines, nonsteroidal anti-inflammatory drugs, antianginal cationic amphiphilic drugs, female sex hormones, CoA depleters such as valproate and salicylate
Krebs cycle	Inhibition of aconitase by superoxide and fluoroacetate, of succinate dehydrogenase by methamphetamine and malonate, of alpha-ketoglutarate dehydrogenase by salicylic acid
Membrane transporters	Inhibition of adenine nucleotide transporter by zidovudine
Permeability transition pore	Opening by reactive oxygen species, reactive nitrogen species, bile acids, thio crosslinkers, atractyloside, betuliniate, lonidamidem various anticancer drugs, to collapse mitochondrial membrane potential and activate mitochondrial apoptotic pathway
Proliferation	Inhibitor of DNA polymerase-gamma (e.g., nucleoside reverse transcriptase inhibitors); inhibition of mitochondrial protein synthesis (e.g., oxazolidinone antibiotics); mitochondrial DNA mutation (e.g., oxidative injury by ethanol)
Oxidative stress	Glutathione depletion (e.g., acetaminophen, bromobenzene, chloroform, allyl alcohol); redox cyclers (see oxidative phosphorylation); reactive metabolites

The occurrence and timing of effects on intracellular ionized calcium concentration, lysosomal mass, oxidative stress or plasma membrane permeability frequently provide additional information indicative of mechanism of toxicity (Table 14.5).

Table 14.5 Cytotoxicity biomarkers and assays [3, 4, 11, 19, 36].

Biomarker	Example
Membrane permeability	Leakage of cell contents (e.g., lactate dehydrogenase) and entry of extracellular dyes (e.g., Trypan blue, DNA stains such as TOTO-3)
Proliferation	Cell number; frequency distribution of nuclear DNA content of cell population, protein content, protein synthesis (e.g., 14C-labeled methionine incorporation), DNA synthesis (e.g., tritiated thymidine incorporation), DNA stains (e.g., Hoechst 33 342; 4′,6-diamidino-2-phenylindole, DAPI; picogreen); mass tracker dyes (e.g., LysoTracker green for lysosomes, MitoTracker deep red for mitochondria, ER-Tracker blue–white DPX for endoplasmic reticulum)
Mitochondria and energy homeostasis	Dye oxidation (e.g., tetrazolium reductase activity with 3-[4,5-dimethylthiazol-2-yl]-2,5-diphenyl tetrazolium bromide, MTT; 2-[4-iodophenyl]-3-[4-nitrophenyl]-5-[2,4-disulfophenyl]-2H tetrazolium monosodium salt, WST-1; 3-(4,5-carboxymethoxyphenyl)-2-(4-sulfophenyl)-2H-tetrazolium, MTS; 2,3-bis(2-methoxy-4-nitro-5-sulfophenyl)-2H-tetrazolium-5-carboxanilide inner salt, XTT; 2,2′-di-p-nitrophenyI-5,5′-diphenyl-3,3′-(3,3′-dimethoxy-4,4′-diphenylene)-ditetrazolium chloride, NBT), Alamar blue assays, ATP concentration (e.g., luciferase assay), oxygen consumption (e.g., oxygen electrodes, phosphorescent oxygen-sensitive dyes), mitochondrial protein and nucleic acid synthesis; mitochondrial mass (e.g., mitotracker dyes); mitochondrial membrane potential (e.g., tetramethylrhodamine methyl ester, TMRM; tetramethylrhodamine ethyl ester, TMRE)
Oxidative stress	Oxidant production (e.g., dihydroethidium, dichlorofluorescein), antioxidant changes (e.g., glutathione = monochlorobimane), antioxidant system enzyme, resistance to dye oxidation (e.g., total antioxidant status), macromolecular oxidation byproducts (e.g., malondialdehyde, hydroxynonenal, 8-hydroxyguanosine)
Lysosomes	Phospholipidosis (e.g., Nile red, lysotracker dyes, electron microscopy of lysosomal multilamellar bodies), vacuolization, autophagy, lysosomal uptake assays for cell viability (e.g., neutral red)
Nuclear and cell shape and size	Cytoskeleton injury, blebbing, shrinkage in apoptosis; increased size in mitosis; nuclear size: contraction with apoptosis and swelling with cell cycle inhibition

Table 14.5 (Continued)

Biomarker	Example
Ca	Ionized and total calcium concentration
Cell signals	Cytoplasmic–nuclear translocation (e.g., proportioning of immunocytochemical stain for NFKB with inflammation and AP-1 and NRF2 with oxidative stress)
Induction	Antioxidant system, compensatory enzymes
Apoptosis	Nuclear condensation and lobulation, caspase activation, phosphatidyl serine externalization, annexin, immuno-cytochemistry, DNA fragmentation and labeled-dUTP incorporation by terminal deoxynucleotidyl transferase
Metabolism	Bench-top or automated chemistry analyzer assays of cell lysates for key enzymes of intermediary metabolism, antioxidant system, ion transport
Function	Cell-based, efficacy, live-cell assays in which assessment of efficacy is based on a cellular function that might be inhibited by cytotoxicity

There are specific fluorescent dyes for specific pathologies created by specific drug classes, such as phospholipidosis from cationic amphiphilic drugs [18, 19], mitochondrial DNA depletion by nucleoside reverse transcriptase inhibitors that also inhibit mitochondrial DNA polymerase gamma and redox cyclers that produce reactive oxygen species. The complex mechanism of statin-induced toxicity is demonstrated with early sublethal effects on apoptosis, mitochondrial function and calcium homeostasis [20].

14.5.4.5 Need for Validation with Human Toxicity Data

One of the largest limitations of *in vitro* assays is their lack of full validation and determination of their sensitivity and specificity for the prediction of human toxicity potential. Assays need to be applied to a large set of marketed drugs that produce toxicity by numerous and different mechanisms for assessment of correlation with human toxicity. This enables determination of the concordance between *in vitro* and *in vivo* results. Typically, such assays show high specificity, in excess of 90%. When compounds react positively in the cytotoxicity evaluation, this is associated with *in vivo* toxicity. The major concern though, is the sensitivity with which the toxic potential is assessed. In a comparison of seven conventional cytotoxicity assays applied to 600 compounds with single end points m measurement in an acute exposure experiment, only glutathione had significant sensitivity (19%). Measures of mitochondrial reductive capacity and DNA synthesis were half as sensitive. Caspase induction, synthesis, protein synthesis, superoxide production and membrane integrity were of negligible value [4, 11].

14.6
High Effectiveness of An HCA Cell Model in Predictive Toxicology

14.6.1
Background on HCA

HCA refers to the application of a recently developed technology that consolidates and automates microscopy, cytochemistry, imaging and bioinfomatics. These are applied to cells in various microtiter plate formats or on glass slides. Multiple morphologic features and fluorescence signals can be measured simultaneously. The measurements can be made at various levels from that of subcellular organelles, to single cells, cell populations and even tissues. They can be made on either fixed cells or on live cells that are incubated under physiological conditions. They can be made in end point assays or kinetically, in real time. Compared to previous manual methods, automation provides a marked improvement in the capacity for sample and experiment throughput, the precision of measurement and in the sheer number and diversity of parameters measureable for an experiment. Consolidation of the technical capabilities allows unparalleled within-experiment, cross-comparisons of biochemical, morphological and functional parameters. Compared to flow cytometry it offers substantially greater analytic capability for morphometric and kinetic parameters, although for substantially lower numbers of cells.

Numerous recent publications demonstrated the above advantages and effectiveness of using HCA in drug discovery toxicology for the assessment of chromosomal toxicity potential using *in vitro* micronuclei testing [21–23] and for target organ toxicity potential using cytotoxicity testing [4, 11, 15, 16, 24–29]. Of these, a comprehensive validation using human toxicants demonstrated the HCA approach to be substantially more effective than conventional cytotoxicity approaches and *in vivo* regulatory animal studies [4].

14.6.2
Idiosyncratic Hepatotoxicity

Idisosyncratic hepatotoxicity is probably the most unpredicted and important cause of the safety attrition of marketed drugs. The use of human hepatocytes with potential for drug metabolism is important for screening for hepatotoxicity potential, as numerous drugs produce this effect by their hepatic metabolites. Drugs producing idiosyncratic hepatotoxicity and/or toxicity by their metabolites [30, 31] were detected with HepG2 cells in an HCA-based assay as effectively as drugs producing toxicity directly. This high concordance contrasted remarkably with the 15% concordance of seven other conventional assays in which a 50% effect at 30 μM was considered positive for changes in any of the seven readouts: DNA synthesis, protein synthesis, glutathione depletion, superoxide secretion, caspase-3 activity, membrane integrity and mitochondrial reductive activity [4, 11]. The basis for this difference in sensitivity was not determined but may relate in part to the induction of metabolic competence over the three days of exposure during the HCS assay. Whereas HepG2 cells may have low levels of cytochrome P450 enzymes for drug metabolism, many of these are inducible [32].

14.6.3
Characteristic Pattern and Sequence of Cytotoxic Changes

Determination of the concentration producing cytotoxicity in an HCA cytotoxicity assay was assessed by 12-point dose–response curves [4]. A toxic effect was defined as the point when values for the parameter departed from the baseline and negative controls by more than two coefficients of variation. The pattern and sequence of changes in the different parameters frequently reflected the mechanism of toxicity. For example, for fenofibrate, there was nuclear swelling and inhibition of cell proliferation, followed by mild increases in intracellular calcium with some loss of mitochondrial membrane potential and an increase in membrane permeability, followed by overt oxidative stress with mitochondrial biogenesis. This pattern contrasted with that of cerivastatin, where first there was nuclear shrinkage and increased mitochondrial membrane potential, followed by increased intracellular ionized calcium. At higher concentrations, calcium progressively increased, mitochondrial potential progressively fell and membrane permeability increased [20].

14.6.4
Safety Margin

Virtually all drugs and chemicals cause toxicity at high enough concentrations. Thus, it is critical to assess toxicity at concentrations relevant to those that are used for drug efficacy. Efficacious concentration, as defined as the maximal serum concentration of drug used for treatment (C_{max}), is highly variable, ranging over 10 000 000-fold in one study of 187 marketed human drugs (from 100 pM to 2 mM), with 90% values less than 100 µM, 60% less than 10 µM, 37% less than 1 µM and 12% less than 100 nM. Most human hepatotoxic drugs (94% of 102 tested) are cytotoxic in the sublethal HCA cytotoxicity assay at concentrations less than 100-fold C_{max}, whereas most nontoxic drugs (96% of 23 tested) are cytotoxic in this assay at concentrations more than 100-fold C_{max} [4, 33].

14.6.5
Hormesis

Hormesis, in which compensatory adaptive changes precede and occur at lower doses than degenerative changes, was detected for half of the toxic drugs for cell proliferation, cell morphology and mitochondria [4, 33]. Hormesis could not be assessed for parameters that normally have low values, such as intracellular calcium measured by fluo4 or membrane permeability measured by toto-3, because assay methods were not sufficiently sensitive. However, for calcium, more sensitive dyes, with calcium dissociation constants closer to the physiologic concentration of ionized calcium, detected biphasic effects on resting calcium [34].

14.6.6
Implementation of HCA Cytotoxicity Testing in Drug Discovery

Data from the HCA cytotoxicity assay would not be used for go/no go decision-making but for compound prioritization and optimization during *in vitro* screening cascades and in the context of efficacy, bioavailability and off-target pharmacologic data. Early ranking of compounds for their progression is important for early initiation of potential hazard identification and for flagging up compounds needing follow-up safety assessment and early development of risk management strategies [4, 22, 29].

The significance of the cytotoxic signals should be interpreted in terms of the ratio of cytotoxic concentration to the concentration causing efficacy. The latter was estimated by comparing with the maximal total concentration of the drug in human serum that is associated with administration of the drug at an efficacious dose. However, the degree of plasma protein binding was not considered in this study. As there is only one-tenth as much plasma protein in the *in vitro* system compared to *in vivo*, significant protein binding would be expected to result in an overestimate of the circulating free drug compared to *in vitro*, with consequent proportionate underestimate of the safety margin and overestimate of the toxicity potential. For example, rosiglitazone's safety margin was underestimated without consideration of the high plasma protein binding. Thus, this ratio should be considered an estimate of the minimal safety margin. Finally, in this context, the best estimates of safety margin for most drugs should be based on drug exposure to free concentration per unit time (i.e., area under the concentration time curve; AUC). However, these values were not available for *in vitro* studies. The risk associated with a low safety margin needs to be considered with respect to both the indication and the dose being used. Lower safety margins are accepted for drugs intended for treatment of life-threatening diseases for which there are no equivalent alternatives. Lower safety margins may also be accepted for drugs in which the ingestion is limited by the bulk required for toxicity or by side-effects such as vomiting. It may also be relevant to interpret the significance of the signal based on the degree of change and the number of parameters affected and the mechanism and the steepness of the concentration–response curve.

Recent studies indicate the concentration of drug needed for assessment of human toxicity potential [4, 33]. At a concentration of 30 µM, 60% of drugs with human toxicity potential were identified, whereas 100 µM identified about 80%. These concentrations are considerably lower, that is, the assay is more sensitive than previous reported assays [12, 15, 16, 35]. Assessment of toxicity potential was more accurate when the concentration of drug tested was based on multiples of the total efficacious concentration (C_{max} for marketed drugs), with 80% of cytotoxicities being detected at a concentration of 30 times the efficacious concentration, C_{max}.

14.6.7
Limitations of HCA Cytotoxicity Testing in Drug Discovery

Whereas drug-induced cytotoxicity may indicate potential for *in vivo* human hepatotoxicity, it is not predictive of such. Cytotoxic effects *in vivo* may be limited or even aggravated, compared to those occurring *in vitro*. Cytotoxicity models are limited by their incomplete modeling of the cell type's structure and function as it occurs *in vivo*, by their incomplete modeling of other cell types, cell functions and interactions with other cells in a tissue, organ, systems and whole body [4, 11, 36], for example: (i) drug properties, concentrations, protein binding and transport may differ *in vivo*; (ii) pharmacokinetic characteristics of absorption, distribution, metabolism and excretion can have a major influence on which target organ is affected and the severity of toxicity; (iii) toxicities may occur at the tissue or organ level such as cholestasis, cataractogenesis and myelotoxicity which cannot be effectively predicted from single-cell systems; (iv) toxicities may occur secondarily to direct cytotoxicity and due to the interaction of organs and systems and other processes such as inflammation, immune-mediated hypersensitivity, plasma volume expansion and endocrine effect; (v) toxicities may be produced by drugs' effects on specific proteins such as channels and transporters not found in hepatocytes or found at very low activity such as the calcium channel toxicity of ryanodine, potassium channel toxicity of astemizole and terfenadine, renal toxicity of zomepirac, dermatotoxicity of isoxicam and hematologic toxicity of vincamine.

Metabolic competence of HepG2 human hepatoblastoma cells depends on the source and culture conditions. They have both Phase I and II metabolizing enzymes. Cytochrome P450 enzymes are found in much lower levels in HepG2 cells than in primary human hepatocytes but many of these enzymes are inducible, including CYP1A1, 1A2, 2B6, 2E1 and 3A4. The latter metabolizes approximately 50% of drugs currently on the market [32].

In the sublethal HCS assay, sensitivity and specificity for identification of human hepatotoxicant drugs were 94 and 96%, respectively, when testing only hepatotoxicant drugs and nontoxic drugs [4]. However, when testing other drugs that produce other organ toxicities (e.g., kidney, heart, bone marrow, muscle, pancreas) their cytotoxic effects were not distinguishable from those of drugs causing hepatotoxicity. Thus, cytotoxicity in the HCS assay was concordant with human toxicity but not specific for liver toxicity (Table 14.6).

14.7
Future Impact of Cytotoxicity Testing

As occurred with the introduction of *in vitro* testing for adverse pharmacokinetic properties, implementation of *in vitro* cytotoxicity testing in drug discovery is likely to reduce later attrition in drug development by an order of magnitude. An indispensable tool will be HCA and a cytotoxicity model similar to that described above. Attendance at the numerous annual industry conferences on HCA indicates that

Table 14.6 Specific applications of HCS cytotoxicity assay.

Application	Comment
Screening	First-tier screen for potential for human target organ toxicity
Chromosomal toxicity	Replacement of manual *in vitro* miconuclei test
Mechanisms of toxicity	Characterize and develop mechanistic understanding of a toxicity
Biomarkers	Translational safety biomarkers (e.g., mitochondrial toxicity can be detected *in vitro* and *in vivo*), phospholipidosis [37]
Cardiotoxicity	Assessment of human cardiotoxicity potential – human embryonic stem cell derived cardiomyocytes and ion and membrane potential dyes (also neurotoxicity, nephrotoxicity, myelotoxicity potential)
Zebrafish, stem cell	Required tool

many pharmaceutical companies already have HCA cytotoxicity assessments. As indicated above, HCA cytotoxicity testing will be tiered and closely associated with other safety assessments, including multiple *in silico* and *in vitro* strategies, such as outlined in Table 14.1, but also with later *in vivo* toleration studies. These drug discovery approaches will lead not only to enhanced detection of human toxicity potential but also to enhanced understanding of the pathophysiological mechanisms by which toxicities occur [38]. For toxicities that must inevitably accompany drug therapy, such as for cancer and infectious diseases, HCA will likely become an indispensable tool for the early detection, monitoring and control of the toxicity using translational safety biomarkers for cytotoxicity [37].

References

1 Kola, I. and Landis, J. (2004) Can the pharmaceutical industry reduce attrition rates? *Nature Reviews. Drug Discovery*, **3**, 711–715.

2 Fung, M., Thornton, A., Mybeck, K., Hsiao-Hui, W., Hornbuckle, K. and Muniz, E. (2001) Evaluation of the characteristics of safety withdrawal of prescription drugs from worldwide pharmaceutical markets – 1960–1999. *Drug Information Journal*, **35**, 293–317.

3 Dykens, J.A. and Will, Y. (2007) The significance of mitochondrial toxicity testing in drug development. *Drug Discovery Today*, **12**, 777–785.

4 O'Brien, P.J., Irwin, W., Diaz, D., Howard-Cofield, E., Krejsa, C.M., Slaughter, M.R., Gao, B., Kaludercic, N. et al. (2006) High concordance of drug-induced human hepatotoxicity with *in vitro* cytotoxicity measured in a novel cell-based model using high content screening. *Archives of Toxicology*, **80**, 580–604.

5 Olson, H., Betton, G., Robinson, D., Thomas, K., Monro, A., Kolaja, G., Lilly, P., Sanders, J. et al. (2000) Concordance of the toxicity of pharmaceuticals in humans and in animals. *Regulatory Toxicology and Pharmacology*, **32**, 56–67.

6 Kramer, J.A., Sagartz, J.E. and Morris, D.L. (2007) The application of discovery toxicology and pathology towards the design of safer pharmaceutical lead candidates. *Nature Reviews. Drug Discovery*, **6**, 637–649.

7 Hughes, J.D., Blagg, J., Price, D.A., Bailey, S., DeCrescenzo, G.A., Devraj, R.V., Ellsworth, E., Fobian, Y.M. et al. (2008) Physiochemical drug properties associated with *in vivo* toxicological outcomes. *Bioorganic and Medicinal Chemistry Letters*, **18** (17), 4872–4875.

8 Muster, W., Breidenbach, A., Fischer, H., Kirchner, S., Muller, L. and Pahler, A. (2008) Computational toxicology in drug development. *Drug Discovery Today*, **13**, 303–310.

9 Spielmann, H., Balls, M., Dupuis, J., Pape, W.J.W., Pechovitch, G., De Silva, O., Holzhütter, H.G., Clothier, R. et al. (1998) EU/COLIPA "*In vitro* phototoxicity" validation study, results of phase II (blind trial), part 1: the 3T3 NRU phototoxicity test. *Toxicology In Vitro: An International Journal Published in Association with BIBRA*, **12**, 305–327.

10 Chen, W.G., Zhang, C., Avery, M.J. and Fouda, H.G. (2001) Reactive metabolite screen for reducing candidate attrition in drug discovery. *Advances in Experimental Medicine and Biology*, **500**, 521–524.

11 Xu, J.J., Diaz, D. and O'Brien, P.J. (2004) Applications of cytotoxicity assays and pre-lethal mechanistic assays for assessment of human hepatotoxicity potential. *Chemico-Biological Interactions*, **150**, 115–128.

12 Pohjala, L., Tammela, P., Samanta, S.K., Yli-Kauhaluoma, J. and Vuorela, P. (2007) Assessing the data quality in predictive toxicology using a panel of cell lines and cytotoxicity assays. *Analytical Biochemistry*, **362**, 221–228.

13 Repetto, G., del Peso, A. and Zurita, J.L. (2008) Neutral red uptake assay for the estimation of cell viability/cytotoxicity. *Nature Protocols*, **3**, 1125–1131.

14 Slaughter, M.R., Thakkar, H. and O'Brien, P.J. (2002) Effect of diquat on the antioxidant system and cell growth in human neuroblastoma cells. *Toxicology and Applied Pharmacology*, **178**, 63–70.

15 Schoonen, W.G.E.J., Westerink, W.M.A., de Roos, J.A.D.M. and Debiton, E. (2005a) Cytotoxic effects of 100 reference compounds on HepG2 and HeLa cells and of 60 compounds on ECC-1 and CHO cells. I. Mechanistic assays on ROS, glutathione depletion and calcein uptake. *Toxicology In Vitro: An International Journal Published in Association with BIBRA*, **19**, 505–516.

16 Schoonen, W.G.E.J., Westerink, W.M.A., de Roos, J.A.D.M. and Debiton, E. Cytotoxic effects of 110 reference compounds on HepG2 and for 60 compounds on HeLa, ECC-1 and CHO cells. I. Mechanistic assays on NAD(P)H, ATP, and DNA contents. *Toxicology In Vitro: An International Journal Published in Association with BIBRA*, (2005b), **19**, 491–503.

17 Miret, S., De Groene, E.M. and Klaffke, W. (2007) Comparison of *in vitro* assays of cellular toxicity in the human hepatic cell line HepG2. *Journal of Biomolecular Screening*, **11**, 184–193.

18 Morelli, J.K., Buehrle, M., Pognan, F., Barone, L.R., Fieles, W. and Ciaccio, P.J. (2006) Validation of an *in vitro* screen for phospholipidosis using a high-content biology platform. *Cell Biology and Toxicology*, **22** (1), 15–27.

19 Davila, J.C., Xu, J.J., Hoffmaster, K.A., O'Brien, P.J. and Storm, S.C. (2007) Chapter 1 Current *in vitro* models to study drug-induced liver injury, in *Hepatotoxicity: From Genomics to In Vitro and In Vivo Models* (ed. S. Sahu), John Wiley & Sons, pp. 3–55.

20 Diaz, D. and O'Brien, P.J. (2006) Defining the sequence of events in cerivastatin toxicity using a high-content multi-parametric cytotoxicity assay. *European Biopharmaceutical Review*, **11**, 38–45.

21 Styles, J.A., Clark, H., Festing, M.F.W. and Rew, D.A. (2001) Automation of mouse micronucleus genotoxicity assay by Laser

Scanning Cytometry. *Cytometry*, **44**, 153–155.

22 Lang, P., Yeow, K., Nichols, A. and Scheer, A. (2006) Cellular imaging in drug discovery. *Nature Reviews: Drug Discovery*, **5**, 343–356.

23 Diaz, D., Scott, A., Carmichael, P., Shi, W. and Costales, C. (2007) Evaluation of an automated *in vitro* micronucleus assay in CHO-K1 cells. *Mutation Research*, **630**, 1–13.

24 Haskins, J.R., Rowse, P., Rahbari, R. and de La Iglesia, F.A. (2001) Thiazolidinedione toxicity to isolated hepatocytes revealed by coherent multiprobe fluorescence microscopy and correlated with multiparameter flow cytometry of peripheral leukocytes. *Archives of Toxicology*, **75**, 425–438.

25 Abraham, V.C., Taylor, L. and Haskins, J.R. (2004) High content screening applied to large-scale cell biology. *Trends in Biotechnology*, **22**, 15–72.

26 Perlman, Z.E., Slack, M.D., Feng, Y., Mitchison, T.J., Wu, L.F. and Altschuler, S.J. (2004) Multidimensional drug profiling by automated microscopy. *Science*, **306**, 1194–1198.

27 Starkuviene, V. and Pepperkok, R. (2007) The potential of high-content high-throughput microscopy in drug discovery. *British Journal of Pharmacology*, **152**, 62–71.

28 Loo, L.-H., Wu, L.-F. and Altschuler, S.J. (2007) Image-based multivariate profiling of drug responses from single cells. *Nature Methods*, **4**, 445–453.

29 Abraham, V.C., Towne, D.L., Waring, J.F., Warrior, U. and Burns, D.J. (2008) Application of a high-content multiparameter cytotoxicity assay to prioritize compounds based on toxicity potential in humans. *Journal of Biomolecular Screening*, **13**, 527–537.

30 Kalgutkar, A.S., Gardner, I., Obach, R.S., Shaffer, C.L., Callegari, E., Henne, K.R., Mutlib, A.E., Dalvie, D.K. *et al.* (2005) A comprehensive listing of bioactivation pathways of organic functional groups. *Current Drug Metabolism*, **6**, 161–225.

31 Kaplowitz, N. (2005) Idiosyncratic drug hepatotoxicity. *Nature Reviews. Drug Discovery*, **4** (6), 489–499.

32 Westerink, W.M.A. and Schoonen, W.G.E.J. (2007) Cytochrome P450 enzyme levels in HepG2 cells and cryopreserved primary human hepatocytes and their induction in HepG2 cells. *Toxicology In Vitro*, **21**, 1581–1591.

33 O'Brien, P.J. (2008) Chapter 13: High content analysis of sublethal cytotoxicity in human HepG2 hepatocytes for assessing potential and mechanism for chemical and drug-induced human toxicity, in *High Content Screening: Science, Techniques and Applications* (ed. S.A. Haney), John Wiley & Sons, Hoboken, NJ, pp. 293–316.

34 O'Brien, P.J., Kalow, B.I., Ali, N., Lassaline, L.A. and Lumsden, J.H. (1990) Compensatory increase in calcium extrusion activity of untreated lymphocytes from swine susceptible to malignant hyperthermia. *American Journal of Veterinary Research*, **51**, 1038–1043.

35 Bugelski, P.J., Atif, U., Molton, S., Toeg, I., Lord, P.G. and Morgan, D.G. (2000) A strategy for primary high throughput cytotoxicity screening in pharmaceutical toxicology. *Pharmaceutical Research*, **17**, 1265–1272.

36 O'Brien, P. and Haskins, J.R. (2007) *In vitro* cytotoxicity assessment. *Methods in Molecular Biology*, **356**, 415–425.

37 O'Brien, P.J. and Domingos, M.C. (2009) Use of high content analysis in toxicologic clinical pathology for identification and monitoring of translational safety biomarkers. *American Drug Discovery* (in press).

38 Houck, K.A. and Kavlock, R.J. (2008) Understanding mechanisms of toxicity: insights from drug discovery research. *Toxicology and Applied Pharmacology*, **227** (2), 163–178.

15
Predicting Drug-Induced Hepatotoxicity: In Vitro, In Silico and In Vivo Approaches

Jinghai J. Xu, Amit S. Kalgutkar, Yvonne Will, James Dykens, Elizabeth Tengstrand, and Frank Hsieh

15.1
Introduction

Hepatotoxicity is a frequent cause of drug candidate failure and contributes to the length and attrition rate of the drug discovery and development process [1]. Drug-induced liver injury or DILI, is the most common reason for postmarketing regulatory actions by the United States Food and Drug Administration (FDA) [2]. Benoxaprofen, bromfenac and troglitazone were withdrawn from the market following reports of rare but severe hepatotoxicity. Strong warning labels of possible adverse hepatic reactions are provided for acetaminophen, felbamate, ketoconazole, leflunomide, nefazodone, nevirapine, pemoline, pyrazinamide, rifampin, terbinafine, tolcapone, valproic acid and zafirlukast [3]. Early predictive technologies including mechanism-based assays, predictive algorithms, and biomarkers for drug-induced hepatotoxicity that could help reduce the risk of hepatotoxicity before it occurs in the clinic is a critical need for the successful development of future pharmaceuticals. In the hit-to-lead stage of the drug discovery process, a better rationale in compound selection to improve success rates regarding hepatic safety is the topic of this chapter.

Liver injury is clinically defined as an increase of serum alanine amino transferase (ALT) levels of more than three times the upper limit of normal and a total bilirubin level of more than twice the upper limit of normal [4]. The clinical patterns of liver injury can be characterized as hepatocellular (with a predominant initial elevation of ALT), cholestatic (with an initial elevation of alkaline phosphatase) or mixed. The mechanisms of drug-induced hepatotoxicity include excessive generation of reactive metabolites, mitochondrial dysfunction, oxidative stress and inhibition of bile salt efflux protein [5]. Better understandings of these mechanisms in the past decades led to the development of assays and models suitable for studying such toxic mechanisms and for selecting better leads in the drug discovery stage.

Hit and Lead Profiling. Edited by Bernard Faller and Laszlo Urban
Copyright © 2009 WILEY-VCH Verlag GmbH & Co. KGaA, Weinheim
ISBN: 978-3-527-32331-9

15.2
Reactive Metabolites

The concept of drug metabolism to electrophilic reactive intermediates that covalently modify proteins and/or DNA leading to toxicity in a manner similar to procarcinogens was first demonstrated in the 1970s with the anti-inflammatory agent acetaminophen by Brodie et al. at the National Institutes of Health [6–8]. The finding that cytochrome P450-mediated bioactivation of acetaminophen to a reactive quinone-imine intermediate (NAPQI) [9], capable of depleting levels of the endogenous anti-oxidant glutathione (GSH) and binding covalently to liver macromolecules has served as a paradigm for drug toxicity assessment over the decades. It is important to make a distinction upfront between agents that exhibit dose-dependent and dose-independent hepatotoxicity. The hepatotoxic effects of acetaminophen in humans are dose-dependent and can be replicated in animals. In contrast, drugs such as troglitazone causes non-dose-dependent hepatotoxicity with a rare incidence of about 1 per 1000 patient-years [10].

While the downstream consequences of reactive metabolite formation as it relates to hepatotoxicity (in particular its idiosyncratic nature) are poorly understood, several hypotheses are proposed to explain this phenomenon. The basic hypothesis that links bioactivation with toxicity is the process of haptenization wherein low molecular weight (<1000 Da) drugs/reactive metabolites are converted to immunogens via binding to high molecular weight carrier biomacromolecules [11]. The best understood idiosyncratic adverse reactions are β-lactam-induced anaphylactic reactions. It is clear that specific immunoglobulin (IgE) antibodies against β-lactams such as penicillin mediate these reactions [12]. The haptenization process involves non-enzymatic β-lactam ring scission by cysteinyl and/or terminal lysine residue(s) in proteins, leading to the acylation of these amino acid nucleophiles [13]. Some examples of drugs associated with haptenization include the hepatotoxins halothane [14], tienilic acid [15] and dihydralazine [16], all of which are bioactivated to reactive metabolites. Interestingly, antibodies detected in sera of patients exposed to these drugs specifically recognize cytochrome P450 isozymes that are responsible for the bioactivation of these drugs and also are targets for covalent adduction [15, 17].

Several risk factors are also proposed to explain the idiosyncratic nature of drug-induced toxicity, of which genetic variability is perhaps the most important one. For example, polymorphism of the N-acetyltransferase 2 gene differentiates fast from slow acetylators; the latter have increased susceptibility to toxicity of certain aniline-containing drugs such as isoniazid, sulfamethoxazole and procainamide [18]. The major route of elimination of these drugs in humans involves N-acetylation of the aniline moiety by NAT2. In a NAT2-deficient population, the aniline functionality is biotransformed by P450 enzymes to yield cytotoxic and reactive metabolites that covalently adduct with GSH and/or proteins [19]. Genetic polymorphisms in glutathione-S-transferase (GST) isozymes, which catalyze GSH conjugation to reactive metabolites, are also considered risk factors for hepatotoxicity caused by several drugs [20]. It is possible that patients deficient in GST isozymes are most at risk towards liver injury because of ineffective scavenging of the reactive metabolites derived from the oxidative bioactivation of these drugs. There is also a strong possibility that components of ingested foods including herbal supplements can modulate drug metabolism and therefore increase the risk of hepatotoxicity. For example, chronic alcohol abuse increases the risk of acetaminophen hepatotoxicity by inducing P4502E1, which predominantly catalyzes acetaminophen bioactivation to NAPQI [21].

15.2.1
Assays and *In Silico* Knowledge to Assess Bioactivation Potential

Whether bioactivation will occur for any given molecule *in vivo* depends on three key factors: (i) does the molecule possess a functionality and/or chemical architecture (referred to as structural alert/toxicophore) that is susceptible to bioactivation; (ii) is there an alternative (higher affinity but innocuous) route of metabolism within the molecule that minimizes the potential bioactivation of the toxicophore; (iii) are there parallel competing detoxification pathways that scavenge the reactive metabolite or its precursor. The presence or absence of a structural alert/toxicophore can be inspected visually or via the use of DEREK software. DEREK for Windows is a knowledge-based expert system that predicts the toxicity of a chemical from its structure. Its predictions are based in part on alerts that describe structural features or toxicophores associated with toxicity [22]. To date, there are no *in silico* tools that have been successfully utilized to predict the occurrence of a bioactivation pathway (and ensuing toxicity) with a drug candidate. While *in silico* tools such as MetaSite have been used to predict metabolic pathways of drug candidates with some success [23], the utility of such software in predicting bioactivation has not been exploited in drug discovery, partly due to lack of validation of such an approach. Electrochemical tools are used to mimic oxidative drug metabolism, including the formation of reactive metabolites [24]. However, this approach requires experimental validation.

15.2.1.1 *In Vitro* Reactive Metabolite Trapping Studies
With the possible exception of some acyl glucuronides and cyclic iminium ions, most reactive metabolites are generally short-lived and are not usually detectable in circulation. Therefore, qualitative *in vitro* assessment of reactive metabolite formation involves "trapping" studies conducted with hepatocytes or NADPH-supplemented human liver microsomes or S-9 fractions and GSH. Analysis of the resulting metabolites by liquid chromatography–tandem mass spectrometry and NMR spectroscopy is employed for structural elucidation of GSH conjugates, which in turn provides insight into the reactive metabolite structure. The presence of the soft nucleophilic sulfydryl group in GSH ensures efficient conjugation with soft electrophilic centers (e.g., Michael acceptors, epoxides, arene oxides, alkyl halides), yielding stable sulfydryl conjugates [25, 26]. It is noteworthy to point out that not all reactive metabolites can be trapped with GSH. Hard electrophiles including DNA-reactive metabolites (e.g., electrophilic carbonyl compounds) preferentially react with hard nucleophiles such as amines (e.g., semicarbazide and methoxylamine), amino acids (e.g., lysine) and DNA bases (e.g., guanine and cytosine) [27]. Likewise, the cyanide

anion is a "hard" nucleophile that can be used to trap electrophilic iminium species that are generated via metabolism of tertiary amines [28].

15.2.1.2 Covalent Binding Determinations

Quantitative assessment of the amount of *in vitro* metabolism-dependent covalent binding to hepatic tissue (e.g., liver microsomes, S-9, hepatocytes) is possible if radiolabeled drug is available [29]. The assay, however, does not provide information about the nature of covalently modified macromolecules. Covalent binding studies can also be performed *in vivo*. Either tissue or blood/plasma can be examined for the degree of covalent binding. However, covalent binding may require multiple dosing to establish the true impact of the compound. Reactive metabolites formed after the first dose may be efficiently trapped by GSH and eliminated from the body. Once GSH is depleted, the extent of covalent binding with cellular macromolecules may increase rapidly, resulting in toxicity.

15.2.2
Utility of Reactive Metabolite Trapping and Covalent Binding Studies in Drug Discovery

Reactive metabolite trapping and/or covalent binding studies can provide valuable insights into the bioactivation pathway(s) of drugs associated with toxicity. Such studies can influence the rational design of successor drug candidates devoid of the bioactivation liability, as illustrated with the anticonvulsant felbamate. Evidence linking felbamate bioactivation to its life-threatening hepatotoxicity and aplastic anemia has been presented by means of *in vivo* characterization of mercapturic acid (downstream metabolites of GSH) conjugates of a highly reactive α β-unsaturated carbonyl derivative 2-phenylpropenal following felbamate administration to rats and human [30]. A mechanism consistent with the conversion of felbamate to 2-phenylpropenal is depicted in Scheme 15.1 and involves esterase-mediated hydrolysis of one of its carbamate groups to afford the primary alcohol metabolite, oxidation of which by alcohol dehydrogenase to the intermediate aldehyde derivative followed by spontaneous β-elimination of the remaining carbamoyl group generates 2-phenylpropenal. Based on this information, fluorofelbamate was specifically designed to eliminate the bioactivation liability of felbamate. Fluorofelbamate does not succumb to bioactivation because the fluorine atom prevents the β-elimination process which leads to the reactive 2-phenylpropenal [31]. Whether absence of bioactivation translates into a reduced risk of idiosyncratic hepatotoxicity or aplastic anaemia remains to be seen. Fluorofelbamate is currently undergoing clinical trials as an anti-epileptic agent [32].

15.2.3
Are Reactive Metabolite Trapping and Covalent Binding Studies Reliable Predictors of Hepatotoxic Potential of Drug Candidates?

While the detection of adducts (GSH, amino, and/or cyano) and covalent binding to hepatic tissue is indicative of the formation of reactive metabolites, the data need to be placed in proper context prior to making a decision on discarding a drug candidate

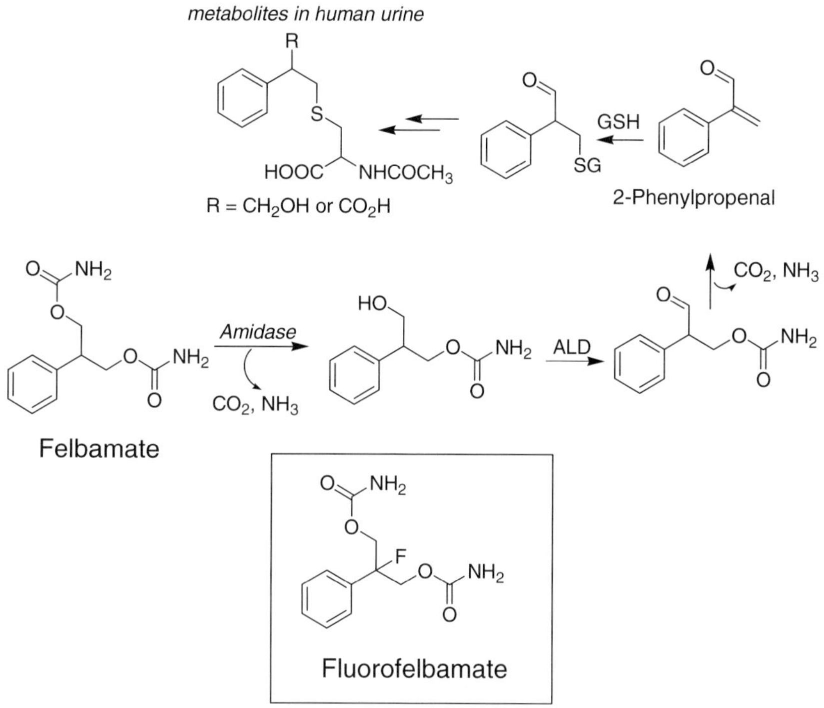

Scheme 15.1 Postulated bioactivation pathways of the anticonvulsant agent felbamate: rational chemical approach to circumvent bioactivation by fluorofelbamate.

associated with this liability. First and foremost, a drug candidate that is devoid of reactive metabolite formation and/or covalent binding to proteins is not a guarantee of its safety. Drugs that mediate toxicity via non-P450-mediated reactive metabolite formation does not display a positive response in assays routinely designed to support a P450-mediated bioactivation process. For instance, despite the *in vivo* observations on felbamate bioactivation, evidence for the *in vitro* metabolism of felbamate to the reactive metabolite 2-phenylpropenal in human hepatic tissue is lacking. At therapeutically relevant concentrations of radiolabeled felbamate incubations with human liver microsomes and human hepatocytes *in vitro*, no GSH adducts (Kalgutkar, unpublished data) and/or covalent binding of felbamate has been discerned [33]. While the reason(s) for this discrepancy remain unclear, in a drug discovery paradigm relying solely on reactive metabolite trapping and liver microsomal covalent binding as means of predicting toxicity potential of drug candidates, felbamate would pass the hurdle with flying colors.

While covalent binding studies have an advantage over the reactive metabolite assay in that they provide a quantitative estimate of covalently bound drug to proteins and therefore an indirect measure of reactive metabolite formation, there are no studies to date which show a correlation between the extent of covalent binding and/or reactive metabolite formed and the probability that a drug is associated with a high incidence of hepatotoxicity. There are numerous examples of blockbuster drugs that are false positives in these assays; that is, they form GSH conjugates and display a degree of protein covalent modification, yet are not associated with a significant incidence of toxicity. The retrospective analysis of the bioactivation potential of the commercial blockbuster drug and selective serotonin reuptake inhibitor paroxetine serves as a notable example of this phenomenon [34]. The NADPH-dependent covalent binding of [^{3}H]-paroxetine to human liver microsomes and liver S-9 fractions is consistent with a bioactivation pathway involving P4502D6-mediated demethylenation of the 1,3-benzdioxozole group in paroxetine to a catechol metabolite followed by two-electron oxidation of this intermediate to reactive ortho-quinonoid intermediates. The characterization of the GSH conjugates of paroxetine-catechol lends credence to this hypothesis

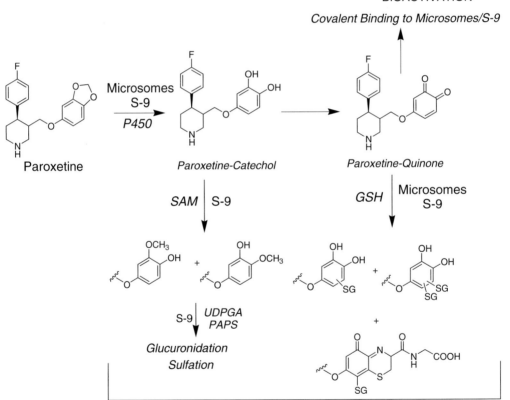

Scheme 15.2 Parallel detoxication pathways that compete with the P450-catalyzed bioactivation pathway of the antidepressant paroxetine as explanation for its wide safety margin.

(Scheme 15.2). Thus, paroxetine fulfills all the obligatory requirements of a molecule prone to bioactivation, and in the absence of any additional metabolism data, such an isolated finding could be interpreted as being a harbinger of a potential toxicological response in the clinic. However, despite decades of clinical use, life-threatening ADRs (e.g., hepatotoxicity) are rarely noted with paroxetine. Plausible reason(s) for this anomaly can be gauged from the additional experimental findings wherein addition of GSH and catechol-O-methyltransferase cofactor S-adenosylmethionine (SAM) to the microsomal and/or S-9 incubations results in a dramatic reduction of covalent binding. The finding that GSH drastically reduces covalent binding of paroxetine is analogous to the case of acetaminophen, where hepatotoxicity is only observed at supra-therapeutic doses (>4 g/day) believed to exceed the capacity of the liver to form GSH adducts with the reactive NAPQI intermediate. The amount of ortho-quinone formed *in vivo* after administration of paroxetine at its daily dose of 20 mg/day may be readily handled by the liver's pool of GSH. In addition, reduction in covalent binding to S-9 in the presence of S-adenosylmethionine is consistent with the known metabolic pathway of paroxetine in humans involving O-methylation of the paroxetine-catechol metabolite to the corresponding guaiacol regioisomers (Scheme 15.2). Overall, the results of these studies indicate that its low daily dose and the efficient scavenging of the catechol and quinone metabolites by S-adenosylmethionine and GSH, respectively, serve as potential explanations for the excellent safety record of paroxetine despite undergoing bioactivation.

15.2.4
Mitigating Factors Against Hepatotoxicity Risks Due to Bioactivation – a Balanced Approach Towards Candidate Selection in Drug Discovery

The availability of methodology to assess bioactivation potential of drugs clearly aided the replacement of a vague perception of a chemical class effect with a sharper picture of individual molecular peculiarity. Information to qualify certain functional groups as structural alerts/toxicophores (Figure 15.1) also was inferred from such studies based on numerous examples of drugs containing these motifs which are bioactivated to reactive metabolites and are associated with various forms of toxicity [25, 26]. There are myriad examples of drugs that are hepatotoxic for which bioactivation mechanisms have been described using reactive metabolite-trapping and/or covalent-binding studies (Figure 15.1).

For many of the drugs associated with hepatotoxicity, there are examples of structurally related drugs which are latent to bioactivation and toxicity because of the absence of the toxicophore or the existence of alternate metabolic pathways. For example, the hepatotoxicity associated with the use of the anti-Parkinson's agent tolcapone does not occur with the structurally related drug entacapone, despite administration at doses similar to tolcapone (200–1000 mg QD). This disparity may be explained in part by the observation that entacapone does not succumb to the bioactivation reactions of tolcapone in humans (Scheme 15.3) [35]. It is also noteworthy that tolcapone but not entacapone is a potent uncoupler of oxidative

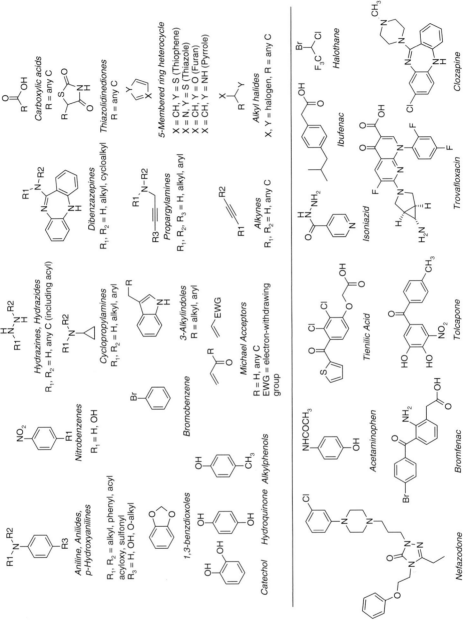

Figure 15.1 Compilation of structural alerts/toxicophores known to undergo bioactivation and examples of hepatotoxic drugs containing the structural alerts.

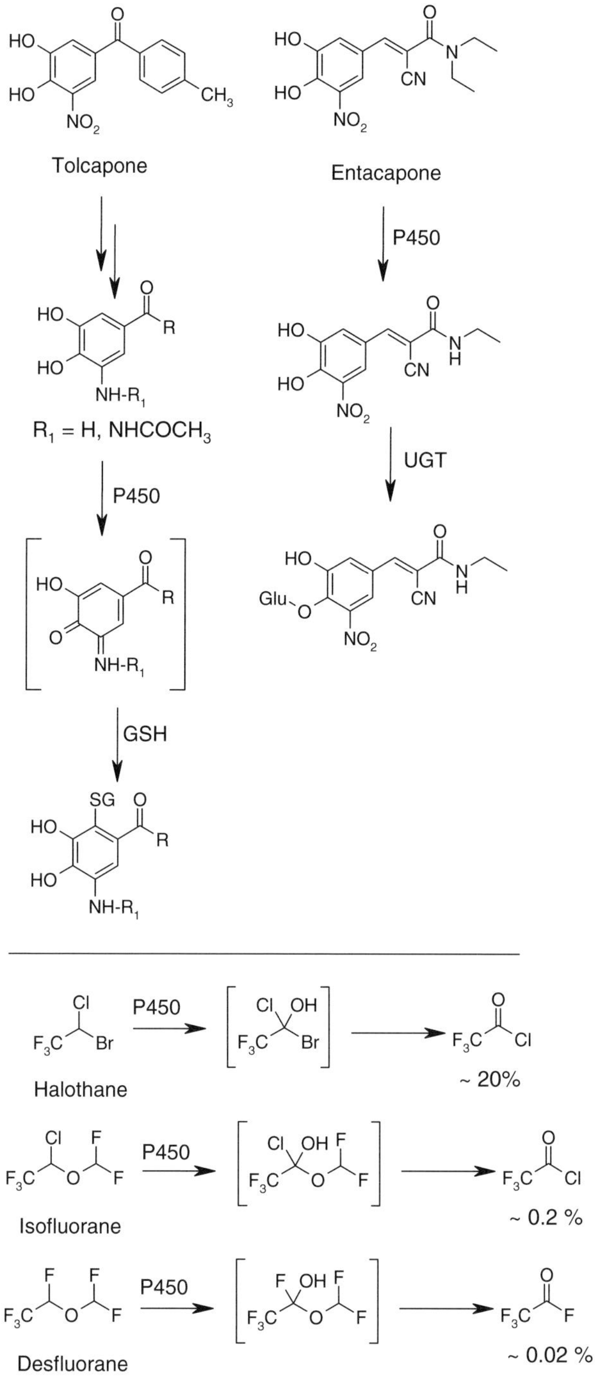

Scheme 15.3 Examples of structure–toxicity relationships.

phosphorylation both *in vitro* and *in vivo* [36]. Thus, in combination with the bioactivation phenomenon, disruption of mitochondrial function by tolcapone may serve as a viable explanation for the differential toxicological response.

An additional example is evident with the inhaled anesthetics. In susceptible patients, halothane, isoflurane and desflurane can produce severe hepatic injury by an immune response directed against reactive acyl halides covalently bound to hepatic biomacromolecules. The relative incidence of hepatotoxicity due to these agents correlates directly with the extent of their conversion to acyl halides by P450, which in turn may be governed by the leaving group ability of the respective substituents within these drugs. As shown in Scheme 15.3, halothane, which exhibits the greatest incidence of hepatotoxicity in the clinic, undergoes the most conversion to reactive acyl chloride, a feature that can be attributed to the presence of bromide substituent, which is a good leaving group. In contrast, isofluorane and desfluorane also undergo oxidative metabolism, resulting in the formation of reactive acyl halides, but the degree to which these anesthetics are bioactivated is significantly lower than halothane [37]. Such a chemical mechanism-based structure–activity relationship (SAR) can be applied during the early drug design and lead identification stage to select safer compounds for further development.

Overall, these examples imply that, by avoiding toxicophores in drug design, one would lessen the odds that a drug candidate will lead to toxicity via a bioactivation mechanism. However, rather than randomly applying such a conservative approach in drug discovery, it is pivotal to consider the above-mentioned factors (alternate metabolic or detoxication pathways) that influence the bioactivation potential for any given molecule. In addition, the daily dose also needs to be considered as a mitigating factor. To the best of our knowledge, there are no examples of drugs dosed at <20 mg/day that caused idiosyncratic adverse effects (whether or not these agents are prone to bioactivation). There are many examples of two structurally related drugs that possess identical toxicophore susceptible to bioactivation, but the one administered at the lower dose is safer than the one given at a higher dose. It is likely that the improved safety of low-dose drugs arises from a marked reduction in the total body burden to reactive metabolite exposure and therefore is unlikely to exceed the threshold needed for toxicity. An illustration of this phenomenon is evident with the anti-diabetic thiazolidinedione (TZD) drugs: troglitazone (Rezulin), rosiglitazone and pioglitazone. Troglitazone was withdrawn from the United States market after numerous reported cases of liver failures requiring immediate liver transplantation or leading to death. In contrast, rosiglitazone and pioglitazone are devoid of much of the hepatotoxicity associated with troglitazone. *In vitro*, troglitazone is bioactivated on its chromane and TZD rings by P4503A4 in NADPH- and GSH-supplemented human liver microsomes, generating several GSH conjugates (Scheme 15.4) [38]. While rosiglitazone and pioglitazone do not contain the chromane ring system found in troglitazone, they do contain the TZD scaffold, which is cleaved to reactive metabolites in a manner similar to troglitazone [39]. While bioactivation of the TZD ring is a common theme in these drugs, a key difference lies in their daily doses – troglitazone (200–400 mg/day) versus rosiglitazone and pioglitazone (<10 mg/day). This factor may offset the bioactivation liability, resulting in an improved safety

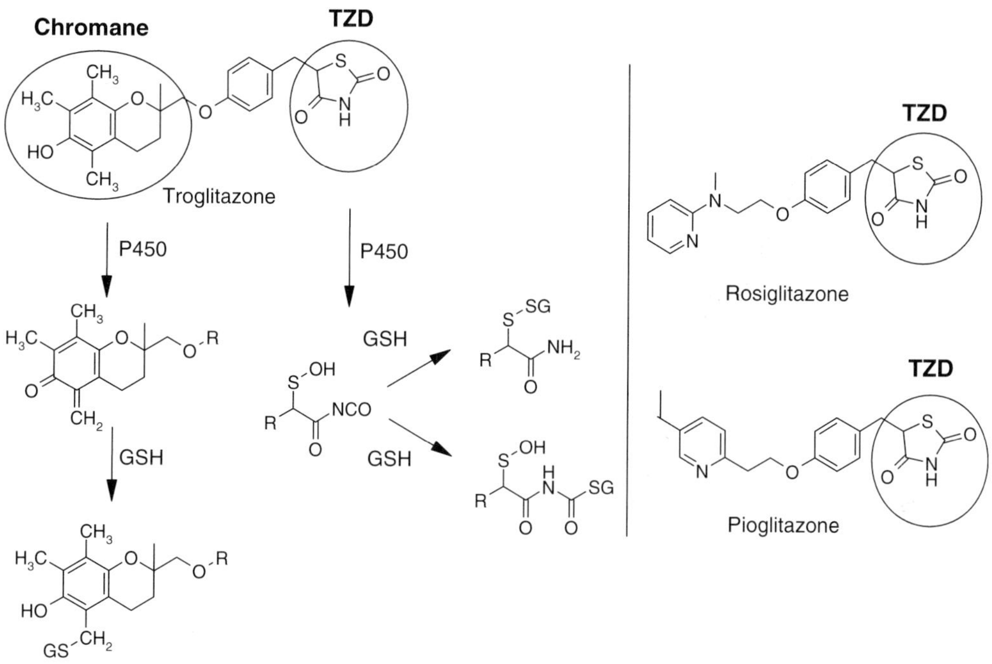

Scheme 15.4 P450-Mediated bioactivation of the thiazolidinedione class of anti-diabetic agents.

profile for the successor agents. Thus SAR modeling effort must take a more holistic approach, that is, predicting not only which functional groups to avoid but also which groups to add to enhance drug potency and bioavailability.

15.2.5
Future Directions

Although much has been learned about the chemistry of reactive metabolite formation and reactivity toward protein nucleophiles, progress in identifying critical protein targets for reactive metabolites of various protoxins has been much slower. Towards this end, proteomics may provide some insights into the identification of protein targets with structurally diverse reactive metabolites. With increasing numbers of target proteins becoming known, more commonality in targeting by reactive metabolites from diverse chemical agents may be discerned. Such commonality may help to separate toxicologically significant covalent-binding events from a background of covalent binding that is toxicologically inconsequential. Idiosyncratic hepatotoxicity is too complex to duplicate in a test tube and the idiosyncratic nature by itself precludes both prospective clinical studies and the development of animal models of hepatotoxicity. Since genetic factors appear to have a crucial role in the induction of hepatotoxic response, a fruitful approach may therefore lie in focused and well controlled phenotype/genotype studies of the rare patients who survive this type of injury. For instance, results of single nucleotide polymorphism (SNP) analysis in patients associated with abacavir hypersensitivity reaction suggest that the known HLA-B gene region could be identified with as few as 15 cases and 200 population controls in a sequential analysis [40]. Until we develop a better understanding of the risk of toxicity arising from the formation of reactive metabolites, a strategy for identifying and minimizing their formation seems appropriate. The bioactivation potential of a new drug candidate or chemical series should be investigated as early as possible, preferentially during the lead optimization stage. The information from such an analysis will provide insights into the structural features within molecules that lead to reactive metabolite formation. This information can be then used in the subsequent design of analogs devoid of bioactivation issue. In practice, attempts to eliminate bioactivation liability in a rational fashion is by no means a trivial exercise; structural alterations that successfully eliminate the propensity of new chemical leads to undergo bioactivation can also confer a detrimental effect on the desired pharmacological (possible changes in agonist/antagonist behavior and/or subtype selectivity for target receptor or enzyme) and pharmacokinetic attributes. It is very important to emphasize that bioactivation is only one aspect of the overall risk/benefit assessment for advancing a drug candidate into development. Consequently, data from reactive metabolite trapping and covalent binding studies need to be placed in a proper and broader context with previously discussed factors such as the daily dose and alternate routes of metabolism/detoxication. Likewise, appropriate consideration needs to be given for drug candidates for potential treatment options for unmet and urgent medical needs.

15.3
Mitochondrial Toxicity

There is compelling evidence that mitochondrial dysfunction contributes to drug-induced liver injury (DILI) [41, 42]. This rapidly evolving field is yielding novel models of organ toxicity where mitochondrial dysfunction can be caused either by the parent molecule, or by a reactive metabolite and where drugs of many important classes can undermine mitochondrial function via direct and indirect effects [43]. The former arise acutely via direct interference with mitochondrial function and the latter arise over longer periods via interference with mitochondrial transcription/translation and/or acceleration of free radical production. Much progress has been made in understanding the different mechanisms that can cause mitochondrial dysfunction [44–46] and the current state of this area has been reviewed [47].

Mitochondria generate 95% of the cell's energy. This occurs in the electron transport chain, which contains four oxidative phosphorylation (OXPHOS) complexes and an ATPase that phosphorylates ADP to ATP. Normally, the respiratory system is coupled with proton translocation that generates a steep voltage difference across the inner membrane, typically 220 mV, inside negative. Maintaining and capitalizing on this potential energy depends on the impermeability of the inner membrane to protons. As such, inner membrane contains a host of specific exchange carriers for respiratory substrates, inorganic phosphate, ADP and ATP.

Oxidizible substrates from glycolysis, fatty acid or protein catabolism enter the mitochondrion in the form of acetyl-CoA, or as other intermediaries of the Krebs cycle, which resides within the mitochondrial matrix. Reducing equivalents in the form of NADH and FADH pass electrons to complex I (NADH-ubiquinone oxidoreductase) or complex II (succinate dehydrogenase) of the electron transport chain, respectively. Electrons pass from complex I and II to complex III (ubiquinol–cytochrome c oxidoreductase) and then to complex IV (cytochrome c oxidase) which accumulates four electrons and then tetravalently reduces O_2 to water. Protons are pumped into the inner membrane space at complexes I, II and IV and then diffuse down their concentration gradient through complex V (F_0F_1-ATPase), where their potential energy is captured in the form of ATP. In this way, ATP formation is coupled to electron transport and the formation of water, a process termed oxidative phosphorylation (OXPHOS).

Under ideal circumstances, all the electrons entering electron transport system (ETS) tetravalently reduce oxygen to water at complex IV. However, electrons can "leak" from several sites along ETS, predominantly complexes I and III and ubiquinone, resulting in univalent reduction of O_2 to form the superoxide radical O_2^- which can spontaneously dismutate to form hydrogen peroxide H_2O_2, or more rapidly dismutate in the reaction catalyzed by superoxide dismutase (SOD). Indeed, mitochondria contain SOD activity based on Mn that is quite different from the cytosolic and extracellular Cu/Zn enzyme. In the presence of transition metal cations, particularly Fe^{2+} and Cu^+, hydrogen peroxide reacts non-enzymatically in the Fenton reaction, yielding the extremely reactive hydroxyl radical $HO^\bullet$. Estimates of ETS superoxide production vary over 1–6%, but it is clear that such reactive oxygen species (ROS) production increases when ETS is blocked "downstream" of the sites capable of auto-oxidizing; and many drugs and other xenobiotics elicit this reaction.

Mitochondria also produce reactive nitrogen species (RNS) such as nitric oxide; and the ensuing chemistry when ROS and RNS interact is complex [48]. Despite high reactivity and potential cellular injury or death, mitochondrial ROS and RNS also function as signaling molecules to modulate ETS reversibly [49]. All aero-tolerant cells maintain a suite of antioxidant mechanisms to moderate ROS, thereby moderating oxidative stress and preventing subsequent cell injury or death, via either necrotic or apoptotic pathways. Among others, these include low molecular weight antioxidants such as vitamin C, vitamin E and the enzymatic systems to regenerate antioxidant potential, reduced pyridine nucleotides NADH and NADPH, as well as reduced glutathione (GSH). Importantly, normal mitochondrial GSH exceeds cytosolic levels, underscoring the importance of antioxidant potential there.

Much progress has been made in understanding the different mechanisms that can cause mitochondrial dysfunction, such as: (i) uncoupling of electron transport from ATP synthesis by undermining integrity of inner membrane; (ii) direct inhibition of electron transport system components; (iii) opening of the mitochondrial permeability transition pore leading to irreversible collapse of the transmembrane potential and release of pro-apoptotic factors; (iv) inhibition of the mitochondrial DNA polymerase, thereby depleting mtDNA-encoded key proteins; (v) inhibition of fatty acid β-oxidation or depletion of CoA. Less often targeted by drugs, but equally important, are the following: (i) inhibition of the Krebs cycle; (ii) inhibition of mitochondrial transporters; (iii) intramitochondrial oxidative stress caused by redox-cycling drugs, glutathione depletion and reactive metabolites. Selected examples for mechanisms i–v are discussed below.

15.3.1
Uncouplers of Mitochondrial Respiration

In functional mitochondria, the flow of electrons is accompanied by the extrusion of protons from the mitochondrial matrix into the intermembrane space, generating a transmembrane potential. The flow of electrons (also called respiration) increases or decreases to maintain this potential. Acidic compounds and carboxylic acids can facilitate re-entry of the protons from the intermembrane space that circumvents generation of ATP leading to an increase in respiration; respiration is no longer coupled to ATP generation. Such uncoupling is induced by many non-steroidal anti-inflammatory drugs (NSAIDS), including nimesulide, diclofenac, indomethacin, piroxicam and meloxicam [50]. The nitrocatechol drug tolcapone, which was used to treat Parkinson's Disease, also uncouples oxidative phosphorylation; and it was withdrawn from the Canadian and European markets in 1998 because of unacceptably high incidence of hepatic failure. It remains on the United States market with severely limited usage, as mandated by the FDA [36, 51].

15.3.2
Drugs that Inhibit OXPHOS Complexes

The antihyperlipidemic drugs, such as clofibrate, fenofibrate, bezafibrate, ciprofibrate and gemfibrozil are associated with liver toxicity and hepatomegaly in some patients. Fenofibrate inhibits complex I and to lesser extent complex V, whereas clofibrate inhibits predominantly complex V. Gemfibrozil also inhibits complex I, even more potently than fenofibrate [52, 53].

Another class of compounds that directly inhibits electron transport are the biguanidines, including metformin, buformin and phenformin, which were developed for the management of hyperglycaemia in type 2 diabetes mellitus patients. The side effects of these drugs include gastrointestinal symptoms and lactic acidosis, the latter causing market withdrawal of phenformin in 1977 and buformin in 1978. In contrast, metformin was found to cause 20-fold less lactic acidosis than phenformin. The antidiabetic effect of these biguanides as well as the lactic acidosis have been attributed to complex I inhibition [54]. However, this effect occurs only at supra-pharmacological concentrations and/or only after preincubation of isolated mitochondria, suggesting that bioaccumulation of metformin driven by membrane potential could be increasing its localized concentration. Indeed, with a membrane potential of -180 mV, thermodynamic considerations would predict a 1000-fold accumulation of metformin within the mitochondria.

However, such complex I inhibition would be self-limiting, as the accumulating metformin would decrease the mitochondrial potential and so moderate further metformin uptake, unless complex II fuels are present to bypass complex I impairment [55].

The thiazolidinediones, such as pioglitazone, rosiglitzone, darglitazone, ciglitazone and troglitazone, are thought to improve insulin sensitivity and lower blood glucose levels via activation of the peroxisome proliferator-activated receptor (PPAR). Troglitazone was withdrawn due to idiosyncratic hepatotoxicity in 1997. Brunnmair et al. [52] reported complex I inhibition at 100 µM in liver homogenates by troglitazone, rosiglitazone, and to a lesser amount, by pioglitazone. This was corroborated by Nadanaciva et al. [53], who noted that more potent targets for the thiazolidinediones are complexes IV and V.

Flutamide, an antiprostate cancer drug, is another example where inhibition of ETS, primarily at complex I, is associated with hepatotoxicity [56, 57]. Nefazodone, an antidepressant, also inhibits complex I activity and was discontinued in 2004 due to idiosyncratic hepatotoxicity [58].

15.3.3
Drugs that Induce the Mitochondrial Permeability Transition Pore (MPT)

The MPT is defined as a sudden non-selective increase in the permeability of the inner mitochondrial membrane to solutes <1500 Da. This collapses the mitochondrial membrane potential and results in osmotic organelle swelling that can lead to rupture of the outer membrane. The MPT is composed of multiple proteins, some integral to the inner membrane, such as the adenine translocase (ANT), or the outer membrane, such as the voltage gated anion channel (VDAC). Discussion continues as to which proteins comprise the pore versus those that serve regulatory roles, but it is clear that inhibition of cyclosporine A is pathomnemonic [59]. MPT formation is potentiated by free radicals and excess Ca^{2+} influx into the mitochondria and repressed by ATP and a host of xenobiotics including the thistle toxin atractyloside.

Betulinic acid, an anticancer drug, the NSAID diclofenac and the cyclo-oxygenase 2 inhibitor nimesulide have all been shown to trigger MPT, leading to hepatotoxicity. In addition to its effects on OXPHOS, troglitazone has also been shown to induce MPT [41].

15.3.4
Drugs Inhibiting mtDNA Synthesis and Mitochondrial Protein Synthesis

Mitochondria contain the only extranuclear genomic DNA (mtDNA) and it encodes 13 proteins using a genetic code different from that in the nucleus. These proteins are key components of OXPHOS I, III, IV and V, but not complex II, which is solely encoded by nuclear DNA (nuDNA). Inhibition of mtDNA transcription as well as expression of mitochondrial proteins will therefore lead to loss of OXPHOS function. Probably the best known drugs that inhibit mtDNA synthesis are the nucleotide reverse transcriptase inhibitors (NRTIs), such as zalcitabine, didanosine and stavudine, all of which cause hepatic DNA depletion. Zidovudine also occasionally causes liver toxicity [60, 61]. Inhibition of mitochondrial protein synthesis was impaired by antibiotics, including erythromycins and chloramphenicol, members of the oxazolidinones among others, which block protein translation by binding to mitochondrial ribosomes [62, 63].

15.3.5
Inhibition of Fatty Acid β-Oxidation or Depletion of CoA

Impairment of mitochondrial β-oxidation leads to accumulation of fat, resulting in steatosis. Examples are various tetracycline derivatives, valproic acid (used to treat seizures) and overdoses of aspirin [64–66]. Certain NSAIDs such as ibuprofen, ketoprofen and naproxen also have the ability to inhibit β-oxidation [67–69].

It is important to mention at this point that most drugs have more than one mechanism of impairing mitochondrial function. For example, troglitazone not only inhibits the OXPHOS complexes IV and V but also induces MPT.

15.3.6
In Vitro and *In Vivo* Assessment of Drug-Induced Mitochondrial Dysfunction

Drugs that impair mitochondrial replication, either via inhibition of DNA replication or protein expression, gradually erode the aerobic capacity until a critical bioenergetic threshold is reached, whereupon cell viability is imperiled. Similarly, drugs that directly and acutely impair mitochondrial function evoke the same pathology, albeit over different time scales, depending on potency and the tissue that is affected. If widespread within a given organ, such losses of viability or diminished capacity for cell stress response and the resulting pathology eventually becomes apparent systemically. For example, to compensate for diminished aerobic OXPHOS capacity, cells accelerate carbon flux though glycolysis, thereby generating lactate. As such, regardless of whether the impairment is caused by repression of function or biomass, one of the hallmark symptoms of mitochondrial dysfunction is elevated serum lactate and this, for example, led to the withdrawal of phenformin and buformin from the market in 1977–1978. Although an elevated lactate level is a late-stage index of mitochondrial failure, it still provides clinical insight and can help monitor HAART treatment against AIDS [70], whether alone or in combination therapies [71].

Similarly, monitoring the amount of mtDNA, usually via the mtDNA:nuDNA ratio [72], provides a more sensitive index of diminishing mitochondrial biomass and much of this work focuses on peripheral blood samples because they are readily available. In fibroblasts treated with ddC for 4 weeks, mtDNA dropped by 80% within the first week and the lactate/pyruvate ratio lagged behind, but was pathologically elevated after 3 weeks. A 4-week wash-out treatment then showed that mtDNA returned to 90% of the initial value within 3 weeks and lactate/pyruvate ratio gradually normalized over 4 weeks. It bears reiteration in this context that elevated glucose in many cell culture media engenders aerobic glycolysis and correspondingly reduces reliance on OXPHOS, which may be one reason why lactate/pyruvate ratios do not track with mtDNA more tightly. Nevertheless, similar patterns are seen in the clinic where mtDNA in peripheral blood mononuclear cells (PBMCs) declined prior to increases in serum lactate and discontinuation of antiretroviral therapy leads to a statistically significant increase in the ratio of mitochondrial to nuclear DNA [72].

Comparison studies in HepG2 cells indicate that the potency of the NRTIs to reduce mtDNA varies, with ddC > ddI > d4T > AZT > ABC = 3TC = TDF [73]; and this is in accord with their observed toxicity in the clinic. It should also be noted that HIV infection per se also significantly lowered mtDNA in PMBCs independent of NRTI exposures [74].

Recent advances in antibody technology provide simple dip-stick methods that can monitor mitochondrial protein expression compared to a nuclear-encoded protein. For example, the amount or activity of complex IV that has three proteins encoded by mtDNA and translated via mt-ribosomes can be compared to frataxin that is encoded by nuDNA, translated in the cytoplasm and then imported into the mitochondria. Repression of the ratio between complex IV and frataxin can be detected within five cell doublings after HepG2 cells are exposed to chloramphenicol or linezolid and the sample can be blood or even epithelial cells obtained via cheek swap. Dipsticks are commercially available (www.mitosciences.com) for either amount or activity of complexes I and IV and pyruvate dehydrogenase and for amounts of frataxin, apoptosis-inducting protein and the mitochondrial trifunctional protein that is central to the β-oxidation of long chain fatty acids. Such technology has utility in the clinic, but also in preclinical drug development where potential drug toxicity needs to be detected and circumvented.

Mitochondrial function and potential drug effects such as uncoupling and inhibition of OXPHOS are most directly studied by monitoring oxygen consumption or membrane potential, using polarographic electrodes and fluorescent dyes, respectively, but other techniques are available, as noted below.

Oxygen consumption provides an index of function that incorporates several parameters, including inner membrane impermeability and OXPHOS integrity. Such observations are often performed on mitochondrial isolated from tissue or cultured cells where substrate availability is readily manipulated, but respiration by intact cells can also be informative. For example, many cells in culture are grown in high-glucose media, which reduces the frequency of refreshing it. However, under these conditions, cells tend to rely on aerobic glycolysis to generate ATP, slighting OXPHOS. This independence from mitochondrial function renders most cultured cells resistant to mitochondrial toxicants [57]. This can be directly detected via monitoring the O_2 consumption of intact cells before and after replacing glucose in the media with galactose. This forces the cells to use OXPHOS for ATP generation and consequently renders them susceptible to mitotoxicants [57]. One problem with monitoring mitochondrial function in the drug development arena using polarographic electrodes is that the through-put is quite low; each drug dose typically takes 10–20 min. To circumvent this bottleneck, higher-throughput assays were developed for 96-well plate readers that use time-resolved phosphorescent probes to report media oxygen concentration [75]. Such probes can be used with isolated mitochondria as well as with intact cells (www.luxcel.com). Mitochondrial impairment in cells causes subsequent acidification as cells try to generate energy through increased glycolyisis. This can be measured using pH sensors, as developed by Luxcel (www.luxcel.com) and Seahorse (www.seahorsebio.com). A decrease in mitochondrial membrane potential also provides an insightful index of mitochondrial function. Because of the net negative charge in the matrix, mito-permeant cationic dyes accumulate there as a function of the Nernst equation [76]. A number of such fluorescent dyes with a variety of spectral characteristics have been developed and most are readily monitored in standard fluorescent microscopes (www.invitrogen.com). Loss of membrane potential, due to either uncoupling or inhibition of electron transport, is detected via corresponding loss of signal intensity. Membrane potential can also be monitored using a TPP+ (tetraphenyl phosphonium) electrode [77] and experiments where simultaneous monitoring of mitochondrial Ca^{2+} uptake and oxygen consumption illuminates much mitochondrial physiology [78].

Non-invasive assessments of mitochondrial function *in vivo* typically reflect the techniques to monitor it in cells or isolated organelles. Direct calorimetry, organismal oxygen consumption, CO_2 production and a host of other techniques all provide insight into mitochondrial capacity, albeit with confounding factors of movement and physical training of the subject.

More recently, advances in nuclear magnetic resonance (NMR) techniques have interrogated mitochondrial function *in situ* using intact tissues and organisms. For example, ^{31}P NMR resolves the three peaks associated with ATP, plus creatine phosphate (or another analog, depending on species) and inorganic phosphate. When the muscle is exogenously paced aggressively, or subjected to hypoxia, the ATP and phosphate peaks decline. The recovery rate once stimulation ceases, or normoxia is restored, directly reflects mitochondrial capacity. Studies using NMR surface coils and other stable isotopes such as ^{13}C and 1H, can also resolve mitochondrial function in animals. When combined with nuclear magnetic imaging, the techniques can detect mitochondrial dysfunction despite normal muscle contractility [79]. Stable isotopes are also being evaluated as non-invasive probes of mitochondrial function in the clinic. For example, hepatic mitochondrial function is being evaluated using ^{13}C methionine, which is preferentially transmethylated to yield α-ketobutyrate in the liver. Monitoring the rate of ^{13}C in exhaled CO_2 provides insight into mitochondrial capacity [80] and the effects of long-term HAART [80, 81].

The growing understanding of "off-target" deleterious mitochondrial drug effects has prompted development of preclinical models and screens to detect it and hence ways to circumvent it. Early preclinical vigilance, combined with animal models that resolve liver lesions previously only detected in the clinic [82], will surely reduce late-stage attrition and incidence of side effects that are caused by mitochondrial impairment.

15.4
Oxidative Stress

Oxidative stress has increasingly been recognized as a key mechanism of DILI [83, 84]. Clinically, DILI is typically delayed by weeks or months. Among other factors, both increasing age and polymorphisms in key enzymes that protect the organism from damage by oxidative stress are risk factors [85]. In mice lacking anti-oxidative protection mechanisms such as superoxide dismutase 2 (Sod2($+/-$)), the animals exhibit increased sensitivity to idiosyncratic hepatotoxic drugs, including troglitazone [82] and nimesulide [85]. Oxidative stress is also involved in animal models of delayed onset DILI and anti-oxidant treatments such as resveratrol have consistently demonstrated *in vivo* protection in this model [86, 87]. In addition, oxidative stress is implicated in cholestatic liver disorders and hepatitis C infections [88, 89] and these pre-existing conditions are known to sensitize the liver to additional drug-induced damage. It is therefore hypothesized that many "idiosyncratic" drug reactions may cause subtle prelethal oxidative insults to the liver that are typically masked by a "normal" oxidative threshold of this highly adaptable organ. Only when such a "normal" threshold is genetically or epigenetically altered does liver toxicity emerge [90–93].

15.4.1
Sources of Oxidative Stress

In mammalian cells, the mitochondrion is the major intracellular source of reactive oxygen species (ROS), which are mainly generated at Complex I and III of the respiratory chain, as part of the normal physiological process (see Section 15.3). Cells have evolved a myriad ways of surviving under normal levels of ROS. However, excessive ROS production can lead to oxidation of macromolecules and has been implicated in mtDNA mutations, aging and cell death. Mitochondrion-generated ROS play an important role in the release of cytochrome c and other pro-apoptotic proteins, which can trigger caspase activation and apoptosis. Conversely, mitochondrial antioxidant enzymes protect the cells from apoptosis [94]. Several toxins and drugs have been shown to increase intracellular oxidative stress by perturbing the balance between oxidative and antioxidative processes [95–97]. From a host's perspective, patients have been identified with genetic mutations and/or disease conditions that result in defective antioxidant systems [98, 99]. The aging process also adds yet another burden of pro-oxidative state [100]. The current working hypothesis is that these patients may be at an increased risk for drug- and toxin-induced oxidative damage.

15.4.2
Measurements of Oxidative Stress

Since oxidative stress is the result of an abnormal balance between pro-oxidative and anti-oxidative processes involving many enzymes and signaling molecules, whole cell assay systems are typically used for the measurement of the "net" oxidative stress. Traditionally, a decrease in GSH concentration, increase of GSSG levels and increase of the GSSG/GSH ratio are considered "gold standard" markers of oxidative stress, both *in vitro* [101] and *in vivo* [102]. Recently, a panel of fluorescent probes, each with different specificity and versatility, has been successfully used in primary hepatocyte cultures or continuously dividing hepatic cell lines [103]. These probes exhibit significantly increased fluorescence in the presence of excessive intracellular oxidative species and hence can be measured by rapid fluorometer-based microplate readers, automated epifluorescent microscopic imagers, or laser scanning cytometers. One of these probes, CM-H_2DCFDA, can be combined with other fluorescent probes such as TMRM, DRAQ5 and mBCl to measure mitochondrial membrane potential, nuclei and intracellular lipids and GSH respectively [104]. This simultaneous multiparametric imaging technology sheds significant light on the putative mechanisms of many drugs that cause idiosyncratic hepatotoxicity in humans.

15.4.3
Critical Review: Is There Sufficient Clinical, Pre-Clinical and *In Vitro* Data to Substantiate the Link Between Oxidative Stress and Idiosyncratic Liver Injury?

The best evidences are studies from preclinical animal models [86, 87, 105], or knockout animals lacking appropriate anti-oxidative pathways [106]. For example, Balb/c mice administered a variety of anti-oxidants in their chow were protected from acetaminophen hepatotoxicity [107]. Rats fed with the anti-oxidant melatonin were protected from cholesterol mediated oxidative liver damage [108]. The best clinical evidence that oxidative stress is a key player in a variety of liver injury diseases is the beneficial application of silymarin in these disease indications [109]. Silymarin is a polyphenolic plant flavonoid (a mixture of flavonoid isomers such as silibinin, isosilibinin, silidianin and silichristin) derived from Silymarin marianum that has antioxidative, antilipid peroxidative, antifibrotic and anti-inflammatory effects [109, 110].

There is a general consensus in the scientific community that too much oxidative stress in a prolonged drug exposure setting is not conducive to the long-term health of an important organ such as the liver. However, the challenge thus far has been to decide how much oxidative stress, tested at what drug concentration and for how long, should be considered a truly toxicologically significant signal. To establish such a threshold is especially important since cells do endogenously generate a baseline level of oxidative stress as by-products of normal metabolism. To address this, we have taken both an experimental and statistical approach [104]. Our investigations resulted in the selection of 100-fold of the drug's therapeutic C_{max} as a toxicologically relevant concentration for the liver for an orally administered drug. When applied to over 300 drugs and chemicals including many that caused rare and idiosyncratic liver toxicity in humans, such a testing strategy has a true-positive rate of 50–60% and an exceptionally low false-positive rate of 0–5%. Mitochondrial damage, oxidative stress and intracellular glutathione, all measured by high content cellular imaging in primary human hepatocyte cultures, are the three most important features contributing to the hepatotoxicity prediction. Such a combined imaging test can identify idiosyncratic human hepatotoxic drugs such as nimesulide, telithromycin, nefazodone, troglitazone, tetracycline, sulindac, zileuton, labetalol, diclofenac, chlorzoxazone, dantrolene and many others (Table 15.1). These findings not only provide insight to key DILI mechanisms, but also suggest a new approach in hepatotoxicity testing of pharmaceuticals [104].

15.5
Inhibition of Bile Salt Efflux Protein and Drug-Induced Cholestasis

Cholestatic liver disorders account for a large proportion of chronic liver ailments in adults, children and infants and are among the leading indications for liver transplantation in all age groups [89]. Cholestasis is defined as a decrease in bile flow and a decrease in the clearance of bile constituents (e.g., bile acids, bilirubin glucuronides, GSH conjugates, sulfate conjugates, drugs and drug metabolites). The generation of bile and the regulation of bile flow is one of the fundamental functions of the liver involving several key enzymes and hepatobilirary transporters [89]. In addition to their key role in determining hepatic drug exposure and clearance, the coordinated action of these enzymes and hepatobilirary transporters is essential for bile formation and the biliary secretion of cholephilic compounds and xenobiotics. There is increasing evidence that cholestatic forms of drug-induced liver damage result from a drug- or metabolite-mediated inhibition of hepatobiliary transporter systems [111]. A drug-mediated functional disturbance of these processes can potentially lead to an intracellular accumulation of harmful levels of bile constituents and result in the development of cholestatic liver cell damage [111]. One of these hepatobiliary transporters, bile salt efflux protein (BSEP, aka ABCB 11), has been shown to be the rate-limiting step of bile acid efflux [112]. Hence, drug or drug metabolite mediated inhibition of BSEP has been given much attention in recent years.

15.5.1
In Vitro and *In Vivo* Assays to Measure BSEP Inhibition

Inhibition of bile acid transport across Na+/taurocholate cotransporting polypeptide (SLC10A1) and bile salt export pump (ABCB 11)-coexpressing LLC-PK1 cells has been demonstrated by several well-known cholestasis-inducing drugs, including rifampicin, rifamycin SV, glibenclamide and cyclosporin A [113]. The vectorial transport of bile acid can be monitored by ^{3}H-labeled taurocholate, or aminofluorescein-tagged bile acids. These fluorescent bile acid analogs, chenodeoxycholylglycylamidofluorescein and cholylglycylamidofluorescein, were substrates of both NTCP and BSEP and their basal-to-apical transport rates across coexpressing cell monolayers were 4× to 5× those of the vector control, although smaller than for the native substrate, taurocholate [113].

Table 15.1 The high content cellular imaging data from the primary human hepatocyte cultures, upon overnight treatment by a panel of 30 selected drugs.

Drug	DILI label	Nuclei count (<0.4 = positive)	Nuclei area (<0.4 = positive)	ROS intensity (>2.5 = positive)	TMRM intensity (<0.4 = positive)	Lipid intensity (>2.5 = positive)	GSH content (<0.4 = positive)	GSH area (<0.65 = positive)	GSH average pixel intensity (<0.4 = positive)	HH imaging final score (logical OR of 8 measures)	Human_C_{max} (μg/ml)
0.1% DMSO	N	1.00	1.00	1.00	1.00	1.00	1.00	1.00	1.00	N	
Perhexiline	P	0.82	0.91	0.00	0.00	1.48	0.01	0.02	1.08	P	0.6
Troglitazone	P	0.71	0.85	0.00	0.01	2.90	0.01	0.02	1.08	P	2.82
Nefazodone	P	0.45	0.52	0.00	0.04	1.81	0.01	0.03	2.10	P	0.4
Tetracycline	P	1.04	1.06	430	0.10	2.90	1.13	0.82	1.97	P	9.3
Nimesulide	P	0.96	0.92	27.3	1.43	2.86	0.88	0.98	0.87	P	6.5
Sulindac	P	1.14	1.08	14.2	0.69	0.79	0.63	0.81	0.66	P	11.4
Zileuton	P	1.08	1.01	4.83	1.32	3.46	0.92	0.67	2.16	P	3.1
Labetalol	P	0.89	0.81	4.88	0.70	5.10	1.41	0.97	1.89	P	0.88
Diclofenac	P	0.61	0.70	35.3	0.98	1.86	1.91	1.22	1.00	P	2.4
Chlorzoxazone	P	0.48	0.74	8.39	0.78	1.70	1.01	1.65	1.31	P	0.5
Dantrolene	P	0.72	0.78	8.54	1.23	1.58	1.57	1.17	0.98	P	1.24
Amitriptyline	N	0.96	1.00	0.30	1.26	1.36	1.06	0.97	0.96	N	0.03
Pioglitazone	N	1.13	1.11	0.88	1.69	1.38	0.57	0.87	0.87	N	1.1
Rosiglitazone	N	0.66	0.79	0.44	1.04	1.66	1.52	1.38	1.13	N	0.4
Primidone	N	0.96	0.91	0.62	0.90	1.19	0.75	0.95	0.91	N	1
Penicillin	N	0.91	0.98	0.29	1.31	1.32	0.67	1.07	0.61	N	2.7
Melatonin	N	0.97	0.96	0.68	0.95	0.93	0.91	1.00	1.00	N	0.006
Nadolol	N	0.95	0.99	0.44	2.07	0.92	0.91	1.04	0.89	N	0.1
Ketotifen	N	1.02	1.01	0.60	1.00	0.88	0.90	0.94	1.00	N	0.0004

Table 15.1 (continued)

Drug	DILI label	Nuclei count (<0.4 = positive)	Nuclei area (<0.4 = positive)	ROS intensity (>2.5 = positive)	TMRM intensity (<0.4 = positive)	Lipid intensity (>2.5 = positive)	GSH content (<0.4 = positive)	GSH area (<0.65 = positive)	GSH average pixel intensity (<0.4 = positive)	HH imaging final score (logical OR of 8 measures)	Human_C_{max} (g/ml)
Paromomycin	N	1.00	1.02	1.02	1.66	0.93	1.23	0.99	0.99	N	23
Sumatriptan	N	1.13	1.10	0.26	1.18	0.86	0.76	0.87	0.85	N	0.08
Famotidine	N	1.20	1.15	0.47	1.15	0.89	0.96	0.84	0.91	N	0.1
Tacrine	N	0.86	0.91	0.48	1.14	1.30	1.14	1.08	0.84	N	0.02
Simvastatin	N	0.72	0.84	0.02	0.81	1.46	1.35	1.32	0.96	N	0.01
Aspirin	N	1.04	1.00	0.58	1.25	0.87	0.62	0.94	0.50	N	1
Fluoxetine	N	1.05	1.07	1.46	0.79	0.84	0.59	0.91	0.83	N	0.015
Propranolol	N	1.12	1.05	0.50	1.08	0.89	0.76	0.87	0.70	N	0.05
Raloxifene	N	1.15	1.04	0.17	0.76	0.89	1.10	0.83	1.06	N	0.0005
Paroxetine	N	1.12	1.04	0.38	0.83	0.85	0.72	0.90	0.77	N	0.02
Buspirone	N	0.99	1.00	1.02	1.13	0.98	0.68	0.98	1.14	N	0.002

The binary heat map was produced by thresholds that best differentiated the DILI negative from positive drugs (the threshold used was listed under the heading for each measurement). The numbers in italic black indicate that the imaging measurements are within the DILI negative threshold, while numbers in bold red indicate that they fall outside of the DILI negative threshold (i.e. become positive). The second rightmost column indicates the combined human hepatocyte (HH) imaging test score, using a logical OR of the 8 previous measurements (P means DILI positive, N means DILI negative). This procedure assigned a DILI positive label to a compound if any single imaging measurement falls outside of the DILI negative threshold. All of these drugs were tested at 100-fold of human therapeutic C_{max} in sandwiched primary human hepatocyte cultures. The C_{max} values for these drugs are listed in the rightmost column. For more on the experimental details and the rationale behind choosing 100-fold human therapeutic C_{max} as a relevant concentration for in vitro hepatotoxicity testing, please refer to Xu et al. [104].

A limitation of this method, which utilizes a polarized kidney cell line, the LLC-PK1, is that it is often not the parent drug but the conjugated metabolite that is the most potent inhibitor of BSEP. For example, troglitazone sulfate is a much more potent inhibitor of BSEP than the parent troglitazone [114]. To overcome this limitation, researchers are in the process of developing and characterizing longer-term polarized human hepatocyte cultures that maintain phases 0 (uptake transporters), 1 (cytochrome p450s), 2 (conjugation enzymes) and 3 (efflux transporters). One of the more promising models recently is by Khetania and Bhatia at MIT, who used a miniaturized, multiwell culture system for human hepatocytes with optimized microscale architecture that maintains differentiated hepatocellular functions for several weeks [115]. Using gene expression profiles, they demonstrated phase I and II metabolism, canalicular transport, secretion of liver-specific products and expected susceptibility to different hepatotoxins. Recently, the use of cryopreserved human hepatocytes in sandwiched culture to form intact bile canaliculi and to exhibit functional uptake and efflux transport was successfully demonstrated [116]. It is expected that, with increased perfection and industrialization of these optimal hepatocyte cultures, researchers will be able to order and receive adult human hepatocytes with sufficient level of activities in phases 0–3 for the evaluation of not only the parent but also metabolite-mediated effects on important liver enzymes and transporters.

In vivo, measuring bile acids in plasma and urine should be revived as potential biomarkers in the modern metabolomic era. Then the first-order scientific question will become: whether early and time-controlled fasting-level measurement of bile acid concentration in plasma and urine can become a sensitive and specific biomarker for drug-induced cholestasis and ultimately liver injury at later time-points [117]? Clinical trials should be conducted to evaluate whether such bile acid measurements can be used as part of a predictive panel to identify patients who are at increased risk of drug-induced cholestasis.

15.5.2
Critical Review: Is There a Link between BSEP Inhibition, Drug-Induced Cholestasis and Idiosyncratic Liver Injury?

The best clinical evidence that BSEP is involved in hepatotoxicity is provided by human genetic studies which found four highly conserved non-synonymous mutations in two hepatobiliary transporters (BSEP and MDR3) that were specific for drug-induced liver injury [118]. Recently, a consortium of investigators identified a remarkable 82 different ABCB11 mutations in 109 families that caused severe BSEP deficiency [119]. It is therefore expected that at least some of these genetic mutations and polymorphisms will put patients at an increased risk of drug-induced cholestasis. Does this justify the implementation of a simple BSEP inhibition screen for all new chemical entities? The answer is not quite that simple.

The reason is that an acute inhibition of BSEP will lead to an elevated bile acid concentration both inside the hepatocytes as well as in the plasma compartment. But bile acids are, by themselves, signaling molecules that can upregulate their own hepatobiliary transporters and other proteins, including BSEP. Indeed, bile acids act via farnesoid X receptor (FXR), which downregulates CYP7A1, the rate-limiting enzyme of bile acid biosynthesis, upregulates BSEP and downregulates NTCP. MRP2 is upregulated by both FXR and pregnane X receptor (PXR), which upregulates CYP3A [120, 121]. Most of the chemical inducers acting on canalicular transporter levels are well-known to upregulate some hepatic drug metabolizing enzymes, suggesting a coordinated regulation of liver detoxifying proteins in response to these compounds. So there is a well-characterized adaptive or feedback mechanism to minimize the injury cased by a transient increase in bile acid concentration. Indeed, a transient increase in serum bile acid concentration *per se* should not be interpreted as a signal of liver injury, since serum bile acid levels fluctuate dramatically throughout the day and are heavily dependent on food intake.

Another case in point is that the same drug may be an inhibitor of BSEP in an acute setting, but also an inducer of BSEP in a chronic setting. This may be related to the adaptive mechanism discussed earlier, and/or the drugs or drug metabolites by themselves are acting via PXR and PXR/FXR. One such example is rifampicin, which inhibits both uptake and efflux transporters [113], but was also reported to be capable of inducing BSEP via the PXR mechanism [122]. Another consideration is the balanced activity between bile acid uptake transporter, NTCP and BSEP. Inhibition of rat Ntcp leads to increased serum bile acids without hepatic injury in rats or humans [113, 123]. Therefore, an elevation of serum bile acid without elevation of serum transaminases could be a result of more potent inhibition of NTCP than BSEP, which is not hepatotoxic [113, 123]. Hence, blindly screening for every drug candidate for BSEP inhibition without putting data into proper context can be problematic. A better approach at the current stage is to use this on drugs that are primarily cleared by the biliary route in pre-clinical animal species, that is, reserved for those more likely to interact with the hepatobiliary transport system. Even so, both a short-term and a long-term assessment of the BSEP function in culture and both BSEP and NTCP inhibition potency are needed to avoid generating false-positive signals for drugs that actually could be quite safe *in vivo*.

15.6
Biomarkers

Serum chemistry markers play an important role in hepatotoxicity evaluation in human and animal safety studies. The classic markers of hepatotoxicity are alanine aminotransferase (ALT), aspartate aminotrasnferase (AST) and alkaline phosphatase (ALP) [124–127]. Drug-induced hepatotoxicity can be difficult to assess in some circumstances. Hepatotoxic responses can be intrinsic (predictable, dose-related) or idiosyncratic (unpredictable, non-dose-related). ALT, AST and ALP are generally not useful for predicting idiosyncratic responses. The administration of some drugs, such as isoniazid, can lead to a high incidence of ALT elevation, but are tolerated by most patients without severe hepatotoxicity. Adverse drug reactions can be masked by elevated serum ALT levels in patients with an underlying liver injury or disease. It may also be difficult to distinguish between true hepatotoxicity and a transient adaptive response. The symptoms of drug-induced hepatotoxicity may not arise or be difficult to interpret prior to wide postmarketing exposure. The integration of classical methods in toxicology with predictive biomarkers would help reduce the risk of hepatotoxicity before it occurs in the clinic.

15.6.1
Hepatocellular Injury

Serum ALT and AST are the classic markers of hepatocelluar damage [124, 128, 129]. Aminotransferases play an important role in amino acid biosynthesis and the metabolic interchanges between liver and skeletal muscle (i.e., the Cori cycle). They are abundantly expressed in the liver, skeletal muscle and kidney. In humans, the ALT and AST activities in liver are ∼3000-fold and 7000-fold higher than in serum, respectively [130]. Two ALT isozymes (ALT1, ALT2) have been identified. In the liver, both ALT isoforms are expressed specifically by hepatocytes [131]. ALT and AST are leaked from hepatocytes during hepatocellular necrosis, injury or regenerative/reparative activity. Serum ALT activity is affected by gender, age, body mass index (BMI), exercise and muscular injury [124]. Cardiovascular disease, such as right heart failure and hypotension, can cause ischemic hepatitis and a >10 000-fold increase in aminotransferase levels [125]. Additional serum chemistry markers used to evaluate hepatocellular injury include lactate dehydrogenase (LDH), sorbitol dehydrogenase (SDH), glutamate dehydrogenase (GDH), α-glutathione-(S)-transferase (α-GST), F protein and arginase I [132].

15.6.2
Cholestatic Injury

Serum ALP and total bilirubin (unconjugated and conjugated fractions) are traditionally used to monitor cholestatic injury. The ALP families of enzymes are zinc metalloproteases that are present in nearly all tissues. In the liver, ALP is immunolocalized to the microvili of the bile canaliculus [124]. Increased synthesis of ALP and its release into the circulation occurs within hours of cholestatic injury [129]. Serum assays of 5'-nucleotidase (5'-NT) or γ-glutamyltransferase activity (GGT) are used to confirm the liver as the specific origin for the elevation of ALP. Increases in serum bilirubin or bile acids are usually the result of bile retention subsequent to impaired bile flow, increased production associated with accelerated erythrocyte destruction, or altered bilirubin metabolism [129].

15.6.3
Application of Serum Chemistry Markers

The traditional approach for assessing hepatotoxicity integrates clinical chemistry markers, histopathology evaluation, cytochrome P450 enzyme induction, in-life observations, metabolism data and knowledge of pharmacologic class effects [133, 134]. The potential risk of toxicity in humans is initially derived from studies performed in animals. The FDA white paper "Nonclinical assessment of potential hepatotoxicity in man" describes the traditional approach to assess hepatotoxicity in animals [133, 134]. The FDA draft guidance document "Drug-induced liver injury: premarketing clinical evaluation" describes the approach to assess the potential for a drug to cause severe liver injury in the clinic [125]. Similar guidance documents are in development in Europe [126] and Canada [127]. Hy's law is one of the observations used to assess a drug's risk of causing serious hepatotoxicity. It is based on the observations that drug-induced jaundice caused by hepatocellular injury, without a significant obstructive component (cholestatic injury), has a high rate of adverse outcomes, at 10–50% mortality (or transplant) [135, 136]. The three requirements of Hy's law are:

1. Evidence that a drug causes hepatocellular injury, as shown by a serum ALT $\geq 3\times$ the upper limit of normal (ULN).
2. Evidence of increased serum total bilirubin ($\geq 2\times$ ULN) with no evidence of intra- or extra-hepatic bilirubin obstruction (elevated serum ALP) or Gilberts' syndrome.
3. No evidence of another cause of hepatocellular injury, such as viral hepatitis, marked hypotension, or congestive heart failure.

15.6.4
Need for New Biomarkers

Drug-induced hepatotoxicity can present in variable manifestations, such as cell death (necrosis, apoptosis), inflammation, degeneration (steatosis), fibrosis/cirrhosis and the development of tumors. The manifestations of drug toxicity may not be mutually exclusive and may occur sequentially, or in combination. ALT and ALP can be used to generally classify the pattern of liver injury as either hepatocellular (ALT $\geq 3\times$ ULN), cholestatic (ALP $\geq 2\times$ ULN, ALT/ALP ≤ 2) or mixed (elevated ALP and ALT). The successful monitoring of hepatotoxicity would identify cases before irreversible injury occurs. The activity levels of ALT, AST and ALP only increase after hepatic or cholestatic injury has occurred. Waiting for activity levels to exceed the established thresholds may be too late [3]. New biomarkers are needed to monitor/predict the specific sequence of events for different classes of hepatotoxic compounds.

A significant portion of acute liver failures ($\sim 10\%$) are due to unexpected genetic sensitivities (allergic or non-allergic idiosyncratic reactions). Changes in the levels of ALT, AST and ALP are not generally useful for predicting/monitoring idiosyncratic responses. Animal models of allergic hepatotoxicity have yet to be developed. To date, no genetic, metabolic or other characteristic has been found to predict the occurrence of severe drug-induced liver injury in humans [3].

Many patients have underlying liver disease with liver function abnormalities. It may be difficult to determine superimposed drug-induced liver injury in patients with viral hepatitis, passive congestion of the liver from heart failure, fatty liver disease secondary to obesity or diabetes and alcoholic liver disease [137]. Liver diseases can affect drug absorption, disposition (pharmacokinetics), efficacy and safety. Clinically useful biomarkers to predict pharmacokinetics/dynamics (PK/PD) and toxicokinetics/dynamics (TK/TD) in patients with hepatic injury are not available [138].

Changes in serum ALT may not always be indicative of a true hepatotoxic response. Mild dose-related ALT elevations ($2\times$ to $3\times$ ULN) are observed in some patients taking lovastatin as a result of an adaptive response [139]. As another example, isoniazid, an anti-tuberculosis agent, leads to a high incidence of ALT and AST elevations, but is tolerated chronically without severe hepatotoxicity. This suggests that more specific and sensitive biomarkers are still needed to predict serious liver injury.

15.6.5
Biomarker Discovery Efforts

The FDA and the National Institutes of Health (NIH) recently expanded their efforts to identify biomarkers to reduce the risk of hepatotoxicity before it occurs; so has the pharmaceutical industry in hopes of improving success rates and reducing costs. The FDA National Center for Toxicological Research (NCTR) has launched a liver toxicity biomarker study (LTBS). The objective of the study is to develop a preclinical test that can be used in the initial stages of the drug development process. The test will also be used to identify patients most likely to suffer from liver toxicity [140]. The NIH launched a network (DILIN) to develop a systematic way of classifying DILI and to establish a registry of patients who have experienced severe DILI. Also within the NIH, the Digestive Diseases Interagency Coordinating Committee released an "action plan for liver disease research". The major goals of the action plan for drug-induced liver injury research are: (i) to establish a means of predicting the likelihood of drug-induced liver injury; (ii) to improve diagnostic ability; (iii) to develop a means to prevent and treat liver cell injury. The action plan outlines several goals centered on the development of biomarker signatures that could be employed for diagnostic use and to predict hepatotoxicity before it occurs [141].

15.6.6
Approaches for Biomarker Discovery

There are two complementary approaches for biomarker discovery. The knowledge-driven strategy involves monitoring specific SNPs, proteins and/or endogenous metabolites based on the existing literature related to drug-induced hepatotoxicity. The second approach makes use of overall profiling strategies (i.e., toxicogenomics, proteomics or metabolomics) to reveal unknown mechanisms of toxicity. Toxicogenomics is the evaluation of gene expression for understanding and predicting toxic events [142–145].

Proteomics is the assessment protein expression levels and can be used to monitor mRNA processing and posttranslational modifications [146, 147]. Metabonomics is an approach to measure time-related endogenous metabolic responses to pathophysiological stimuli [148, 149]. The different approaches should be integrated with PK/PD data and traditional methods in toxicology to identify sensitive and specific biomarkers of hepatotoxic response.

15.6.6.1 Development of *In Vivo* Biomarkers

The development of new biomarkers is based on an understanding of the physiologic functions of the liver and its response to injury. Drug exposure can alter the function of the liver and elicit injurious effects through different mechanisms. These mechanisms are becoming better understood and have been reviewed [3–5, 150, 151]. A panel of *in vivo* biomarkers that reflects the different mechanisms of toxicity and that could be used to predict drug response in tissue would be invaluable in hepatotoxicity risk assessment.

As an example, acetaminophen (APAP) in overdose has been used by several groups to identify hepatotoxicity biomarkers in mice. APAP-induced hepatotoxicity is characterized by hepatic centrilobular necrosis and hepatitis. APAP biotransformation by Phase I enzymes leads to the formation of the reactive metabolite N-acetyl-p-benzoquinone (NAPQI), which can deplete glutathione and form adducts with hepatic proteins (see Section 15.2). Protein adduction primes the hepatocytes for cytokines released by activated macrophages (Kupffer cells) and/or destructive insults by reactive nitrogen species. Although necrosis is recognized as the mode of cell death in APAP overdose, the precise mechanisms are still being elucidated [152].

Toxicogenomic signatures in mice suggest that MAP kinases, including members of the Jnk signaling pathway (Traf2, Mapk8ip3, Dusp10), are positively associated with APAP-induced liver necrosis and confirm that neutrophil chemotaxis (i.e., Fcgr3, Itgb2, Fcer1g) is one of the significant biological processes induced by APAP [153]. Proteomics studies using fluorescence 2D-DIGE, in-gel proteolysis with mass spectrometry, have revealed protein targets of APAP covalent modification and changes in protein expression related to hepatotoxicity [154, 155]. Metabolomic studies have identified new APAP metabolites and ophthalmate in mouse serum and liver extracts as potential new biomarkers of APAP-induced oxidative stress [156, 157]. The change in metabolic signature seen after drug treatment can be correlated with the magnitude of pathologic change, as described in toxicity studies by Baronas *et al.* and Hsieh *et al.* [148, 158].

15.6.6.2 Development of *In Vitro* Biomarkers

The use of *in vitro* methods can help reduce time, costs and the number of animals that are used in safety evaluation. Rat hepatocytes and liver slices are accepted *in vitro* systems to study the biotransformation, cytochrome P450 enzyme induction and hepatotoxicity of drug compounds. Boess *et al.* [159] used microarray technology to characterize the gene expression in two rat cell lines (BRL3A, NRL clone 9), in primary hepatocytes and liver tissue slices. The results suggested that knowledge of system-related differences (i.e., inflammatory reactions in liver slices, isolation stress in primary cell culture models) is required for the comparison and interpretation of gene and protein expression data between models. The potential applications for *in vitro* biomarker test systems include preliminary drug hepatotoxicity assessments (prescreens), complementary testing to gain mechanistic information and evaluate findings across species and surrogate tests to help in the refinement, reduction and replacement of animals used for testing methods [144, 145].

15.6.6.3 Biomarker Validation

New biomarkers will be useful in hepatotoxicity risk assessment if the data quality and validity can be established. The FDA defines a valid biomarker as one that can be measured in an analytical test system with well-established performance characteristics and has an established scientific framework or body of evidence that elucidates the significance of the test results [160]. Although there is no formerly agreed upon path, biomarker validation should include appropriate end-points for study (i.e., toxicology, histopathology, bioanalytical chemistry, etc.) and dose- and time-dependent measurements. An assessment of species, sex and strain susceptibility is also important to evaluate across species differences. More specific considerations for validation of gene and protein expression technologies are reviewed by Corvi *et al.* and Rifai *et al.* [144, 147].

Conventional methods can be used to validate new biomarkers in accordance with existing regulatory guidance. For example, Suter *et al.* used gene expression analysis to examine the effect of two 5-HT6 receptor antagonists on the rat liver [145]. The identified candidate biomarkers were amenable to testing by PCR. Similarly, protein biomarkers can be validated using immunoassays. Endogenous metabolites can be validated through LC-MS/MS. System suitability testing (linearity, accuracy, precision, specificity) should be required to confirm that the test system functions properly [134]. The performance specifications for the known valid biomarkers (i.e., ALT, AST, ALP) are reviewed by Dufour *et al.* [130]. The target values for performance goals for total error in ALT and AST activity measurements are 15–20% [161].

15.6.7
Future Biomarker Directions

Drug discovery and development is a resource laden and lengthy process with a high failure rate. Biomarker analysis, including the elucidation of toxicology biological pathways, would help provide a stronger rationale for selecting compounds to advance to development. Some of the potential applications where valid biomarkers can play future roles in hepatotoxicity evaluation include:

- Sensitive and early detection of hepatotoxic response;
- Toxicity mechanism of action and site of injury studies;
- Across-species toxicity and susceptibility analysis;
- Prediction of injury before it occurs;
- Optimization of drug safety windows and dose scheduling;
- Compound selection and benefit/risk assessment.

As an example, Hsieh et al. identified toxicodynamic biomarkers in monkey serum that demonstrated a quantitative relationship with drug exposure (C_{max}, AUC) and related pathological events [148]. The biomarkers were used for a more precise calculation of the no observed adverse effect level (NOAEL). The safety of three different dosing schedules was predicted using pharmacokinetic pharmacodynamic (PKPD) modeling and biomarker analysis.

A predictive biomarker approach can help reduce resources and the number of animals that are used in drug safety assessment. There are modifier genes in various species or strains that can affect the action of a drug through metabolism or during the processes of injury and repair [162]. Biomarker analysis can help identify even more relevant animal models for the prediction of human toxicity. Potential toxic liabilities can be identified sooner in the drug discovery and development process. Biomarkers can also be employed to reveal on-target versus off-target toxicological responses during drug treatment. The understanding of the mechanisms of drug-induced hepatotoxicity will improve as toxicogenomics, proteomics and metabolomics databases are developed more fully. The combination of traditional methods in hepatotoxicity evaluation and predictive biomarker analysis would better determine the benefit/risk ratio of potentially hepatotoxic drugs.

15.7
Conclusions

Despite being one of the top reasons of drug attrition, the statistics of drug development failures due to hepatotoxicity have not changed significantly in the past decade. Recently, much progress has been made in the development, evaluation and "validation" of *in vitro* assays targeting key mechanisms of hepatotoxicity. At the present time, several major research-based pharmaceutical companies have characterized and/or adopted some collections of *in vitro* assays in the drug discovery stage to minimize the downstream failure due to hepatotoxicity. These assays include: reactive metabolites, mitochondrial damage, oxidative stress and most recently, inhibition of BSEP. It is important for the healthy progression of the field for pharmaceutical researchers to publish how they score a drug as "positive" versus "negative" in these assays and what is the rationale and predictivity of their scoring criteria. It is possible that since there is not a singular mechanism leading to hepatotoxicity, a rational combination of better characterized assays could provide the best predictor for positive versus negative drugs. In this regard, a recent publication by Pfizer researchers provided a key proof of concept that well-characterized cell culture models and rationally combined assays can augment the prediction of drug-induced liver injury in the drug discovery and development process [104]. Since drug-induced liver injury has been recognized as a "national and global problem" [163], even more focused efforts in evaluating and validating predictive methodologies including imaging, biomarkers analysis, *in silico* SAR and PKPD modeling will be needed to address this important public health concern.

References

1 Schuster, D., Laggner, C. and Langer, T. (2005) Why drugs fail–a study on side effects in new chemical entities. *Current Pharmaceutical Design*, **11** (27), 3545–3559.

2 Giacomini, K.M. et al. (2007) When good drugs go bad. *Nature*, **446** (7139), 975–977.

3 Kaplowitz, N. (2005) Idiosyncratic drug hepatotoxicity. *Nature Reviews. Drug Discovery*, **4** (6), 489–499.

4 Navarro, V.J. and Senior, J.R. (2006) Drug-related hepatotoxicity. *The New England Journal of Medicine*, **354** (7), 731–739.

5 Lee, W.M. (2003) Drug-induced hepatotoxicity. *The New England Journal of Medicine*, **349** (5), 474–485.

6 Jollow, D.J. et al. (1973) Acetaminophen-induced hepatic necrosis. II. Role of covalent binding *in vivo*. *Journal of Pharmacology and Experimental Therapeutics*, **187** (1), 195–202.

7 Mitchell, J.R. et al. (1973) Acetaminophen-induced hepatic necrosis. I. Role of drug metabolism. *Journal of Pharmacology and Experimental Therapeutics*, **187** (1), 185–194.

8 Mitchell, J.R. et al. (1973) Acetaminophen-induced hepatic necrosis. IV. Protective role of glutathione. *Journal of Pharmacology and Experimental Therapeutics*, **187** (1), 211–217.

9 Dahlin, D.C. et al. (1984) N-acetyl-p-benzoquinone imine: a cytochrome P-450-mediated oxidation product of acetaminophen. *Proceedings of the National Academy of Sciences of the United States of America*, **81** (5), 1327–1331.

10 Graham, D.J., Drinkard, C.R. and Shatin, D. (2003) Incidence of idiopathic acute liver failure and hospitalized liver injury in patients treated with troglitazone. *The American Journal of Gastroenterology*, **98** (1), 175–179.

11 Ju, C. and Uetrecht, J.P. (2002) Mechanism of idiosyncratic drug reactions: reactive metabolite formation, protein binding and the regulation of the immune system. *Current Drug Metabolism*, **3** (4), 367–377.

12 Padovan, E. et al. (1997) Penicilloyl peptides are recognized as T cell antigenic determinants in penicillin allergy. *European Journal of Immunology*, **27** (6), 1303–1307.

13 Wagner, E.S. and Gorman, M. (1971) The reaction of cysteine and related compounds with penicillins and cephalosporins. *Journal of Antibiotics*, **24** (9), 647–650.

14 Satoh, H. et al. (1989) Human anti-endoplasmic reticulum antibodies in sera of patients with halothane-induced hepatitis are directed against a trifluoroacetylated carboxylesterase. *Proceedings of the National Academy of Sciences of the United States of America*, **86** (1), 322–326.

15 Lecoeur, S., Andre, C. and Beaune, P.H. (1996) Tienilic acid-induced auto-immune hepatitis: anti-liver and-kidney microsomal type 2 autoantibodies recognize a three-site conformational epitope on cytochrome P4502C9. *Molecular Pharmacology*, **50** (2), 326–333.

16 Bourdi, M. et al. (1992) Anti-liver microsomes autoantibodies and dihydralazine-induced hepatitis: specificity of autoantibodies and inductive capacity of the drug. *Molecular Pharmacology*, **42** (2), 280–285.

17 Bourdi, M. et al. (1990) Anti-liver endoplasmic reticulum autoantibodies are directed against human cytochrome P-450IA2. A specific marker of dihydralazine-induced hepatitis. *Journal of Clinical Investigation*, **85** (6), 1967–1973.

18 Blum, M. et al. (1991) Molecular mechanism of slow acetylation of drugs and carcinogens in humans. *Proceedings of the National Academy of Sciences of the United States of America*, **88** (12), 5237–5241.

19 Cribb, A.E. et al. (1991) Reactions of the nitroso and hydroxylamine metabolites of sulfamethoxazole with reduced glutathione. Implications for idiosyncratic toxicity. *Drug Metabolism and Disposition: The Biological Fate of Chemicals*, **19** (5), 900–906.

20 Ueda, K. et al. (2007) Glutathione S-transferase M1 null genotype as a risk factor for carbamazepine-induced mild hepatotoxicity. *Pharmacogenomics*, **8** (5), 435–442.

21 Buckley, N.A. and Srinivasan, J. (2002) Should a lower treatment line be used when treating paracetamol poisoning in patients with chronic alcoholism?: a case for. *Drug Safety*, **25** (9), 619–624.

22 Dearden, J.C. (2003) In silico prediction of drug toxicity. *Journal of Computer-Aided Molecular Design*, **17** (2–4), 119–127.

23 Cruciani, G. et al. (2005) MetaSite: understanding metabolism in human cytochromes from the perspective of the chemist. *Journal of Medicinal Chemistry*, **48** (22), 6970–6979.

24 Madsen, K.G. et al. (2007) Development and evaluation of an electrochemical method for studying reactive phase-I metabolites: correlation to *in vitro* drug metabolism. *Chemical Research in Toxicology*, **20** (5), 821–831.

25 Kalgutkar, A.S. et al. (2005) A comprehensive listing of bioactivation pathways of organic functional groups. *Current Drug Metabolism*, **6** (3), 161–225.

26 Kalgutkar, A.S. and Soglia, J.R. (2005) Minimising the potential for metabolic activation in drug discovery. *Expert Opinion on Drug Metabolism and Toxicology*, **1** (1), 91–142.

27 Henderson, A.P. et al. (2004) 2,6-diarylaminotetrahydropyrans from reactions of glutaraldehyde with anilines: models for biomolecule cross-linking. *Chemical Research in Toxicology*, **17** (3), 378–382.

28 Argoti, D. et al. (2005) Cyanide trapping of iminium ion reactive intermediates followed by detection and structure identification using liquid chromatography-tandem mass spectrometry (LC-MS/MS). *Chemical Research in Toxicology*, **18** (10), 1537–1544.

29 Evans, D.C. et al. (2004) Drug-protein adducts: an industry perspective on minimizing the potential for drug bioactivation in drug discovery and development. *Chemical Research in Toxicology*, **17** (1), 3–16.

30 Dieckhaus, C.M. et al. (2002) Mechanisms of idiosyncratic drug reactions: the case of felbamate. *Chemico-Biological Interactions*, **142** (1–2), 99–117.

31 Parker, R.J. et al. (2005) Stability and comparative metabolism of selected felbamate metabolites and postulated fluorofelbamate metabolites by post-mitochondrial suspensions. *Chemical Research in Toxicology*, **18** (12), 1842–1848.

32 Roecklein, B.A. et al. (2007) Fluorofelbamate. *Neurotherapeutics*, **4** (1), 97–101.

33 Leone, A.M. et al. (2007) Evaluation of felbamate and other antiepileptic drug toxicity potential based on hepatic protein covalent binding and gene expression. *Chemical Research in Toxicology*, **20** (4), 600–608.

34 Zhao, S.X. et al. (2007) NADPH-dependent covalent binding of [3H] paroxetine to human liver microsomes and S-9 fractions: identification of an electrophilic quinone metabolite of paroxetine. *Chemical Research in Toxicology*, **20** (11), 1649–1657.

35 Smith, K.S. et al. (2003) *In vitro* metabolism of tolcapone to reactive intermediates: relevance to tolcapone liver toxicity. *Chemical Research in Toxicology*, **16** (2), 123–128.

36 Nissinen, E. et al. (1997) Entacapone, a novel catechol-O-methyltransferase inhibitor for Parkinson's disease, does not impair mitochondrial energy production. *European Journal of Pharmacology*, **340** (2–3), 287–294.

37 Njoku, D. et al. (1997) Biotransformation of halothane, enflurane, isoflurane, and

desflurane to trifluoroacetylated liver proteins: association between protein acylation and hepatic injury. *Anesthesia and Analgesia*, **84** (1), 173–178.

38 Kassahun, K. et al. (2001) Studies on the metabolism of troglitazone to reactive intermediates *in vitro* and *in vivo*. Evidence for novel biotransformation pathways involving quinone methide formation and thiazolidinedione ring scission. *Chemical Research in Toxicology*, **14** (1), 62–70.

39 Alvarez-Sanchez, R. et al. (2006) Thiazolidinedione bioactivation: a comparison of the bioactivation potentials of troglitazone, rosiglitazone, and pioglitazone using stable isotope-labeled analogues and liquid chromatography tandem mass spectrometry. *Chemical Research in Toxicology*, **19** (8), 1106–1116.

40 Mallal, S. et al. (2008) HLA-B*5701 screening for hypersensitivity to abacavir. *The New England Journal of Medicine*, **358** (6), 568–579.

41 Pessayre, D. and Fromenty, B. (2005) NASH: a mitochondrial disease. *Journal of Hepatology*, **42** (6), 928–940.

42 Pessayre, D. et al. (1999) Hepatotoxicity due to mitochondrial dysfunction. *Cell Biology and Toxicology*, **15** (6), 367–373.

43 Wallace, K.B. (2009) Mitochondrial off targets of drug therapy. *Trends in Pharmacological Sciences*, in press.

44 Amacher, D.E. (2005) Drug-associated mitochondrial toxicity and its detection. *Current Medicinal Chemistry*, **12** (16), 1829–1839.

45 Wallace, K.B. and Starkov, A.A. (2000) Mitochondrial targets of drug toxicity. *Annual Review of Pharmacology and Toxicology*, **40**, 353 388.

46 Zhou, S. and Wallace, K.B. (1999) The effect of peroxisome proliferators on mitochondrial bioenergetics. *Toxicological Sciences*, **48** (1), 82–89.

47 Dykens, J.a.W.Y. (2008) *Drug-Induced Mitochondrial dysfunction*, John Wiley and Sons.

48 Goldstein, S. and Merenyi, G. (2008) The chemistry of peroxynitrite: implications for biological activity. *Methods in Enzymology*, **436**, 49–61.

49 Dykens, J.A. (2007) RedOx Targets: Enzyme Systems and Drug Development Strategies for Mitochondrial Dysfunction, in *Comprehensive Medicinal Chemistry II* (eds D.J. Triggle and J.B. Taylor), Elsevier, Oxford, pp. 1053–1087.

50 Moreno-Sanchez, R. et al. (1999) Inhibition and uncoupling of oxidative phosphorylation by nonsteroidal anti-inflammatory drugs: study in mitochondria, submitochondrial particles, cells, and whole heart. *Biochemical Pharmacology*, **57** (7), 743–752.

51 Haasio, K. et al. (2002) Effects of entacapone and tolcapone on mitochondrial membrane potential. *European Journal of Pharmacology*, **453** (1), 21–26.

52 Brunmair, B. et al. (2004) Fenofibrate impairs rat mitochondrial function by inhibition of respiratory complex I. *Journal of Pharmacology and Experimental Therapeutics*, **311** (1), 109–114.

53 Nadanaciva, S. et al. (2007) Mitochondrial impairment by PPAR agonists and statins identified via immunocaptured OXPHOS complex activities and respiration. *Toxicology and Applied Pharmacology*, **223** (3), 277–287.

54 Owen, M.R., Doran, E. and Halestrap, A.P. (2000) Evidence that metformin exerts its anti-diabetic effects through inhibition of complex 1 of the mitochondrial respiratory chain. *The Biochemical Journal*, **348** (Pt. 3), 607–614.

55 Marroquin, L.D., dykens, J.D., Nadanaciva, S., Jamieson, J. and Will, Y. (2008) Biguanide-induced mitochondrial dysfunction increases lactate production and reduces viability of aerobically poised HepG2 and human hepatocytes in culture. *The Toxicologist*, **2008**, 903.

56 Fau, D. et al. (1994) Toxicity of the antiandrogen flutamide in isolated rat hepatocytes. *Journal of Pharmacology and*

Experimental Therapeutics, **269** (3), 954–962.
57 Marroquin, L.D. *et al.* (2007) Circumventing the Crabtree effect: replacing media glucose with galactose increases susceptibility of HepG2 cells to mitochondrial toxicants. *Toxicological Sciences*, **97** (2), 539–547.
58 Dykens, J.A. *et al.* (2008) In vitro assessment of mitochondrial dysfunction and cytotoxicity of nefazodone, trazodone and buspirone. *Toxicological Sciences*, 10.1093/toxsci/kfn056.
59 Juhaszova, M. *et al.* (2008) The identity and regulation of the mitochondrial permeability transition pore: where the known meets the unknown. *Annals of the New York Academy of Sciences*, **1123**, 197–212.
60 Chariot, P. *et al.* (1999) Zidovudine-induced mitochondrial disorder with massive liver steatosis, myopathy, lactic acidosis, and mitochondrial DNA depletion. *Journal of Hepatology*, **30** (1), 156–160.
61 Walker, U.A. *et al.* (2004) Depletion of mitochondrial DNA in liver under antiretroviral therapy with didanosine, stavudine, or zalcitabine. *Hepatology*, **39** (2), 311–317.
62 Anandatheerthavarada, H.K. *et al.* (1999) Physiological role of the N-terminal processed P4501A1 targeted to mitochondria in erythromycin metabolism and reversal of erythromycin-mediated inhibition of mitochondrial protein synthesis. *Journal of Biological Chemistry*, **274** (10), 6617–6625.
63 De Vriese, A.S. *et al.* (2006) Linezolid-induced inhibition of mitochondrial protein synthesis. *Clinical Infectious Diseases*, **42** (8), 1111–1117.
64 Deschamps, D. *et al.* (1991) Inhibition by salicylic acid of the activation and thus oxidation of long chain fatty acids. Possible role in the development of Reye's syndrome. *Journal of Pharmacology and Experimental Therapeutics*, **259** (2), 894–904.
65 Labbe, G. *et al.* (1991) Effects of various tetracycline derivatives on in vitro and in vivo beta-oxidation of fatty acids, egress of triglycerides from the liver, accumulation of hepatic triglycerides, and mortality in mice. *Biochemical Pharmacology*, **41** (4), 638–641.
66 Ponchaut, S., van Hoof, F. and Veitch, K. (1992) In vitro effects of valproate and valproate metabolites on mitochondrial oxidations. Relevance of CoA sequestration to the observed inhibitions. *Biochemical Pharmacology*, **43** (11), 2435–2442.
67 Bravo, J.F., Jacobson, M.P. and Mertens, B.F. (1977) Fatty liver and pleural effusion with ibuprofen therapy. *Annals of Internal Medicine*, **87** (2), 200–201.
68 Dutertre, J.P., Bastides, F., Jonville, A.P., De Muret, A., Sonneville, A. Larrey, D. and Autret, E. (1991) Microvesicular steatosis after ketoprofen administration. *European Journal of Gastroenterology and Hepatology*, **3**, 953–954.
69 Victorino, R.M. *et al.* (1980) Jaundice associated with naproxen. *Postgraduate Medical Journal*, **56** (655), 368–370.
70 Moyle, G.J., Dutta, D., Mandalia, S., Morlese, J., Asboe, D. and Gazzard, B.G. (2002) Hyperlactataemia and lactic acidosis during antiretroviral therapy: relevance, reproducibility and possible risk factors. *AIDS*, **16** (10), 1341–1349.
71 Lafeuillade, A., Hittinger, G. and Chadapaud, S. (2001) Increased mitochondrial toxicity with ribavirin in HIV/HCV coinfection. *Lancet*, **357** (9252), 280–281.
72 Côté, H.C., Brumme, Z.L., Craib, K.J., Alexander, C.S., Wynhoven, B., Ting, L., Wong, H., Harris, M., Harrigan, P.R., O'Shaughnessy, M.V. and Montaner, J.S. (2002) Changes in mitochondrial DNA as a marker of nucleoside toxicity in HIV-infected patients. *The New England Journal of Medicine*, **346** (11), 811–820.
73 de Baar, M.P., de Rooji, E., Smolders, K.G., van Schijndel, H.B., Timmermans,

E.C. and Bethell, R. (2007) Effects of apricitabine and other nucleoside reverse transcriptase inhibitors on replication of mitochondrial DNA in HepG2 cells. *Antiviral Research*, **76** (1), 68–74.

74 Casula, M., Bosboom-Dobbelaer, I., Smolders, K., Otto, S., Bakker, M., de Baar, M.P., Reiss, P. and de Ronde, A. (2005) Infection with HIV-1 induces a decrease in mtDNA. *Journal of Infectious Diseases*, **191** (9), 468–471.

75 Hynes, J., Marroquin, L., Ogurtsov, V.I., Christiansen, K.N., Stevens, G.J., Papkovsky, D.B. and Will, Y. (2006) Investigation of drug-induced mitochondrial toxicity using fluorescence-based oxygen-sensitive probes. *Toxicological Sciences*, **92** (1), 186–200.

76 Dykens, J.A. and Stout, A.K. (2001) Fluorescent dyes and assessment of mitochondrial membrane potential in FRET Modes. Fluorescent dyes and assessment of mitochondrial membrane potential in FRET modes. *Methods in Cell Biology*, **65**, 285–309.

77 Kamo, N., Muratsugu, M., Hongoh, R. and Kobatake, Y., (1979) Membrane potential of mitochondria measured with an electrode sensitive to tetraphenyl phosphonium and relationship between proton electrochemical potential and phosphorylation potential in steady state. *Journal of Membrane Biology*, **49** (2), 105–121.

78 Wingrove, D.E., Amatruda, J. and Gunter, T.E. (1984) Glucagon effects on the membrane potential and calcium uptake rate of rat liver mitochondria. *Journal of Biological Chemistry*, **259** (15), 9390–9394.

79 Kemp, G., Crowe, A.V., Anijeet, H.K.I., Gong, O.Y., Bimson, W.E., Frostick, S.P., Bone, J.M., Bell, G.M. and Roberts, L.N. (2004) Abnormal mitochondrial function and muscle wasting, but normal contractile efficiency, in haemodialysed patients studied non-invasively, *in vivo*. *Nephrology, Dialysis, Transplantation*, **19**, 1520–1527.

80 Milazzo, L., Piazza, M., Sangaletti, O., Gatti, N., Cappelletti, A., Adorni, F., Antinori, S., Galli, M., Moroni, M. and Riva, A. (2005) [13C]Methionine breath test: a novel method to detect anti-retroviral drug-related mitochondrial toxicity. *Journal of Antimicrobial Chemotherapy*, **55** (1), 84–89.

81 Banasch, M., Goetze, O., Hollborn, I., Hochdorfer, B., Bulut, K., Schlottmann, R., Hagemann, D., Brockmeyer, N.H., Schmidt, W.E. and Schmitz, F. (2005) 3C-methionine breath test detects distinct hepatic mitochondrial dysfunction in HIV-infected patients with normal serum lactate. *Journal of Acquired Immune Deficiency Syndromes*, **40** (2), 149–152.

82 Ong, M.M., Latchoumycandane, C. and Boelsterli, U.A. (2007) Troglitazone-induced hepatic necrosis in an animal model of silent genetic mitochondrial abnormalities. *Toxicological Sciences*, **97** (1), 205–213.

83 Balasubramaniyan, V., Kalaivani Sailaja, J. and Nalini, N. (2003) Role of leptin on alcohol-induced oxidative stress in Swiss mice. *Pharmacological Research*, **47** (3), 211–216.

84 Bhattacharyya, A. *et al.* (2007) Black tea-induced amelioration of hepatic oxidative stress through antioxidative activity in EAC-bearing mice. *Journal of Environmental Pathology, Toxicology and Oncology*, **26** (4), 245–254.

85 Boelsterli, U.A. and Lim, P.L. (2007) Mitochondrial abnormalities–a link to idiosyncratic drug hepatotoxicity? *Toxicology and Applied Pharmacology*, **220** (1), 92–107.

86 Kasdallah-Grissa, A. *et al.* (2007) Resveratrol, a red wine polyphenol, attenuates ethanol-induced oxidative stress in rat liver. *Life Sciences*, **80** (11), 1033–1039.

87 Saravanan, N., Rajasankar, S. and Nalini, N. (2007) Antioxidant effect of 2-hydroxy-4-methoxy benzoic acid on ethanol-induced hepatotoxicity in rats. *Journal of*

Pharmacy and Pharmacology, **59** (3), 445–453.

88 Choi, J. and Ou, J.H. (2006) Mechanisms of liver injury. III. Oxidative stress in the pathogenesis of hepatitis C virus. *American Journal of Physiology. Gastrointestinal and Liver Physiology*, **290** (5), G847–G851.

89 Sokol, R.J. et al. (2006) "Let there be bile"–understanding hepatic injury in cholestasis. *Journal of Pediatric Gastroenterology and Nutrition*, **43** (Suppl 1), S4–S9.

90 Li, A.P. (2002) A review of the common properties of drugs with idiosyncratic hepatotoxicity and the "multiple determinant hypothesis" for the manifestation of idiosyncratic drug toxicity. *Chemico-Biological Interactions*, **142** (1–2), 7–23.

91 Watkins, P.B. (2005) Idiosyncratic liver injury: challenges and approaches. *Toxicologic Pathology*, **33** (1), 1–5.

92 Ulrich, R.G. (2007) Idiosyncratic toxicity: a convergence of risk factors. *Annual Review of Medicine*, **58**, 17–34.

93 Uetrecht, J. (2008) Idiosyncratic drug reactions: past, present, and future. *Chemical Research in Toxicology*, **21** (1), 84–92.

94 Ott, M. et al. (2007) Mitochondria, oxidative stress and cell death. *Apoptosis: An International Journal on Programmed Cell Death*, **12** (5), 913–922.

95 Lee, C.H. et al. (2007) Protective mechanism of glycyrrhizin on acute liver injury induced by carbon tetrachloride in mice. *Biological & Pharmaceutical Bulletin*, **30** (10), 1898–1904.

96 Li, J. et al. (2007) Role of Nrf2-dependent ARE-driven antioxidant pathway in neuroprotection. *Methods in Molecular Biology (Clifton, NJ)*, **399**, 67–78.

97 Xu, Z. et al. (2008) Ghrelin prevents doxorubicin-induced cardiotoxicity through TNF-alpha/NF-kappaB pathways and mitochondrial protective mechanisms. *Toxicology*, **247** (2–3), 133–138.

98 Ozata, M. et al. (2000) Defective antioxidant defense system in patients with a human leptin gene mutation. *Hormone and Metabolic Research*, **32** (7), 269–272.

99 Robertson, R.P. et al. (2003) Glucose toxicity in beta-cells: type 2 diabetes, good radicals gone bad, and the glutathione connection. *Diabetes*, **52** (3), 581–587.

100 Pang, C.Y., Ma, Y.S. and Wei, Y.U. (2008) MtDNA mutations, functional decline and turnover of mitochondria in aging. *Frontiers in Bioscience: a Journal and Virtual Library*, **13**, 3661–3675.

101 Castilla, R. et al. (2004) Dual effect of ethanol on cell death in primary culture of human and rat hepatocytes. *Alcohol and Alcoholism (Oxford, Oxfordshire)*, **39** (4), 290–296.

102 Grezzana, T.J. et al. (2004) Oxidative stress, hepatocellular integrity, and hepatic function after initial reperfusion in human hepatic transplantation. *Transplantation Proceedings*, **36** (4), 843–845.

103 Lautraite, S. et al. (2003) Optimisation of cell-based assays for medium throughput screening of oxidative stress. *Toxicology In Vitro*, **17** (2), 207–220.

104 Xu, J.J. et al. (2009) Cellular imaging predictions of clinical drug-induced liver injury. *Toxicological Sciences, in press.*

105 Tayal, V. et al. (2007) Hepatoprotective effect of tocopherol against isoniazid and rifampicin induced hepatotoxicity in albino rabbits. *Indian Journal of Experimental Biology*, **45** (12), 1031–1036.

106 Aleksunes, L.M. and Manautou, J.E. (2007) Emerging role of Nrf2 in protecting against hepatic and gastrointestinal disease. *Toxicologic Pathology*, **35** (4), 459–473.

107 Oz, H.S. et al. (2004) Diverse antioxidants protect against acetaminophen hepatotoxicity. *Journal of Biochemical and Molecular Toxicology*, **18** (6), 361–368.

108 Balkan, J. et al. (2004) Melatonin improved the disturbances in hepatic

prooxidant and antioxidant balance and hepatotoxicity induced by a high cholesterol diet in C57BL/6J mice. *International Journal for Vitamin and Nutrition Research*, **74** (5), 349–354.

109 Pradhan, S.C. and Girish, C. (2006) Hepatoprotective herbal drug, silymarin from experimental pharmacology to clinical medicine. *The Indian Journal of Medical Research*, **124** (5), 491–504.

110 Kiruthiga, P.V. et al. (2007) Silymarin protection against major reactive oxygen species released by environmental toxins: exogenous H2O2 exposure in erythrocytes. *Basic & Clinical Pharmacology & Toxicology*, **100** (6), 414–419.

111 Pauli-Magnus, C. and Meier, P.J. (2006) Hepatobiliary transporters and drug-induced cholestasis. *Hepatology (Baltimore, Md)*, **44** (4), 778–787.

112 Stieger, B., Meier, Y. and Meier, P.J. (2007) The bile salt export pump. *Pflugers Archiv: European Journal of Physiology*, **453** (5), 611–620.

113 Mita, S. et al. (2006) Inhibition of bile acid transport across Na+/taurocholate cotransporting polypeptide (SLC10A1) and bile salt export pump (ABCB 11)-coexpressing LLC-PK1 cells by cholestasis-inducing drugs. *Drug Metabolism and Disposition: The Biological Fate of Chemicals*, **34** (9), 1575–1581.

114 Funk, C. et al. (2001) Troglitazone-induced intrahepatic cholestasis by an interference with the hepatobiliary export of bile acids in male and female rats. Correlation with the gender difference in troglitazone sulfate formation and the inhibition of the canalicular bile salt export pump (Bsep) by troglitazone and troglitazone sulfate. *Toxicology*, **167** (1), 83–98.

115 Khetani, S.R. and Bhatia, S.N. (2008) Microscale culture of human liver cells for drug development. *Nature Biotechnology*, **26** (1), 120–126.

116 Bi, Y.A., Kazolias, D. and Duignan, D.B. (2006) Use of cryopreserved human hepatocytes in sandwich culture to measure hepatobiliary transport. *Drug Metabolism and Disposition: The Biological Fate of Chemicals*, **34** (9), 1658–1665.

117 Nunes de Paiva, M.J. and Pereira Bastos de Siqueira, M.E. (2005) Increased serum bile acids as a possible biomarker of hepatotoxicity in Brazilian workers exposed to solvents in car repainting shops. *Biomarkers: Biochemical Indicators of Exposure, Response, and Susceptibility to Chemicals*, **10** (6), 456–463.

118 Lang, C. et al. (2007) Mutations and polymorphisms in the bile salt export pump and the multidrug resistance protein 3 associated with drug-induced liver injury. *Pharmacogenet Genomics*, **17** (1), 47–60.

119 Strautnieks, S.S. et al. (2008) Severe bile salt export pump deficiency: 82 different ABCB11 mutations in 109 families. *Gastroenterology*, **134** (4), 1203–1214.

120 Fardel, O. et al. (2001) Regulation of biliary drug efflux pump expression by hormones and xenobiotics. *Toxicology*, **167** (1), 37–46.

121 Takikawa, H. (2002) Hepatobiliary transport of bile acids and organic anions. *Journal of Hepatobiliary and Pancreatic Surgery*, **9** (4), 443–447.

122 Jigorel, E. et al. (2006) Differential regulation of sinusoidal and canalicular hepatic drug transporter expression by xenobiotics activating drug-sensing receptors in primary human hepatocytes. *Drug Metabolism and Disposition: The Biological Fate of Chemicals*, **34** (10), 1756–1763.

123 Leslie, E.M. et al. (2007) Differential inhibition of rat and human Na+-dependent taurocholate cotransporting polypeptide (NTCP/SLC10A1) by bosentan: a mechanism for species differences in hepatotoxicity. *Journal of Pharmacology and Experimental Therapeutics*, **321** (3), 1170–1178.

124 Boone, L., Meyer, D., Cusick, P., Ennulat, D., Provencher Bollinger, A.,

Everds, N., Meador, V., Elliot, G., Honor, D., Bounous, D. and Jordan, H. (2005) Selection and interpretation of clinical pathology indicators of hepatic injury in preclinical studies. *Veterinary Clinical Pathogy*, 34 (3), 182–188.
125 FDA (2007) Guidance for Industry Drug-Induced Liver Injury: Premarketing Clinical Evaluation (draft document).
126 EMEA (2008) Non-clinical Guideline on Drug-Induced Hepatotoxicity, http://www.emea.europa.eu/pdfs/human/swp/15011506en.pdf.
127 Canada, H. (2004) Draft Recommendations from the Scientific Advisory Panel Sub-groups on Hepatotoxicity: Hepatotoxicity of Health Products.
128 Ozer, J.R.M., Shaw, M., Wendy, B. and Schomaker, S. (2009) The current state of serum biomarkers of hepatotoxicity. *Toxicology, in press*.
129 Ramaiah, S. (2007) A toxicologist guide to the diagnosic interpretation of hepatic biochemical parameters. *Food and Chemical Toxicology*, 45, 1551–1557.
130 Dufour, D.R.L.J., Nolte, F.S., Gretch, D.R., Koff, R.S. and Seeff, L.B. (2003) Diagnosis and monitoring of hepatic injury. I. Performance characteristics of laboratory tests. *Clinical Chemistry*, 46 (12), 2027–2049.
131 Lindblom, P., Rafter, I., Copley, C., Andersson, U., Hedberg, J., Berg, A.L., Samuelsson, A., Hellmold, H., Cotgreave, I. and Glinghammar, B. (2007) Isoforms of alanine aminotransferases in human tissues and serum-differential tissue expression using novel antibiotics. *Archives of Biochemistry and Biophysics*, 466, 66–77.
132 Crawford, J. (2003) *Chapter 16: The Liver and the Biliary Tract, Robbins Basic Pathology*, Philadelphia, Pennsylvania, pp. 591–633.
133 FDA (2000) Nonclinical Assessment of Potential Hepatotoxicity in Man.
134 FDA (2000) Draft Guidance for Industry: Analytical Procedures and Methods Validation: Chemistry, Manufacturing, and Controls Documentation.
135 Kaplowitz, N. (2006) Rules and laws of drug hepatotoxicity. *Pharmaco-epidemiology and Drug Safety*, 15, 231–233.
136 Temple, R. (2006) Hy's law: predicting serious hepatotoxicity. *Pharmaco-epidemiology and Drug Safety*, 15 (4), 241–243.
137 Bleibel, W., Kim, S., D'Silva, K. and Lemmer, E.R. (2007) Drug-induced liver injury: review article. *Digestive Disease and Sciences*, 52, 2463–2471.
138 FDA (2003) Pharmacokinetics in Patients with Impaired Hepatic Function: Study Design, Data Analysis, and Impact on Dosing and Labeling.
139 Tolman, K. (2002) The liver and lovastatin. *The American Journal of Cardiology*, 89 (12), 1374–1380.
140 FDA (2006) FDA Proposes Labeling Changes to Over-the-Counter Pain Relievers. FDA News, http://www.fda.gov/bbs/topics/NEWS/2006/NEW01533.html (accessed May 28th, 2007).
141 US Department of Health, Human Services, N.I.o.H. (2004) Action Plan for Liver Disease Research.
142 Albertini, S.S.-D.L., Ruepp, S. and Weiser, T. (2004) Toxicogenomics: How predictive is toxicogenomics for toxicity in animal and man? 7th International Society for the Study of Xenobiotics Meeting, Vancouver.
143 Collins, C.D., Purohit, S., Podolsky, R.H., Zhao, H.S., Schatz, D., Eckenrode, S.E., Yang, P., Hopkins, D., Muir, A., Hoffman, M., McIndoe, R.A., Rewers, M. and She, J.X. (2006) The application of genomic and proteomic technologies in predictive, preventive and personalized medicine. *Vascular Pharmacology*, 45, 258–267.
144 Corvi, R., Ahr, H., Albertini, S., Blakey, D.H., Clerici, L., Coecke, S., Douglas, G.R., Gribaldo, L., Groten, J.P., Haase, B., Hamernik, K., Hartung, T., Inoue, T., Indans, I., Maurici, D., Orphanides, G., Rembges, D., Sansone, S.A., Snape, J.R.,

Toda, E., Tong, W., van Delft, J.H., Weis, B. and Schechtman, L.M. (2006) Validation of toxicogenomics-based test systems: ECVAM-ICCVAM/NICEATM considerations for regulatory use. *Environmental Health Perspectives*, **114**, 420–429.

145 Suter, L., Babiss, L. and Wheeldon, E.B. (2004) Toxicogenomics in predictive toxicology in drug development. *Chemistry and Biology*, **11**, 161–171.

146 Issaq, H.J., Xiao, Z. and Veenstra, T.D. (2007) Serum and plasma proteomics. *Chemical Reviews*, **107**, 3601–3620.

147 Rifai, N., Gillette, M. and Carr, S.A. (2006) Protein biomarker discovery and validation: the long and uncertain path to clinical utility. *Nature Biotechnology*, **24** (8), 971–983.

148 Hsieh, F.Y., Tengstrand, E., Lee, J.W., Li, L.Y., Silverman, L., Riordan, B., Miwa, G., Milton, M., Alden, C. and Lee, F. (2007) Drug safety evaluation through biomarker analysis – a toxicity study in the Cynomolgus monkey using an antibody-cytotoxic conjugate against ovarian cancer. *Toxicology and Applied Pharmacology*, **224**, 12–18.

149 Lindon, J.C., Keun, H., Ebbels, T.M.D., Pearce, J.M.T., Holmes, E. and Nicholson, J.K. (2005) The Consortium for Metabonomic Toxicology (COMET): aims, activities and achievements. *Pharmacogenomics*, **6** (7), 691–699.

150 Park, B.K., Kitteringham, N., Maggs, J.L., Pirmohamed, M. and Williams, D.P. (2005) The role of metabolic activation in drug-induced hepatotoxicity. *Annual Review of Pharmacology and Toxicology*, **35**, 177–202.

151 Trienen-Molsen, M. (2001) Chapter 13: Toxic Repsonses of the Liver. *Casarett & Doull's Toxicology: The Basic Science of Poisons*, McGraw-Hill Medical Publishing Division, New York, pp. 471–489.

152 Xu, J.J. et al. (2008) Multiple effects of acetaminophen and p38 inhibitors: towards pathway toxicology. *FEBS Letters*, **582** (8), 1276–1282.

153 Beyer, R.P., Fry, R., Lasarev, M.R., McConnachie, L.A., Meira, L.B., Palmer, V.S., Powell, C.L., Ross, P.K., Bammler, T.K., Bradford, B.U., Cranson, A.B., Cunningham, M.L., Fannin, R.D., Higgins, G.M., Hurban, P., Kayton, R.J., Kerr, K.F., Kosyk, O., Lobenhofer, E.K., Sieber, S.O., Cliet, P.A., Weis, B.K., Wolfinger, R., Woods, C.G., Freedman, J.H., Linney, E., Kaufmann, W.K., Kavanagh, T.J., Paules, R.S., Rusyn, I., Samson, L.D., Spencer, P.S., Suk, W., Tennant, R.J., Zarbl, H. and members of the Toxicogenomics Research Consortium (2007) Multicenter study of acetaminophen hepatotoxicity reveals the importance of biological endpoints in genomic analyses. *Toxicological Sciences*, **99** (1), 326–337.

154 Amacher, D.E., Alder, R., Herath, A. and Townsend, R.R. (2005) Use of proteomic methods to identify serum biomarkers associated with rat liver toxicity or hypertrophy. *Clinical Chemistry*, **51** (10), 1796–1803.

155 Kikkawa, R., Fujikawa, M., Yamamoto, T., Hamada, Y., Yamada, H. and Horii, I. (2006) *In vivo* hepatotoxicity study of rats in comparison with *in vitro* hepatotoxicity screening system. *Journal of Toxicological Sciences*, **31** (1), 23–34.

156 Chen, C., Krausz, K. Idle, J. and Gonzalez, F.J. (2008) Identification of novel toxicity-associated metabolites by metabolomics and mass isotopomer analysis of acetaminophen metabolism in wild-type and Cyp2e1-null mice. *Journal of Biological Chemistry*, **238** (8), 4543–4559.

157 Soga, T., Baran, R., Suematsu, M., Ueno, Y., Ikeda, S., Sakurakawa, T., Kakazu, Y., Ishikawa, T., Robert, M., Nishioka, T. and Tomita, M. (2006) Differential metabolomics reveals ophthalmic acid as an oxidative stress biomarker indicating hepatic glutathione consumption. *Journal of Biological Chemistry*, **281** (24), 16768–16776.

158 Baronas, E.T., Lee, J., Alden, C. and Hsieh, F.Y. (2007) Biomarkers to monitor drug-induced phospholipidosis. *Toxicology and Applied Pharmacology*, **218**, 72–78.

159 Boess, F., Kamber, M., Romer, S., Gasser, R., Muller, D., Albertini, S. and Suter, L. (2003) Gene expression in two hepatic cell lines, cultured primary hepatocytes, and liver slices compared to the *in vivo* liver gene expression in rats: possible implications for toxicogenomics use of *in vitro* systems. *Toxicological Sciences*, **73**, 386–402.

160 FDA (2005) Guidance for Industry: Pharmacogenomic Data Submissions.

161 Biochemistry, N.A.o.C (2000) Laboratory Guidelines for Screening, Diagnosis, and Monitoring of Hepatic Injury. National Academy of Clinical Biochemistry, Washington, DC, USA.

162 Paules, R. (2003) Phenotypic anchoring: linking cause and effect. *Environmental Health Perspectives*, **111** (6), A338–A339.

163 FDA, http://www.fda.gov/cder/livertox/ accessed May 28th, 2007.

16
Should Cardiosafety be Ruled by hERG Inhibition? Early Testing Scenarios and Integrated Risk Assessment

Dimitri Mikhailov, Martin Traebert, Qiang Lu, Steven Whitebread, and William Egan

16.1
Introduction

Drug safety has been a recent focus of pharmaceutical industry and regulatory agencies worldwide as one of the major causes for clinical attrition and postmarketing drug failures. Cardiac safety is the biggest challenge facing drug discovery, accounting for 8.7% of reported drug withdrawals between 1960 and 1999 [1]. Up until the late 1980s, cases of sudden death due to ventricular arrhythmias were not uncommon. This issue was highlighted by the Framingham study [2]. This was soon followed by the removal from the market of the first drugs linked to deaths caused by Torsades de Pointes (TdP) arrhythmia, for example, prenylamine in 1988 and terodiline in 1991 [1]. At the same time, the cardiac arrhythmia suppression trial (CAST) identified an increased risk of death with encainide and flecainide and called into question the clinical utility of class III antiarrhythmic agents, such as dofetilide, E-4031 and sotalol [3].

While the underlying mechanisms of cardiac toxicity are generally complex [4], the link between the inhibition of the IKr potassium current by blocking the potassium channel encoded by human ether-a-go-go-related gene (hERG) and cardiac arrhythmia in man is well known. The hERG gene was discovered in 1994 [5]; later, the group of M. Keating revealed the link between TdP, the hERG potassium channel and IKr, based on evidence from patients with inherited and acquired long QT (LQT) syndrome [6, 7].

The hERG channel conducts the rapid component of the delayed rectifier potassium current, IKr, which is crucial for repolarization of cardiac action potentials. Hereditary LQT syndromes are caused by a reduction in hERG current due to genetic defects, while blockade of the channel (or its trafficking) by a drug leads to acquired LQT syndrome. This is characterized by action potential prolongation, lengthening of the QT interval on the surface electrocardiogram (ECG) and an increased risk for TdP arrhythmia – a rare event that can cause sudden death. As a consequence, multiple drugs with the mechanism of action linked to hERG blockade have been pulled off the market in the past decade for causing arrhythmia-related deaths.

Hit and Lead Profiling. Edited by Bernard Faller and Laszlo Urban
Copyright © 2009 WILEY-VCH Verlag GmbH & Co. KGaA, Weinheim
ISBN: 978-3-527-32331-9

While TdP is the relevant clinical endpoint, both hERG blockade and LQT represent pro-arrhythmic risks, especially when combined with other factors such as heart disease, bradycardia and disturbances of cation homeostasis [8]. Therefore, the consequence of positive preclinical findings for either potent hERG blockade or statistically significant LQT (>10% prolongation of QT interval) can result in a requirement for a thorough QT/QTc (TQTS) study in man as part of clinical safety trials. This could be an additional hurdle preventing otherwise promising compounds from progressing into the clinic. Hence, there is a pragmatic need to design out cardiosafety liability during lead selection and lead optimization phases of drug discovery [8].

The hERG channel is particularly vulnerable to inhibition by small molecules due to its drug-like pharmacophore [9]. According to some reports 20–30% of drug discovery projects have hERG liabilities, which implies a significant negative impact by hERG on the whole pharmaceutical industry [10]. In addition, a low concentration of inhibitor (equivalent to about 10% inhibition) is often sufficient for a significant change of QT interval in man [11]. Consequently, many drug discovery projects are affected by positive hERG signals and must work to develop strategies to remove the hERG blockade [12], requiring additional chemistry resources and resulting in longer project time lines.

While a significant risk factor, hERG blockade does not always translate to LQT and subsequently to arrhythmia [13]. Hence, there is a strong requirement for early integrated risk assessment to minimize unnecessary de-prioritization of chemical scaffolds and to reduce potentially negative impact on early chemistry projects. These and other factors together drive the need for early testing strategies to assess the risk of cardiotoxicity due to hERG inhibition [14]. Traditionally, the manual patch clamp technique using recombinant human cell lines, has been used to measure hERG inhibition. This method is considered the "gold standard" assay, offering high reproducibility and control of experimental conditions (temperature, voltage protocol). However, manual patch clamp assay is not suitable for screening larger numbers of compounds produced in the early phases of drug discovery projects. Over the past five years, a battery of *in vitro* assays have become available to test for hERG inhibition. These range from high-throughput binding assays to more sophisticated automated patch clamp systems. Based on the volume of data produced by these higher-throughput assays, *in silico* models have been devised to help predict hERG inhibition before a molecule has even been synthesized. Both computational and experimental methods are reviewed in the subsequent sections.

No single assay is 100% accurate in the prediction of arrhythmias in humans. Furthermore, significant variation may occur in assay results because of poor physicochemical properties of the test compounds, for example, low solubility or low cell permeability, especially in the micromolar range where hERG inhibition is typically found for most discovery compounds. A strategy needs to be devised for assessing risk in the widest context considering possible assay artifacts and uncertainties. Analysis of all available data is recommended: hERG results, physicochemical and PK properties, including these of major metabolites, program-related information such as the indication, proposed route of administration and potency at the primary target. Based on this assessment, compounds can be selected for further development with a higher degree of confidence for the level of LQT risk related to hERG.

Although the hERG channel has been shown to be the most significant of the risk factors that cause LQT, the full mechanism of TdP arrhythmia is more complex [13, 15] and the range of relevant biological targets linked with other cardiac toxicities is much broader [4]. Other ion channels involved in regulating cardiac action potential are also known to cause cardiotoxicity. For example, the Nav1.5 and Cav1.2 channels regulate initial depolarizing current responsible for the upstroke and the depolarizing current that sustains and modulates cardiac action potential plateau, respectively (reviewed below). Safety profiling assays for these targets should be part of a cardiosafety strategy and provide useful tools for mechanistic studies [16]. *In vitro* cardiac action potential assays using isolated cardiomyocytes, Purkinje fibers, ventricular wedge preparations or isolated rabbit heart account for the interplay of multiple currents and commonly used for exploratory preclinical studies. These lower-throughput methods are briefly discussed in subsequent sections.

In addition, other target classes such as kinases and GPCRs, have also been linked to human cardiotoxicity, and these are reviewed in the literature [4, 16, 17] and in another chapter.

16.2
Role of Ion Channels in Heart Electrophysiology

The vital function of the heart strongly relies on its normal electrophysiological behavior, a result of the orchestrated propagation of excitatory stimulations. Such orchestration comes from the orderly action of each cardiac cell, controlled by electrophysiological means: the generation and propagation of the action potential. This results in contraction and relaxation of heart muscle, forming the basis for cardiac rhythm. However, failing to generate or propagate action potentials, or alteration of the duration or configuration of such potentials among individual cardiac cells in various regions in the heart causes a disordered cardiac rhythm or arrhythmia.

What then lies under all the electrophysiological behavior of the heart? Among all the contributors, voltage-gated ion channels are major family that determines "excitability" of all "excitable cells" (i.e., cells that generate and propagate action potentials) such as cardiomyocytes. It is the diversity in the voltage dependence and the ion selectivity of those channels that make the complex behavior of cardiac action potential [18]. While there are some minor differences between different regions in cardiac tissue in terms of electrophysiological activities, a typical ventricular action potential is shown in Figure 16.1.

Genetic studies have identified at least six separate genes that, if mutated, can cause congenital long-QT syndrome. By far, the most described channel involved is encoded by the human ether-a-go-go-related gene (hERG). This is a potassium channel protein that regulates a major repolarizing potassium current, IKr (phase 3

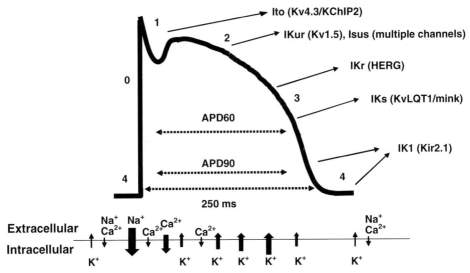

Figure 16.1 Typical ventricular action potential. Corresponding ion channels and electric currents at phases 0–4 are labeled. The contributions and directionality (influx vs efflux) of each ion current at corresponding time points are indicated at the bottom. APD60 and APD90 is the action potential duration at 60% and 90% of repolarization respectively. (Reprinted from [19], with permission from Elsevier).

in Figure 16.1). Blocking (or loss-of-function mutation) of this channel reduces IKr, resulting in prolongation of action potentials in individual cells, causing the congenital long-QT syndrome. In contrast, virtually all drugs that prolong the QT interval and cause TdP also block IKr [7]. Detailed structural and modeling analysis indicated that comparing with all other potassium channels, there are totally eight (instead of four) aromatic amino acid residues (Tyr652 and Phe656, in tetrameric configuration) lining the aqueous phase of the pore of hERG channel, making it more vulnerable to the binding of small molecules [20].

However, the reverse is not necessarily true: all compounds that block the hERG channels do not prolong action potentials. Part of the reason lies in the fact that many compounds have a mixed effect on ion channels, particularly due to the blocking effect on both hERG and the L-type calcium channel [21], which is responsible for phase 2 of the cardiac action potential (Figure 16.1). Examples for such dual-blockers include bepridil, verapamil and mibefradil [22], all blocking hERG and L-type calcium channels at the therapeutic concentrations. However, only verapamil has nearly no cardiac liabilities.

The apparent liability of bepridil and mibefradil seems to result from their additional blocking effect on another important ion channel, KvLQT1/minK [23], which is responsible for phase 3 of the action potential (Figure 16.1). Indeed, the IKs blockers prolong the cardiac APD and QT interval and suppress electrically induced ventricular tachyarrhythmias in animals with acute coronary ischemia and exercise superimposed on a healed myocardial infarction [24].

Other potassium channels also play important roles here. For example, Kv4.3/KChIP complex conducts the transient outward current, Ito, responsible for the descending phase 1 of the cardiac action potential, whereas Kv1.5 is underlying the ultra rapid delayed rectifying current, IKur, responsible for descending phase 2. Finally, inward rectifier potassium channel (Kir2 family) is responsible for IK1 current, which maintains the action potential close to or at the resting level (phase 4).

For the ascending phases caused by the influx of cations, Nav1.5 is responsible for the initial depolarization of the action potential (phase 0). Mutations in SCN5A, the gene that encodes Nav1.5, result in multiple cardiac arrhythmia syndromes [25] A large number of mutations leading to loss of Nav1.5 channel function can result in Brugada syndrome (BrS; OMIM 601144) [26], with an estimated 5–50 cases per 10 000 individuals [27]. However, mutations leading to a gain-of-function of the channel cause long QT syndrome type 3 (LQT3; OMIM 603830) [28]. Gain-of-function mutations in Nav1.5 result in an increase in the late component of the Na + current, resulting in a slow and constant entry of Na + in the plateau phase of the action potential, leading to a prolonged QT interval on the electrocardiogram (ECG) [29].

Among all the cardiac ion channels, hERG seems to generate the biggest impact because its blockade by small molecules causes serious clinical consequences and therefore it is the main focus of subsequent sections.

16.3
hERG Profiling Assays

The CAST study [3] directly influenced an insightful investigation by the group of Chadwick *et al.* which paved the way to the first high-throughput method to identify hERG inhibitors [30]. They realized that, whereas radioligands for the calcium and sodium channels were known and they had facilitated the characterization of drug interactions at these channels, there were no radioligands available to study drug interactions with potassium channels. The antiarrhythmic agents tested by CAST were known to block the rapidly activating delayed rectifier K + currents (IKr). [^{3}H] Dofetilide was chosen as a probe for the potassium channel responsible for these currents due to its higher affinity (0.005–1 µM reported). Ventricular cardiomyocytes isolated from male guinea pigs, dogs and rats were chosen for the study. High affinity binding sites were found in the guinea pig (Kd = 70 nM, Bmax = 300 fmol/mg protein), but not in the rat. The dog also had high affinity binding, but at a much lower level. This group was also the first to demonstrate a correlation between binding affinity and functional activity (IKr block in guinea pig cardiomyocytes) of [^{3}H]dofetilide and known antiarrhythmic drugs (Figure 16.2). Several studies using [^{3}H]dofetilide followed [31–35].

The spate of drug withdrawals due to TdP made it imperative to screen for hERG inhibition during the drug discovery phase in high-throughput format. The available manual electrophysiology patch clamp techniques, while ideal for late-stage testing,

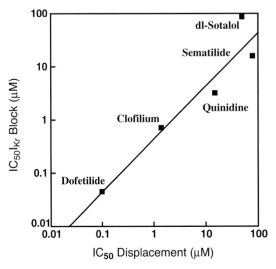

Figure 16.2 Correlation between [^{3}H]dofetilide binding affinity and IKr block in guinea pig myocytes. (Reprinted from [30], with permission).

were too slow and expensive for early screening. The pioneering work on [^{3}H] dofetilide provided the first opportunity to set up such a high-throughput assay, but some cellular, non-electrophysiological assays were soon also developed [14]. At the same time, several attempts were being made to automate the patch clamp assay, and these are now proving successful. This section focuses on high-throughput methods, though lower-throughput techniques are also briefly discussed at the end.

16.3.1
Cell-Free Competition Binding Assays

Competition binding experiments have been used for many years to characterize receptor proteins and to discover novel compounds interacting with such proteins. Typically a detection marker (label), such as a radioactive isotope or fluorescent molecule, is incorporated into a known high affinity ligand. The specific binding of such a ligand (tracer) to the protein of interest can then be measured. The binding is reversible, so any other unlabeled compound which can bind to the same receptor will be able to compete with the tracer for the available binding sites. Keeping the concentration of tracer constant and increasing the concentration of competitor will result in a concentration-dependent drop in signal in a typically sigmoidal fashion. From such concentration response curves, the affinity of the competing unlabeled ligand can be calculated.

The key to these assays is to find a suitable method by which the bound labeled ligand can be measured, separate from the unbound fraction. Three separate methods have been used to measure hERG binding: filtration through glass fiber filters [36, 37], scintillation proximity assay (SPA) technology [38] and fluorescence polarization (FP) [39, 40]. All use cell membranes prepared from cells over-expressing recombinant hERG. Critical for both SPA and FP is a cell line with a very high level of hERG expression. Binding is very sensitive to the potassium concentration in the medium [33, 36]. Typically 10 mM potassium chloride is used, although higher concentrations (up to 60 mM) can increase both the affinity of the radioligand and the maximum concentration of binding sites [36].

16.3.1.1 Radioligand Binding

Several radioligands have been used to measure hERG binding, but the one most commonly used is [^{3}H]dofetilide, as pioneered by Chadwick [30]. Additional radioligands which have been reported are [^{3}H]astemizole [41, 42], [^{3}H]MK499 [43], [^{35}S]MK499 [44, 45] and [^{125}I]BeKm [46]. BeKm is a scorpion toxin which does not bind to the intracellular "dofetilide" binding site, but to an extracellular site on the channel pore [47]. It cannot therefore be used for screening purposes to predict for dofetilide-like inhibitory activities in a hERG patch clamp assay.

Typically, filtration is used to separate bound from free using 96-well plates in a total volume of 200 µL, but SPA technology using yttrium silicate wheatgerm agglutinin-coated beads in 384-well plates and a total volume of 60 µL has also been used [43].

16.3.1.2 Fluorescence Polarization

More recently, a nonradioactive binding assay was developed using fluorescence polarization (FP) technology [40, 48]. One difficulty with setting up an FP assay is to find a suitable fluorescent ligand [40]. Typically, fluorescent labels are large, relative to the size of the parent ligand, and so the binding characteristics of a fluorescently labeled ligand are often very different and can result in a large drop in affinity. Another problem with FP assays is the phenomenon of light scattering. Membrane particles have to be very fine and homogeneous to reduce this effect. Heavy precipitation of poorly soluble compounds in the assay could also give problems for this reason. But, FP assays have the advantage of avoiding the safety and waste regulations when working with radioactivity.

16.3.2
Non-Electrophysiological Functional Cellular Assays

16.3.2.1 Rubidium Efflux and Thallium Influx

The rubidium assay uses the observation that rubidium (Rb+) has a high permeability through K+ channels. hERG-expressing cells are first loaded for 3–4 h with rubidium, which enters the cells via Na/K ATPases. After excess extracellular rubidium is removed, test compounds are added to the cell medium. The rubidium loaded inside the cell then passes back into the extracellular compartment through the open hERG K+ channels after depolarization with high (50 mM) potassium. Compounds which are able to block the hERG channels prevent this process. The assay is quantified by measuring the amount of rubidium remaining in the cells, either by radioactive measurement if [^{86}Rb] is used [49], or by flame atomic absorption spectroscopy (AAS) analysis [50, 51].

This is a long, but fairly cheap and high-throughput assay to run. However, several groups have reported that, when compared to patch clamp and [^{3}H]dofetilide binding data, it is rather insensitive and not ideally suited for preclinical screening of hERG blockers [52, 53].

Thallium is a surrogate for potassium ions and it freely moves through open hERG and other potassium channels. Thallium is detected through specific thallium detection dyes such as benzothiazole coumarin acetoxymethyl ester (BTC-AM) [54, 55], which requires Cl-free media, or FluxOR (Invitrogen), a new dye which fluoresces upon binding to thallium. Plates can be read on fluorometric imaging plate readers such as Flipr and FlexStation (Molecular Devices) or the FDSS (Hamamatsu). Little has been published so far demonstrating how well thallium flux hERG assays compare with other methods.

16.3.2.2 Membrane Potential-Sensitive Fluorescent Dyes

First attempts to reach a higher throughput with cell-based assays to assess hERG inhibition used membrane potential-sensitive fluorescent dyes such as the oxonol-based dyes bis-(1,3-dibutylbarbituric acid)-trimethine oxonol (DiBAC4(3)) and FMP, which partition across the cell membrane in a voltage-dependent manner. Like the thallium-sensitive dyes, these have to be read on a fluorometric imaging plate reader due to the kinetic readout. Due to compounds interacting with the dyes and other nonspecific effects, these assays gave high false hit rates [51]. An adaptation of the method using the same oxonol dyes was used to create an endpoint assay which could be read on a conventional fluorescent plate reader [14]. This assay provided a considerably greater throughput than the kinetic readout assays, but a rather poor correlation with a manual patch clamp assay was obtained [56].

16.3.3
Higher-Throughput Planar Patch Technologies

There are currently two main types of plate-based planar patch instruments: those which produce giga-Ohm seals, as in conventional patch clamp (e.g., PatchXpress, QPatch) and those producing <100 mega-Ohm seals as a compromise to allow a higher throughput (e.g., IonWorks HT, IonWorks Quattro) [57, 58].

The IonWorks HT and the IonWorks Quattro are similar systems from the same manufacturer. They differ in the number of pores per well on which cells can attach. The IonWorks HT has just one pore per well, resulting in a lower success rate (~65%), but slightly better seals (~100 mega-Ohm) than the IonWorks Quattro. The latter has 64 pores or cells per well (population patch), resulting in a much higher success rate (>95%) but only 30–50 mega-Ohm seals. For the measurement of hERG inhibition, the performance of early tests were not better than that of the rubidium flux assay, primarily due to compound-specific potency shifts [50], but consequent efforts minimized the shifts by using lower cell count [59].

The giga-Ohm seals achieved by the PatchXpress (Molecular Devices) [60, 61] and QPatch (Sophion Biosciences) [62] make them the higher-throughput patch clamp instruments of choice for hERG inhibition screening as they are more comparable with the manual patch clamp technology. Both instruments employ a single pore per well, with 16 channels run in parallel, or 48 channels for an HT version of QPatch (Sophion Biosciences). The advantages of the true giga-Ohm seal obtained through PatchExpress or QPatch for cardiac channel measurement lie in the fact that they can bear higher fidelity in the membrane potential controls, especially for the fast channels such as Nav1.5. In addition, the all-glass based system such as QPatch has a significant higher correlation in compound pharmacology better comparable to the gold-standard manual patch-clamp.

For the manual patch clamp technique, considerable electrophysiology expertise is required to set up and run the assays. That said, there are advantages of this technique with currently no alternative by any automated recording techniques. For example, the recording from primary cells such as cardiac myocytes is only available through manual recordings (voltage or current clamp), partly due to low availability of cells (tens of millions cells are required by automated recording per experiment) and partly due to the heterogeneity of the cells. Another unique feature that is currently only available with manual recording is a sophisticated temperature control system, from recording chamber to compound incubation, in order to address the need for characterizing compound/cell performance in more physiological conditions (e.g., 37 °C). Finally, for GLP purposes, outflow fractions of each test condition have to be collected for quantitative measurement of the true compound concentrations. This can currently be only achieved in the manual setup.

16.3.4
Non-hERG Ion Channel Assays Related to Cardiotoxicity

The calcium L-type channel Cav1.2 and cardiac sodium channel Nav1.5 are two important cardiac ion channels which are relatively rare targets of small molecules, but their blockade can cause cardiotoxicity and they must also be monitored [16]. They are much less promiscuous than hERG and therefore screening is at a lower rate. The calcium L-type channel pharmacology is quite complex, as there are several different subunits making up the channel. Splice variants are known and the different calcium blockers using this channel as a drug target have different binding sites [63, 64]. Radioligand binding assays have been available for many years to study binding to these channels, using [^{3}H]nitrendipine for the dihydropyridine site, [^{3}H]diltiazem for the benzothiazepine site and [^{3}H]desmethoxyverapamil for the phenylalkylamine site [65–68]. Usually, these assays use rat brain cortex membranes in a 96-well filtration format and their relevance to the human clinical situation needs to be explored better. Mason *et al.* recently showed a positive correlation between the IC$_{50}$ found in the [^{3}H]diltiazem binding assay and the side effect "palpitations" reported for drugs on the market [69]. Both the Cav1.2 and the Nav1.5 can however be run using human recombinant cell lines on the high-throughput patch clamp systems described in the previous section.

There are of course many other targets which are known to mediate cardiovascular side-effects, for example, the serotonin 5HT2b receptor, but these are beyond the scope of this section and are reviewed in another chapter.

16.3.5
Nonclinical Cardiosafety Assays in Early Drug Development

Nonclinical assessment of cardiac safety must be performed for a compound to qualify to be submitted to the health authorities to begin studies in man. For this purpose the regulatory bodies require that the cardiosafety assays should follow the principles of GLP wherever possible. The following assays/technologies are frequently used to predict potential clinical QT liability.

The manual hERG patch clamp assay (GLP) applies whole cell technique to measure hERG current amplitude of stably transfected mammalian cells. Usually the assay is conducted at 37 °C and drugs are tested up to the solubility limit or the occurrence of cytotoxic effects. Based on the changes at different concentrations of the peak outward hERG tail current, an IC_{50} value is determined. The final drug concentration in the bath solution is determined frequently by analytical chemistry. For many mechanistic studies, cardiomyocytes are isolated from guinea pig atria or ventricles. For the isolation process, the heart is removed and retrogradely perfused via the aorta with enzyme cocktail to disconnect and separate the cardiomyocytes. Theoretically, every ion channel involved in the generation of the cardiac action potential can be analyzed by using the manual patch clamp technique. Thus isolated cardiomyocytes are a valuable option to measure ion channels for which the human isoform is not available in a transfected mammalian cell line. However, some ionic currents can only be measured in the presence of specific blockers or using a special voltage protocols [70, 71].

A next-level assay is usually an isolated heart/cardiac tissue preparation. The canine Purkinje fiber assay (GLP) measures several action potential parameters, like resting membrane potential, upstroke velocity, action potential duration and shape, but also if a drug acts reverse-use dependently [72]. Based on changes of the action potential shape it is possible to conclude which ion channels are modulated (e.g., L-type calcium channel block would abolish the plateau phase). The papillary muscle assay (e.g., guinea pigs) determines similar parameters [73].

The isolated, paced rabbit heart method (Langendorff preparation) [74] is a very powerful tool to identify compounds with proarrhythmic potential based on the observance of compound-induced triangulation (triangle-shaped action potential) and instability of the monophasic action potential (high variability in APD from beat to beat), ectopic beats, and reverse-use dependence of prolongation of the APD (greater effects at lower stimulation rates). These indices taken together indicate different proarrhythmic risk depending on the context in which they develop. Triangulation associated with APD prolongation (Figure 16.3a) indicates a potential QT liability (+/− torsadogenicity), while triangulation associated with APD shortening is indicative of a profibrillatory risk (Figure 16.3b).

Additionally, the isolated heart can be used to measure chronotropic or inotropic effects. There are several additional *ex vivo* assays like the sinoatrial node preparation [76], left ventricular wedge preparation [77] available which address specific questions. All of the *ex vivo* studies mentioned above with the

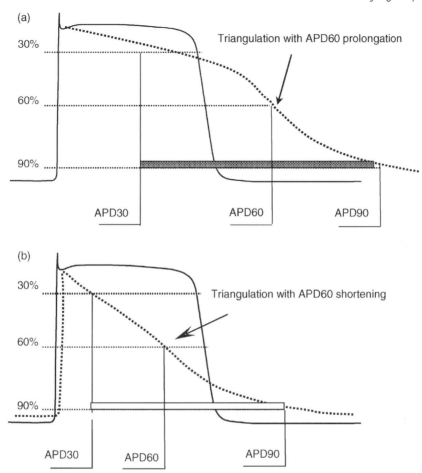

Figure 16.3 Schematic representation of monophasic action potentials (MAP) recorded in the isolated rabbit heart system, showing MAP duration changes: Triangulation with APD60 prolongation (a) and triangulation with APD60 shortening (b). Triangulation is calculated by the difference in ms between MAP duration at 90% (APD90) and MAP duration at 30% (APD30) of repolarization. APD30, APD60 and APD90 are same as described in Figure 16.1. (Reprinted from [75], with permission from Elsevier).

exception of the Purkinje fiber and papillary muscle assay are usually not performed in GLP compliance.

Beagle dogs [78] and cynomolgus monkeys [79] are frequently used telemetered to collect arterial blood pressure, heart rate and ECG information. These are usually GLP-compliant single-dose studies including the determination of toxicokinetic parameters. All possible ECG variations can be captured. The QT interval is corrected for heart rate influence by using usually Bazett, Fridericia, van de Water [80–82] or an individualized correction formula. It is empowered to detect QT interval changes of 5–10 ms.

16.4
Computational Models for hERG

In silico models can help deal with hERG issues in several ways. First, they can be used to estimate hERG affinity of a set of virtual molecules, thus permitting chemists to prioritize which molecules to synthesize first. Second, *in silico* models can be used to help understand the cause of hERG affinity in already synthesized molecules and suggest design approaches to reduce hERG affinity. Three types of computational models have been used to predict the affinity of a molecule for the hERG channel: pharmacophore, homology docking, QSAR models.

16.4.1
Pharmacophore Models

A number of pharmacophore models for hERG binding ligands have been published. An early pharmacophore for Class III antiarrhythmics was proposed by Morgan and Sullivan in 1992 which contained a tertiary or quaternary amine plus two or three substituted aromatic rings [83]. Ekins *et al.* used a small dataset of anti-psychotics and other literature compounds to generate a Catalyst pharmacophore [84]. The resulting pharmacophore contained five features: four hydrophobic features and one positive ionizable feature (a four-sided pyramid). Cavalli *et al.* fit a CoMFA model (a 3-D QSAR approach) to 37 molecules with known hERG activity [85]. The resulting pharmacophore contained four features: three aromatic rings and a tertiary amine. The authors noted that not all features were contained in each molecule. Aronov [86, 87] proposed a family of hERG pharmacophores containing three to four features in linear, V-shaped, or pyramidal configurations. The features are aromatic rings plus a basic amine, although the basic amine is not always required. The aromatic rings in the majority of molecules used to create all of these pharmacophore models were phenyl rings.

It is common practice to enlarge the largest common denominator pharmacophore to include features which provide great potency but are not present in all active molecules. This is misleading. Examination of the published literature shows that molecules with only two of three pharmacophoric features can cause significant hERG block.

Figure 16.4 shows the chemical structures of a variety of molecules with potent activity against the hERG channel, including withdrawn drugs and Class III antiarrhythmics. Below are some examples of different structures associated with hERG inhibition.

Ficker *et al.* [88] demonstrated that C10-tetraethylammonium (C10-TEA) has an IC_{50} of 3.6 µM against hERG. C10-TEA has only an aliphatic (hydrophobic) tail attached to a quarternary amine which is of course permanently positively charged [88]. Clofilium is a Class III antiarrhythmic that was designed based on the observation that quaternary amines like TEA inhibit potassium channels [83]. It has highly potent hERG activity ($IC_{50} = 7$ nM in patch clamp experiment). Clofilium has one phenyl ring in addition to two aliphatic linkers off the amine.

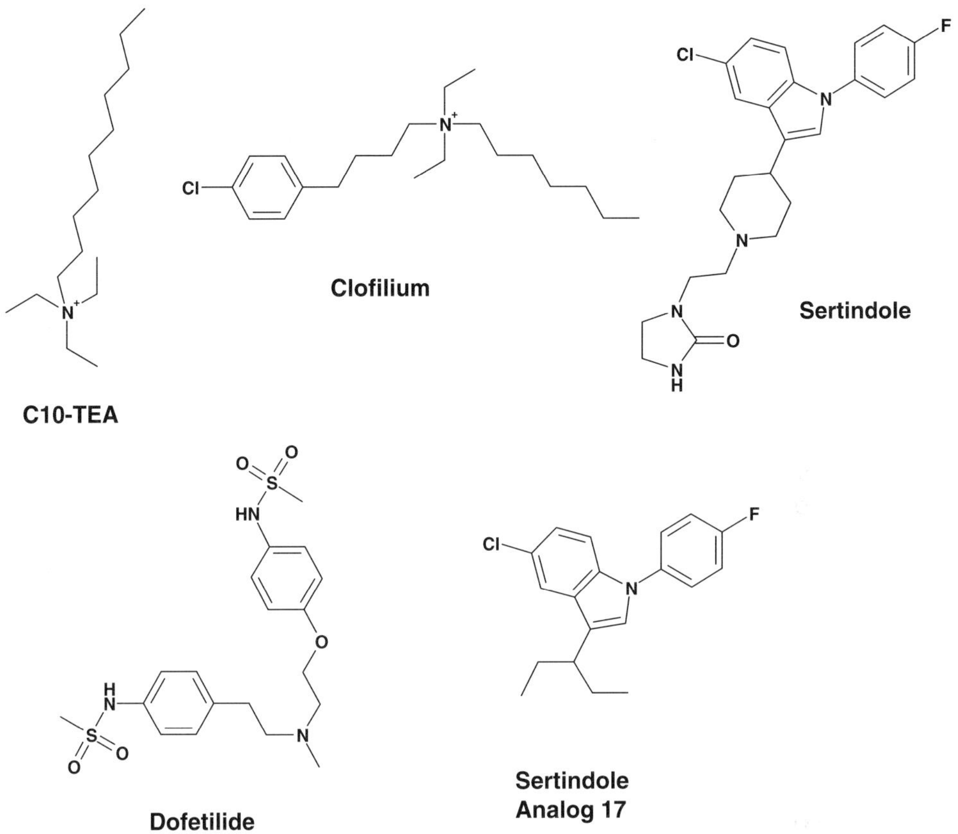

Figure 16.4 Examples of potent hERG blockers.

Sertindole was withdrawn from the market due to arrhythmias and deaths and has a hERG IC$_{50}$ of 3 nM. Sertindole has two aromatic rings in a "V" conformation with a basic amine in the tail of the molecule. Pearlstein *et al.* demonstrated that an analog of sertindole (analog 17) made by removal of the tail of the molecule containing the basic amine still possessed potent hERG activity (IC$_{50}$ = 1.48 μM) [89].

Dofetilide, a Class III antiarrhythmic with nanomolar hERG activity, is commonly used as a standard in competitive binding assays for hERG inhibition (see Section NaN). Dofetilide is only slightly larger with a core of two phenyl rings linked across an amine which is positively charged at physiological pH.

16.4.2
Docking to Homology Models

At present, there is no crystal structure of the hERG channel. However, homology models have been built using crystal structures of bacterial potassium channels (e.g., MthK, KcsA [90, 91]). Blockers must cross the cell membrane and enter the channel in the open state to inhibit function. The channel is a tetramer with each of the four subunits containing a pair of aromatic residues, Phe656 and Tyr652, considered by many researchers to form crucial binding interactions. These two residues are not commonly found in other potassium channels, which contain Ile or Val residues at those positions. Mutagenesis studies also indicate other residues such as Thr623 and Ser624 play a role in binding of some compounds, although mutagenesis can cause allosteric effects on the channel which cloud interpretation of those experiments.

Pearlstein and coworkers [9, 89] conducted a series of insightful docking studies on the hERG channel, using MthK and KvAP structures. Their work using induced fit docking into the open KvAP structure was particularly interesting. The model showed a crown-shaped hydrophobic volume in the intracellular pore formed mainly by the eight Phe656 and Tyr652 aromatic side chains (10.3–12.0 Å in diameter). A propeller-shaped hydrophilic volume was located between the intracellular base of the selectivity filter and the extracellular side of the crown-shaped hydrophobic volume.

Induced fit docking of clofilium predicted interactions with seven of the eight aromatic side chains: all four Tyr652 and three of four Phe656 side chains. The charged quarternary amine partially occupies the propeller-shaped hydrophilic volume. The purpose of the hERG channel is to move K+ cations, and the propeller-shaped region is consistent with that functionality. Zhu et al. [92] have reported that the addition of a carboxylic acid group (–COOH) to many molecules generally reduces measured hERG inhibition by a significant amount. A –COO– anion would clash with the electronic preference of the channel.

Six molecules with strong hERG binding were docked using induced fit and all six had multiple ring stacking and hydrophobic interactions with the Tyr652 and Phe656 side chains. This suggests the promiscuity of the channel is in part due to its large size (ability to accommodate a wide variety of molecular size/shapes) and in part due to the combinatorial possibilities for interactions of one to three aromatic rings/hydrophobic chains on a ligand with eight aromatic side chains in the channel.

16.4.3
QSAR Models

Waring and Johnstone published an extensive study of the relationship of hERG inhibition as measured using high-throughput electrophysiology with log D and c Log P using logistic regression models [93]. An increased probability of hERG inhibition with both basic and more lipophilic molecules was observed. They suggest that if a relationship is established for a chemical series between log P and hERG activity, lipophilicity be reduced to <3. If such a reduction is not possible, or is accomplished but hERG activity still remains, they caution that specific structural modification is necessary. Shamovsky et al. [94] demonstrated the use of lipophilicity-adjusted hERG potency to reduce hERG liability in a chemokine receptor antagonist project.

Complex field-based 3-D QSAR models have also been applied to the problem of predicting hERG activity. Cavalli et al. [85] used a CoMFA model, as previously discussed. Pearlstein et al. [89] modeled a set of sertindole analogs using comparative molecular similarity analysis (CoMSiA), another 3-D QSAR approach. Both approaches require significant work to align the molecules being used. Alignment-independent approaches such as GRIND have also been applied to the hERG problem, although with limited success ($q^2 = 0.35$, pIC_{50} SSEcv $= 0.71$) [95].

Multivariate models using neural networks, support vector machines and least median squares regression have been used to predict hERG activity [96–98]. These types of models function more as computational "black box" assays.

16.5
Integrated Risk Assessment

16.5.1
Cardiosafety Assessment of Early Discovery Projects

Cardiosafety risk assessment in early drug discovery projects focuses on hERG as the most frequently hit and well validated target linked to TdP. In pharmaceutical settings, it is common to use a combination of *in silico* and high-throughput experimental assays to assess LQT risk for larger numbers of compounds [8, 14].

In our experience, it is crucial for a project team to be aware of hERG inhibition as the main LQT risk factor during the early phases of drug discovery and to have easy access to training materials and internal experts if consultation is needed. During lead selection, use of appropriate hERG assays and early LQT risk assessments must be done in the context of a lead series represented by at least ten compounds (Figure 16.5).

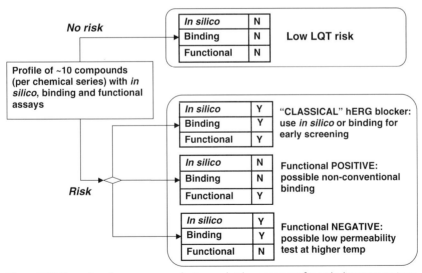

Figure 16.5 Examples of proper assay selection and risk assessment for early discovery projects.

Selecting proper assays is key at this stage. For example, if a project team has access to an *in silico* hERG model, data sources used for training of the model have to be carefully considered. For example, a QSAR model trained on patch clamp data will likely perform differently from one trained on radioligand binding data. Also, novel scaffolds not recognized by a model as potential hERG inhibitors may have positive results in *in vitro* and *in vivo* tests. Models will often fail or succeed by scaffold. Therefore, testing performance of an *in silico* model for further use to guide SAR is crucial at the lead selection phase. The decision is based on the experimental data: good correlation enables the project to use the *in silico* model for SAR, thus saving time and cost. In an ideal situation, *in silico* models can predict if a compound will block the hERG channel and a biochemical assay such as radioligand binding will provide the potency. If a project team establishes good correlation between binding and functional assays (Figure 16.6a) what remains is to spot check with a cellular patch clamp assay to confirm functional blockage.

In other cases, the high-throughput binding assays might miss functional chemotypes and early reliance on a high-throughput functional assay is needed for adequate data interpretation. The latter also requires proper understanding of factors that might affect assay performance. For example, low solubility or low permeability can produce false negatives.

It is common to have poorly soluble compounds in early drug discovery projects. Though issues are rarely raised with primary pharmacological target assays that normally screen compounds at the nanomolar concentration range, profiling for hERG is done at much higher concentrations, in the mid- to high-micromolar range

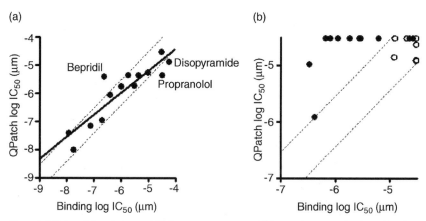

Figure 16.6 Correlation between hERG radioligand binding and QPatch functional assays could be used for proper assay selection and risk assessment. Dotted lines indicate 3× acceptable variation between the assays. (a) Example of good correlation between hERG radioligand binding IC_{50} and functional hERG QPatch IC_{50}. Functional assay could be used to spot check results of higher throughput binding assay. (b) Example of systematic shift to less potent hERG IC_{50} values in QPatch functional assay for compounds with low permeability (filled circles). Results of functional assay would have to be properly interpreted together with results of cell free binding assay.

to establish safety margins. Some compounds might precipitate at higher concentrations and result in lower than the "real" potency, making assay data interpretation challenging. Yet, functional assays can be affected by several additional factors such as cell batch variation, temperature and voltage protocol [99]. Permeability is another important factor as most compounds block the channel from inside the cell. Therefore, compounds must first penetrate the cell membrane to induce functional blockade. Compounds with low cell permeability will tend to have less potent IC_{50} values in a functional assay when compared to a noncellular binding assay (Figure 16.6b). Hence, both solubility and permeability *in vitro* data must be available to properly interpret results of hERG profiling.

Once a project team establishes relevant experimental and *in silico* tools, an early strategy to dial out hERG activity can be developed. Having such a strategy in place early does not have to be viewed as a go/no go decision point for a project. An early hERG strategy can help project teams better assess the need for extra resources and the possibility of longer timelines during the lead optimization phase. Medicinal chemistry approaches for reducing hERG activity have been highlighted above and extensively described in the literature [12]. It is important to optimize out hERG inhibition relative to *in vitro* primary target potency in early phases and using relevant PK data (C_{max}) at the point of selecting a clinical candidate in order to establish an acceptable safety margin.

16.5.2
Cardiosafety Assessment of Preclinical Positive Signals

If a drug is about to enter the clinical phase, an integrated safety assessment is necessary to evaluate its risk to induce a QT prolongation in man. Such an integrated preclinical cardiosafety assessment is influenced by both internal (corporate cardiac testing strategies) and regulatory guidelines (e.g., ICH S7B, ICH E14 [100, 101]). The ICH S7B, The Nonclinical Evaluation of the Potential for Delayed Ventricular Repolarization (QT Interval Prolongation) By Human Pharmaceuticals, describes a nonclinical testing strategy for assessing the potential of a test substance to delay ventricular repolarization. This guideline includes information concerning nonclinical assays and possible integrated risk assessments.

Data from all available assays (*in silico, in vitro, in vivo*) must be considered in an integrated preclinical risk assessment. Because none of the assays is predictive enough by themselves, the package should contain at least a GLP hERG channel study combined with an GLP *in vivo* nonrodent ECG study (usually telemetered dogs or monkeys). Additionally, the results from mechanistic repolarization assay in isolated tissue preparations (e.g., isolated rabbit heart, Purkinje fibers, etc.) can be very important to bridge the gap between *in vitro* and *in vivo* studies. However, at the moment the results of such *ex vivo* studies are regarded as "mechanistic studies" by the regulatory bodies who leave it to the pharmaceutical industry to employ them or not. One key element of each preclinical cardiosafety assessment is the calculation of a therapeutic index (TI) or safety margin, that is, the free plasma concentration of the drug required for the undesired effect divided by the efficacious free plasma concentration (EFPC) of the drug. The concentration for the undesired effect is reflected for example by an IC_{50} value (e.g., hERG channel inhibition) and the concentration of the desired effect is expressed ideally as the free therapeutic plasma concentration or its estimate.

In early phases of drug development, the information on therapeutic concentrations is not available. Therefore, for internal guidance, it can be replaced by EC_{50} or IC_{50} values from robust cellular pharmacological assays. In a detailed analysis, Redfern *et al.* [11] showed that most drugs associated with TdP in humans are also associated with hERG channel block at concentrations close to or the same as free plasma concentrations found in clinical use. Based on the analysis of 52 drugs covering a broad range of therapeutic classes, the authors found a 30-fold margin between the maximal therapeutic free plasma level (C_{max}) and the hERG IC_{50} to provide an acceptable degree of safety for arrhythmogenicity. Hence, a hERG IC_{50} value $<1\,\mu M$ or $<30\times$ free therapeutic plasma concentration is regarded as a positive *in vitro* signal whereas for the *in vivo* cardiovascular studies a 10% increase in the corrected QTc interval or statistically significant increase are regarded as reasons for concern. In clinical studies, a positive signal is defined by a maximum group mean QTc increase (placebo/baseline subtracted) >5 ms.

When data for the integrated risk assessment are analyzed in a wider context its complexity may appear as discrepancies across similar assays (e.g., hERG binding assay vs hERG electrophysiology, as described in previous section) or between different *in vitro* and/or *in vivo* assays. The latter inconsistencies should be addressed proactively with appropriate mechanistic assays or additional studies (e.g., testing of metabolites or testing for myocardial accumulation of the drug). Although a compound might be expected to block solely hERG channel activity, prolong action potential duration *in vitro* and translate into a prolongation of the QT interval at comparable free drug plasma levels, this simple and direct relationship can only be observed in a minority of cases. Interactions with multiple ion channels involved in the generation of the cardiac action potential can either mitigate or exacerbate the QT interval prolongation resulting from hERG channel inhibition, for example, hERG channel blockers are equally active at channels carrying inward current like the L-type calcium channel, leading to hERG blockers that do not prolong APD [102].

The results of the core battery can be refined by additional studies, in particular assays on isolated cardiac tissues determining changes in cardiac action potential duration, shape and variability over time [100]. These assays are also able to show if a drug induces early after-depolarizations or even TdP. Adverse drug effects on cardiac electrophysiological function, in particular impulse formation and conduction, are usually evaluated through changes in ECG, generally recorded in dogs, pigs or monkeys. TdP-related arrhythmias are detected very seldom in healthy dogs or monkeys but the triggering of arrhythmia could be investigated for example under hypokalemic conditions with artificially created bradycardia [4]. Adverse drug effects on cardiac electrophysiological function, in particular impulse formation and conduction, are usually evaluated through changes in ECG, generally recorded in dogs, pigs or monkeys. However, depending on compound availability and/or tolerability, other smaller species like guinea pigs or rabbits can be considered. Changes in cardiac contractility occurring either as a primary effect of the drug on cardiac function or as a consequence of cardiac lesions can be investigated in telemetered or anaesthetized animals in which cardiac contractility is evaluated by measurement of left ventricular pressure. In addition, echocardiography would also allow the measurement of drug-induced changes in ventricular wall movements and cardiac haemodynamics indicative of effects on contractility.

There are, of course, a variety of other reasons for surprise outcomes and "false positive" results in *in vivo* studies. The formation of species-specific metabolites can frequently lead to a situation where the parent drug has low hERG activity but produces QT interval prolongation at low plasma exposures in a dog model or even in clinical studies. Another factor can be partitioning of the parent drug or active metabolites into cardiac tissue [103] resulting in a compound accumulation in cardiac tissue and a much higher cardiac concentration than in the plasma. This can sometimes explain the disconnect between the electrophysiological QT data and pharmacokinetic data obtained in plasma samples. Additionally, QT prolongation may even occur by influencing the trafficking of the hERG channel protein to the cardiac cell membrane, thus leading to a decrease in toal hERG current [104]. Indirect effects of drugs that modulate the autonomic tone or the systemic hemodynamics may also lead to conflicting results because the complex relationship between QT and RR intervals is influenced by these two parameters [105]. The challenge here is to try to understand the mechanistic basis of the effects caused by these compounds and determine whether viable preclinical assays can be put in place to detect them. Ideally, at the end of the investigations the complicating factors manifesting only in an animal model have to be identified.

Finally, if a drug is eventually given to patients during clinical trials or postmarketing, there are number of potential drug–drug interactions and differences in genetic background that could produce effects on the QT interval despite a "safe" nonclinical profile.

16.6 Summary

Recent scientific discussion has developed to question if QT interval prolongation is the appropriate endpoint to focus on. An action potential prolongation and a QT interval prolongation can in fact be antiarrhythmic. It precipitates only under certain circumstances into life-threatening events like Torsades de Pointes. The torsadogenic potential of drugs may not necessarily be proportional to their ability to prolong the QT interval. It is a dynamic combination of multiple predisposing factors and components rather than a single particular event that can trigger this particular tachycardia [106]. The main problem in cardiac safety pharmacology today is still how to combine the capabilities of different methodologies with their strengths and limitations in order to detect the potential of one molecular entity to induce a lethal arrhythmia of very low clinical incidence. Despite all the efforts described above, there will still be compounds that might prolong the QT interval in clinical studies but bear a significant potential benefit for patients with serious illnesses, such as terminal cancer, prevention of rejection in transplantation and other life-threatening diseases.

In conclusion, an integrated preclinical cardiosafety assessment of a drug is based on the results of *in vitro* tests, with overall moderate to high throughput and *in vivo* experiments which have to be put into relationship to the estimated or real free therapeutic plasma concentration in man. In any case, it would be prudent to select at least drug candidates with no hERG activity or with the largest possible therapeutic index to hERG IC_{50} values and effects in other nonclinical models because these margins may later reduce. However it becomes increasingly important to think outside the hERG paradigm and to test with appropriate tools if new pharmaceutical drugs have a multi-ion channel liability or mediate other targets relevant for cardiosafety.

Acknowledgments

The authors want to acknowledge Laszlo Urban, Mats Holmqvist, Berengere Dumotier and John Davies for reviewing this chapter.

References

1 Fung, M. (2001) Evaluation of the characteristics of safety withdrawal of prescription drugs from worldwide pharmaceutical markets-1960 to 1999. *Drug Information Journal*, **35**, 293–317.

2 Kannel, W.B., Cupples, L.A. and D'Agostino, R.B. (1987) Sudden death risk in overt coronary heart disease: The Framingham Study. *American Heart Journal*, **113**, 799–804.

3 CAST (1989) Preliminary report: effect of encainide and flecainide on mortality in a randomized trial of arrhythmia suppression after myocardial infarction. The cardiac arrhythmia suppression trial (CAST) investigators. *The New England Journal of Medicine*, **321**, 406–412.

4 Hanton, G. (2007) Preclinical cardiac safety assessment of drugs. *Drugs R D*, **8**, 213–228.

5 Warmke, J.W. and Ganetzky, B. (1994) A family of potassium channel genes related to eag in drosophila and mammals. *Proceedings of the National Academy of Sciences of the United States of America*, **91**, 3438–3442.

6 Curran, M.E., Splawski, I., Timothy, K.W., Vincen, G.M., Green, E.D. and Keating, M.T. (1995) A molecular basis for cardiac arrhythmia: HERG mutations cause long QT syndrome. *Cell*, **80**, 795–803.

7 Sanguinetti, M.C., Jiang, C., Curran, M.E. and Keating, M.T. (1995) A mechanistic link between an inherited and an acquird cardiac arrthytmia: HERG encodes the IKr potassium channel. *Cell*, **81**, 299–307.

8 Pollard, C.E., Valentin, J.P. and Hammond, T.G. (2009) Strategies to reduce the risk of drug-induced QT interval prolongation: a pharmaceutical company perspective. *British Journal of Pharmacology*, in press.

9 Pearlstein, R., Vaz, R. and Rampe, D. (2003) Understanding the structure-activity relationship of the human ether-a-go-go-related gene cardiac $K+$ channel. A model for bad behavior. *Journal of Medicinal Chemistry*, **46**, 2017–2022.

10 Witchel, H.J. (2007) The hERG potassium channel as a therapeutic target. *Expert Opinion on Therapeutic Targets*, **11**, 321–336.

11 Redfern, W.S., Carlsson, L., Davis, A.S., Lynch, W.G., MacKenzie, I., Palethorpe, S., Siegl, P.K.S., Strang, I., Sullivan, A.T., Wallis, R., Camm, A.J. and Hammond, T.G. (2003) Relationships between preclinical cardiac electrophysiology, clinical QT interval prolongation and torsade de pointes for a broad range of drugs: evidence for a provisional safety margin in drug development. *Cardiovascular Research*, **58**, 32–45.

12 Jamieson, C., Moir, E.M., Rankovic, Z. and Wishart, G. (2006) Medicinal chemistry of hERG optimizations: Highlights and hang-ups. *Journal of Medicinal Chemistry*, **49**, 5029–5046.

13 Hoffmann, P. and Warner, B. (2006) Are hERG channel inhibition and QT interval prolongation all there is in drug-induced torsadogenesis? A review of emerging trends. *Journal of Pharmacological and Toxicological Methods*, **53**, 87–105.

14 Netzer, R., Bischoff, U. and Ebneth, A. (2003) HTS techniques to investigate the potential effects of compounds on cardiac ion channels at early-stages of drug discovery. *Current Opinion in Drug Discovery & Development*, **6**, 462–469.

15 Shah, R.R. (2005) Drug-induced QT dispersion: does it predict the risk of Torsade de Pointes? *Journal of Electrocardiology*, **38**, 10–18.

16 Whitebread, S., Hamon, J., Bojanic, D., Urban, L. and Hamon, J. (2005) In vitro safety pharmacology profiling: an essential tool for successful drug development. *Drug Discovery Today*, **10**, 1421–1433.

17 Force, T., Krause, D.S. and Van Etten, R.A. (2007) Molecular mechanisms of cardiotoxicity of tyrosine kinase inhibition. *Nature Reviews. Cancer*, **7**, 332–344.

18 Antzelevitch, C. and Dumaine, R. (2002) Electrical heterogeneity in the heart: physiological, pharmacological and clinical implications, in *Handbook of Physiology. The Cardiovascular System. The Heart*, **1**, American Physiological Society, Bethesda, MD, p. 654.

19 Ten Eick, R.E., Baumgarten, C.M. and Singer, D.H. (1981) Ventricular dysrhythmia: Membrane basis or of currents, channels, gates, and cables. *Progress in Cardiovascular Diseases*, **24**, 157–188.

20 Farid, R., Day, T., Friesner, R.A. and Pearlstein, R.A. (2006) New insights about HERG blockade obtained from protein modeling, potential energy mapping, and docking studies. *Bioorganic & Medicinal Chemistry*, **14**, 3160–3173.

21 Splawski, I., Timothy, K.W., Decher, N., Kumar, P., Sachse, F.B., Beggs, A.H., Sanguinetti, M.C. and Keating, M.T. (2005) Severe arrhythmia disorder caused by cardiac L-type calcium channel mutations. *Proceedings of the National Academy of Sciences of the United States of America*, **102**, 8089–8096.

22 Chouabe, C., Drici, M.D., Romey, G., Barhanin, J. and Lazdunski, M. (1998) HERG and KvLQT1/IsK, the cardiac K+ channels involved in long QT syndromes, are targets for calcium channel blockers. *Molecular Pharmacology*, **54**, 695–703.

23 Sanguinetti, M.C., Curran, M.E., Zou, A., Shen, J., Spector, P.S., Atkinson, D.L. and Keating, M.T. (1996) Coassembly of K(v) LQT1 and minK (IsK) proteins to form cardiac I-Ks potassium channel. *Nature*, **384**, 80–83.

24 Busch, A.E., Suessbrich, H., Waldegger, S., Sailer, E., Greger, R., Lang, H.J., Lang, F., Gibson, K.J. and Maylie, J.G. (1996) Inhibition of I-Ks in guinea pig cardiac myocytes and guinea pig I-sK channels by the chromanol 293B. *Pflugers Archiv- European Journal of Physiology*, **432**, 1094–1096.

25 Keating, M.T. and Sanguinetti, M.C. (2001) Molecular and cellular mechanisms of cardiac arrhythmias. *Cell*, **104**, 569–580.

26 Chen, Q.Y., Kirsch, G.E., Zhang, D.M., Brugada, R., Brugada, J., Brugada, P., Potenza, D., Moya, A., Borggrefe, M., Breithardt, G., Ortiz-Lopez, R., Wang, Z., Antzelevitch, C., O'Brien, R.E., Schulze-Bahr, E., Keating, M.T., Towbin, J.A. and Wang, Q. (1998) Genetic basis and molecular mechanism for idiopathic: ventricular fibrillation. *Nature*, **392**, 293–296.

27 Antzelevitch, C. (2005) Brugada syndrome, report of the Second Consensus Conference (vol 2, pg 429, 2005). *Heart Rhythm*, **2**, 905.

28 Wang, Q., Shen, J.X., Li, Z.Z., Timothy, K., Vincent, G.M., Priori, S.G., Schwartz, P.J. and Keating, M.T. (1995) Cardiac sodium-channel mutations in patients with long Qt syndrome. An inherited cardiac-arrhythmia. *Human Molecular Genetics*, **4**, 1603–1607.

29 Bennett, P.B., Yazawa, K., Makita, N. and George, A.L. (1995) Molecular mechanism for an inherited cardiac-arrhythmia. *Nature*, **376**, 683–685.

30 Chadwick, C.C., Ezrin, A.M., O'Connor, B., Volberg, W.A., Smith, D.I., Wedge, K.J., Hill, R.J., Briggs, G.M., Pagani, E.D. and Silver, P.J. (1993) Identification of a specific radioligand for the cardiac rapidly activating delayed rectifier K+ channel. *Circulation Research*, **72**, 707–714.

31 Chadwick, C.C., Krafte, D.S., Oconnor, B., Volberg, W.A., Ezrin, A.M., Johnson, R.E. and Silver, P.J. (1995) Evidence for multiple antiarrhythmic binding-sites on the cardiac rapidly activating delayed rectifier K+ channel. *Drug Development Research*, **34**, 376–380.

32 Duff, H.J., Feng, Z.P. and Sheldon, R.S. (1995) High- and low-affinity sites for [3H] Dofetilide binding to guinea pig myocytes. *Circulation Research*, **77**, 718–725.

33 Duff, H.J., Feng, Z.P., Fiset, C., Wang, L., Lees-Miller, J. and Sheldon, R.S. (1997) [3H]Dofetilide binding to cardiac myocytes: modulation by extracellular potassium. *Journal of Molecular and Cellular Cardiology*, **29**, 183–191.

34 Fiset, C., Feng, Z.P., Wang, L., Sheldon, R.S. and Duff, H.J. (1996) [H-3]Dofetilide binding: Biological models that manifest solely the high or the law affinity binding site. *Journal of Molecular and Cellular Cardiology*, **28**, 1085–1096.

35 Geonzon, R., Exner, D.V., Woodman, R.C., Wang, L., Feng, Z.P. and Duff, H.J. (1998) A high affinity binding site for [H-3]-dofetilide on human leukocytes. *Journal of Molecular and Cellular Cardiology*, **30**, 1691–1701.

36 Diaz, G.J., Daniell, K., Leitza, S.T., Martin, R.L., Su, Z., McDermott, J.S., Cox, B.F. and Gintant, G.A. (2004) The [3H] dofetilide binding assay is a predictive screening tool for hERG blockade and proarrhythmia: Comparison of intact cell and membrane preparations and effects of altering [K+]o. *Journal of Pharmacological and Toxicological Methods*, **50**, 187–199.

37 Finlayson, K., Turnbull, L., January, C.T., Sharkey, J. and Kelly, J.S. (2001) [H-3] dofetilide binding to HERG transfected membranes: a potential high throughput preclinical screen. *European Journal of Pharmacology*, **430**, 147–148.

38 Cook, N.D. (1996) Scintillation proximity assay: A versatile high-throughput screening technology. *Drug Discovery Today*, **1**, 287–294.

39 Burke, T.J., Loniello, K.R., Beebe, J.A. and Ervin, K.M. (2003) Development and application of fluorescence polarization assays in drug discovery. *Combinatorial Chemistry & High Throughput Screening*, **6**, 183–194.

40 Singleton, D.H., Boyd, H., Steidl-Nichols, J.V., Deacon, M., de Groot, M.J., Price, D., Nettleton, D.O., Wallace, N.K., Troutman, M.D., Williams, C. and Boyd, J.G. (2007) Fluorescently labeled analogues of dofetilide as high-affinity fluorescence polarization ligands for the human ether-a-go-go-related gene (hERG) channel.

Journal of Medicinal Chemistry, **50**, 2931–2941.

41 Au, E., Vu, A., Ly, J.Q., Misner, D.L., Kondru, R.K. and Martin, R.S. (2006) Interactions at the human ether a go-go (hERG) potassium channel investigated through multiple radioligands. *The FASEB Journal*, **20**, A1112.

42 Chiu, P.J.S., Marcoe, K.F., Bounds, S.E., Lin, C.H., Feng, J.J., Lin, A., Cheng, F.C., Crumb, W.J. and Mitchell, R. (2004) Validation of a [H-3]astemizole binding assay in HEK293 cells expressing HERG K+ channels. *Journal of Pharmacological Sciences*, **95**, 311–319.

43 Greengrass, P.M., Stewart, M. and Wood, C.M. (2003) Affinity-Assay for the Human ERG Potassium Channel. WO/2003/021271.

44 Raab, C.E., Butcher, J.W., Connolly, T.M., Karczewski, J., Yu, N.X., Staskiewicz, S.J., Liverton, N., Dean, D.C. and Melillo, D.G. (2006) Synthesis of the first sulfur-35-labeled hERG radioligand. *Bioorganic & Medicinal Chemistry Letters*, **16**, 1692–1695.

45 Wang, J., la Penna, K., Wang, H., Karczewski, J., Connolly, T.M., Koblan, K.S., Bennett, P.B. and Salata, J.J. (2003) Functional and pharmacological properties of canine ERG potassium channels. *American Journal of Physiology. Heart and Circulatory Physiology*, **284**, H256–H267.

46 Angelo, K., Korolkova, Y., Grunnet, M., Grishin, E., Pluzhnikov, K., Klaerke, D., Knaus, H.G., Møller, M. and Olesen, S.P. (2003) A radiolabeled peptide ligand of the hERG channel, [125I]-BeKm-1. *Pflügers Archiv European Journal of Physiology*, **447**, 55–63.

47 Korolkova, Y.V., Bocharov, E.V., Angelo, K., Maslennikov, I.V., Grinenko, O.V., Lipkin, A.V., Nosyreva, E.D., Pluzhnikov, K.A., Olesen, S.P., Arseniev, A.S. and Grishin, E.V. (2002) New binding site on common molecular scaffold provides HERG channel specificity of scorpion toxin BeKm-1. *The Journal of Biological Chemistry*, **277**, 43104–43109.

48 Piper, D.R., Duff, S.R., Eliason, H.C., Frazee, W.J., Frey, E.A., Fuerstenau-Sharp, M., Jachec, C., Marks, B.D., Pollok, B.A., Shekhani, M.S., Thompson, D.V., Whitney, P., Vogel, K.W. and Hess, S.D. (2008) Development of the predictor hERG fluorescence polarization assay using a membrane protein enrichment approach. *ASSAY and Drug Development Technologies*, **6**, 213–223.

49 Cheng, C.S., Alderman, D., Kwash, J., Dessaint, J., Patel, R., Lescoe, M.K., Kinrade, M.B. and Yu, W. (2002) A High-throughput HERG potassium channel function assay: An old assay with a new look. *Drug Development and Industrial Pharmacy*, **28**, 177–191.

50 Sorota, S., Zhang, X.S., Margulis, M., Tucker, K. and Priestley, T. (2005) Characterization of a hERG screen using the IonWorks HT: comparison to a hERG rubidium efflux screen. *ASSAY and Drug Development Technologies*, **3**, 47–57.

51 Tang, W., Kang, J., Wu, X., Rampe, D., Wang, L., Shen, H., Li, Z., Dunnington, D. and Garyantes, T. (2001) Development and evaluation of high throughput functional assay methods for hERG potassium channel. *Journal of Biomolecular Screening*, **6**, 325–331.

52 Chaudhary, K.W., O'Neal, J.M., Mo, Z.L., Fermini, B., Gallavan, R.H. and Bahinski, A. (2006) Evaluation of the rubidium efflux assay for preclinical identification of hERG blockade. *ASSAY and Drug Development Technologies*, **4**, 73–82.

53 Rezazadeh, S., Hesketh, J.C. and Fedida, D. (2004) Rb+ Flux through hERG channels affects the potency of channel blocking drugs: correlation with data obtained using a high-throughput Rb+ efflux assay. *Journal of Biomolecular Screening*, **9**, 588–597.

54 Hougaard, C., Eriksen, B.L., Jorgensen, S., Johansen, T.H., Dyhring, T., Madsen, L.S., Strobak, D. and Christophersen, P. (2007) Selective positive modulation of

the SK3 and SK2 subtypes of small conductance Ca2+-activated K+ channels. *British Journal of Pharmacology*, **151**, 655–665.

55 Weaver, C.D., Harden, D., Dworetzky, S.I., Robertson, B. and Knox, R.J. (2004) A thallium-sensitive, fluorescence-based assay for detecting and characterizing potassium channel modulators in mammalian cells. *Journal of Biomolecular Screening*, **9**, 671–677.

56 Dorn, A., Hermann, F., Ebneth, A., Bothmann, H., Trube, G., Christensen, K. and Apfel, C. (2005) Evaluation of a high-throughput fluorescence assay method for hERG potassium channel inhibition. *Journal of Biomolecular Screening*, **10**, 339–347.

57 Dunlop, J., Bowlby, M., Peri, R., Vasilyev, D. and Arias, R. (2008) High-throughput electrophysiology: an emerging paradigm for ion-channel screening and physiology. *Nature Reviews. Drug Discovery*, **7**, 358–368.

58 Wood, C., Williams, C. and Waldron, G.J. (2004) Patch clamping by numbers. *Drug Discovery Today*, **9**, 434–441.

59 Bridgland-Taylor, M.H., Hargreaves, A.C., Easter, A., Orme, A., Henthorn, D.C., Ding, M., Davis, A.M., Small, B.G., Heapy, C.G., bi-Gerges, N., Persson, F., Jacobson, I., Sullivan, M., Albertson, N., Hammond, T.G., Sullivan, E., Valentin, J.P. and Pollard, C.E. (2006) Optimisation and validation of a medium-throughput electrophysiology-based hERG assay using IonWorks(TM) HT. *Journal of Pharmacological and Toxicological Methods*, **54**, 189–199.

60 Guo, L. and Guthrie, H. (2005) Automated electrophysiology in the preclinical evaluation of drugs for potential QT prolongation. *Journal of Pharmacological and Toxicological Methods*, **52**, 123–135.

61 Tao, H., Santa Ana, D., Guia, A., Huang, M., Ligutti, J., Walker, G., Sithiphong, K., Chan, F., Guoliang, T., Zozulya, Z., Saya, S., Phimmachack, R., Sie, C., Yuan, J., Wu, L., Xu, J. and Ghetti, A. (2004) Automated tight seal electrophysiology for assessing the potential hERG liability of pharmaceutical compounds. *ASSAY and Drug Development Technologies*, **2**, 497–506.

62 Mathes, C. (2006) QPatch: the past, present and future of automated patch clamp. *Expert Opinion on Therapeutic Targets*, **10**, 319–327.

63 Barrett, T.D., Triggle, D.J., Walker, M.J.A. and Maurice, D.H. (2005) Mechanism drug action in the cardiovascular system. *Molecular Interventions*, **5**, 84–93.

64 Striessnig, J. (1999) Pharmacology, structure and function of cardiac L-type Ca2+ channels. *Cellular Physiology and Biochemistry*, **9**, 242–269.

65 Ehlert, F.J., Roeske, W.R., Itoga, E. and Yamamura, H.I. (1982) The binding of [H-3]-Labeled nitrendipine to receptors for calcium-channel antagonists in the heart, cerebral-cortex, and ileum of rats. *Life Sciences*, **30**, 2191–2202.

66 Gould, R.J., Murphy, K.M.M. and Snyder, S.H. (1982) [3H]Nitrendipine-labeled calcium channels discriminate inorganic calcium agonists and antagonists. *Proceedings of the National Academy of Sciences of the United States of America*, **79**, 3656–3660.

67 Reynolds, I.J., Snowman, A.M. and Snyder, S.H. (1986) (−)-[3H] desmethoxyverapamil labels multiple calcium channel modulator receptors in brain and skeletal muscle membranes: differentiation by temperature and dihydropyridines. *The Journal of Pharmacology and Experimental Therapeutics*, **237**, 731–738.

68 Schoemaker, H. and Langer, S.Z. (1985) [H-3] diltiazem binding to calcium-channel antagonists recognition sites in rat cerebral-cortex. *European Journal of Pharmacology*, **111**, 273–277.

69 Mason, J.S., Migeon, J., Dupuis, P. and Otto-Bruc, A. (2008) Use of broad biological profiling as a relevant descriptor to describe and differentiate compounds: structure-*In Vitro*

(Pharmacology-ADME)-*In Vivo* (Safety) relationships, in *Antitargets* (eds R.J. Vaz and T. Klabunde), Wiley-VCH, Weinheim, pp. 23–52.

70 Christ, T., Wettwer, E., Wuest, M., Braeter, M., Donath, F., Champeroux, P., Richard, S. and Ravens, U. (2008) Electrophysiological profile of propiverine – relationship to cardiac risk. *Naunyn-Schmiedebergs Archives of Pharmacology*, **376**, 431–440.

71 Lee, S.Y., Kim, Y.J., Kim, K.T., Choe, H. and Jo, S.H. (2006) Blockade of HERG human K+ channels and I-Kr of guinea-pig cardiomyocytes by the antipsychotic drug clozapine. *British Journal of Pharmacology*, **148**, 499–509.

72 Gintant, G.A., Limberis, J.T., McDermott, J.S., Wegner, C.D. and Cox, B.F. (2001) The canine Purkinje fiber: An *in vitro* model system for acquired long QT syndrome and drug-induced arrhythmogenesis. *Journal of Cardiovascular Pharmacology*, **37**, 607–618.

73 Hayashi, S., Kii, Y., Tabo, M., Fukuda, H., Itoh, T., Shimosato, T., Amano, H., Saito, M., Morimoto, H., Yamada, K., Kanda, A., Ishitsuka, T., Yamazaki, T., Kiuchi, Y., Taniguchi, S., Mori, T., Shimizu, S., Tsurubuchi, Y., Yasuda, S., Kitani, S., Shimada, C., Kobayashi, K., Komeno, M., Kasai, C., Hombo, T. and Yamamoto, K. (2005) QT PRODACT: A multi-site study of *in vitro* action potential assays on 21 compounds in isolated guinea-pig papillary muscles. *Journal of Pharmacological Sciences*, **99**, 423–437.

74 Valentin, J.P., Hoffmann, P., De Clerck, F., Hammond, T.G. and Hondeghem, L. (2004) Review of the predictive value of the Langendorff heart model (Screenit system) in assessing the proarrhythmic potential of drugs. *Journal of Pharmacological and Toxicological Methods*, **49**, 171–181.

75 Dumotier, B.M., Deurinck, M., Yang, Y., Traebert, M. and Suter, W. (2008) Relevance of *in vitro* SCREENIT results for drug-induced QT interval prolongation *in vivo*: A database review and analysis. *Pharmacology & Therapeutics*, **119**, 152–159.

76 Zhao, D. and Ren, L.M. (2003) Electrophysiological responses to imidazoline/alpha(2)-receptor agonists in rabbit sinoatrial node pacemaker cells. *Acta Pharmacologica Sinica*, **24**, 1217–1223.

77 Antzelevitch, C. (2004) Arrhythmogenic mechanisms of QT prolonging drugs: Is QT prolongation really the problem? *Journal of Electrocardiology*, **37**, 15–24.

78 Chezalvielguilbert, F., Davy, J.M., Poirier, J.M. and Weissenburger, J. (1995) Mexiletine antagonizes effects of sotalol on qt interval duration and its proarrhythmic effects in a canine model of torsade-de-pointes. *Journal of the American College of Cardiology*, **26**, 787–792.

79 Authier, S., Tanguay, J.F., Gauvin, D., Fruscia, R.D. and Troncy, E. (2007) A cardiovascular monitoring system used in conscious cynomolgus monkeys for regulatory safety pharmacology: Part 2: Pharmacological validation. *Journal of Pharmacological and Toxicological Methods*, **56**, 122–130.

80 Bazett, H.C. (1920) An analysis of the time-relations of electrocardiograms. *Heart*, **7**, 353–370.

81 Fridericia, L.S. (1920) The duration of systole in the electrocardiogram of normal subjects and of patients with heart disease. *Acta Medica Scandinavica*, **53**, 469–486.

82 Vandewater, A., Verheyen, J., Xhonneux, R. and Reneman, R.S. (1989) An improved method to correct the Qt interval of the electrocardiogram for changes in heart-rate. *Journal of Pharmacological Methods*, **22**, 207–217.

83 Morgan, J. and Sullivan, M.E. (1992) An overview of class III electrophysiological agents: A new generation of antiarrhythmic therapy, in *Progress in Medicinal Chemistry*, Vol. 29 (ed. G.P. Ellis), Elsevier, pp. 65–108.

84 Ekins, S., Crumb, W.J., Sarazan, R.D., Wikel, J.H. and Wrighton, S.A. (2002)

Three-dimensional quantitative structure-activity relationship for inhibition of human ether-a-go-go-related gene potassium channel. *The Journal of Pharmacology and Experimental Therapeutics*, **301**, 427–434.

85 Cavalli, A., Poluzzi, E., De Ponti, F. and Recanatini, M. (2002) Toward a pharmacophore for drugs inducing the long QT syndrome: Insights from a CoMFA study of HERG K+ channel blockers. *Journal of Medicinal Chemistry*, **45**, 3844–3853.

86 Aronov, A.M. and Goldman, B.B. (2004) A model for identifying HERG K+ channel blockers. *Bioorganic & Medicinal Chemistry*, **12**, 2307–2315.

87 Aronov, A.M. (2006) Common pharmacophores for uncharged human ether-a-go-go-related gene (hERG) blockers. *Journal of Medicinal Chemistry*, **49**, 6917–6921.

88 Ficker, E., Obejero-Paz, C.A., Zhao, S. and Brown, A.M. (2002) The binding site for channel blockers that rescue misprocessed human long QT syndrome type 2 ether-a-gogo-related gene (HERG) mutations. *The Journal of Biological Chemistry*, **277**, 4989–4998.

89 Pearlstein, R.A., Vaz, R.J., Kang, J.S., Chen, X.L., Preobrazhenskaya, M., Shchekotikhin, A.E., Korolev, A.M., Lysenkova, L.N., Miroshnikova, O.V., Hendrix, J. and Rampe, D. (2003) Characterization of HERG potassium channel inhibition using CoMSiA 3D QSAR and homology modeling approaches. *Bioorganic & Medicinal Chemistry Letters*, **13**, 1829–1835.

90 Mitcheson, J.S., Chen, J., Lin, M., Culberson, C. and Sanguinetti, M.C. (2000) A structural basis for drug induced long QT syndrome. *Proceedings of the National Academy of Sciences*, **97**, 12329–12333.

91 Sanguinetti, M.C. and Mitcheson, J.S. (2005) Predicting drug-hERG channel interactions that cause acquired long QT syndrome. *Trends in Pharmacological Sciences*, **26**, 119–124.

92 Zhu, B.Y., Jia, Z.J., Zhang, P.L., Su, T., Huang, W.R., Goldman, E., Tumas, D., Kadambi, V., Eddy, P., Sinha, U., Scarborough, R.M. and Song, Y.H. (2006) Inhibitory effect of carboxylic acid group on hERG binding. *Bioorganic & Medicinal Chemistry Letters*, **16**, 5507–5512.

93 Waring, M.J. and Johnstone, C. (2007) A quantitative assessment of hERG liability as a function of lipophilicity. *Bioorganic & Medicinal Chemistry Letters*, **17**, 1759–1764.

94 Shamovsky, I., Connolly, S., David, L., Ivanova, S., Norddn, B., Springthorpe, B. and Urbahns, K. (2008) Overcoming undesirable hERG potency of chemokine receptor antagonists using baseline lipophilicity relationships. *Journal of Medicinal Chemistry*, **51**, 1162–1178.

95 Cianchetta, G., Li, Y., Kang, J.S., Rampe, D., Fravolini, A., Cruciani, G. and Vaz, R.J. (2005) Predictive models for hERG potassium channel blockers. *Bioorganic & Medicinal Chemistry Letters*, **15**, 3637–3642.

96 Johnson, S.R., Yue, H.W., Conder, M.L., Shi, H., Doweyko, A.M., Lloyd, J. and Levesque, P. (2007) Estimation of hERG inhibition of drug candidates using multivariate property and pharmacophore SAR. *Bioorganic & Medicinal Chemistry*, **15**, 6182–6192.

97 Seierstad, M. and Agrafiotis, D.K. (2006) A QSAR model of hERG binding using a large, diverse, and internally consistent training set. *Chemical Biology & Drug Design*, **67**, 284–296.

98 Jia, L. and Sun, H. (2008) Support vector machines classification of hERG liabilities based on atom types. *Bioorganic & Medicinal Chemistry*, **16**, 6252–6260.

99 Yao, J.A., Du, X., Lu, D., Baker, R.L., Daharsh, E. and Atterson, P. (2005) Estimation of potency of HERG channel blockers: Impact of voltage protocol and temperature. *Journal of*

Pharmacological and Toxicological Methods, **52**, 146–153.

100 ICH (2005b) S7B: the nonclinical evaluation of the potential for delayed ventricular repolarization (QT interval prolongation) by human pharmaceuticals. 2005.

101 ICH (2005) E14: the clinical evaluation of QT/QTc interval prolongation and proarrhythmic potential for non-antiarrhythmic drugs.

102 Martin, R.L., McDermott, J.S., Salmen, H.J., Palmatier, J., Cox, B.F. and Gintant, G.A. (2004) The utility of hERG and repolarization assays in evaluating delayed cardiac repolarization: Influence of multi-channel block. *Journal of Cardiovascular Pharmacology*, **43**, 369–379.

103 Titier, K., Canal, M., Deridet, E., Abouelfath, A., Gromb, S., Molimard, M. and Moore, N. (2004) Determination of myocardium to plasma concentration ratios of five antipsychotic drugs: comparison with their ability to induce arrhythmia and sudden death in clinical practice. *Toxicology and Applied Pharmacology*, **199**, 52–60.

104 Ficker, E., Kuryshev, Y.A., Dennis, A.T., Obejero-Paz, C., Lu, W., Hawryluk, P., Wible, B.A. and Brown, A.M. (2004) Mechanisms of arsenic-induced prolongation of cardiac repolarization. *Molecular Pharmacology*, **66**, 33–44.

105 Fossa, A.A., Wisialowski, T., Magnano, A., Wolfgang, E., Winslow, R., Gorczyca, W., Crimin, K. and Raunig, D.L. (2005) Dynamic beat-to-beat modeling of the QT-RR interval relationship: Analysis of QT prolongation during alterations of autonomic state versus human ether a-go-go-related gene inhibition. *The Journal of Pharmacology and Experimental Therapeutics*, **312**, 1–11.

106 Ahmad, K. and Dorian, P. (2007) Drug-induced QT prolongation and proarrhythmia: an inevitable link? *Europace*, **9**, 16–22.

17
Hematotoxicity: *In Vitro* and *Ex Vivo* Compound Profiling
David Brott and Francois Pognan

17.1
Introduction

The pharmaceutical industry spent approximately U.S. $ 35 billion in 2007 for research and development. This is an approximate 12-fold increase from the 1980 level, but the number of new chemical entities (NCE) remained flat over this time period. This decreased productivity is a major concern and could be due to several factors, including late-stage attrition rate increasing from 50 to 89% during drug development [1]. The majority of safety-related attrition occurs preclinically with approximately 30% of attrition being due to toxicology and clinical safety [2]. Significant focus of the industry has been to improve compound selection during discovery to decrease preclinical and clinical attrition, most noticeably by perfecting pharmacological efficacy and drug disposition and pharmacokinetics parameters. A new trend is now emerging in which assays to profile toxicity side effects may also be used for this early compound selection. Here we will call "front-loading" this concept of using *in vitro* assays that mimic *in vivo* known and observed toxicities for the profiling and selection of chemical series or specific chemicals within a series. Additional tools such as *in silico* expert systems for the prediction of toxicity, based on *in vitro* and *in vivo* observations, are also used to the same end. *In vitro* compound profiling and *in silico* expert systems may lead to the discovery of potential biomarkers which can be used after some validation in preclinical and clinical studies.

The main target organs for compound toxicity leading to either drug withdrawal or arrest of compound development as estimated in various studies [3], are classically pointing at liver, the cardiovascular system and bone marrow (hematotoxicity). Cardiovascular and hepatotoxicity were discussed in previous chapters and this chapter focuses on hematotoxicity.

Hematotoxicity, defined as drug-induced altered production of peripheral blood cells, is most commonly associated with antiproliferative oncology compounds but is also caused by drugs for various indications, covering a wide pharmacology and chemical structure diversity (Table 17.1). This vast variety of chemical structures makes it difficult to predict hematotoxicity by *in silico* approaches and to model

Hit and Lead Profiling. Edited by Bernard Faller and Laszlo Urban
Copyright © 2009 WILEY-VCH Verlag GmbH & Co. KGaA, Weinheim
ISBN: 978-3-527-32331-9

Table 17.1 Compounds from different therapy areas, pharmacological classes and structures that induce hematotoxicity [59–63].

Therapy area	Compounds
Analgesic and anti-inflammatory	Acetylsalicylic acid, aminopyrine, benoxaprofen, dipyrone, bucillamine diclofenac, diflunisal, fenoprofen, ibuprofen, indomethacin, mefenamic acid, mesalazine, naproxen, pentazocine, phenylbutazone, piroxicam, quinine, sulindac, tolmetin
Anticonvulsant	Carbamazepine, ethosuximide, lamotrigine, mesantoin, phenytoin, trimethadione, valproic acid
Antipsychotics, antidepressants	Amitriptyline, chlordiazepoxide, chlorpromazine, clomipramine, clozapine, cyanamide, desipramine, diazepam, dothiepin, doxepin, fluoxetine, haloperidol, imipramine, indalpine, levomepromazine, maprotiline, meprobamate, methotrimeprazine, mianserin, mirtazapine, olanzapine, perazine, phenothiazines, phenelzine, quetiapine, remoxipride risperidone, thioridazine, thiothixene, tiapride, trazodone, ziprasidone
Anti-infectives	Abacavir, amodiaquine, amoxicillin-clavulanic acid, ampicillin, carbenicillin, cefamandole, cefepime, cefotaxime, ceftriaxone, cefuroxime, cephalexin, cephalothin, cephapirin, cephradine, chloramphenicol, chlorogunide, clarithromycine, clindamycin, cloxacillin, dapsone, doxycyclin, flucytosine, fusidic acid, gentamicin, griseofulvin, hyrdorxycloroquine, imipenem-cilastatin, indinavir, isoniazid, levamisol, lincomycine linozilide, mebendazole, mietronidazole minocycline, nafcillin, nifuroxazide, nitrofurantoin, norfloxacin, novobiocin, oxacillin, penicillin G, pernicillin G-procaine, piperacillin, pyrimethamine, quinine, ristocetin, rifampin, streptomycine, terbinafine, thiacetazone, ticarcillin, trimethoprim-sulfamethoxazole, vancomycin, zidovudine
Cardiovascular	Acetyldigosin, ajmaline, amiodarone, aprindine, bepridil, bezafibrate, captopril, dinepazide, clopidogrel, coumarins, diazoxide, digoxin, dipyridamole, disopyramide, doxazosin, enalapril, flurbiprofen, furoxemide, hydralazine, lisinopril methyldopa, metolazone, nifedipine, phenindione, procainamide, propanolol, propafenone, quinidine, ramapril, spironolactone, thiazide diuretics, ticlopidine, vesnarinone
Gastrointestinal	Cimetidine, famotidine, mesalazine, metiamide, metoclopramide, omeprazole, pirenzepine, ranitidine
Antihistamine	Brompheniramine, cimetidine, methapheniline, methylthiouracil, mianserin, ranitidine, thenalidine, tripelennamine
Antithyroid	Carbimazole, mithimazole, potassium perchlorate, potassium thiocyanate, propylthiouracil
Other drugs	Acetazolamide, acetosulfone, acetylcysteine, acitretin, allopurinol, aminoglutehimide, benzafibrate, brompheniramine, calcium dobesilate, chlorpheniramine, chlorpropamide, colchicine, deferiprone, dapsone, flutamide, glibenclamide, hydroxychloroquine, mebhydrolin, meprobamate, metapyrilene, methazolamide, metochlopramide, prednisone, promethazine, retinoic acid, riluzole, ritodrine, tolbutamide, yohimbine

predictive *in vitro* assays. Therefore, historically, hematotoxic potential of compounds were first evaluated during drug candidate nomination *in vivo* studies by microscopic evaluation of bone marrow cellularity from decalcified bone smears, hematology and in some cases bone marrow differentials. Identification of bone marrow toxicity in these *in vivo* studies may result in late-stage nonclinical attrition when clinical indications may not tolerate such untoward effects or when the safety margin between the therapeutic effect and the first observed bone marrow side effects are too narrow. For example, a drug for asthma must have very stringent toxicity criteria, while an anticancer treatment could tolerate much higher risk. However, even anticancer drugs are now improving their whole range of undesirable side effects and it is clear that, all other parameters being equal, an anticancer molecule with a better hematotoxicity profile is favored by the pharmaceutical industry as well as by the regulatory authorities, clinicians and patients.

This late-stage attrition due to bone marrow toxicity can be reduced if chemical compounds in early stages of research can be profiled with relative confidence before reaching development. For clear reasons of throughput, material quantities, cost and reduction of animal use issues, *in vivo* studies are not convenient for such a hematotoxicity front-loading. Hence, the solution can only be in the use of *in vitro* assays reflecting more or less accurately the *in vivo* biology of bone marrow. Therefore, prior to developing front-loading assays to evaluate target-related or chemistry-induced hematotoxicity, the general pathophysiological pathways of hematopoiesis must be understood. Hematopoiesis, the production of blood cells, is a continuum of blood-forming cells from pluripotent stem cells to multipotent stem cells and ending with the mature blood cells from the following lineages: lymphocytes, myelocytes (neutrophils, eosinophils, basophils), monocytes, nonnucleated red blood cells and megakaryocytes that produce platelets. This continuum of cells in the various lineages entails cellular proliferation, maturation and interactions with stromal cells, cytokines and hormones, and depending on duration and severity, interruption with any of these processes can result in hematotoxicity. The next paragraphs describe compounds known to induce clinical hematotoxicity and various potential mechanisms.

17.2
Known Compounds with Hematotoxic Potential

The goal in profiling compounds early in drug discovery is to predict clinical outcome also known as adverse drug reaction (ADR) for compounds. In clinical studies, bone marrow toxicity is quantified by hematology analysis of peripheral blood with the major toxicities being agranulocytosis/neutropenia, thrombocytopenia and anemia [4]. Therefore, screening assays and cascade should predict these clinical hematology changes. Prior to developing such assays, pharmacological and structural characteristics of compounds that induce hematotoxicity and the various mechanisms of these compounds need to be understood. The most recognized class of compounds that induce clinical bone marrow toxicity are the antiproliferative oncology compounds, since these general cytotoxins destroy proliferating cells and bone marrow is a highly proliferative tissue. However, some non-antiproliferative (non-oncology) compounds are also known to induce bone marrow toxicity in the clinical setting.

Table 17.1 lists non-oncology compounds from diverse therapeutic, chemical, pharmacological areas and structures that induce clinical hematotoxicity. This demonstrates that bone marrow toxicity is not restricted to a small number of pharmacological or structural classes, thereby making it more difficult to understand specific mechanisms of toxicity. However, there are three classes of mechanisms of hematotoxicity, including antiproliferative, immune-mediated and other. Immune-mediated hematotoxicity and other indirect toxicities (e.g., a decrease of erythropoietin in kidney, leading to an impeded red cell production in the bone marrow) are not discussed in detail in this chapter as it requires involvement of the immune system or remote interactions and *in vitro* profiling assays have not been developed to detect these mechanisms.

Antiproliferative compounds are easily detected using cell line or colony-forming unit (CFU) assays. Some of the potential mechanisms of non-antiproliferative compounds leading to bone marrow toxicity include mitochondrial dysfunction [5, 6], aromatic hydrocarbon receptor (AhR) activation, receptor-mediated, altered receptor expression [7] and reactive intermediates [8, 9], but this list may grow with additional research as the mechanism(s) leading to bone marrow toxicity is still unknown for many compounds and will require significant amount of effort to elucidate. The next paragraphs briefly describe these potential mechanisms.

In many ways, mitochondria resemble bacteria; for example, the mitochondrial ribosomal RNA genes of all eukaryotes have been traced back to the eubacteria [10]. This can explain why some antibacterial compounds with the target of inhibiting bacterial protein synthesis also inhibit mitochondrial protein synthesis [6, 11, 12], resulting in hematotoxicity. Tetracycline, chloramphenicol and some oxazolidinone antibiotics have been shown to induce hematotoxicity by inhibiting mitochondrial protein synthesis [13].

The AhR is expressed in bone marrow stromal cells [14] and human hematopoietic stem cells [15] and upon agonist binding the receptor translocates to the nucleus, resulting in altered transcriptional expression such as increased CYP1A1 [16] and resulting in reactive oxygen species [17]. Nonpharmaceutical compounds such as TCDD, benzo(a)pyrene and benzene have been shown to induce hematotoxicity using this mechanism *in vivo* and *in vitro* [18, 19].

In addition to oxygen free radicals, other compounds such a clozapine, olanzapine and procainamide induce reactive intermediates [8, 9]. Clozapine and olanzapine bioactivation is thought to occur through a nitrenium ion [20]; however clozapine but not olanzapine induce toxicity to neutrophils. This can lead to an immune-mediated depletion of neutrophils and their precursors (CFU-GM) [21]. Also, nonsteroidal anti-inflammatory drugs (NSAIDs) have pro-oxidant radicals that when metabolized could cause oxidative stress [22].

Primary or secondary pharmacology can influence hematopoiesis because hematopoietic and stromal cells express many different receptors that are also therapeutic targets, such as neurotransmitters [23–25]. In the mouse, an H1 receptor agonist antagonized the H2-induced increase of CFU-GM by its off-target effect at the latter receptor [26]. Albeit this is not an example of direct hematotoxicity, it does demonstrate that therapeutic drugs bind to targets on hematopoietic and stromal cells and influence hematopoiesis.

The last potential mechanism to be discussed in this chapter is drug-induced altered receptor expression. Hematopoiesis is a very intricate process that is regulated by cytokines and cell–cell interactions. Interruption with any of these processes can result in hematotoxicity. For example, zidovudine (AZT) decreases Epo [27], GM-CSFα and to lesser extent IL-3 receptor expression [7]. Decrease in the expression of the above receptors seems to lead to anemia and neutropenia, by decreasing the number of CFU-E and CFU-GM, respectively.

Although not a mechanism of hematotoxicity, polymorphic metabolism of a compound needs to be discussed since polymorphism can be associated with clinical hematotoxicity. For several compounds [28–39], one of the polymorphic enzymes increases exposure to the toxic form of the compound and thereby induces hematotoxicity in the patient, due to higher exposure levels and not due to a specific mechanism of toxicity within the patient populations.

17.3
Tiered Cascade of Testing

Over the past years *in vitro* assays, such as the colony-forming unit (CFU) assay, have been qualified for predicting *in vivo* toxicity and these assays now permit front-loading evaluation of bone marrow toxicity potential of compounds. The different CFU assays described below, present many advantages, not least that they utilize primary bone marrow cells, have a relatively good validation history and gained popularity in the pharmaceutical industry. Nonetheless several drawbacks, most noticeably the low throughput and the need for experts and their relative objectivity for reading the assays, made it necessary to develop more advanced and complementary techniques.

The next paragraphs describe several assays of various throughput and automation, using cell lines and primary cells of various species used in toxicology, able to deliver complementary information, as well as more mechanistic methods based on *in vivo* material, developed by the present authors and others. For the optimal use of these techniques, we have ordered them in a three-tiered logical cascade from "high throughput–low information" to "low throughput–high information." This approach for evaluating hematotoxicity from target identification through candidate nomination is discussed in detail in the following sections, together with the limited validation compound set used for assessing their viability and predictive value.

17.3.1
Tier 1 Tests

To screen for bone marrow toxicity early in drug discovery, assays must be able to evaluate hundreds of compounds, be inexpensive, report results within two weeks (in order to impact chemistry cycle times) and be able to detect toxicity irrespective of cytotoxic or cytostatic mechanisms. Only cell line-based assays can meet all of these various criteria.

Brott et al. [40, 41] evaluated bone marrow toxicity to myeloid, erythroid and stromal lineages using mouse cell lines. Several cell lines were actually evaluated and the present authors selected the M1 myeloid line (ATCC TIB-192), the HCD57 erythroid line (a generous gift from Dr. Hankins [42]), the lymphoid line M-NFS-60 (ATCC CRL-1838) and the stromal line M2-10B4 (ATCC CRL-1972). The nonhematopoietic line HepG2 (ATCC HB-8065) was used to evaluate general cytotoxicity and as a control to enhance the predictive value of the assay. The concentration that decreased the cell number by 50% (IC_{50}) was calculated for each of the cell lines and used to determine whether a compound was a bone marrow toxicant. A compound was deemed negative if it had an $IC_{50} > 100\,\mu M$ for all cell lines; a "potentially positive" compound had an $IC_{50} \geq 1\,\mu M$ and $< 100\,\mu M$ for at least one bone marrow cell lineage; and a "positive" compound had an $IC_{50} < 1\,\mu M$ for at least one cell lineage. The goal of the assay was to influence chemistry until a best possible compound(s) or series of compounds could be progressed by the project team. However, if a project must progress a "potentially positive" or a "positive" compound, then this compound must be evaluated in tier 2 assays to determine species specificity and relevance of tier 1 results using primary bone marrow cells.

When developing a medium- or high-throughput assay, the method by which the assay is quantified is extremely important. For the various mouse cell lines in the medium-throughput bone marrow tier 1 assay, there was linearity between cell line number and luminescence evaluated using the ATP reagent CellTiter Glo at the time of culture initiation and at 24, 48 and 72 h of culture for each cell line (Figure 17.1). Optimal assay culture time for each cell line was based on cell line doubling times with increased luminescence between culture initiation and harvest time. The assay parameters for each cell line are shown in Table 17.2.

Tier 1 assay qualification entailed: (i) evaluating compounds known to induce lineage specific hematotoxicity; (ii) comparing the results from the myeloid tier 1 assay to the mouse CFU-GM assay; (iii) comparing the results from the erythroid tier 1 assay to reduction in peripheral blood reticulocytes.

The tier 1 assay accurately predicted *in vivo* lineage specific hematotoxicity and general cytotoxicity (Table 17.3) with the erythroid cell line having the lowest IC_{50} value for the erythrotoxicant chloramphenicol and the myeloid cell line having the lowest IC_{50} values for the myelotoxicant methotrexate. These results documented that the cell lines did not detect general cytotoxicity, but were able to quantify lineage specific toxicity similar to *in vivo*. In addition, compounds were evaluated several times within the assay and showed good reproducibility (Figure 17.2) for a medium-throughput screening assay.

Table 17.2 Tier 1 assay conditions. Cell lines and optimal culture conditions for evaluating bone marrow toxicity potential of compounds early in drug discovery. The adherent cell lines M2-10B4 and HepG2 are allowed to adhere to plates (preculture time) prior to addition of test compound. Relative cell number within a well is evaluated after the culture time using CellTiter Glo.

Lineage	Cell line	Media	Media additives	Cells seeded	Type	Preculture	Culture time
Myeloid	M1	RPMI-1640	10%FBS, Pen/Strep	4000/well	Non-adherent	0 h	72 h
Erythroid	HCD57	IMDM	30% FBS, Pen/Strep, L-glutamine, 100 pg/mL rmEpo, 20 μM β-ME	5000/well	Non-adherent	0 h	72 h
Lymphoid	MNFS60	RPMI-1640	10%FBS, Pen/Strep, 62 ng/mL rhM-CSF, 50 μM β-ME	2800/well	Non-adherent	0 h	48 h
Stromal	M2-10B4	RPMI-1640	10%FBS, Pen/Strep	2000/well	Adherent	24 h	72 h
Nonhematopoietic	HepG2	DMEM	10%FBS, Pen/Strep	2000/well	Adherent	24 h	72 h

Abbreviations: β-ME: beta mercaptoethanol; DMEM: Dulbecco's modified Eagle's medium; FBS: fetal bovine serum; IMDM: Iscove's modified Dulbecco's medium; Pen/Strep: 1× penicillin/streptomycin; rhM-CSF: recombinant human macrophage-colony stimulating factor; rmEpo: recombinant murine erythropoietin.

Table 17.3 Tier 1 assay qualification using compounds known to induce lineage specific toxicity. The five compounds are evaluated using the optimal culture conditions for each of the cell lines ($n = 3$ experiments with triplicate wells within each experiment). The lowest IC_{50} for each compound corresponds to the expected BM toxicity.

Compound	Expected BM toxicity	Micromolar inhibitory concentration 50% (IC_{50})				
		Myeloid	Erythroid	Lymphoid	Stromal	Nonhematopoietic
Acebutolol hydrochloride	None	>100	>100	>100	>100	>100
Methotrexate	Myeloid	0.005	>100	0.2	0.05	>100
Chloramphenicol	Erythroid	>100	8	>100	81	>100
Taxol	Myeloid	0.009	2	0.03	0.9	40
Camptothecin	general	<0.003	0.7	0.04	0.06	0.9

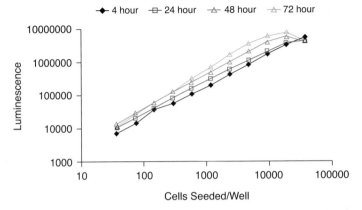

Figure 17.1 Correlation of cell number with luminescence and expansion of cells over 72 hours. Various number of myeloid (M1) cells were seeded at $t = 0$ and evaluated using CellTiter Glo at the designated times. There was a linear correlation between cell number seeded and luminescence (4 h time point) indicating CellTiter Glo is adequate to evaluate relative number of cells in a well. Luminescence increased between 4 and 72 h at almost all seeding densities. $N = 3$ experiments with triplicate wells in each experiment. Although not shown, the erythroid (HCS57), lymphoid (M-NFS-60), stromal (M2-10B) and non-hematopoietic (HepG2) cell lines had similar results.

To further qualify the myeloid tier 1 assay, the myeloid cell line IC_{50} values were compared with the mouse CFU-GM IC_{50} values using compounds of very diverse structures and targets (Figure 17.3). The mouse CFU-GM assay was used as the comparator since this assay is known to detect compounds that will induce neutropenia, decreased number of peripheral blood myeloid cells. The two assays correlated well ($r^2 = 0.80$), indicating the tier 1 myeloid assay was able to quantify the potential of compounds to induce neutropenia. However, this was done with compounds that had very diverse structures and targets and during drug discovery the assay would be used to rank many compounds from one target and with potentially similar core chemistry. To determine whether the myeloid tier 1 assay was able to distinguish hematotoxicity of similar chemistries, 13 compounds with similar core chemistry were evaluated in both the tier 1 and the mouse CFU-GM assays (Figure 17.4). The two assays correlated well ($r^2 = 0.74$), qualifying the tier 1 myeloid assay for evaluating compounds of similar chemistry early in drug discovery.

Qualification of the erythroid tier 1 assay was more difficult as there are fewer compounds known to induce *in vivo* erythrotoxicity and the CFU-E assay has not been used to predict *in vivo* toxicity potential of compounds. Instead, the erythroid tier 1 assay was qualified by comparing IC_{50} values with the percent peripheral blood reticulocyte reduction using 16 AstraZeneca compounds with similar core chemistry (Figure 17.5). When plotting the results from 15 compounds, $r^2 = 0.83$.

Qualification of the tier 1 assays with the limited number of compounds indicated that the cell lines were able to predict the *in vivo* hematotoxicity potential of compounds, but further qualification using more compounds and specifically noncytotoxic compounds are still required.

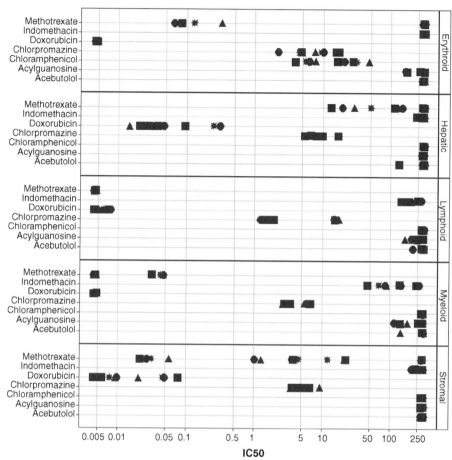

Figure 17.2 Reproducibility of compound concentration that decreases relative cell number by 50% (IC$_{50}$). Each data point is based on the IC$_{50}$ from a 12-point titration curve of each compound. $N \geq 3$ experiments with triplicate wells within each experiment.

As powerful or predictive as these assays can be, an ordinate and ingenious use of them is necessary for optimal impact on drug development. As described above, the mouse cell line screening assay allows a fast and relative prediction of bone marrow toxicity of known toxicants *in vivo* (positive controls of the validation set). More interestingly, it allows to rank order chemical series and chemicals within a series. The simplicity of the assay itself, the low cost, its possible automation and the fast turnaround of data generation makes it an ideal tool to profile large numbers of compounds. Hence, this step can be used at relatively early stages of drug discovery. The whole assay can be streamlined with automatic cell culture and maintenance, linked to robotic stations and multiplate reader analysis to measure the ATP content

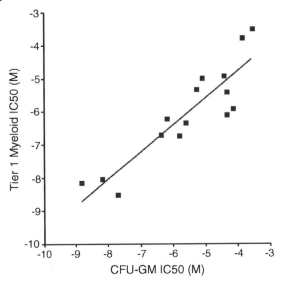

Figure 17.3 Tier 1 myeloid assay (M1 cell line) qualification using known hematotoxicants of different chemical pharmacology and structure. Fifteen compounds with either known colony-forming unit granulocyte-macrophage (CFU-GM) IC_{50} values from literature or evaluate in-house were compared to IC_{50} from level 1 myeloid cell assay. $n = 3$ experiments with triplicate wells within each experiment. The linear regression line is plotted showing the correlation between the two assays.

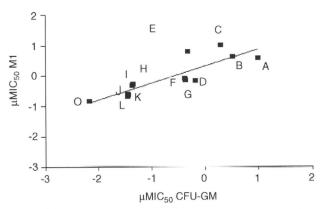

Figure 17.4 Tier 1 myeloid assay (M1 cell line) qualification using compounds of similar chemical pharmacology and structure. Thirteen compounds from a single core structure were evaluated in the tier 1 myeloid assay ($n = 1$ experiment with triplicate conditions) and 35 mm dish CFU-GM assay ($n = 1$ experiment with triplicate plates). The linear regression line is plotted showing the correlation between the two assays.

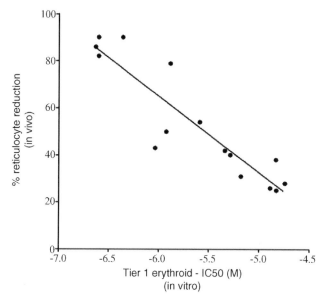

Figure 17.5 Tier 1 erythroid assay qualification using compounds of similar chemical pharmacology and structure. Fifteen compounds from a single pharmacological class were evaluated in the tier 1 erythroid assay and *in vivo* measuring absolute number of peripheral blood reticulocytes. $r^2 = 0.83$. Tier 1 erythroid IC_{50} values are the average from triplicate wells ($n = 1$ experiment); reticulocyte counts were based on results from an Advia hematology analyzer ($n = 1$).

by luminescence. With such a set up, a large volume of data can be generated rapidly enough to orientate the chemistry in one direction or another. This process can be iterative, back-and-forth between bone marrow toxicity profiling and new chemistry synthesis. This should in principle allow sufficient refining of the drug candidates to be devoid of hematotoxicity if not directly linked to pharmacology, or at least to a tolerable level and not impede further drug development up to the patients.

Interestingly, it is not unusual for chemical series to be fairly toxic on the erythroid cell line, for example, while having no effect at all on the white cell lineages, or the stromal lineage, or any other combination. However, while optimizing the chemistry to reduce the erythroid lineage toxicity, other lineage toxicity might arise. Hence, it can be difficult to choose the proper chemical structures to avoid overall bone marrow toxicity as, for the same project, every series may have its own hematotoxicity specificity not acceptable for progressing those compounds. A choice has often to be made in the function of therapeutic indication, usually in collaboration with clinicians, where perhaps a mild erythropenia might be more tolerable than neutropenia. Equally interesting is the possibility of having series that do not display hematotoxicity but which are toxic in the nonhematopoietic general toxicity cell line (HepG2). One can assume that this is the ideal case and therefore move forward such chemicals. However, this might be an indication of a possible hepatotoxicity issue, although HepG2s are poor predictors of liver toxicity.

The specificity (rate of false positives) and the sensitivity (rate of false negatives) are difficult to calculate with the limited number of chemicals that have been so far tested both in this system and *in vivo* in animals and human. False negatives, though, are more acceptable than false positives at early stages of drug discovery. Indeed, false negatives would be spotted during regular GLP *in vivo* animal studies and would not reach the human population more than they currently do. However, false positives may lead to the rejection of a good chemical series that could have ended up as a useful drug for patients. Hence, increasing the level of confidence of the tier 1 assay is essential, which is in part the role of the tier 2 assay.

17.3.2
Tier 2 Tests

Despite displaying a fair predictive value, the tier 1 assay is based on simple cytotoxicity measurement of cell lines, not primary cells, which may have lost a number of primitive characteristics. Therefore, the trust level of this assay to embrace a wide range of predictable events is not as high as it is for the CFU assay. It is then advisable to confirm some key findings of the tier 1 stage, by the more elaborated and more validated CFU assay [43–49].

The 35 mm dish assay most frequently used was for the myeloid lineage (CFU-GM), but there are also assays for erythroid (CFU-E/BFU-E), lymphoid (CFU-L), stromal (CFU-F) and megakaryocyte (CFU-Meg) lineages. All of these assays are available to evaluate human bone marrow and several of these assays are also available for evaluating toxicity in mouse, rat, dog [50] and monkey in order to determine species-specificity. Hence, this is extremely useful to determine whether a positive result in tier 1 on mouse cell lines also holds in other species of higher interest, like man. Our recommendation is to check some of the worst toxicants as determined in tier 1 in the CFU assays, to confirm the results and to gradually build up the confidence into the predictivity of the tier 1 cell line assay. If this does indeed corroborate the tier 1 assessment, the development of chemical series or chemicals within a series can be stopped and the chemistry refined following the structures of the less-toxic compounds (Figure 17.6). Equally some of the best compounds (nonhematotoxic) in tier 1 should be controlled in the CFU assay for confirmation of their innocuousness in the species of interest (Figure 17.6 – "Spot-check"). Such compounds would be the leading structures for even further refinement, if needed.

It is relatively obvious that CFU assays cannot be used for wide profiling and that a careful choice of some of the compounds tested in tier 1 should be tested on tier 2. Therefore, a constant exchange of data and information between the profiler and the chemist is essential.

The 35 mm dish assay detects compounds that are cytotoxic to or alter proliferation of the multipotent stem cells, but the main limitation of the 35 mm dish CFU assay is the need to microscopically identify and count the colonies to determine the compound concentration that decreased the number of colonies by 50% (IC_{50}) or 90% (IC_{90}). The European Community for Validation of Alternative Methods (ECVAM) supported the recommendation of using the mouse and human CFU-GM IC_{90} with

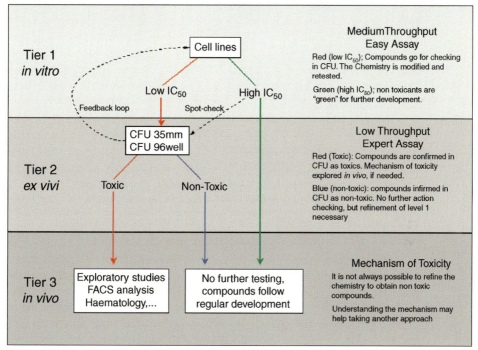

Figure 17.6 Hematotoxicity screening cascade. Assays used during drug discovery with tier 1 as the early discovery front-loading assay.

the concentration that induced neutropenia *in vivo* in the mouse to calculate the expected human maximum tolerated dose (MTD), in respect to bone marrow ADR (Figure 17.7) [45, 46]. However, the assay used in these studies is labor-intensive, low-throughput and requires highly trained staff. Several manuscripts have been published attempting to increase the throughput of these assays. For example, an algorithm was written to automatically count CFU-GM colonies [51]. This decreased subjectivity of colony counting increases reproducibility and generates a permanent record of the colonies, but the 35 mm dish assays still need to be scanned, which takes a significant amount of time. Malerba *et al.* [52] modified the assay into a 96-well format, but still required microscopic identification and counting of the colonies. The largest improvement was the development of multiwell CFU assays [53] where the relative number of colonies was quantified using luminescence. This automatable format greatly increases the possibility of checking tier 1 results in tier 2, as the throughput is much higher than with 35 mm dishes. If the cost of such an assay decreased enough, then it could possibly replace the tier 1 cell line assay. One possibility is to build up a homemade platform, as the current authors did; however, the main limitation still remains the cost and availability of the cytokines necessary for the differentiation and growth of the different lineages.

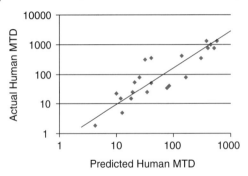

Figure 17.7 Predicted versus observed human in vivo MTD using colony forming unit (CFU) assay. The mouse CFU-GM IC$_{50}$, human CFU-GM IC$_{50}$ and mouse maximum tolerated dose (MTD) were used to calculate predicted human MTD based on the European Community for Validation of Alternative Methods (ECVAM). The data plotted are based on published results [45, 46]. The linear regression line is plotted showing the correlation between the two assays.

The "homemade assay," modified from Horowitz et al. [54], is a semiautomated 96-well assay with 50 μL of primary bone marrow cells in methylcellulose containing cytokines and 50 μL of compound titrated in DMSO and diluted in media (0.1% DMSO final concentration). Relative cell number was analyzed using 100 μL of CellTiter Glo at the end of the culture period, one week for mouse and two weeks for human. At least 40 compounds could be evaluated in any given experiment using robotics to titrate and dilute compounds and then to add the diluted compounds to replicate plates that contain the tier 1 cells. The 96-well semiautomated mouse CFU-GM assay was qualified by comparing to the standard 35 mm dish CFU-GM assay using compounds with diverse structure and targets (Figure 17.8; $r^2 = 0.77$).

The other limitation of the CFU assay in either format is that it remains an in vitro environment where distant interactions, like liver metabolism (either detoxifying the compounds or producing toxic metabolites) or immunomodulation, are absent. Investigating the mechanism of toxicity in animals for some carefully chosen compounds after being characterized in the two previous assays, can provide valuable information for the whole series, allow further refinement of the in vitro assays (e.g., addition of S9 for metabolism) and give an early indication of which biomarkers could be used in later GLP studies.

17.3.3
Tier 3 Tests

Tier 3 is the evaluation of bone marrow after in vivo exposure to determine in vivo applicability of the in vitro results (tiers 1 and 2) and predict clinical target- and chemistry-related toxicities. Historically, the bone marrow toxicity potential of compounds was evaluated by microscopic assessment of rat bone marrow cellularity from decalcified sternum bone slides, hematology and in some cases bone marrow differentials [55] only when a compound reached development.

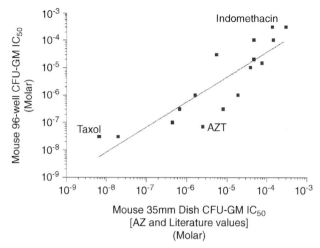

Figure 17.8 Mouse 35 mm dish versus mouse 96-well colony-forming unit granulocyte/macrophage (CFU-GM) assays. Each compound was evaluated in the 96-well CFU-GM assay, 12-point titration curve with triplicate samples while the 35 mm dish results were based on literature results or a twelve point titration curve with duplicate 35 mm dish results. The linear regression line is plotted showing the correlation between the two assays.

Decrease in hematology parameters requires careful evaluation as it can result from drug-induced hematotoxicity or from increased cell loss. For example, microvascular hemorrhage from the gastrointenstinal tract results in decreased peripheral red blood cell numbers due to blood loss, even though the bone marrow is functioning adequately. There are a few limitations with bone marrow differentials that require highly trained clinical pathologists to do 200 or more cell differentials, but more importantly the differential only yields a percentage of cells without respect to the absolute cell number. This can lead to misinterpretation of the results. For example, decreased percentage of a cell type with an elevated absolute number of total cells could yield a normal absolute cell number. To circumvent this limitation, a flow cytometric method was developed that reported the absolute numbers of lymphoid, immature myeloid, maturing myeloid, immature erythroid and maturing nucleated erythroid cells in rat, dog and monkey bone marrow [56]. This assay can screen the *in vivo* bone marrow hematotoxicity potential of compounds, but slides for cytology were always prepared in case a compound interfered with staining. The advantage of this and other flow cytometric methods developed [57, 58] include: (i) differential based on at least 10 000 cells; (ii) reporting absolute cell numbers; (iii) results reported within a few days (compared to weeks for doing 200 cell microscopic differentials); (iv) bone marrow toxicity irrespective of the general pathophysiological pathway: proliferation, maturation and/or stromal cell interactions. Compounds inhibiting proliferation decrease the number of immature myeloid or erythroid cells. Compounds that inhibit maturation are detected by decreased maturing cells and altered hematology. Stromal cell interactions are not directly evaluated by this assay but stromal cells support hematopoiesis and so inhibition of stromal cell function or

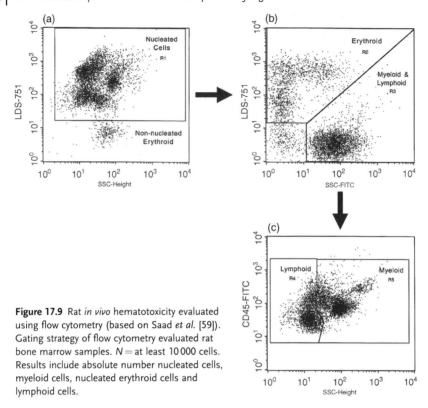

Figure 17.9 Rat *in vivo* hematotoxicity evaluated using flow cytometry (based on Saad *et al.* [59]). Gating strategy of flow cytometry evaluated rat bone marrow samples. N = at least 10 000 cells. Results include absolute number nucleated cells, myeloid cells, nucleated erythroid cells and lymphoid cells.

stromal cell loss results in decreased proliferation and/or maturation of the hematopoietic cells.

The tier 3 assay used was modified from Saad *et al.* [59]. This flow cytometric method distinguishes between nucleated and nonnucleated cells, based on side scatter and LDS-751 staining. LDS-751 is a nucleic acid stain (Figure 17.9). On our flow cytometer, bone marrow reticulocytes (polychromatic erythrocytes) were within the LDS-751 positive population, as was demonstrated when evaluating isolated nonnucleated cells by sepharose column (Figure 17.10). Therefore a slightly modified gating strategy for data analysis was used to quantify nonnucleated cells, reticulocytes and nucleated erythroid cells separately, in addition to the myeloid and lymphoid populations (Figure 17.11).

17.4
Triggers for Hematotoxicity Testing

There is a high prevalence of bone marrow toxicity with antiproliferative oncology compounds that also occurs with many non-antiproliferative compound classes but at a much lower prevalence. It is these non-antiproliferative compounds that are of greatest

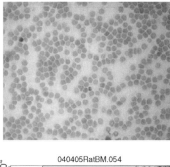
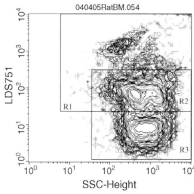

Figure 17.10 Flow cytometric method does not differentiate between nucleated erythroid cells and reticulocytes, on some instruments. Non-nucleated erythroid cells were isolated using cellulose fractionation. Part of the sample was stained with Wright-Giemsa and reticulocytes and mature nucleated cells quantified by trained medical technologists. Rest of the sample was stained using the method by Saad et al. [59]. There are two non-nucleated erythroid populations based on LDS751 staining (LDS751$^-$ and LDS751^{dim}). Additional stains (results not shown) indicate the LDS751^{dim} cells are reticulocytes and the LDS751$^-$ cells are mature non-nucleated erythrocytes.

importance to evaluate early in drug discovery to influence chemistry, but it is typically not possible to evaluate all of these compounds within the company library or compounds generated by the chemists. Hence, three possible approaches are attempted.

The first consists of selecting a handful of representative compounds which cover the chemical space of a series and testing only those. If there are some alerts, then further compounds can be tested. This can be done systematically for all series of all projects. However, this absorbs a fair amount of resources for a potentially limited return on investment.

The second approach necessitates a mechanism to identify compounds or chemical series from a project that enter the screening cascade. These triggers may include target-related information, previous experience and *in silico* analysis of compounds.

One of the roles of a toxicologist involved in early discovery as a project team representative can be to generate a list of potential and likely toxicities deduced from target-related information such as tissue expression, similarity to other targets, precedent described in literature and sometimes chemical structure similarity. When

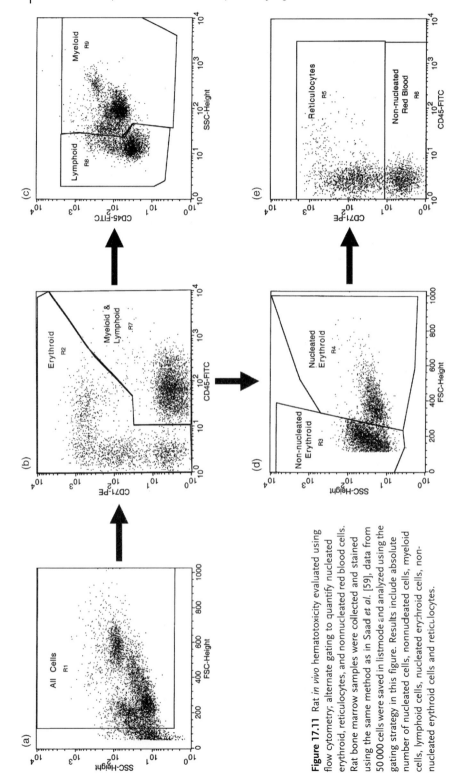

Figure 17.11 Rat *in vivo* hematotoxicity evaluated using flow cytometry; alternate gating to quantify nucleated erythroid, reticulocytes, and nonnucleated red blood cells. Rat bone marrow samples were collected and stained using the same method as in Saad *et al.* [59], data from 50 000 cells were saved in listmode and analyzed using the gating strategy in this figure. Results include absolute number of nucleated cells, nonnucleated cells, myeloid cells, lymphoid cells, nucleated erythroid cells, nonnucleated erythroid cells and reticulocytes.

reasonable theoretical concerns can be formulated, then project compounds need to be evaluated using the proposed cascade, to assess the reality of those potential BM toxicities. Furthermore, it is sometimes possible to determine whether bone marrow toxicity is due to pharmacology and/or formulate a structure–activity relationship. By using this targeted approach, one can limit compound-profiling activities to areas of high likelihood of BMT and optimize the cost-effectiveness of such screening.

However, when hematotoxicity are observed *in vivo* for initial lead compounds or projects, then backups or next generation projects have an easy trigger to justify a thorough profiling of follow-up compounds through the whole cascade very early in discovery.

The third potential trigger of the cascade is *in silico* that can evaluate thousands of compounds generated by the chemists for all projects, but the authors are not aware of any such *in silico* models at this time. However, some models are under development and should be implemented within the next couple years as more compounds are evaluated using this BMT profiling cascade. Five different bone marrow toxicity *in silico* models are needed as some compounds are toxic to only some of the lineages (myeloid, erythroid, lymphoid, megakaryocyte/platelet, stromal) while other compounds are toxic to all five lineages. It is hoped that a thorough and constant use of the described assays could feed the training sets of such *in silico* systems for better prediction. Hence, with time, more and more triggers are likely to be due to *in silico* warnings.

17.5
Conclusions

Hematotoxicity is an ADR with varying incidence clinically and consists of drug-induced agranulocytosis/neutropenia, thrombocytopenia and anemia. There are at least several mechanisms of drug-induced hematotoxicity still unknown for most compounds. A cascade of assays was developed and qualified to permit evaluation of various compounds from a pharmacological target and similar chemical structures. The tier 1 assay is medium-throughput and allows a fast screening of small amounts of compounds early in drug discovery. Tier 2 assays are lower-throughput, but enable the assessment of species-specificity and should be used to check tier 1 results. The tier 3 assay evaluates the hematotoxicity potential of compounds by flow cytometry after *in vivo* dosing. This cascade is used successfully, but still needs further qualification using non-antiproliferative compounds and verifying the ability of the cascade to predict clinical BMT ADR.

References

1 Vangala, S. and Tonelli, A. (2007) Biomarkers, metabonomics, and drug development: can inborn errors of metabolism help in understanding drug toxicity? *AAPS Journal*, **9**, E284–E297.

2 Kola, I. and Landis, J. (2004) Can the pharmaceutical industry reduce attrition rates? *Nature Reviews. Drug Discovery*, **3**, 711–715.

3 Fung, M., Thornton, A., Mybeck, K., Wu, J.H., Kornbuckle, K. and Muniz, E. (2001) Evaluation of characteristics of safety withdrawal of prescription drugs from worldwide pharmaceutical markets – 1960 to 1999. *Drug Information Journal*, **35**, 293–317.

4 Lubran, M.M. (1959) Hematologic side effects of drugs. *Annals of Clinical and Laboratory Science*, **19**, 114–121.

5 Zhu, H., Li, Y. and Trush, M.A. (1995) Characterizatoin of benzo[a]pyrene quinine-induced toxicity to primary cultured bone marrow stromal cells from DBA/2 mice: potential role of mitochondrial dysfunction. *Toxicology and Applied Pharmacology*, **130**, 108–120.

6 McKee, E.E., Furguson, M., Bentley, A.T. and Marks, T.A. (2006) Inhibition of mammalian mitochondrial protein synthesis by oxazolidinones. *Antimicrob Agents Chemotherapy*, **50**, 2042–2049.

7 Chitnis, S., Mondal, D. and Agrawal, K.C. (2002) Zifovudine (AZT) treatment suppresses granulocyte-monocyte colony stimulating factor receptor type alpha (GM-CSFRa) gene expression in murine bone marrow cells. *Life Sciences*, **71**, 967–978.

8 Siraki, A.G., Deterding, L.J., Bonini, M.G., Jian, J., Ehrenshaft, M., Tomer, K.B. and Mason, R.P. (2008) Procainamide, but not N-Acetylprocainamide, induces protein free radical formation on myeloperoxidase: a potential mechanism of agranulocytosis. *Chemical Research in Toxicology*, **21**, 1143–1153.

9 Pereira, A. and Dean, B. (2006) Clozapine bioactivation induces dose-dependent, drug-specific toxicity of human bone marrow stromal cells: a potential *in vitro* system for the study of agranulocytosis. *Biochemical Pharmacology*, **72**, 783–793.

10 Gray, M.W., Cedergren, R., Abel, Y. and Sankoff, D. (1989) On the evolutionary origin of the plan mitochondrion and its genome. *Proceedings of the National Academy of Sciences of the United States of America*, **86**, 2267–2271.

11 Riesbeck, K., Bredberg, A. and Forsgren, A. (1990) Ciprofloxacin does not inhibit mitochondrial functions but other antibiotics do. *Antimic Agents Chemther*, **34**, 167–169.

12 Kroon, A.M., Donje, B.H., Holtrop, M. and Van Den Bogert, C. (1984) The mitochondrial genetic system as a target for chemotherapy: tetracyclines as cytostatics. *Cancer Letters*, **24**, 33–40.

13 Scatena, R., Bottoni, P., Botta, G., Martorana, G.E. and Giardina, B. (2007) The role of mitochondria in pharmacotoxicology: a reevaluation of an old, newly emerging topic. *American Journal of Physiology. Cell Physiology*, **293**, C12–C21.

14 Lavin, A.L., Hahn, D.J. and Gasiewicz, T.A. (1998) Expression of functional aromatic hydrocarbon receptor and aromatic hydrocarbon nuclear translocator proteins in murine bone marrow stromal cells. *Archives of Biochemistry and Biophysics*, **352**, 9–18.

15 van Grevenynghe, J., Bernard, M., langouet, S., Le Berre, C., Fest, T. and Fardel, O. (2005) Human CD34-positive hematopoietic stem cells constitute targets for carcinogenic polycyclic aromatic hydrocarbons. *The Journal of Pharmacology and Experimental Therapeutics*, **314**, 693–702.

16 Pendurthi, U.R., Okino, S.T. and Tukey, R.H. (1993) Accumulation of the nuclear dioxin (Ah) receptor and transcriptional activation of the mouse cyp1a-1 and cyp1a-2 genes. *Archives of Biochemistry and Biophysics*, **306**, 65–69.

17 Yoon, B.I., Hirabayashi, Y., Kaneko, T., Kodama, Y., Kano, J., Yodoi, J., Kim, D.Y. and Inoue, T. (2001) Transgene expression of thioredoxin (TRX-ADF) protects against 2,3,7,8-tetrachlorodibenzo-p-dioxin (TCDD)-induced hematotoxicity. *Archives of Environmental Contamination and Toxicology*, **41**, 232–236.

18. Yoon, B.I., Hirabayashi, Y., Kawasaki, Y., Kodama, Y., Kaneko, T., Kanno, J., Kim, D.Y., Fujii-Kuriyama, Y. and Inoue, T. (2002) Aryl hydrocarbon receptor mediates benzene-induced hematotoxicity. *Toxicological Sciences*, **70**, 150–156.
19. Galvan, N., Teske, D.E., Zhou, G., Moorthy, B., MacWilliams, P.S., Czuprynski, C.J. and Jefcoate, C.R. (2005) Induction of CYP1A1 and CYP1B1 in liver and lung by benzo(a)pyrene and 7,12dimthylbenz(a)anthracene do not affect distribution of polycylic hydrocarbons to target tissue: role of AhR and CYP1B1 in bone cytotoxicity. *Toxicology and Applied Pharmacology*, **202**, 244–257.
20. Garndner, I., Zahid, N., MacCrimmon, D. and Uetrecht, J.P. (1998) A comparison of the oxidation of clozapine and olanzapine to reactive metabolites and the toxicity these metabolites to human leukocytes. *Molecular Pharmacology*, **53**, 991–998.
21. Pisciotta, A.V., Konings, S.A., Ciesemier, L.L., Cronkite, C.E. and Lieberman, J.A. (1992) On the possible and predictability of clozapine-induced agranulocytosis. *Drug Safety*, **7** (suppl 1), 33–44.
22. Galati, G., Tafazoli, S., Sabzevari, O., Chan, T.S. and O'Brien, P.J. (2002) Idiosyncratic NSAID drug induced oxidative stress. *Chemico-Biological Interactions*, **142**, 25–41.
23. Pereira, A., McLaren, A., Bell, W.R., Copolov, D. and Dean, B. (2003) Potential clozapine target sites on peripheral hematopoietic cells and stromal cells of the bone marrow. *The Pharmacogenomics Journal*, **3**, 227–234.
24. Broome, C.S., Whetton, A.D. and Miyan, J.A. (2000) Neuropeptide control of bone marrow neutrophil production is mediated by both direct and indirect effects on CFU-GM. *British Journal of Haematology*, **108**, 140–150.
25. Liu, C., Ma, X., Jiang, X., Wilson, S.J., Hofstra, C.L., Blevitt, J., Byati, J., Li, X., Chai, W., Carruthers, N. and Lovenbert, T.W. (2001) Cloning and pharmacological characterization of a fourth histamine receptor (H(4)) expressed in bone marrow. *Molecular Pharmacology*, **59**, 420–426.
26. Corbel, S., Schneider, E. and Lemoine, F. (1995) Dy, Murine hematopoietic progenitors are capable of both histamine synthesis and update. *Blood*, **86**, 531–539.
27. Gogu, S.R., Malter, J.S. and Agrawal, K.C. (1992) Zidovudine-induced blockade of the expression and function of the erythropoietin receptor. *Biochemical Pharmacology*, **44**, 1009–1012.
28. Wadelius, M., Stjernberg, E., Wiholm, B.E. and Rane, A. (2000) Polymorphisms of NAT2 in relation to sulphasalazine-induced agranulocytosis. *Pharmacogenetics*, **10**, 35–41.
29. Sebbag, L., Boucher, P., Davelu, P., Boissonnat, P., Champsaur, G., Ninet, J., Dureau, G., obadia, J.F., Vallon, J.J. and Delaye, J. (2000) Thiopurine s-methyltransferase gene polymorphism is predictive of azathioprine-induced myelosuppression in heart transplant recipients. *Transplantation*, **69**, 1524–1527.
30. Schwab, M., Schaffeler, E., Marx, C., Fischer, C., Lang, T., Behrens, C., Gregor, M., Eichelbaum, M., Zanger, U.U. and Kaskas, B.A. (2002) Azathioprine therapy and adverse drug reactions in patients with inflammatory bowel disease: impact of thiopurine s-methyltransferase polymorphism. *Pharmacogenetics*, **12**, 429–438.
31. Mosyagin, I., Dettling, M., Roots, I., Mueller-Oerlinghausen, B. and Cascorbi, I. (2004) Impact of myeloperoxidase and NADPH-oxidase polymorphisms in drug-induced agranulocytosis. *Journal of Clinical Psychopharmacology*, **24**, 613–617.
32. Kiyotani, K., Mushiroda, T., Kubo, M., Zembutsu, H., Sugiyama, Y. and Nakamura, Y. (2008) Association of genetic polymorphisms in SLCO1B3 and ABCC2 with docataxel –induced leucopenia. *Cancer Science*, **99**, 967–972.
33. Biason, P., Basier, S. and Toffoli, G. (2008) UGT1A*28 and other UGT1A

polymorphisms as determinants of irinotecan toxicity. *Journal of Chemotherapy*, **20**, 158–165.

34 Rha, S.Y., Jeung, H.C., Choi, Y.H., Yang, W.I., Yoo, J.H., Kim, B.S., Roh, J.K. and Chung, H.C. (2007) An association between RRM1 haplotype and gemcitabine-induced neutropenia in breast cancer patients. *Oncologist*, **12**, 622–630.

35 Hor, S.Y., Lee, S.C., Wong, C.I., Lim, Y.W., Lim, R.C., Wang, L.Z., Fan, L., Guo, J.Y., Lee, H.S., Goh, B.C. and Tan, T. (2008) PXR, CAR, and HNF4alpha genotypes and their association with pharmacokinetics and pharmacodynamics of docetaxel and doxorubicin in asian patients. *The Pharmacogenomics Journal*, **8**, 139–146.

36 Mealey, K.L., Fidel, J., Gay, J.M., Imperllizeri, J.A., Clifford, C.A. and Bergman, P.J. (2008) ABCB1-1Delta polymorphism can predict hematologic toxicity in dogs treated with vincristine. *Journal of Veterinary Internal Medicine/American College of Veterinary Internal Medicine*, **22**, 996–1000.

37 Mielke, S. (2007) Individualized pharmacotherapy with paclitaxel. *Current Opinion in Oncology*, **19**, 586–589.

38 Sandvliet, A.S., Huitema, A.D., Copalu, W., Yamada, Y., Tamura, T., Beijnen, J.H. and Schellens, J.H. (2007) Cyp2c9 and cyp2c19 polymorphic forms are related to increased indisulam exposure and higher risk of severe hematologic toxicity. *Clinical Cancer Research*, **13**, 2970–2976.

39 Sakamoto, K., Oka, M., Yoshino, S., hazama, S., Abe, T., Okayama, N. and Hinoda, Y. (2006) Relation between cytokine promoter gene polymorphism and toxicity of 5-fluorouracil plus cisplatin chemotherapy. *Oncology Reports*, **16**, 381–387.

40 Brott, D., Kelly, T., Capobianchi, K., Huggett, T., Goodman, J., Saad, A. and Pognan, F. (2007) Frontloading the evaluation of bone marrow toxicity using a three-tired approach. *The Toxicologist*, **2007**, 1169.

41 Huggett, T., Saad, A., Kelly, T., Pognan, F., Otieno, M. and Brott, D. (2005) Validation of an *in vitro* cell line for screening myelotoxicity. *The Toxicologist*, **2005**, 1626.

42 Hankins, W.D., Chin, K., Dons, R. and Sigounas, G. (1989) Erythropoietin-dependent and erythropoietin-producing cell lines. Implications for research and for leukemia therapy. *Annals of the New York Academy of Sciences*, **554**, 21–28.

43 Erickson-Miller, C.L., May, R.D., Tomaszewski, J., Osborn, B., Murphy, M.J., Page, J.G. and Parchment, R.E. (1997) Differential toxicity of camptothecin, otpotecan and 9-amino-camptothecin to human canine and murine myeloid progenitors (CFU-GM) in vitro. *Cancer Chemotherapy and Pharmacology*, **39**, 467–474.

44 Pessina, A., Malerba, I. and Gribaldo, L. (2005) Hematotoxicity testing by cell clonogenic assay in drug development and preclinical trials. *Current Pharmaceutical Design*, **11**, 1055–1065.

45 Pessina, A., Albella, B., Bueren, J., Brantom, P., Casati, S., Gribaldo, L., Croera, C., Gagliardi, G., Foti, P., Parchment, R., Parent-Massin, D., Sibiril, Y., Schoeters, G. and Van Den Heuvel, R. (2001) Prevalidation of a model for predicting acute neutropenia by colony forming unit granulocyte/macrophage(CFU-GM) assay. *Toxicol in Vitro*, **15**, 729–740.

46 Pessina, A., Albella, B., Bayo, M., Bueren, J., Brantom, P., Casati, S., Croera, C., Gagliardi, G., Foti, R., Parchment, R., Parent-Massin, D., Schoeters, G., Sibiril, Y., Van Den Heuvel, R. and Grialdo, L. (2003) Application of the CFU-GM assay to predict acute drug-induced neutropenia: an interanational blind trial to validate a prediction model of the maximum tolerated dose (MTD) of myelosuppresive xenobiotics. *Toxicol Sciences*, **75**, 355–367.

47 Goldfain-Blanc, R., Wattrelos, O., Casadevall, N., Beamonte, A., Delongeas, J.L. and Claude, N. (2004) Value of *in vitro* models for the assessment of drug-induced haematotoxicity. *Therapie*, **59**, 607–610.

48 Pessina, A., Croera, C., Bayo, M., Malerba, I., Passardi, L., Cavicchini, L., Neri, M.G. and Gribaldo, L. (2004) A methylcellulose microculture assay for the in vitro assessment of drug toxicity on granulocyte/macrophage progenitors (CFU-GM). *Alternatives to Laboratory Animals*, **32**, 17–23.

49 Parchment, R.E. (1998) Alternative testing systems for evaluating noncarcinogenic, hematologic toxicity. *Environmental Health Perspectives*, **106** (Suppl. 2), 541–547.

50 Deldar, A., Lewis, H., Bloom, J. and Weiss, L. (1988) Reproducibile cloning assays for in vitro growth of canine hematopoietic progenitor cells and their potential applications in investigative hematotoxicity. *American Journal of Veterinary Research*, **49**, 1393–1401.

51 Crosta, G.F., Fumarola, L., Malerba, I. and Gribaldo, L. (2007) Scoring CFU-GM colonies in vitro by data fusion: a first account. *Experimental Hematology*, **35**, 1–12.

52 Malerba, I., Casati, S., Diodovich, C., Parent-Massin, D. and Gribaldo, L. (2004) Inhibition of CFU-E/BFU-E and CFU-GM colony growth by cyclophosphamide, 5-fluorouracil and taxol: development of high-throughput in vitro method. *Toxicol in vitro*, **18**, 293–300.

53 Rich, I.N. and Hall, K.M. (2005) Validation and development of a predictive paradigm for hematotoxicology using multifunctional bioluminescence colony-forming proliferation assay. *Toxicol Sciences*, **87**, 427–441.

54 Horowitz, D. and King, A.G. (2000) Colorimetric determination of inhibition of hematopoietic progenitor cells in soft agar. *Journal of Immunological Methods*, **244**, 49–58.

55 Bollinger, A.P. (2004) Cytological evaluation of bone marrow in rats: indications, methods and normal morphology. *Veterinary Clinical Pathology*, **33**, 58–67.

56 Martin, R.A., Brott, D.A., Zandee, J.C. and McKeel, M.J. (1992) Differential analysis of animal bone marrow by flow cytometry. *Cytometry*, **13**, 638–643.

57 Criswell, K.A., Sulkanen, A.P., Hochbaum, A.F. and Bleavins, M.R. (2000) Effects of phenylhydrazine or phlebotomy on peripheral blood, bone marrow and erythropoietin in wistar rats. *Journal of Applied Toxicology*, **20**, 25–34.

58 Weiss, D.J. (2001) Use of monoclonal antibodies to refine flow cytometric differential cell counting of canine bone marrow cells. *American Journal of Veterinary Research*, **62**, 1273–1278.

59 Saad, A., Palm, M., Widell, S. and Reiland, S. (2000) Differential analysis of rat bone marrow by flow cytometry. *Comparative Haem International*, **10**, 97–101.

60 Garbe, E. (2007) Non-chemotherapy drug-induced agranulocytosis. *Expert Opinion on Drug Safety*, **6**, 323–335.

61 Andres, E., Zimmer, J., Affenberger, S., Federici, L., Alt, M. and Maloisel, F. (2006) Idiosyncratic drug-induced agranulocytosis: update of an old disorder. *European Journal of Internal Medicine*, **17**, 529–535.

62 Flanagan, R.J. and Dunk, L. (2008) Haematological toxicity of drugs used in psychiatry. *Human Psychopharmacology-Clinical and Experimental*, **23**, 27–41.

63 Andres, E., Federici, L., Weitten, T., Vogel, T. and Alt, M. (2008) Recognition and management of drug-induced blood cytopenias: the example of drug-induced acute neutropenia and agranulocytosis. *Expert Opinion on Drug Safety*, **7**, 481–489.

18
Profiling Adverse Immune Effects

Wim H. De Jong, Raymond Pieters, Kirsten A Baken, Rob J. Vandebriel, Jan-Willem Van Der Laan, and Henk Van Loveren

18.1
Immunotoxicology

18.1.1
The Immune System and Immunotoxicology

Immunotoxicology is that part of toxicology focused on the study of the effect of xenobiotics including pharmaceuticals on the immune system [1–8]. Components of the immune system are distributed all over the body and comprise multiple organs, with bone marrow and the thymus playing pivotal roles, bone marrow for the generation of new cells and the thymus for maturation and selection of the thymus-dependent T cells. In addition to these central organs, there are the peripheral immune organs such as the spleen and a multitude of lymph nodes and localized areas of lymphoid tissue such as bronchial-associated lymphoid tissue (BALT) in the respiratory tract and gut-associated lymphoid tissue (GALT) including Peyer's patches (PP) in the gastro-intestinal tract.

The primary function of the immune system is to protect the body from invading organisms like bacteria, viruses and parasites. Toxic effects on the immune system may result in reduced immune responses, leading to enhanced incidence or severity of infectious diseases when the system is challenged, and certain forms of neoplasia. Another effect may be immune disregulation that can exacerbate or facilitate the development of allergy or autoimmunity. For direct immunotoxicity or immunosuppression a compound is considered immunotoxic when effects on organs or cells of the immune system are observed at doses that do not induce overt (other) toxicity. In reference to the term immunotoxicity, toxic effects of xenobiotics, including pharmaceuticals may occur with the immune system being a passive target organ. However, immunotoxicology comprises more than just toxicity for immune organs and immune cells. Also effects such as an (excessive) immune response to the xenobiotic itself resulting in clinical allergy and an (excessive) stimulation of the immune system resulting in autoimmune disease belongs to the realm of

Hit and Lead Profiling. Edited by Bernard Faller and Laszlo Urban
Copyright © 2009 WILEY-VCH Verlag GmbH & Co. KGaA, Weinheim
ISBN: 978-3-527-32331-9

immunotoxicology. In this respect special emphasis should be given to the therapeutic use of components of the immune system itself, such as monoclonal antibodies and cytokines, and therapeutics targeted at the immune system. When the immune system is challenged, even low-level immunosuppresssion may be detrimental for the potential development of diseases. A clear example of the effects of immunosuppression are the well known opportunistic infections in human immunodeficiency virus (HIV) patients [9–12], cytomegalus infections in transplant patients treated with immunosuppresssive drugs [13–15], and posttransplant lymphoproliferative disorders [16].

One of the first papers presenting an overview on immunotoxicity was published in 1977 by Vos [17]. This seminal paper was a comprehensive review on a large series of xenobiotics that affect immune reactivity in laboratory animals and hence might influence the health of exposed individuals (Table 18.1). It showed that immunotoxicity should be seriously considered and investigated as part of the whole toxicological investigation of compounds. The complexity of the immune system results in multiple potential target sites and pathological effects for immunotoxic xenobiotics. So far, immunotoxicity is mainly investigated in animal models, usually in a tiered approach [5, 18], which is formalized for pharmaceuticals in the International Conference on Harmonization of Technical Requirements for Registration of Pharmaceuticals for Human Use (ICH) S8 Guidance document as: *Standard Toxicity Studies*; followed by *Additional Immunotoxicity Studies* in cases giving cause for concern [19].

The interactions between the various organs within the immune system limit the possibilities for *in vitro* evaluation of xenobiotics and pharmaceuticals for their potential to interact with the immune system. However, for the identification of direct immunotoxicity some approaches may be used as pretest screening in order to limit animal experiments. *In vitro* testing enables the use of cells and tissues of human origin, which in the field of immunotoxicology means peripheral blood mononuclear cells (PBMC) (and thus also dendritic cells that can be cultured from blood monocytes), which are easily available. The use of human cells increases the relevance of the obtained results and facilitates extrapolation of the observed effects for human risk. In addition, there is an ever increasing knowledge on the immune system and development of tools to characterize immune cells. Mechanistic understanding of the modes of action of (immuno)toxicants has increased using genomics technologies. Important advantages of "omics" technologies are the breadth and depth of analyzing systems without *a priori* knowledge, and the analysis of toxic action not only at the gene but also at the pathway level. Novel developments include profiling not only the messenger ribonucleic acid (mRNA) but also the proteome. In addition, small interfering RNA (siRNA) technology allows the knockdown of single genes to assess or validate the role of specific genes and pathways in immunotoxic action.

In other areas of immunotoxicology such as allergy and autoimmunity non-animal testing is under development but still limited. Both adverse immune responses are dependent on the triggering of an immune response in which the antigen-specific activation of T cells plays a central role. For allergy *in vitro* approaches are being developed, driven by European Union (EU) legislation on the ban of animal

Table 18.1 Chemicals expressing immunotoxicity in animal studies as reviewed by Vos [17].

Chemicals	Main immunotoxic effect (animal)
2,3,7,8-Tetrachlorodibenzo-p-dioxin (TCDD)	Thymus atrophy (rat, mouse, guinea pig)
Di-n-butyltindichloride (DBTC)	Thymus atrophy (rat)
Di-n-octyltindichloride (DOTC)	Thymus atrophy (rat)
Lead acetate/lead nitrate	Increased susceptibility for infection (rat, mouse)
Cadmium acetate	
Cadmium chloride	Reduced antibody responses (mouse, rabbit)
Arsenicals	
Sodium arsenite	Increased susceptibility for infection (mouse)
Arsenic trioxide	
Sodium arsenate	
p-Arsanilic acid	
4-Hydroxy-3-nitrobezenearsonic acid	
Organo metals	
Triethyltin hydroxide	Thymus atrophy (rat, guinea pig)
Triphenyltin hydroxide	Thymus atrophy (guinea pig)
Triphenyltin acetate	Thymus atrophy (guinea pig)
Methylmercury chloride	Reduced antibody responses (mouse)
Mercury chloride	Reduced antibody responses (rabbit)
Cobalt sulfate	Increased susceptibility for infection (mouse)
Nickel acetate	Reduced antibody responses (rat)
Disodium chromate	Reduced antibody responses (rat)
Dichlorodiphenyltrichloroethane (DDT)	Increased susceptibility for infection (chicken, duck)
	Reduced antibody responses (rabbit)
Halogenated biphenyls	
Polychlorinated biphenyls (PCB)	Increased susceptibility for infection (duck)
	Reduced antibody responses (guinea pig, rabbit)
Hexabromobiphenyl	Reduced antibody responses (guinea pig)
Pesticides	
Dieldrin	Reduced antibody responses (rabbit)
Carbaryl	Reduction of thymus cortex (rabbit)
Carbofuran	Reduction of thymus cortex (rabbit)
Methylparathion	Reduction of thymus cortex (rabbit)

experiments for cosmetics, and the implementation of the Registration, Evaluation, Authorization and Restriction of Chemicals (REACH) legislation. However, such approaches are not yet available. The *in silico* approach using (quantitative) structure–activity relationships (SARs) may be useful as part of a weight of evidence approach for allergens, but can so far only be applied to a limited number of specific groups of chemicals. Techniques may become available in the near future that will allow for medium- to high-throughput screening of pharmaceuticals for direct immunotoxic activity. For the more complicated areas like autoimmunity the situation is quite different, although mechanistic knowledge combined with an "omics" approach and determination of individual patient sensitivity may well lead to alternative approaches in the future.

18.1.2
Detection of Immunotoxicity

In vivo toxicity studies for regulatory purposes generally are performed according to Organization for Economic Co-operation and Development (OECD) protocols, either as short term (up to 28 days) studies or longer subchronic (up to 90 days) and chronic (1–2 years) studies. Immunotoxicity as such is not specifically addressed in these studies. However, animal studies performed according to revised OECD guideline 407 of 1995 may result in the first indications for an immunotoxic effect [20]. Besides general parameters such as organ weight, which may indicate a target organ-specific toxicity, the histology of an organ is a prominent method for the detection of toxicity and, in addition to organ weight, may play an important role as a first indicator for the presence of direct immunotoxicity, that is, immunosuppression. In the context of regulatory guidelines, histopathology is routinely performed in the evaluation of adverse effects and determination of no-effect levels in toxicity studies performed in laboratory animals [5, 20, 21]. The differentiation between direct toxicity and toxicity due to an immune response to a compound or an enhanced response to altered self antigens is to a certain extent artificial. Some compounds can exert a direct toxic action on the immune system as well as specifically induce an adverse immune response, an example being heavy metals such as mercury, which shows immunosuppressive activity, hypersensitivity and autoimmunity [1, 22, 23]. Criteria for the evaluation of direct immunotoxicity were published by the World Health Organization(WHO) in an International Program on Chemical Safety(IPCS) monograph [5] and by the regulatory parties in the pharmaceutical field in the ICH S8 Guidance document [19].

For pharmaceuticals the considerations for evaluating the effect on the immune system can be several, one of them being that the drug may have pharmacological properties with direct effects on components of the immune system, for example, anti-inflammatory drugs [19], or may be directed at the immune system itself like cyclosporine-A to induce immunosuppression to prevent organ rejection in transplantation. This warrants a well validated test system in order to select the most promising compounds. However, immunosuppression as an unwanted side effect may seriously hamper the health of an already compromised (sick) patient, which is another cause for concern for pharmaceuticals requesting additional immunotoxicity studies [19]. In order to investigate the induction of direct immunotoxicity by pharmaceuticals it seems obvious to determine the functionality of the immune system by performing immune function assays to demonstrate a decrease in immune reactivity. However, as the interactions with the immune system may be multiple and of varying nature, a so-called tiered approach is the methodology to follow independently whether the investigations are performed in mice or rats [5]. In the first tier (TIER-1) general toxicity studies are performed which includes parameters for detection of toxic effects on the immune system (Table 18.2). The second tier (TIER-2) consists of more in-depth studies to the functionality of various parts

Table 18.2 *In vivo* and ex vivo biomarkers for detection of immune suppression.

In vivo biomarkers

Animal weight
Organ weight
Histopathology of lymphoid organs
Spleen and lymph node cellularity
Bone marrow (BM) cellularity and differentiation
Peripheral blood mononuclear cells (PBMC), cell number and differentiation
Serum immunoglobulins, total IgG, and subclasses IgM, IgG, IgE (Luminex assay, ELISA)
Serum cytokine levels (Luminex assay, ELISA)
Lymphocyte subset analysis: flow cytometry of PMBC and cells of lymphoid organs (spleen, lymph nodes)
Bronchial alveolar lavage fluid (BALF), cell number and differentiation
Bronchial alveolar lavage fluid (BALF), cytokine levels (Luminex assay, ELISA)
Lymphoid cell gene expression (RT-PCR, microarray)
Lymphoid cell protein expression (Luminex assay, antibody array, proteomics)

Ex vivo biomarkers

Cellular proliferation of lymphoid cells (3H-TdR or BrdU incorporation)
Mitogen responses of lymphoid cells (phytohaemagglutinine (PHA), concanavalin A (Con A) as T cell mitogens, lipopolysaccharide (LPS) as B cell mitigen)
Cytokine production by lymphoid cells (Luminex assay, ELISA)
Intracellular cytokine levels (Flow cytometry using fluorescent labels)
Lymphoid cell surface marker expression (Flow cytometry using fluorescent labels)
Lymphoid cell gene expression (RT-PCR, microarray)
Lymphoid cell protein expression (Luminex assay, antibody array, proteomics)

of the immune system [5, 18]. Examples are the routine toxicity studies that are performed like the 28 day toxicity study according to the enhanced OECD 407 protocol. In such studies both organ weight and the extended histopathology can indicate the induction of direct immunotoxicity [20].

18.1.3
Evaluation of the Immune System in Toxicity Studies

The evaluation of direct immunotoxicity in TIER-1 studies focuses on the effect of agents on the various lymphoid organs of the immune system being bone marrow, thymus, spleen, lymph nodes and blood [18]. The immune system is not static. It changes (diminishes) during aging, for example, the decrease in thymus weight, and also changes depending on the functional state, for example, antibody production after infection. This makes the evaluation of for instance organ weights difficult. Weight of spleen and thymus are indicators for systemic direct immunotoxicity [24, 25]. The minimum for routine evaluation of the lymphoid system consists of careful gross examination of the organs of the immune system such as thymus, spleen, draining lymph nodes, and bone marrow *in situ* [8]. In addition to organ weight the microscopic evaluation of these organs is a reliable indicator for local and systemic immunotoxicity [26, 27]. The evaluation of distant lymph nodes that is, distant from the site of entry of the compound, also may be indicative for the occurrence of systemic direct immunotoxicity. In oral toxicity studies (OECD 407) the Peyer's patches (PP) and mesenteric lymph nodes may be evaluated for local immunotoxic effects as these are the first lymphoid organs exposed to the chemical. Systemic immunotoxic effects are evaluated in distant lymph nodes (e.g., popliteal lymph node), spleen and thymus. For the description of possible alterations in immune organs it is necessary to evaluate the separate compartments and cell populations in the various lymphoid organs [3, 4, 8, 28]. Alterations in immune organs after exposure to immunotoxic xenobiotics need to be described and quantified [3, 29]. The methodology consists of a semi-quantitative evaluation of routinely prepared hematoxylin and eosin (HE) stained sections of lymphoid organs. Additionally immunohistochemical techniques detecting specific subsets of immune cells may be useful for the evaluation [4, 30–32]. Each compartment of the various lymphoid organs should be evaluated. Less obvious changes may best be quantified by morphometrical analyses which may be performed after indications observed by routine histology [33]. Part of the immune system can be evaluated by clinical pathology involving routine hematology and clinical chemistry. This may include bone marrow cytology to differentiate between cells of lymphoid, myeloid and erythroid lineage. The histopathology is considered as a first screen for the detection of immunosuppression [26].

The various organs of the immune system such as spleen, lymph nodes, thymus and bone marrow containing the cells involved in the various immune responses offer the possibility to harvest these cells and perform *in vitro* assays for evaluation of effects on the immune system. When part of an *in vivo* animal study this may indicate a direct toxic effect of pharmaceuticals, that is, immunosuppression (Table 18.2). So, it is feasible to obtain cell suspensions for further evaluation such as determination of cellular subsets of T and B leukocytes by fluorescent activated cell sorter analysis (FACS analysis), and determination of natural killer (NK) cell activity of the spleen cell population. An advantage of this approach is that it may lead to identification of a biomarker to be used in clinical studies. In addition, *in vitro* stimulation of spleen cells with mitogens activating specific subsets may indicate potential effects on the functionality of splenic cell populations. Concanavalin A (Con A) and phytohemagglutinin (PHA) activate T cells, while lipopolysaccharide (LPS) activates primarily B cell populations. Blood is collected for total white blood cell (WBC) determination and blood cell differential count. In addition, serum can be obtained for determination of serum immunoglobulins.

It was proposed that an immune function assay which would normally be performed as part of the additional immunotoxicity studies in TIER-2, such as the T cell dependent antibody response assay (TDAR-assay) should be included already in the TIER-1 investigations of a xenobiotic [34]. In 2000 the European Medicines Agency/Committee for Medicinal Products for Human Use (EMEA/CHMP) incorporated the TDAR assay (or the nonfunctional immunotyping of leucocytes) as a routine test in the Note for Guidance on Repeated Dose Toxicity for human pharmaceuticals [7, 21]. Germolec *et al.* [35, 36] evaluated past National Toxicology Program (NTP) studies performed in the mouse using ten chemicals and three positive controls. Thymus, spleen and mesenteric lymph node provided information to aid the quantitative risk assessment for immunotoxicity. The immune function analyses using these compounds indicated that two or three immune tests are sufficient to predict immunotoxic compounds in rodents. The tests with highest association with immunotoxicity were the splenic antibody plaque forming cell assay and cell surface markers analysis, although the latter is essentially not a functional assay [37]. Also the other validation studies concluded that for the functional assays, the most reliable and useful was the "antibody plaque-forming cell" technique, while others such as the mitogen proliferation assay and NK assay showed promise [24, 25].

In the additional functional (TIER-2) studies the immune system is more thoroughly investigated, while the animals are exposed to one or more doses of xenobiotics. Immune responses to several different types of antigens may be determined, including T cell-dependent antigens like tetanus toxoid and ovalbumin, sheep red blood cells (SRBC) [38–41] and T cell-independent antigens like LPS [38, 42]. For keyhole limpet hemocyanine (KLH) both antibody responses and delayed type hypersensitivity (DTH) reactions can be determined [43–45]. In addition several infectious models, including bacterial, viral and parasitic infections may be used to challenge the immune system [18, 46]. As survival and eradication of the infections is the primary function of the immune system, these models provide direct information on the functional status of the immune system. Direct immunotoxic compounds will induce immunosuppression and thus an increase in infection rate and/or severity of the infection. The number of infectious agents (bacteria, parasites, or viral colony-forming units), increased morbidity and mortality are indications for an immunotoxic effect. Also a reduction in specific antibody levels in animals treated with the test compound compared to nontreated controls indicates immunosuppression.

Besides infectious diseases, to some extent tumor formation is also linked to the functionality of the immune system. Macrophages, NK cells and cytotoxic T cells are able to kill tumor cells. Impairment of these cell types may result in enhanced tumor take and/or growth. Thus, tumor models may be used for evaluation of the immune system [43, 44, 47]. Although these infection and tumor models may be of value in demonstrating the functionality of the immune system, contradictory effects including enhancement and reduction in infectivity or tumor growth may occur [43, 44, 47, 48]. Such differences may be explained by the immunotoxic effect on certain subpopulations of cells, and the differences in resistance mechanisms for various types of infections and/or tumor models.

18.1.4
Testing for Induction of Allergy

Chemicals and pharmaceuticals may be tested for their capacity to induce skin sensitization [49]. The potency of a xenobiotic or pharmaceutical compound to induce delayed type hypersensitivity (DTH) or contact dermatitis (CD) may be tested in the so called local lymph node assay (LLNA) in which the induction of an immune response in lymph nodes is determined after local (skin) exposure [49–51]. The induction of cellular proliferation in draining lymph nodes is measured by determining the tritium-thymidine incorporation in the DNA as an indicator for immune stimulation. This assay has replaced almost entirely the previously used guinea pigs assays (Buehler assay, guinea pig maximization test) after extensive validation and evaluation [7, 52–54]. The cellular proliferation after treatment is compared to that of control (vehicle) treated animals, and a so-called stimulation index (treated vs control) is calculated. A compound inducing a stimulation index (SI) of 3 or higher is considered a sensitizer [50, 55]. The effective concentration inducing an SI of 3 (EC3) can be calculated and gives an indication of the potency of chemicals [56, 57]. Based on the EC3 value a ranking of relatively strong (EC3 below 0.1% concentration of the chemical) and relatively weak (EC3 above 10% concentration of the chemical) can be determined in order to select compounds which may have a weak sensitizing potency [58, 59].

For the detection of respiratory sensitizers which generally but not exclusively act via IgE mediated responses after secondary challenge no predicting assay is available yet and compounds are designated respiratory sensitizers based on human data [60]. Only a limited number of chemicals act as respiratory sensitizers while there is an abundant amount of skin sensitizers inducing contact dermatitis. However, the harm induced by respiratory sensitizers can be most serious as it may ultimately result in anaphylactic shock and death, while for skin sensitizers the resulting contact dermatitis is generally manageable.

18.1.5
Testing for Induction of Autoimmunity

18.1.5.1 Introduction
Preclinical testing for autoimmunogenic potential of chemicals is extremely difficult. This is because many inherent as well as environmental (other than the suspected chemical) factors co-determine whether a chemical induces an autoimmune disease and moreover, autoimmune phenomena develop against the background of normally existing autoimmunity [61]. Among the inherent factors genetic polymorphisms like major histocompatibility complex (MHC) haplotype and metabolic traits are important, while microbial insults are examples of environmental factors that predispose for development of clinical autoimmune(-like) diseases, including drug allergy responses. On top of that, clinical phenomena often resolve when exposure to the chemical is stopped on time [62–64].

Many chemicals (including pharmaceuticals but also environmental and occupational chemicals) are known to stimulate the immune system in a way that autoimmune diseases occur [61]. However, because of its multifactorial nature, the occurrence of autoimmune-like (including drug allergic) diseases is rare if considered on a compound-by-compound base. But, in some cases (e.g., in case of HIV or Herpes virus-infected individuals), adverse reactions occur at a higher rate [65, 66].

18.1.5.2 Assays for Testing the Induction of Autoimmunity
Because of the idiosyncratic nature of chemical induced autoimmunity (including drug allergy) it is impossible to predict this phenomenon in routine toxicity studies

that use outbred strains of animals, mostly rats. One particular rat strain, the Brown Norway (BN) rat, has been successfully used to detect autoimmunogenic potential of some compounds (metals like $HgCl_2$, $AuCl_2$, D-penicillamine, nevirapine) [67–70] but again other compounds (captopril, felbamate) [71, 72] were not effective in this strain. Importantly, under normal supposedly healthy conditions BN rats display a high Th2 responsiveness and therefore BN rats have also been used as sensitive strain in food allergy studies [73]. Also in case of mice certain particular strains are more susceptible than others for the development of autoimmune phenomena [74–77]. In view of this it is of particular interest that the antiarrhytmatic drug procainamide, involving both hepatic and extrahepatic bioactivation, is more effective in stimulating the formation antiDNA antibodies in slow acetylating A/J mice than in fast-acetylating C57BL/6 mice [78].

Unresponsiveness to autoimmunity by chemicals may be circumvented by co-exposure to microbial components. For instance, DBA mice do normally not develop autoimmune phenomena as result of HgCl2 exposure, but when co-exposed to $HgCl_2$ and LPS profound increases of autoimmune parameters (e.g., antinucleolar antibodies, anti-thyroglobulin, anti-collagen, glomerulonephritis) are observed [79]. Apparently, innate immune activation (in the case of LPS via TLR4) may predispose for development of an autoimmune disease. Also BN rats become more sensitive to D-penicillamine-induced autoimmune disease when co-exposed to a TLR ligand, polyinosinic:polycytosinic acid (polyI:C) [80].

Some studies have demonstrated that chemicals can increase autoimmune disease in autoimmune-prone mice (e.g., NZB mice) [70, 81, 82]. Together, these and other examples demonstrate that indeed chemical-induced autoimmunity can be induced in animals. However, these examples also show that a chemical may require very specific circumstances to induce autoimmune phenomena. In other words, it may be an illusion that one single animal model will be found or developed that will cover all different chemical-related autoimmune diseases.

18.1.5.3 Alternative Approach for Evaluation of Autoimmunity Potential of Chemicals

To predict a chemical's capacity to cause autoimmune disease an alternative approach to animal testing is to assess whether the chemical modulates certain key processes considered crucial for induction of disease. In this way, a stepwise translational strategy could be designed. For this knowledge on basic mechanisms is needed. Autoimmune phenomena as well as allergy depend on the activation of specific immune responses and thus largely on the adaptive arm of the immune system. But nowadays it is well acknowledged that the adaptive and innate immune system are very much entangled: the innate immune system is needed for optimum activation of the adaptive immune system, and the innate immune system (that supplies the effector arm of the immune system) operates much better in combination with adaptive immunity, that is, with the help of specific T cells.

Two processes are suggested to be of importance in the induction of T cell sensitization by chemicals: (i) the formation of neoantigens (i.e., cryptic epitopes or hapten-carrier conjugates); (ii) the stimulation of innate immune processes (i.e., adjuvant activity or induction of danger signals; reviewed by Uetrecht [64]). The formation of neoantigens, in particular hapten-carrier complexes, often depends on metabolism as to make compounds reactive. Once reactive, chemicals may not only form neoantigens but also cause cell stress and death (apoptosis or necrosis). Cellular stress and cellular remnants may stimulate all kinds of cells, including antigen presenting dendritic cells, for instance via any of the different innate pattern recognition receptors (e.g., Toll-like receptors, scavenger receptors). The dendritic cells may display costimulatory signals that function as adjuvant signals for hapten-specific T cells.

Based on the knowledge of the processes of T cell sensitization by chemicals and the importance of T cells in induction of autoimmune diseases a number of key indicators of autoimmunogenic compounds can be defined. These include the possibility to be subject of metabolic conversion (either intra- or extra-hepatically), the capacity to activate dendritic cells, to induce cytokine production (in any cell type), or the potency to cause cell stress or cell death. Most of these processes can be studied *in vitro*, but none of the available methods have been tested for this purpose and often chemicals may behave completely different *in vitro* than *in vivo*. However, much can be learned from initiatives to design alternative methods for contact allergens, as many of these basic processes that lead to T cell sensitization are similar for allergenic and autoimmunogenic chemicals.

The translation from *in vitro* to disease models can be made via simple straightforward *in vivo* methods such as the popliteal lymph node assay (PLNA) [83]. By using this method the T cell sensitizing capacity of compounds can be easily assessed by detecting T cell activation (proliferation, cytokine production) in response to footpad injection of the compound. Variations of the PLNA include the use of reporter antigens (RA-PLNA) to determine the mechanism of T cell activation more specifically [84, 85]. The mechanism of lymph node activation in the PLNA, includes all processes thought to be of importance in T cell sensitization by chemicals, including co-stimulation [86], neo-antigen formation and hapten-carrier formation [87].

Outcomes of *in vitro* methods or simple *in vivo* methods such as the PLNA, only indicate whether a compound can sensitize the immune system. They do not predict whether a compound can induce an autoimmune disease. For that disease models are warranted. However, most disease models, as mentioned, will often require predisposed animal strains such as systemic lupus erythematosus (SLE)-prone mice [81, 82]. Often models using autoimmune-prone mice or rats (including the BN rat) are considered too sensitive and are for that reason undesired by various stakeholders (i.e., pharmaceutical industries, regulatory agencies).

However, human beings that develop an autoimmune disease as result of chemical exposure, may be prone to get an autoimmune disease as well. Thus characterizing patients genetically (by assessing single nuclear polymorphisms or human leukocyte antigen (HLA)-haplotype) may provide human risk indicators. So by combining simple *in vitro* and *in vivo* methods (PLNA), disease models and information of patients one might eventually come to a predictive translational model to assess hazard and risk of chemicals to induce autoimmune disease or drug allergy (Table 18.3). All steps in a strategic approach have their advantages and disadvantages, but they may all help to at least get a clue as to whether a compound may, under

Table 18.3 Overview of options to detect risk of compounds with regard to induction of autoimmune derangements. *In vitro* and various *in vivo* options may be used in sequential preclinical strategies.

In vitro options	*In vivo* options	
Activation of innate or acquired immunity Chemical interactions with biological systems or biomolecules	**T cell sensitization**	**Clinical outcomes/relevant route of exposure models**
Metabolism (e.g., CYPs, COX, Myeloperoxidase) *Hapten-Carrier formation* (e.g., binding with proteins or aminoacids)	*PLNA* (s.c. injection, indication of possibility to induce systemic allergy) *(read-out: immunological parameters)*	*Susceptible animals:* mouse (e.g., NZB, NOD) or rat (BN, Lewis) strains. *Parameters: for example, autoimmune parameters, histopathology*
Direct activation of T cells (e.g., derived from patients) *Cell damage* (reactive oxygen species, apoptosis, necrosis)	*LLNA* (topical application, indication of hapten-protein conjugation)	*Oral exposure studies* (using bystander or reporter antigens to read out immunosensitization)
Cell activation (e.g., dendritic cells, macrophages, neutrophils)		
Cytokine production (e.g., TNF-α by macrophages)		
Complement activation or inhibition		

particular conditions (such as virus infection) elicit an autoimmune-like disease or drug allergy. Important in this specific area of immunotoxicology is to realize that a chemical is not always a risk for all individuals, that is, the problem might not be the chemical, but the patient.

18.1.6
Structures Associated with Immunotoxicity

Estrogen is one of the compounds known to modulate immune responses. Estrogenic immunosuppression was found to be due to a direct interaction with lymphoid target cells as well as via non lymphoid tissue being the thymic epithelium with its function for lymphoid maturation and selection [88].

For halogenated aromatic hydrocarbons like polychlorinated biphenyls (PCBs), polychlorinated dibenzofurans (PCDFs), and polychlorinated dibenzo-p-dioxins (PCDDs) the binding to the aryl hydrocarbon (Ah) receptor regulates their toxicity [89]. The Ah receptor controls the induction of one of the cytochrome P450 enzymes in the liver. Toxic responses such as thymic atrophy, weight loss, immunotoxicity and acute lethality are associated with the relative affinity of PCBs, PCDFs and PCDDs for the Ah receptor [89]. The quantitative structure–activity relationship (QSAR) models predicting the affinity of the halogenated aromatic hydrocarbons with the Ah receptor describe the electron acceptor capability as well as the hydrophobicity and polarizability of the chemicals [89].

In a recent study on metal compounds, including the platinum group elements titanium and arsenic, the immunotoxicity was suggested to be dependent on speciation of the metals [90].

Especially for sensitization, structural alerts may be important for *in silico* evaluation (see Section 18.2.1).

18.1.7
Immunostimulation by Components of the Immune Systems Used as Therapeutics

The therapeutic use of various components of the immune system itself may result in a variety of adverse effects [91]. This group of therapeutics includes antibodies used as therapeutics agents in diseases such as rheumatoid arthritis, Crohn's disease and several types of cancer and as an immunosuppressant in transplant patients. A specific issue of this new class of therapeutics is the potential induction of a so-called cytokine release syndrome, first observed after administration with OKT3, but more recently and more vigorously with TGN1412. In the 1980s the mouse monoclonal antibodies OKT3 induced adverse events, such as fever and so on. These symptoms appeared to be associated with a strong T cell activation and release of cytokines [92]. The syndrome did not exist after a second injection of the same monoclonal antibody, but the cytokine induced vascular leakage induced by the first injection had a rather severe character. More reports are in literature describing similar phenomena with certain but not all monoclonals [93]. Most recently the "Tegenero case" was reported in which six healthy volunteers became seriously ill and needed intensive care after treatment with TGN1412 [94]. Based on measurements of cytokines in the blood of these volunteers the situation in this case was also designated a cytokine release syndrome [94, 95]. An *in vivo* model was described in mice in which high doses of glucocorticoids prevented the massive cytokine release [96, 97].

Also when the cytokine interleukin 2 (IL-2) was used for cancer treatment, serious adverse effects were noted resulting in the so-called "vascular leak syndrome" (VLS) [98, 99]. VLS is a life-threatening toxicity marked by vasopermeability with hypotension induced during high dose IL-2 treatment of cancer patients [100]. VLS is caused by endothelial activation and can be induced in lungs and liver of mice by IL2 administration [99]. The mechanism of IL-2-induced VLS is still poorly understood and at present there is no specific therapy for VLS. For the investigation of these specific therapeutic applications *in vitro* and *in vivo* screens are under discussion to predict this type of effects.

18.2
Non-Animal Approaches for the Determination of Immunotoxicity

18.2.1
In Silico Approaches

One of the possible methods for an early screening of chemical specific effects (either wanted or unwanted side effects) is by using *in silico* techniques for the evaluation of ADME and Tox analysis by evaluation of structure activity relationships [101]. Both free and commercial software is available be it with certain limitations. The *in silico* evaluations are especially important as an alternative to the animal models that are used to assess sensitizing capacity. Although several *in silico* (QSAR) systems are available, such as DEREK, TOPKAT and TOPS-MODE, none of these three systems performed sufficiently well to act as a stand alone tool to predict sensitizing properties [102]. The major importance of mechanistic chemistry for sensitization strongly suggests that mechanistic applicability domains be used [103–105]. Assignment to such a domain is a critical first step for understanding how chemical properties influence the potency of sensitizers [106]. Sofar, these *in silico* systems for the evaluation of sensitizing capacity of chemicals are only applicable to a limited domain within certain chemical families [107].

18.2.2
In Vitro Approaches to Test Various Aspects of Immunotoxicity

18.2.2.1 Introduction
The immune system is complex, as it is not confined to one or several organs, but rather spread throughout the body. In addition, it involves delicate interactions between different cell types that vary not only between different locations but also in space and time after a toxic or pathologic insult. The various types of immunotoxicity differ considerably in the complexity of the mechanisms they affect. Therefore, also the phase of development of *in vitro* testing differs considerably between the various types of immunotoxicity.

Immunosuppressive activity largely affects thymocytes and (im)mature T-cells and thus lymphocyte cultures are a rather straightforward model to assess immunosuppressive activity. Thymocyte cultures are also used, but may be less amenable to routine *in vitro* testing (Table 18.4).

Although chemical sensitization is a more complex process than immunosuppression, by far most of the efforts on developing *in vitro* assays are in this field. An important reason for this is that from the various fields of immunotoxicity, most of the animals are used for sensitization testing. In fact the number of animals required for sensitization is second only after developmental toxicity testing.

Table 18.4 *In vitro* biomarkers for detection of immunotoxicity.

Parameter	Methodology
Viability/membrane damage	Trypan blue dye exclusion, Lactate Dehydrogenase (LDH) release
Viability/metabolic activity	Alamar blue assay, Tetrazole reduction (MTT, WST assay)
Cell proliferation	Tritium-thymidine (3H-TdR) incorporation, bromodeoxyuridine (BrdU) incorporation
Cytokine production	Enzyme-Linked Immuno Sorbant Assay (ELISA), Luminex assay using multi-analyte profiling beads
Intracellular cytokine levels	Flow cytometry using fluorescent lables
Surface marker expression	Flow cytometry using fluorescent labels
Gene expression	Real-time polymerase chain reaction (RT-PCR), microarray
Protein expression	Luminex assay, antibody array, proteomics
Signal transduction	Gel shift, ELISA

While chemical sensitization involves undesired exposure of chemicals via the skin and airways, another type of allergic response is drug hypersensitivity that involves an allergic response after oral exposure. In case of chemical sensitization the chemical itself is subject of safety assessment, and *in vitro* models are designed to identify its sensitizing capacity (Table 18.5). For drug hypersensitivity, however, not the drug itself but the individual response of certain patients (often a small minority) to the drug is subject of concern. An important cause for these inter-individual differences is the patients' genetic makeup, predominantly polymorphisms in genes involved in metabolism and the immune response (including but not confined to

Table 18.5 *In vitro* assays.

In vitro tests for immune suppression

Stimulation of lymphoid cells in the presence of chemicals/pharmaceuticals
Cytotoxicity by measuring membrane damage or metabolic activity (Table 18.2)
Cellular proliferation of lymphoid cells (3H-TdR or BrdU incorporation)
Mitogen responses of lymphoid cells (Phytohaemagglutinine (PHA), Concanavalin A (Con A) as T cell mitogens, Lipopolysaccharide (LPS) as B cell mitogen)
Cytokine production by lymphoid cells (Luminex assay, ELISA)
Intracellular cytokine levels (Flow cytometry using fluorescent labels)
Lymphoid cell surface marker expression (Flow cytometry using fluorescent labels)
Lymphoid cell gene expression (RT-PCR, microarray)
Lymphoid cell protein expression (Luminex assay, antibody array, proteomics)

In vitro test for allergy

Protein or peptide binding
Cytokine production by keratinocytes
Gene expression of keratinocytes
Cellular maturation of dendritic cells
Mast cell degranulation

HLA). Hence, *in vitro* assays for drug hypersensitivity testing are limited and genotyping of patients prior to drug administration seems to be the way forward. It has to be noted that, when drugs are topically applied (ointments), the assays developed for chemical sensitization testing apply.

For the other types of immunotoxicity (immunoenhancement, autoimmunity, developmental immunotoxicity) little or no efforts have been made regarding *in vitro* testing. These processes are not only complex involving delicately balanced interactions encompassing many tissues, they are often ill understood, and cell systems that may mimic some of the processes involved are difficult to devise. Especially the possible adverse effects of components of the immune system itself, such as (monoclonal) antibodies and cytokines, pose a real challenge in terms of alternative testing. For monoclonal antibodies interacting with the T cell receptor (OKT-3) *in vitro* T-cell activation was investigated to predict the possibility of induction cytokine release syndrome [108]. Whether the Tegenero case (see Section 18.1.7) can be positively detected in these testing systems will probably remain an unanswered question.

18.2.2.2 Immunosuppression

In 2003 a workshop hosted by ECVAM was held in order to review the state-of-the-art in the field of *in vitro* immunotoxicology [109]. Based on its recommendations, an ECVAM-sponsored project was undertaken in which several assays to measure immunosuppression *in vitro* were compared [110]. A follow-up project comprised an inter-laboratory evaluation of a selected combination of cells, stimuli and parameters. This line of research has shown that it is indeed possible to detect immunosuppressive activity *in vitro* (Tables 18.4 and 18.5). Human PBMC, mouse and rat splenocytes were exposed to a dose range of immunosuppressive drugs and chemicals while being stimulated. Cytotoxicity was measured by release of lactate dehydrogenase and was absent at the chemical concentrations tested. Rodent T and B cells were stimulated using concanavalin A and lipopolysaccharide, respectively, while human T cells were stimulated by a combination of antibodies, antiCD3 (stimulation, signal 1) and antiCD28 (co-stimulation, signal 2). Cell proliferation, measured as ^{3}H-thymidine-uptake, and IFN-γ and TNF-α production were taken as endpoints. Also the immunosuppressive activity of cyclophosphamide and benzo(a)pyrene, compounds that require metabolism before exerting this activity could be detected. Importantly, this enables using human PBMC overcoming the drawback of interspecies extrapolation. Although the use of human PBMC introduces inter-donor variability, it is also felt that incorporating this variability significantly improves risk assessment.

A second approach, with a more distant time horizon, is the use of gene profiling in the context of *in vitro* immunosuppression, as exemplified by Baken *et al.* [111] for the immunosuppressive compound bis(tri-*n*-butyltin)oxide. Gene profiling allows understanding the underlying mechanism at the level of affected pathways. In addition, testing a range of compounds should result in more sensitive and robust markers for immunosuppression, compared to the ones currently in use. A further extension of this line of research is to combine, at the genomic level, rodent *in vivo* data with rodent and human *in vitro* data to predict effects in humans (parallelogram approach).

This may be complemented with *ex vivo* gene profiling of PBMC from patients on immunosuppressive drugs. Finally, instead of using fresh human PBMC and rodent splenocytes, cell lines such as the human Jurkat T-cell line and the mouse EL4 thymoma cell line can be used.

18.2.2.3 Chemical Sensitization

Introduction The process of chemical sensitization encompasses various steps. These steps, discussed below, were first put into the perspective of *in vitro* sensitization testing by Jowsey *et al.* [112]. The first four steps (determination of bioavailability/ skin penetration, haptenization, keratinocyte response, dendritic cell maturation) are amenable for *in vitro* testing. Since each assay covering a specific step is highly different from the other ones (biochemical, cell culture) they cannot be put into a single assay. Moreover, the relative contribution of each of these steps (and the predictivity of each of these assays) to the overall sensitization process is still unclear. To assess these relative contributions, chemical databases that relate the outcome of each assay to the overall sensitization potential are required (e.g., using LLNA data). Not only will this knowledge improve hazard identification and risk assessment [113], it can prioritize the key step(s) in the process of developing *in vitro* alternatives to sensitization testing. In fact, it was suggested by Roberts and Aptula [114] that haptenization is the key event in the whole of the sensitization process implicating that it is this step that needs to be modeled and should be the focus of research.

In the context of skin sensitization bioavailability can be seen as the capacity of the compound to reach the viable epidermis, where it interacts with keratinocytes and Langerhans cells. This capacity is dependent on its molecular weight and solubility in polar and apolar solvents [115]. Importantly, potency prediction solely on the basis of cell culture models (steps 3 and 4) does not account for skin penetration rate and may thus wrongly predict potency *in vivo*. Possible *in vitro* approaches to detect allergic capacity of chemicals/pharmaceuticals are presented in Table 18.5.

Protein Binding Small molecular weight chemicals are not recognized by the immune system as such. In order to be recognized they have to bind to proteins (a process called hapten formation or haptenization) and it is (part of) the peptide-hapten complex that is recognized. Haptenization can be measured using a peptide reactivity assay [116]. In this assay, certain peptides as well as glutathione (or only glutathione) [117] are incubated with haptens, and hapten formation is measured. The majority of haptens are electrophilic and therefore react strongly with nucleophiles, such as glutathione or the amino acids cysteine and lysine. On some occasions, haptens need to be metabolized first in order to bind to amino acids, in which case they are called prohaptens. The peptide reactivity assay holds promise in the assessment of sensitizing capacity *in vitro*, since evaluation of 82 chemicals resulted in an accuracy of prediction compared to current *in vivo* methods of 89% [118].

***In Vitro* Cell Culture** Keratinocytes (KC) comprise some 95% of the cells in the skin and are the first cells that come into contact with the allergen. Moreover, KC respond to allergen exposure by producing a set of cytokines (and possibly cell surface proteins) and in this way have the capacity to influence the dendritic cell (DC) response (reviewed by Vandebriel et al. [119]). Therefore, KC should make a suitable assay for *in vitro* sensitization testing. We have shown that KC can indeed be used to detect sensitizers and, moreover, even allow potency determination [120]. We are currently in the process of improving this assay by using gene profiling (Baken et al., unpublished observations). A future extension will be the use of reconstructed skin models (RSM). In these models KC spontaneously form the four skin layers.

Respiratory sensitizers have the lung as target organ and thus *in vitro* models should comprise lung epithelial cells, alveolar macrophages and DC (reviewed by Roggen et al. [121]). A model to identify respiratory sensitizers using these cell types is currently lacking.

Langerhans cell maturation and migration is a key step in the skin immune response to low molecular weight allergens and many investigators have therefore used these cells in an assay to detecting sensitizers. Since Langerhans cells are not readily available in sufficient numbers, DC are used (mostly of human and sometimes of mouse origin). Many groups have indeed shown that sensitizer exposure resulted in DC maturation (reviewed in [122, 123]). Human DC are cultured either from CD34 + cord blood cells (CD34 + DC) or from CD14 + peripheral monocytes (moDC). After exposure to sensitizers (and nonsensitizing controls, including irritants) maturation is analyzed, generally by expression of surface markers (e.g., CD40, CD80, CD83, CD86, HLA-DR) and by production of cytokines (e.g., IL-6, IL-8, IL-12p40, TNF-α). Apparently, CD34 + DC show less inter-donor variability but are also less sensitive than moDC [124].

Although DC maturation can be used to detect sensitizing capacity, major concerns remain on this assay: (i) the limited reproducibility within and between laboratories due to inter-donor variability and variations in cell isolation and culture techniques; (ii) the lack of sensitivity and dynamic range [122]. To circumvent inter-donor variability cell lines such as THP-1, U937, KG-1 and MUTZ-3 have been used. In fact, benzocaine (a weak sensitizer, leading to variable results in the LLNA) can be identified using MUTZ-3 [125].

Several ways to improve on the current DC maturation assays are being investigated. First, DC have been subjected to gene profiling resulting in potential biomarkers of exposure [126, 127]. Second, signal transduction is another parameter that is changed upon sensitizer exposure [128, 129]. Third, using RSM in which CD34 + DC are included topical application of sensitizers induced IL-1β and CD86 mRNA expression, which are both markers of maturating DC [130].

No *in vitro* assays that are based on proliferation of naïve lymphocytes upon sensitizer exposure have been developed as yet. Using haptenized DC, proliferation can be induced but only for strong sensitizers such as trinitrophenol and fluorescein iso-thiocyanate, or with para-phenylenediamine in only a limited proportion of the experiments.

18.2.2.4 Conclusions

Many attempts are underway to devise *in vitro* assays for immunotoxicity testing. The first results will likely comprise assays with limited applicability that may still be very useful in the context of prescreening (e.g., for pharmaceutical companies) and in situations where there is limited information. For immunosuppression testing prevalidation studies are at the brink of being started. For sensitization testing several routes (biochemical, cell culture, *in silico*) are being pursued. For testing other types of immunotoxicity, *in vitro* alternatives are not foreseen within the next decade.

Taken together, it is unclear which non-animal assay(s) will be the one(s) of choice. A likely order to perform non-animal tests is the order desk top analysis to laboratory work, taking into account time and cost, being QSAR models, peptide reactivity assays and cell culture assays. As indicated before we do not know which (combination) of these models is predicting *in vivo* sensitization testing best. In case of limited information, risk assessors should know which combinations of limited information (also including physico-chemical and human data) are sufficient for risk assessment. Initiatives such as the EU OSIRIS project (http://www.osiris-reach.eu) are underway to provide a weight-of-evidence approach to meet this goal.

18.2.3
Toxicogenomics

18.2.3.1 Introduction

Toxicogenomics studies the adverse effects of xenobiotics by means of gene expression profiling. Microarray analysis, which allows simultaneous measurement of the activity of thousands of genes in a given sample, is nowadays a widely applied technique to obtain gene expression profiles. In short, total RNA is isolated from control and compound-exposed samples, labeled with fluorescent dyes and hybridized onto microarray slides comprising multiple copies of DNA segments representing specific genes. Scanning the slides yields intensity values for all genes evaluated, from which (after processing and statistics) a set of differentially expressed genes can be derived. Clustering of genes showing similar expression patterns and pathway analysis are then applied to evaluate effects of toxicant exposure [131]. Since the function of many gene products is known and the expression patterns presumably correlate with the amount of active product produced, gene expression profiling provides insight into the mechanisms of action of xenobiotics.

18.2.3.2 Immunotoxicogenomics

Examples of immunotoxicogenomic studies that have appeared in the literature (reviewed by Baken *et al.* [132] and Burns-Naas *et al.* [133]) show that microarray analysis is able to detect known and novel effects of a wide range of immunomodulating agents, but they also indicate several pitfalls. The impact of duration of exposure and dose level on the outcome of microarray analysis was for instance illustrated by a series of experiments on the immunosuppressive model compound bis(tri-*n*-butyl)tinoxide (TBTO). Induction of thymocyte apoptosis by TBTO appeared to precede inhibition of cell proliferation, since the former was found after short exposure times *in vitro*, whereas the latter was the main finding at later time points during *in vitro* and *in vivo* studies [111]. Administration of a high dose of TBTO to mice resulted in significant regulation of gene expression in the thymus, whereas absence of overt gene expression changes was found in rat thymus after exposure to a somewhat lower dose, even though immunotoxic effects were observed as indicated by the involution of this organ [134].

The use of both low and high doses in a study on hexachlorobenzene (HCB) by Ezendam *et al.* [135] revealed the complexity of cells and mediators that participate in the response to this compound. Such approaches may provide valuable insight into gene expression changes in the presence and absence of pathological or cellular effects.

18.2.3.3 Interpretation of Results

Correct interpretation of gene expression profiles in terms of functional effects is often challenging in toxicogenomics. Changes in expression of genes mediating a certain process do not always all point to the same direction, for example, and not all genes taking part in a certain pathway will necessarily be regulated. Furthermore, induction of an immune response may be required for immunomodulators to exert their effects, which may therefore be more easily detected after stimulation by antigens or mitogens. The interpretation of *in vivo* microarray results may also be complicated by the effect of changes in cell populations on gene expression profiles. When assessing effects in spleen, influx of cells via the blood (possibly as a result of xenobiotic exposure) may cause altered abundance of certain mRNAs and thus altered gene expression profiles, as was for instance seen after exposure to a high dose of HCB [135]. Furthermore, effects of xenobiotics may differ per cell type, and when effects of several xenobiotics are compared in the same organ, different compounds may affect different cell types.

For a correct interpretation of genomic results anchoring of gene expression profiles to pathological and functional endpoints is important [132, 136]. It is equally important to establish correlation of absence of changes in gene expression with functional effects, since effects may only be observable in specific experimental settings or at other levels than the transcriptome, such as posttranscriptional or posttranslational. Results of *in vitro* approaches should most ideally be confirmed with *in vivo* effects, since functional differences may exist between cells in culture or *in vivo*, and *in vitro* designs lack interaction of various different cell types [131].

18.2.3.4 Toxicogenomics for Prediction of Effects

In addition to elucidating mechanisms of action, gene expression profiling might aid in characterizing the classes of compounds and identifying biomarkers for the prediction of specific toxic effects [137–139]. This approach is based on the assumption that exposures leading to the same endpoint will share changes in gene expression and is supported by several proof of principle studies with well characterized chemicals [140–143]. Pharmaceutical and biotechnical industries therefore apply predictive toxicogenomics to identify small sets of biomarkers that may be sufficient to indicate early toxic effects of their products and can be used for high-throughput screening [144, 145].

In order to identify biomarkers for immunotoxicity, overlapping transcriptional effects of model compounds were studied by Baken et al. [146]. Microarray analysis was performed in mouse spleens after exposure to TBTO, cyclosporin A (CsA), benzo[a]pyrene (B[a]P), and acetaminophen (APAP). The process that was most significantly affected by all toxicants was cell division, and it was concluded that the immunosuppressive properties of the model compounds appeared to be mediated by cell cycle arrest. Since highly proliferating immune cells will be particularly sensitive to effects on cell division, evaluation of cell proliferation thus remains a valuable tool to assess immunosuppression. Patterson and Germolec [147] examined gene expression changes induced by the prototype immunosuppressive agents 2,3,7,8-tetrachlorodibenzo-p-dioxin (TCDD), cyclophosphamide, diethylstilbestrol (DES) and dexamethason in mouse thymus and spleen. Preliminary data showed that, although most transcriptional effects were compound-specific, some genes were regulated by all compounds. These genes were mainly involved in apoptosis, immune cell activation, antigen presentation and processing and again cell proliferation. Although the specificity and predictivity of inhibition of cell division for immunotoxicity in general should be confirmed by testing a larger range of compounds, both studies show that microarray analysis offers opportunities to discover gene expression changes that may be indicative of immunosuppression.

18.2.3.5 Target Organs and Cells for Immunotoxicity

Several of the studies described above have shown that the spleen is a suitable organ for detection of immunosuppression by gene expression profiling. This is a promising finding with respect to development of screening assays since effects in this organ are presumably reflected in peripheral lymphocytes that can easily be obtained from human blood. Inter-species comparison may thereby become superfluous. For the screening of chemicals for sensitizing properties, dendritic cells, which play an important role in the development of an immune response towards allergens, can be routinely obtained (by culture) from human peripheral blood. Transcript changes identified by microarray analyses in dendritic cells (either derived from human precursor cells or dendritic cell-like cell lines) such as performed by Gildea et al. [126] and the group of Schoeters [127] may very well serve as new markers for allergenicity. The sensitivity, specificity, and robustness demonstrated in these and other studies show that *in vitro* methods relying on microarray analysis have the potential to uncover sensitizing effects of compounds [132, 148].

18.2.3.6 Conclusions

Although toxicogenomics may not yet be able to replace the current methods for assessment of immunotoxicity, the examples described above show that it offers opportunities for development of *in vitro* screening assays for immunotoxicity by identifying molecular markers that may already be detected after relatively short exposure periods. This merit of toxicogenomics is also recognized within drug discovery research [149]. Current efforts to analyze a wider range of immunotoxic compounds and cell types are expected to yield specific biomarkers. The implementation of advanced techniques such as RNA silencing and proteomics within this research area will improve the interpretation and functional validation of effects detected at the gene expression level. Immunotoxicogenomics is thus a valuable addition to methods available for hazard identification of existing and novel compounds.

18.3
Summary

In view of the complexity of the immune system the safety evaluation of possible harmful effects of xenobiotics, including pharmaceuticals, is primarily based on various *in vivo* assays. Special attention is needed for those therapeutics that are targeted at the immune system or are essentially components of the immune system itself. For preclinical screening, however, several possible alternatives are available. For immunosuppression *in vitro* assays are available that may give a first indication for an adverse effect on the various cells of the immune system. Similarly screening assays for induction of allergic potential are under development. These latter include QSAR evaluation, protein binding and the cellular responses of both keratinocytes and dendritic cells after *in vitro* exposure. For evaluation of possible induction or promotion of autoimmunity a single assay is not available and a translational approach is preferable. For autoimmunity even patient evaluation may be more relevant than evaluation of the pharmaceutical itself. As for other areas of toxicological evaluation also in immunotoxicity genomics may be applied.

The limitation of all these approaches is that they are not (yet) validated. However, they can be a useful tool for preclinical screening. The results of this screening may then be used for further development of specific pharmaceuticals and/or point at the immune system as an area needing specific attention in the safety evaluation to be performed before marketing a product.

References

1 Lawrence, D., Mudzinski, S., Rudofsky, U. and Warner, A. (1987) Mechanisms of metal induced immunotoxicity, in *Immunotoxicology* (eds A. Berlin, J. Dean, M.H. Draper and F. Spreafico), Martinus Nijhoff, Dordrecht, The Netherlands, pp. 293–307.
2 Luster, M.I., Munson, A.E., Thomas, P.T., Holsapple, M.P., Fenters, J.D., White, K.L. Jr, Lauer, L.D., Germolec, D.R., Rosenthal, G.J. and Dean, J.H. (1988) Development of a testing battery to assess chemical induced immunotoxicity: National toxicology program's guidelines for immunotoxicity evaluation in mice. *Fundamental and Applied Toxicology*, **10**, 2–19.
3 Schuurman, H.-J., Kuper, C.F. and Vos, J.G. (1994) Histopathology of the immune system as a tool to assess immunotoxicity. *Toxicology*, **86**, 187–212.
4 Kuper, C.F., Schuurman, H.-J. and Vos, J.G. (1995) Pathology in immunotoxicology, in *Methods in Immuntoxicology*, Vol. 1 (eds G.R. Burleson, J.H. Dean and A.E. Munson), Wiley-Liss, New York, USA, pp. 397–436.
5 WHO (1996) International Programme on Chemical Safety, Principles and methods for assessing direct

immunotoxicity associated with exposure to chemicals, *Environmental Health Criteria 180*, WHO, Geneva, Zwitserland.
6 Hinton, D.M. (2000) US FDA "Redbook II" immunotoxicity testing guidelines and research in immunotoxicity evaluations of food chemicals and new food proteins. *Toxicologic Pathology*, 28, 467–478.
7 Putman, E., Van Der Laan, J.W. and Van Loveren, H. (2003) Assessing immunotoxicity: guidelines. *Fundamental & Clinical Pharmacology*, 17, 615–626.
8 Haley, P., Perry, R., Ennulat, D., Frame, S., Johnson, C., Lapointe, J.-M., Nyska, A., Snyder, P.W., Walker, D. and Walter, G. (2005) STP position paper: best practice guideline for the routine pathology evaluation of the immune system. *Toxicologic Pathology*, 33, 404–407.
9 Kaplan, J.E., Hanson, D., Dworkin, M.S., Frederick, T., Bertolli, J., Lindegren, M.L., Holmberg, S. and Jones, J.L. (2000) Epidemiology of human immunodeficiency virus-associated opportunistic infections in the United States in the era of highly active antiretroviral therapy. *Clinical Infectious Diseases*, 30, S5–S14.
10 Nagappan, V. and Kazanjian, P. (2005) Bacterial infections in adult HIV-infected patients. *HIV Clinical Trials*, 6, 213–228.
11 Bower, M., Palmieri, C. and Dhillon, T. (2006) AIDS related malignancies: changing epidemiology and the impact of highly active antiretroviral therapy. *Current Opinion in Infectious Diseases*, 19, 14–19.
12 Tang, H.J., Liu, Y.C., Yen, M.Y., Chen, Y.S., Wann, S.R., Lin, H.H., Lee, S.S., Lin, W.R., Huang, C.K., Su, B.A., Chang, P.C., Li, C.M. and Tseng, H.H. (2006) Opportunistic infections in adults with acquired immunodeficienct syndrome: a comparison of clinical and autopsy findings. *Journal of Microbiology, Immunology and Infection*, 39, 310–315.
13 Rowshani, A.T., Bemelman, F.J., Van Leeuwen, E.M., Van Lier, R.A. and Ten Berge, I.J. (2005) Clinical and immunological aspects of cytomegalovirus infection in solid organ transplant recipients. *Transplantation*, 79, 381–386.
14 Strippoli, G.F., Hodson, E.M., Jones, C. and Craig, J.C. (2006) Preemptive treatment for cytomegalovirus viraemia to prevent cytomegalovirus disease in solid organ transplant recipients. *Transplantation*, 81, 139–145.
15 Tan, H.H. and Goh, C.L. (2006) Viral infections affecting the skin in organ transplant recipients: epidemiology and current management strategies. *American Journal of Clinical Dermatology*, 7, 13–29.
16 Vial, T. and Descotes, J. (2003) Immunosuppressive drugs and cancer. *Toxicology*, 185, 229–240.
17 Vos, J.G. (1977) Immune suppression as related to toxicology. *CRC Critical Reviews in Toxicology*, 5, 67–101.
18 De Jong, W.H. and Van Loveren, H. (2007) Screening of xenobiotics for direct immunotoxicity in an animal study. *Methods (San Diego, Calif)*, 41, 3–8.
19 International Conference on Harmonization (2005) www.ich.org.
20 OECD (1995) OECD guideline for the testing of chemicals 407. Repeated dose 28-day oral toxicity study in rodents. OECD, Paris, France.
21 European Medicines Agency (2000) Note for Guidance on Repeated Dose Toxicity, www.emea.europa.eu.
22 Moszczynski, P. (1997) Mercury compounds and the immune system: a review. *International Journal of Occupational Medicine and Environmental Health*, 10, 247–258.
23 Silbergeld, E.K., Silva, I.A. and Nyland, J.F. (2005) Mercury and autoimmunity: implications for occupational and environmental health. *Toxicology and Applied Pharmacology*, 207, 282–292.
24 ICICIS (1998) Report of validation study of assessment of direct immunotoxicity in the rat. The ICICIS group investigators. international collaborative immunotoxicity study. *Toxicology*, 125, 183–201.

25. Schulte, A., Althoff, J., Ewe, S. and Richter-Reichhelm, H.-B. (2002) BGVV group investigators, two immunotoxicity ring studies according to OECD TG 407 comparison of data on cyclosporin A and hexachlorbenzene. *Regulatory Toxicology and Pharmacology*, **36**, 12–21.
26. Basketter, D.A., Bremmer, J.A., Buckley, P., Kammüller, M.E., Kawabata, T., Kimber, I., Loveless, S.E., Magda, S., Stringer, D.A. and Vohr, H.-W. (1995) Pathology considerations for, and subsequent risk assessment of, chemicals identified as immunosuppressive in routine toxicology. *Food and Chemical Toxicology: An International Journal Published for the British Industrial Biological Research Association*, **33**, 239–243.
27. Maronpot, R.R. (2006) A monograph on histomorphologic evaluation of lymphoid organs. *Toxicologic Pathology*, **34**, 407–408.
28. De Jong, W.H., Kuper, C.F., Van Loveren, H. and Vos, J.G. (2009) Histopathology in immunotoxicity evaluation. *Perspectives in Experimental Clinical Immunotoxicology*, in press.
29. Gopinath, C. (1996) Pathology of toxic effects on the immune system. *Inflammation Research*, **45**, S74–S78.
30. Ward, J.M., Uno, H. and Frith, C.H. (1993) Immunohistochemistry and morphology of reactive lesions in lymph nodes and spleen of rats and mice. *Toxicologic Pathology*, **21**, 199–205.
31. Mitsumori, K., Takegawa, K., Shimo, T., Onodera, H., Yasuhara, K. and Takahashi, M. (1996) Morphometric and immunohistochemical studies on atrophic changes in lympho-hematopoietic organs of rats treated with piperonyl butoxide or subjected to dietary restriction. *Archives of Toxicology*, **70**, 809–814.
32. Kuper, C.F., De Heer, E., Van Loveren, H. and Vos, J.G. (2002) Chapter 39 immune system, in *Handbook of Toxicologic Pathology* (eds W. Haschek, C.G. Rousseaux and M.A. Wallig), Academic Press, San Diego, pp. 585–646.
33. De Jong, W.H., Kroese, E.D., Vos, J.G. and Van Loveren, H. (1999) Detection of immunotoxicity of benzo[a]pyrene in a subacute toxicity study after oral exposure in rats. *Toxicological Sciences*, **50**, 214–220.
34. Putman, E., Van Loveren, H., Bode, G., Dean, J., Hastings, K., Nakamura, K., Verdier, F. and Van Der Laan, J.W. (2002) Assessment of the immunotoxic potential of human pharmaceuticals: a workshop report. *Drug Information Journal*, **36**, 417–427.
35. Germolec, D.R., Nyska, A., Kashon, M., Kuper, C.F., Portier, C., Kommineni, C., Johnson, K.A. and Luster, M.I. (2004) Extended histopathology in immunotoxicity testing: interlaboratory validation studies. *Toxicological Sciences*, **78**, 107–115.
36. Germolec, D.R., Kashon, M., Nyska, A., Kuper, C.F., Portier, C., Kommineni, C., Johnson, K.A. and Luster, M.I. (2004) The accuracy of extended histopathology to detect immunotoxic chemicals. *Toxicological Sciences*, **82**, 504–514.
37. Luster, M.I., Portier, C., Pait, D.G., White, K.L. Jr, Gennings, C., Munson, A.E. and Rosenthal, G.J. (1992) Risl assessment in immunotoxicology. I. Sensitivity and predictability of immune tests. *Fundamental and Applied Toxicology*, **18**, 200–210.
38. Vos, J.G., De Klerk, A., Krajnc, E.I., Kruizinga, W., Van Ommen, B. and Rozing, J. (1984) Toxicity of bis(tri-n-butyltin)oxide in the rat. II. Suppression of thymus dependent immune responses and of parameters of non-specific resistance after short term exposure. *Toxicology and Applied Pharmacology*, **75**, 387–408.
39. Van Loveren, H., Verlaan, A.P. and Vos, J.G. (1991) An enzyme linked immunosorbent assay of anti-sheep red blood cell antibodies of the classes M, G and A in the rat. *International Journal of Immunopharmacology*, **13**, 689–695.

40 Smialowicz, R.J., Luebke, R.W. and Riddle, M.M. (1992) Asessment of the immunotoxic potential of the fungicide dinocap in mice. *Toxicology*, **75**, 235–247.

41 Houben, G.F., Penninks, A.H., Seinen, W., Vos, J.G. and Van Loveren, H. (1993) Immunotoxic effects of the color additive caramel color III: immune function studies in rats. *Fundamental and Applied Toxicology*, **20**, 30–37.

42 Vos, J.G., Krajnc, E.I. and Beekhof, P. (1982) Use of the enzyme-linked immunosorbent assay (ELISA) in immunotoxicity testing. *Environmental Health Perspectives*, **43**, 115–121.

43 Burns, L.A., Bradley, S.G., White, K.L., McCay, J.A., Fuchs, B.A., Stern, M., Brown, R.D., Musgrove, D.L., Holsapple, M.P. and Luster, M.I. (1994) Immunotoxicity of 2,4-diaminotoluene in female B6C3F1 mice. *Drug and Chemical Toxicology*, **17**, 401–436.

44 Burns, L.A., White, K.L., McCay, J.A., Fuchs, B.A., Stern, M., Brown, R.D., Musgrove, D.L., Holsapple, M.P., Luster, M.I. and Bradley, S.G. (1994) Immunotoxicity of mono-nitrotoluene in female B6C3F1 mice: II. Meta-nitrotoluene. *Drug and Chemical Toxicology*, **17**, 359–399.

45 Roth, D.R., Roman, D., Ulrich, P., Mahl, A., Junker, U. and Perentes, E. (2006) Design and evaluation of immunotoxicity studies. *Experimental and Toxicologic Pathology*, **57**, 367–371.

46 Van Loveren, H., De Jong, W.H., Vanndebriel, R.J., Vos, J.G. and Garssen, J. (1998) Risk assessment and immunotoxicology. *Toxicology Letters*, **102–103**, 261–265.

47 Karrrow, N.A., Guo, T.L., Zhang, L.X., McCay, J.A., Musgrove, D.L., Peachee, V.L., Germolec, D.R. and White, K.L. Jr (2003) Thalidomide modulation of the immune response in female B6C3F1 mice: a host resistance study. *International Immunopharmacology*, **3**, 1447–1456.

48 Holsapple, M.P., White, K.L. Jr, McCay, J.A., Bradley, S.G. and Munson, A.E. (1988) An immnotoxicological evaluation of 4,4-thiobis-(6-t-butyl-m-cresol) in female B6C3F1 mice.2. Humoral and cell-mediated immunity, macrophage function, and host resistance. *Fundamental and Applied Toxicology*, **10**, 701–716.

49 WHO (1999) International Programme on Chemical Safety, Principles and methods for assessing allergic hypersensitization associated with exposure to chemicals, *Environmental Health Criteria 212*, WHO, Geneva, Zwitserland.

50 Kimber, I. and Weisenberger, C. (1989) A murine local lymph node assay for the identification of contact allergens. Assay development and results of an initial validation study. *Archives of Toxicology*, **63**, 274–282.

51 EMEA Note for Guidance on non-clinical local tolerance testing of human pharmaceuticals. http://www.emea.europa.eu/pdfs/human/swp/214500en.

52 Dean, J.H., Twerdok, L.E., Tice, R.R., Sailstad, D.M., Hattan, D.G. and Stokes, W.S. (2001) ICCVAM evaluation of the murine local lymph node assay. II Conclusions and recommendations of an independent scientific peer review panel. *Regulatory Toxicology and Pharmacology*, **34**, 258–273.

53 Haneke, K.E., Tice, R.R., Carson, B.L., Margolin, B.H. and Stokes, W.S. (2001) ICCVAM evaluation of the murine local lymph node assay. III Data analysis completed by the national toxicology program interagency center for the evaluation of alternative toxicological methods. *Regulatory Toxicology and Pharmacology*, **34**, 274–286.

54 Sailstad, D.M., Hattan, D., Hill, R.N. and Stokes, W.S. (2001) ICCVAM evaluation of the murine local lymph node assay. I The ICCVAM review process. *Regulatory Toxicology and Pharmacology*, **34**, 249–257.

55 Basketter, D.A., Clapp, C., Jefferies, D., Safford, B., Ryan, C.A., Gerberick, F., Dearman, R.J. and Kimber, I. (2005)

Predictive identification of human skin sensitization thresholds. *Contact Dermatitis*, **53**, 260–267.

56 Basketter, D.A., Lea, L.J., Cooper, K., Stocks, J., Dickens, A., Pate, I., Dearman, R.J. and Kimber, I. (1999) Threshold for classification as a skin sensitizer in the local lymph node assay: a statistical evaluation. *Food and Chemical Toxicology: An International Journal Published for the British Industrial Biological Research Association*, **37**, 1167–1174.

57 Basketter, D.A., Lea, L.J., Dickens, A., Briggs, D., Pate, I., Dearman, R.J. and Kimber, I. (1999) A comparison of statistical approaches to the derivation of EC3 values from local lymph node assay dose responses. *Journal of Applied Toxicology*, **19**, 261–266.

58 Van Och, F.M.M., Slob, W., De Jong, W.H., Vandebriel, R.J. and Van Loveren, H. (2000) A quantitative method for assessing the sensitizing potency of low molecular weight chemicals using a local lymph node assay: Employment of a regression method that includes determination of the uncertainty margins. *Toxicology*, **146**, 49–59.

59 De Jong, W.H., Van Och, F.M.M., Den Hartog Jager, C.F., Speikstra, S.W., Slob, W., Vandebriel, R.J. and Van Loveren, H. (2002) Ranking of allergenic potency of rubber chemicals in a modified local lymph node assay. *Toxicological Sciences*, **66**, 226–232.

60 Arts, J.H.E. and Kuper, C.F. (2007) Animal models to test respiratory allergy of low molecular weigth chemicals: a guidance. *Methods (San Diego, Calif)*, **41**, 61–71.

61 WHO (2006) International Programme on Chemical Safety, Principles and methods for assessing autoimmunity associated with exposure to chemicals, *Environmental Health Criteria 236*, WHO, Geneva, Zwitserland.

62 Kammüller, M.E., Bloksma, N. and Seinen, S. (1989) Immune disregulation induced by drugs and chemicals, in *Autoimmunity and Toxicology* (eds M.E. Kammuller, N. Bloksma and W. Seinen), Academic Press, San Diego, pp. 3–34.

63 Griem, P., Wulferink, M., Sachs, B., Gonzalez, J.B. and Gleichmann, E. (1998) Allergy and autoimmune reactions to xenobiotics: how do they arise? *Immunology Today*, **19**, 133–141.

64 Uetrecht, J. (2008) Idiosyncratic drug reactions: past, present, and future. *Chemical Research in Toxicology*, **21**, 84–92.

65 Pirmohamed, M. and Park, B.K. (2001) HIV and drug allergy. *Current Opinion in Allergy & Clinical Immunology*, **1**, 311–316.

66 Hashimoto, K., Yasukawa, M. and Tohyama, M. (2003) Human herpesvirus 6 and drug allergy. *Current Opinion in Allergy & Clinical Immunology*, **3**, 255–260.

67 Tournade, H., Pelletier, L., Pasquier, R., Vial, M.C., Mandet, C. and Druet, P. (1990) D-penicillamine-induced autoimmunity in Brown-Norway rats. Similarities with $HgCl_2$-induced autoimmunity. *Journal of Immunology (Baltimore, Md: 1950)*, **144**, 2985–2991.

68 Tournade, H., Guery, J.C., Pasquier, R., Nochy, D., Hinglais, N., Guilbert, B., Druet, P. and Pelletier, L. (1991) Experimental gold induced autoimmunity. *Nephrology, Dialysis, Transplantation*, **6**, 621–630.

69 Shenton, J.M., Teranishi, M., Abu-Asab, M.S., Yager, J.A. and Uetrecht, J.P. (2003) Characterization of a potential animal model of an idiosyncratic drug reaction: nevirapine-induced skin rash in the rat. *Chemical Research in Toxicology*, **16**, 1078–1089.

70 Rowley, B. and Monestier, M. (2005) Mechanisms of heavy metal-induced autoimmunity. *Molecular Immunology*, **42**, 833–838.

71 Donker, A.J., Venuto, R.C., Vladutiu, A.O., Brentjens, J.R. and Andres, G.A. (1984) Effects of prolonged administration of D-penicillamine or captopril in various strains of rats. Brown-Norway rats treated with D-penicillamine develop autoantibodies, circulating

72 Popovic, M., Nierkens, S., Pieters, R. and Uetrecht, J. (2004) Investigating the role of 2-phenylpropenal in felbamate-induced idiosyncratic drug reactions. *Chemical Research in Toxicology*, **17**, 1568–1576.

73 Knippels, L.M., Houben, G.F., Spanhaak, S. and Penninks, A.H. (1999) An oral sensitization model in Brown Norway rats to screen for potential allergenicity of food proteins. *Methods (San Diego, Calif)*, **19**, 78–82.

74 Robinson, C.J., Balazs, T. and Egorov, I.K. (1986) Mercuric chloride, gold sodium thiomalate, and D-penicillamine-induced antinuclear antibodies in mice. *Toxicology and Applied Pharmacology*, **86**, 159–169.

75 Mirtcheva, J., Pfeiffer, C., De Bruijn, J.A., Jacquesmart, F. and Gleichmann, E. (1989) Immunological alterations inducible by mercury compounds. III. H-2A acts as an immune response and H-2E as an immune "suppression" locus for HgCl2-induced antinucleolar autoantibodies. *European Journal of Immunology*, **19**, 2257–2261.

76 Monestier, M., Novick, K.E. and Losman, M.J. (1994) D-penicillamine- and quinidine-induced antinuclear antibodies in ASW (H-2s) mice: similarities with autoantibodies in spontaneous and heavy metal-induced autoimmunity. *European Journal of Immunology*, **24**, 723–730.

77 Wooley, P.H., Sud, S., Whalen, J.D. and Nasser, S. (1998) Pristane-induced arthritis in mice. V. Susceptibility to pristane-induced arthritis is determined by the genetic regulation of the T cell repertoire. *Arthritis and Rheumatism*, **41**, 2022–2031.

78 Goebel, C., Vogel, C., Wulferink, M., Mittman, S., Sachs, B., Scraa, S., Abel, J., Degen, G., Uetrecht, J. and Gleichmann, E. (1999) Procainamide, a drug causing lupus, induces prostaglandin H synthase-2 and formation of T-cell sensitizing drug metabolites in mouse macrophages. *Chemical Research in Toxicology*, **12**, 488–500.

79 Abedi-Valugerdi, M., Nilsson, C., Zargari, A., Gharibdoost, F., DePierre, J.W. and Hassan, M. (2005) Bacterial lipopolysaccharide both renders resistant mice susceptible to mercury-induced autoimmunity and exacerbates such autoimmunity in susceptible mice. *Clinical and Experimental Immunology*, **141**, 238–247.

80 Sayeh, E. and Uetrecht, J.P. (2001) Factors that modify penicillamine-induced autoimmunity in Brown Norway rats: failure of the Th1/Th2 paradigm. *Toxicology*, **163**, 195–211.

81 Pollard, K.M., Pearson, D.L., Hultman, P., Hildebrandt, B. and Kono, D.H. (1999) Lupus-prone mice as models to study xenobiotic-induced acceleration of systemic autoimmunity. *Environmental Health Perspectives*, **107**, 729–735.

82 Shaheen, V.M., Satoh, M., Richards, H.B., Yoshida, H., Shaw, M., Jennette, J.C. and Reeves, W.H. (1999) Immunopathogenesis of environmentally induced lupus in mice. *Environmental Health Perspectives*, **107**, 723–727.

83 Ravel, G. and Descotes, J. (2005) Popliteal lymph node assay: facts and perspectives. *Journal of Applied Toxicology*, **25**, 451–458.

84 Albers, R., Broeders, A., van der Pijl, A., Seinen, W. and Pieters, R. (1997) The use of reporter antigens in the popliteal lymph node assay to assess immunomodulation by chemicals. *Toxicology and Applied Pharmacology*, **143**, 102–109.

85 Gutting, B.W., Schomaker, S.J., Kaplan, A.H. and Amacher, D.E. (1999) A comparison of the direct and reporter antigen popliteal lymph node assay for the detection of immunomodulation by low molecular weight compounds. *Toxicological Sciences*, **51**, 71–79.

86 Nierkens, S., van Helden, P., Bol, M., Bleumink, R., van Kooten, P., Ramdien-

Murli, S., Boon, L. and Pieters, R. (2002) Selective requirement for CD40-CD154 in drug-induced type 1 versus type 2 responses to trinitrophenyl-ovalbumin. *Journal of Immunology (Baltimore, Md: 1950)*, **168**, 3747–3754.
87. Kubicka-Muranyi, M., Kremer, J., Rottmann, N., Lubben, B., Albers, R., Bloksma, N., Luhrmann, R. and Gleichmann, E. (1996) Murine systemic autoimmune disease induced by mercuric chloride: T helper cells reacting to self proteins. *International Archives of Allergy and Immunology*, **109**, 11–20.
88. Luster, M.I., Hayes, H.T., Korach, K., Tucker, A.N., Dean, J.H., Greenlee, W.F. and Boorman, G.A. (1984) Estrogen immunosuppression is regulated through estrogenic responses in the thymus. *Journal of Immunology (Baltimore, Md: 1950)*, **133**, 110–116.
89. Mekenyan, O.G., Veith, G.D., Call, D.J. and Ankley, G.T. (1996) A QSAR evaluation of Ah receptor binding of haloginated aromatic zenobiotiocs. *Environmental Health Perspectives*, **104**, 1302–1310.
90. Di Gioacchino, M., Verna, N., Di Giampaolo, L., Di Claudio, F., Turi, M.C., Perrone, A., Petrarca, C., Mariani-Costantini, R., Sabbioni, E. and Boscolo, P. (2007) Immunotoxicity and sensitizing capacity of metal compounds depend on speciation. *International Journal of Immunopathology and Pharmacology*, **20**, 15–22.
91. Ponce, R. (2008) Adverse consequences of immunostimulation. *Journal of Immunotoxicology*, **5**, 33–41.
92. Sgro, C. (1995) Side-effects of a monoclonal antibody, muromonab CD3/orthoclone OKT3: bibliographic review. *Toxicology*, **105**, 23–29.
93. Wing, M.G., Moreau, T., Greenwood, J., Smith, R.M., Hale, G., Isaacs, J., Waldmann, H., Lachman, P.J. and Compston, A. (1996) Mechanism of first-dose cytokine-relaease Syndrome by Campath 1-H: Involvement of CD 16 (FCγRIII) and CD11a/CD18 (LFA-1) on NK cells. *The Journal of Clinical Investigation*, **98**, 2819–2826.
94. Schneider, C.K., Kalinke, U. and Löwer, J. (2006) TGN1412-a regulator's perspective. *Nature Biotechnology*, **24**, 493–496.
95. Suntharalingam, G., Perry, M.R., Ward, S., Brett, S.J., Castello-Cortes, A., Brunner, M.D. and Panoskaltsis, N. (2006) Cytokine storm in a phase 1 trial of the Anti-CD28 monoclonal antibody TGN1412. *New England Journal of Medicine*, **355**, 1–11.
96. Alegre, M., Depierreux, M., Florquin, S., Najdovski, T., Vandenabeele, P., Abramowicz, D., Leo, O., Deschodt-Lanckman, M. and Goldman, M. (1990) Acute toxicity of Anti-CD3 monoclonal antibody in mice: a model for OKT3 first dose reactions. *Transplantation Proceedings*, **22**, 1920–1921.
97. Alegre, M.L., Vandenabeele, P., Depierreux, M., Florquin, S., Deschodt-Lanckman, M., Flamand, V., Moser, M., Leo, O., Urbain, J. and Fiers, W. (1991) Cytokine release syndrome induced by the 145-1C11 anti-CD3 monoclonal antibody in mice: prevention by high doses of methylprednisolone. *Journal of Immunology* (Baltimore, MD, 1950), **146**, 1184–1191.
98. Cotran, R.S., Pober, J.S., Grimborne, M.A. Jr, Springer, T.A., Wiebke, E.A., Gaspari, A.A., Rosenberg, S.A. and Lotze, M.T. (1988) Endothelial activation during interleukin 2 immunotherapy. A possible mechanism for teh vascular leak syndrome. *Journal of Immunology* (Baltimore, MD, 1950), **140**, 1883–1888.
99. Guan, H., Nagarkatti, P.S. and Nagarkatti, M. (2007) Blockade of hyaluronan inhibits IL-2-induced vascular leak syndrome and maintains effectiveness of IL-2 treatment for metastatic melanoma. *Journal of Immunology* (Baltimore, MD, 1950), **179**, 3715–3723.
100. Baluna, R. and Vitetta, E.S. (1997) Vascular leak syndrome: a side effect of immunotherapy. *Immunopharmacology*, **37**, 117–132.

101 Mohan, C.G., Gandhi, T., Garg, D. and Shinde, R. (2007) Computer-assisted methods in chemical toxicity prediction. *Mini-Reviews in Medicinal Chemistry*, **7**, 499–507.

102 Patlewicz, G., Aptula, A.O., Uriarte, E., Roberts, D.W., Kern, P.S., Gerberick, G.F., Kimber, I., Dearman, R.J., Ryan, C.A. and Basketter, D.A. (2007) An evaluation of selected global (Q)SARs/ expert systems for the prediction of skin sensitisation potential. *SAR and QSAR in Environmental Research*, **18**, 515–541.

103 Aptula, A.O., Patlewicz, G. and Roberts, D.W. (2005) Skin sensitization: reaction mechanistic applicability domains for structure-activity relationships. *Chemical Research in Toxicology*, **18**, 1420–1426.

104 Aptula, A.O. and Roberts, D.W. (2006) Mechanistic applicability domains for nonanimal-based prediction of toxicological end points: general principles and application to reactive toxicity. *Chemical Research in Toxicology*, **19**, 1097–1105.

105 Roberts, D.W., Aptula, A.O., Cronin, M.T., Hulzebos, E. and Patlewicz, G. (2007) Global (Q)SARs for skin sensitisation: assessment against OECD principles. *SAR and QSAR in Environmental Research*, **18**, 343–365.

106 Roberts, D.W., Patlewicz, G., Kern, P.S., Gerberick, F., Kimber, I., Dearman, R.J., Ryan, C.A., Basketter, D.A. and Aptula, A.O. (2007) Mechanistic applicability domain classification of a local lymph node assay dataset for skin sensitization. *Chemical Research in Toxicology*, **20**, 1019–1030.

107 Patlewicz, G., Van Loveren, H., Cockshott, A., Gebel, T., Gundert-Remy, U., De Jong, W.H., Matheson, J., McCarry, H., Musset, L., Selgrade, M.K. and Vickers, C. (2008) Skin sensitization in chemical risk assessment: Report of a WHO/IPCS international workshop focusing on dose–response assessment. *Regulatory Toxicology and Pharmacology*, **50**, 155–199.

108 Revillard, J.P., Robinet, E., Goldman, M., Bain, H., Latinne, D. and Chatenoud, L. (1995) *In vitro* correlates of the acute toxic syndrome induced by some monoclonal antibodies: a rationale for the design of predictive tests. *Toxicology*, **96**, 51–58.

109 Gennari, A., Ban, M., Braun, A., Casati, S., Corsini, E., Dastych, J., Descotes, J., Hartung, T., Hooghe-Peters, R., House, R., Pallardy, M., Pieters, R., Reid, L., Tryphonas, H., Tschirhart, E., Tuschl, H., Vandebriel, R. and Gribaldo, L. (2005) The use of *in vitro* systems for evaluating immunotoxicity: the report and recommendations of an ECVAM Workshop. *Journal of Immunotoxicology*, **2**, 61–83.

110 Carfi, M., Gennari, A., Malerba, I., Corsini, E., Pallardy, M., Pieters, R., Van Loveren, H., Vohr, H.-W., Hartung, T. and Gribaldo, L. (2007) *In vitro* tests to evaluate immunotoxicity: a preliminary study. *Toxicology*, **229**, 11–22.

111 Baken, K.A., Arkusz, J., Pennings, J.L., Vandebriel, R.J. and van Loveren, H. (2007) *In vitro* immunotoxicity of bis(tri-n-butyltin)oxide (TBTO) studied by toxicogenomics. *Toxicology*, **237**, 35–48.

112 Jowsey, I.R., Basketter, D.A., Westmoreland, C. and Kimber, I. (2006) A future approach to measuring relative skin sensitising potency: a proposal. *Journal of Applied Toxicology*, **26**, 341–350.

113 Grindon, C., Combes, R., Cronin, M.T., Roberts, D.W. and Garrod, J.F. (2008) An integrated decision-tree testing strategy for repeat dose toxicity with respect to the requirements of the EU REACH legislation. *Alternatives to Laboratory Animals*, **36**, 93–101.

114 Roberts, D.W. and Aptula, A.O. (2008) Determinants of skin sensitisation potential. *Journal of Applied Toxicology*, **28**, 377–387.

115 Basketter, D.A., Pease, C., Kasting, G., Kimber, I., Casati, S., Cronin, M., Diembeck, W., Gerberick, F., Hadgraft, J., Hartung, T., Marty, J.P., Nikolaidis, E., Patlewicz, G., Roberts, D., Roggen, E.,

Rovida, C. and van de Sandt, J. (2007) Skin sensitisation and epidermal disposition: the relevance of epidermal disposition for sensitisation hazard identification and risk assessment. The report and recommendations of ECVAM workshop 59. *Alternatives to Laboratory Animals*, **35**, 137–154.

116 Gerberick, G.F., Vassallo, J.D., Bailey, R.E., Chaney, J.G., Morrall, S.W. and Lepoittevin, J.P. (2004) Development of a peptide reactivity assay for screening contact allergens. *Toxicological Sciences*, **81**, 332–343.

117 Aptula, A.O., Patlewicz, G., Roberts, D.W. and Schultz, T.W. (2006) Non-enzymatic glutathione reactivity and *in vitro* toxicity: a non-animal approach to skin sensitization. *Toxicology In Vitro: An International Journal Published in Association with BIBRA*, **20**, 239–247.

118 Gerberick, G.F., Vassallo, J.D., Foertsch, L.M., Price, B.B., Chaney, J.G. and Lepoittevin, J.P. (2007) Quantification of chemical peptide reactivity for screening contact allergens: a classification tree model approach. *Toxicological Sciences*, **97**, 417–427.

119 Vandebriel, R.J., Van Och, F.M.M. and Van Loveren, H. (2005) *In vitro* assessment of sensitizing activity of low molecular weight compounds. *Toxicology and Applied Pharmacology*, **207**, 142–148.

120 Van Och, F.M.M., Van Loveren, H., Van Wolfswinkel, J.C., Machielsen, A.J. and Vandebriel, R.J. (2005) Assessment of potency of allergenic activity of low molecular weight compounds based on IL-1alpha and IL-18 production by a murine and human keratinocyte cell line. *Toxicology*, **210**, 95–109.

121 Roggen, E.L., Soni, N.K. and Verheyen, G.R. (2006) Respiratory immunotoxicity: an *in vitro* assessment. *Toxicology In Vitro: An International Journal Published in Association with BIBRA*, **20**, 1249–1264.

122 Casati, S., Aeby, P., Basketter, D.A., Cavani, A., Gennari, A., Gerberick, G.F., Griem, P., Hartung, T., Kimber, I., Lepoittevin, J.P., Meade, B.J., Pallardy, M., Rougier, N., Rousset, F., Rubinstenn, G., Sallusto, F., Verheyen, G.R. and Zuang, V. (2005) Dendritic cells as a tool for the predictive identification of skin sensitisation hazard. The Report and Recommendations of ECVAM Workshop 51. *Alternatives to Laboratory Animals*, **33**, 47–62.

123 Ryan, C.A., Kimber, I., Basketter, D.A., Pallardy, M., Gildea, L.A. and Gerberick, G.F. (2007) Dendritic cells and skin sensitization: biological roles and uses in hazard identification. *Toxicology and Applied Pharmacology*, **221**, 384–394.

124 De Smedt, A.C., Van Den Heuvel, R.L., Van Tendeloo, V.F., Berneman, Z.N., Schoeters, G.E., Weber, E. and Tuschl, H. (2002) Phenotypic alterations and Il-1 neta production in CD34(+) progenitor- and monocyte-derived dendritic cells after exposure to allergens: a comparative analysis. *Archives of Dermatological Research*, **294**, 109–116.

125 Azam, P., Peiffer, J.L., Chamousset, D., Tissier, M.H., Bonnet, P.A., Vian, L., Fabre, I. and Ourlin, J.C. (2006) The cytokine dependent MUTZ-3 cell line as an *in vitro* model for the screening of contact sensitizers. *Toxicology and Applied Pharmacology*, **212**, 14–23.

126 Gildea, L.A., Ryan, C.A., Foertsch, L.M., Kennedy, J.M., Dearman, R.J., Kimber, I. and Gerberick, G.F. (2006) Identification of gene expression changes induced by chemical allergens in dendritic cells: opportunities for skin sensitization testing. *The Journal of Investigative Dermatology*, **126**, 1813–1822.

127 Schoeters, E., Verheyen, G.R., Nelissen, I., Van Rompay, A.R., Hooyberghs, J., Van Den Heuvel, R.L., Witters, H., Schoeters, G.E., Van Tendeloo, V.F. and Berneman, Z.N. (2007) Microarray analyses in dendritic cells reveal potential biomarkers for chemical-induced skin sensitization. *Molecular Immunology*, **44**, 3222–3233.

128 Boislève, F., Kerdine-Römer, S., Rougier-Larzat, N. and Pallardy, M. (2004) Nickel

and DNCB induce CCR7 expression on human dendritic cells through different signalling pathways: role for TNF-alpha and MAPK. *The Journal of Investigative Dermatology*, **123**, 494–502.

129 Ade, N., Antonios, D., Kerdine-Romer, S., Boisleve, F., Rousset, F. and Pallardy, M. (2007) NF-kappaB plays a major role in the maturation of human dendritic cells induced by NiSO(4) but not by DNCB. *Toxicological Sciences*, **99**, 488–501.

130 Facy, V., Flouret, V., Régnier, M. and Schmidt, R. (2005) Reactivity of Langerhans cells in human reconstructed epidermis to known allergens and UV radiation. *Toxicology In Vitro: An International Journal Published in Association with BIBRA*, **19**, 787–795.

131 De Longueville, F., Bertholet, V. and Remacle, J. (2004) DNA microarrays as a tool in toxicogenomics. *Combinatorial Chemistry & High Throughput Screening*, **7**, 207–211.

132 Baken, K.A., Vandebriel, R.J., Pennings, J.L.A., Kleinjans, J.C. and van Loveren, H. (2007) Toxicogenomics in the assessment of immunotoxicity. *Methods (San Diego, Calif)*, **41**, 132–141.

133 Burns-Naas, L.A., Dearman, R.J., Germolec, D.R., Kaminski, N.E., Kimber, I., Ladics, G.S., Luebke, R.W., Pfau, J.C. and Pruett, S.B. (2006) Omics technologies and the immune system. *Toxicology Mechanisms and Methods*, **16**, 101–119.

134 Baken, K.A., Pennings, J.L.A., De Vries, A., Breit, T.M., van Steeg, H. and van Loveren, H. (2006) Gene expression profiling of bis(tri-butyltin)oxide (TBTO)-induced immunotoxicity in mice and rats. *Journal of Immunotoxicology*, **3**, 227–244.

135 Ezendam, J., Staedtler, H., Pennings, J.L.A., Vandebriel, R.J., Pieters, R., Harleman, J.H. and Vos, J.G. (2004) Toxicogenomics of subchronic hexachlorobenzeneexposure in Brown Norway rats. *Environmental Health Perspectives*, **112**, 782–791.

136 Luebke, R.W., Holsapple, M.P., Ladics, G.S., Luster, M.I., Selgrade, M., Smialowicz, R.J., Woolhiser, M.R. and Germolec, D.R. (2006) Immunotoxicogenomics: the potential of geniomics technology in the immunotoxicity risk assessment process. *Toxicological Sciences*, **94**, 22–27.

137 Tugwood, J.D., Hollins, L.E. and Cockerill, M.J. (2003) Genomics and the search for novel biomarkers in toxicology. *Biomarkers: Biochemical Indicators of Exposure, Response, and Susceptibility to Chemicals*, **8**, 79–92.

138 Steiner, G., Suter, L., Boess, F., Gasser, R., De Vera, M.C., Albertini, S. and Ruepp, S. (2004) Discriminating different classes of toxicants by transcript profiling. *Environmental Health Perspectives*, **112**, 1236–1248.

139 Waters, M.D. and Fostel, J.M. (2004) Toxicogenomics and systems toxicology: aims and prospects. *Nature Reviews. Genetics*, **5**, 936–948.

140 Burczynski, M.E., McMillian, M., Ciervo, J., Li, L., Parker, J.B., Dunn, R.T., Hicken, S., Farr, S. and Johnson, M.D. (2000) Toxicogenomics based discrimination of toxic mechanism in HepG2 human hepatoma cells. *Toxicological Sciences*, **58**, 399–415.

141 Thomas, R.S., Rank, D.R., Penn, S.G., Zastrow, G.M., Hayes, K.R., Pande, K., Glover, E., Silander, T., Craven, M.W., Reddy, J.K., Jovanovich, S.B. and Bradfield, C.A. (2001) Identification of toxicologically predictive gene sets using cDNA microarrays. *Molecular Pharmacology*, **60**, 1189–1194.

142 Waring, J.F., Jolly, R.A., Ciurlionis, R., Lum, P.Y., Praestgaard, J.T., Morfitt, D.C., Buratto, B., Roberts, C., Schadt, E. and Ulrich, R.G. (2001) Clustering of hepatotoxins based on mechanism of toxicity using gene expression profiles. *Toxicology and Applied Pharmacology*, **175**, 28–42.

143 Hamadeh, H.K., Bushel, P.R., Jayadev, S., Martin, K., DiSorbo, O., Sieber, S., Bennett, L., Tennant, R., Stoll, R., Barrett, J.C., Blanchard, K., Paules, R.S. and Afshari, C.A. (2002) Gene expression analysis reveals chemical specific profiles. *Toxicological Sciences*, **67**, 219–231.

144 Fielden, M.R. and Kolaja, K.L. (2006) The state of the art in predictive toxicogenomics. *Current Opinion in Drug Discovery & Development*, **9**, 84–91.

145 Mendrick, D.L. (2008) Genomic and genetic biomarkers of toxicity. *Toxicology*, **245**, 175–181.

146 Baken, K.A., Pennings, J.L.A., Jonker, M.J., Schaap, M.M., de Vries, A., van Steeg, H., Breit, T.M. and van Loveren, H. (2008) Overlapping gene expression profiles of model compounds provide opportunities for immunotoxicity screening. *Toxicology and Applied Pharmacology*, **226**, 46–59.

147 Patterson, R.M. and Germolec, D.R. (1076) Gene expression alterationsin immune system pathways following exposure to immunosuppressive chemicals. *Annals of the New York Academy of Sciences*, **2006**, 718–727.

148 Pennie, W.D. and Kimber, I. (2002) Toxicogenomics: transcript profiling and potential application to chemical allergy. *Toxicology In Vitro: An International Journal Published in Association with BIBRA*, **16**, 319–326.

149 Foster, W.R., Chen, S.J., He, A., Truong, A., Bhaskaran, V., Nelson, D.M., Dambach, D.M., Lehman-McKeeman, L.D. and Car, B.D. (2007) A retrospective analysis of toxicogenomics in the safety assessment of drug candidates. *Toxicologic Pathology*, **35**, 621–635.

19
In Vitro Phototoxicity Testing: a Procedure Involving Multiple Endpoints
Laurent Marrot and Jean-Roch Meunier

19.1
Introduction

Some chemicals, even if not toxic by themselves, may become reactive under exposure to environmental sunlight, inducing adverse biological effects. Phototoxicity is of increasing concern in dermatology, since modern lifestyle is often associated with exposure to sunlight. In many cases, skin reactions (sunburn, hyperpigmentation, eczema) can be triggered by daily sunlight, although UVA in the range 320–400 nm is generally regarded as harmless [1, 2]. The various mechanisms involved in photosensitizing effects are well described [3, 4]. After absorption of photons of the appropriate wavelength, a chromophore may reach an excited state and react with biomolecules forming adducts to either DNA (photogenotoxicity) or proteins (possible haptenization, leading to photoallergy). The most commonly reported process is photosensitization via oxidative reactions. The sensitizer in its excited state reacts with oxygen and generates reactive oxygen species (ROS), such as superoxide anion ($O_2^{\bullet-}$) after electron transfer (type I reaction), or singlet oxygen ($^1O_2$) after energy transfer (type II reaction). $O_2^{\bullet-}$ can lead to H_2O_2 after dismutation, and H_2O_2 can produce the highly toxic hydroxyl radical ($OH^{\bullet}$) in the presence of traces of transition metals (such as iron) via the Fenton reaction. In cells, these processes produce local oxidative stress which, in turn, may damage genomic DNA, proteins and lipids within cell membranes (see Figure 19.1, [3]). New pharmaceutical or cosmetic compounds are tested for their phototoxic potential when they absorb light at the wavelengths of sunlight (above 290 nm). In the past, phototoxicity and photosensitization were assessed in *in vivo* models, although phototoxicity is increasingly assessed by a validated *in vitro* test, that is, neutral red uptake by 3T3 fibroblasts in culture (3T3, three of 47 NRU, [5]). This test is recommended by EU test guidelines [6] and is described by the OECD Guideline 432 [7]. However, given the limitations of this test, it may be important to develop other models. Thus, a strategy using complementary tests with increasing complexity may be a relevant approach to characterize the phototoxic potential of substances in order to ensure the safety of consumers.

Hit and Lead Profiling. Edited by Bernard Faller and Laszlo Urban
Copyright © 2009 WILEY-VCH Verlag GmbH & Co. KGaA, Weinheim
ISBN: 978-3-527-32331-9

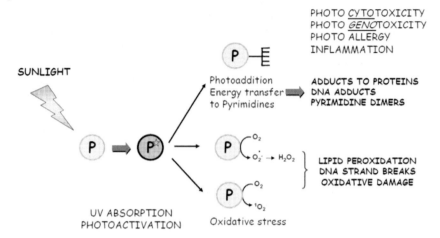

Figure 19.1 Mechanisms involved in sunlight-induced phototoxicity of drugs. Type 1 photosensitization (electron transfer) mainly generates singlet oxygen $O_2^{\cdot-}$, whereas type 2 reaction (energy transfer) leads to adduct formation or singlet oxygen $^1O_2$ production.

19.2
Optical Considerations: Relevant UV Sources and Sunlight Absorption

19.2.1
Working with the Appropriate Artificial Sunlight Source Determines the Relevance of Phototoxicity Screening

The spectrum of sunlight reaching the surface of the earth is composed of different wavebands; those mainly considered with regard to their biological effects are UV at 290–400 nm (dUVB, 290–320 nm; UVA2, 320–340 nm; UVA1, 340–400 nm), visible light at 400–800 nm, and infrared at 800–3000 nm. Phototoxicity is generally studied using light sources emitting in the UV range, although some compounds are photoreactive to visible light, for example, substances used in photodynamic therapy. However, it is assumed that most of the time UV absorption is involved in phototoxic events.

A rigorous and realistic assessment of the phototoxic potential of a substance requires laboratory exposure conditions that resemble solar UV radiation in terms of spectral power distribution (matching of wavelengths distribution and irradiance for each radiation), a task which is difficult to achieve. In the literature, photobiological studies have been performed with various light sources: some provided mainly dUVB, sometimes including wavelengths shorter than those of sunlight, others mainly UVA, generally with a maximum of emission at 365 nm (fluorescent UV tubes). In order to harmonize light sources in validation studies for phototoxicity screening, it was recommended to use either xenon or mercury halide arc lamps combined with appropriate optical filters in order to obtain an emission spectrum comparable with that of sunlight. At present, solar simulators such as those produced by ORIEL (Stratford, USA) or the SOL500 (Dr Hönle, Martinsried, Germany) appear to be good compromises and are generally used in laboratories studying phototoxicity. However, using adequate commercial systems should not prevent from paying special attention to the exposure conditions: for example, an excessive dUVB proportion may produce toxicity and hide effects of test substance-induced photoreactions; insufficient dUVB would miss phototoxicity of substances that mainly absorb in these wavelengths. Moreover, in order to remove infrared radiation that may heat samples, optical filters such as Schott UG5 or UG11 are sometimes used, but considering that these filters also absorb some of the longer UVA wavelengths (380–400 nm), it is preferable to use a dichroic mirror, even if some visible light around 450 nm remains in the emitted spectrum. In our laboratory, we use a solar simulator (ORIEL, Xenon 1600 W short arc lamp) equipped with a specific cut off filter that reproduces the UVR spectrum of sunlight including the entire UVA domain and an attenuated dUVB domain [8]. This UV source is particularly well adapted to phototoxicity assessment under realistic, non-extreme exposure conditions (Figure 19.2).

Another important point is the method of assessing UV doses received by samples. The use of various types of dosimeters, more or less well calibrated, which convert the photonic energy collected in a specific waveband (variable from one device to another) into an electric signal has led to a situation where comparison of experimental conditions in different laboratories is sometimes impossible. The most rigorous approach would be spectro-radiometry measuring genuine spectral irradiance, but this method requires expensive devices. A comprehensive document has been issued

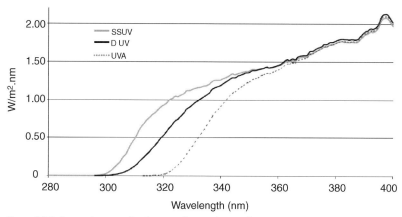

Figure 19.2 Spectral power distribution of UV radiation from a solar simulator (ORIEL): (SSUV) simulated solar zenithal UV (intense solar UVB domain); (DUV) simulated daily UV (attenuated solar UVB domain); (UVA) solar UVA (no UVB).

by COLIPA on the monitoring of UV sources (Colipa, http://www.colipa.com). It is recommended that, at least, each laboratory should provide the spectrum of the light source (that should be regularly checked) and the exposure durations used in the experiments.

19.2.2
When to Study the Phototoxicity of a Substance?

Any light-induced generation of reactive species or of toxic photoproducts requires that the substance absorbs radiation and converts the photonic energy into chemical reactivity (e.g., triplet status). A phototoxic potential is thus linked to light absorption in the sunlight range, that is, from 290 nm (or 300 nm according to some authors) to 800 nm for the visible part of solar spectrum. Considering that short dUVB wavelengths are absorbed by the stratum corneum and by the very first layers of the epidermis, substances which absorb mainly below 300 nm and not above are not expected to be phototoxic *in vivo*. Consequently, it has been recommended (European Community Directive 2000/33, April 2000 [9]) that, for a coefficient of molar extinction (ε) of less than $10\,L\,mol^{-1}\,cm^{-1}$ in the solar domain, phototoxicity has not to be assessed. It should, however, be noticed first that a coefficient of molar extinction is generally defined for pure substances. Therefore, it is difficult to calculate these data for mixtures; furthermore, the degree of absorption may not be proportional to the phototoxic potential: low absorption does not mean low phototoxicity, thus, additional screening methods are necessary, even if ε is only slightly higher than $10\,L\,mol^{-1}\,cm^{-1}$.

19.3
In Silico Methods for Prediction of Phototoxicity – (Q)SAR Models

In silico methods differ depending on various criteria, two major ones being: (i) the way they are constructed (mechanism-based models versus statistical models); (ii) the chemical space they cover (global models built for non-congeneric sets of chemicals versus local models built for specific chemical classes with a common mechanism of action).

Only a limited number of reliable prediction tools are currently available for photoinduced toxicity. This is not surprising since establishing phototoxic potential is a complex task. Phototoxicity can be the consequence of various mechanisms such as photogeneration of reactive oxygen species, production of toxic photoproducts or sensitization of DNA damage by energy transfer. In addition, so far, there are no available universal descriptors (indicators) to predict the photodynamic potency of chemicals.

19.3.1
Global Models

A limited number of reliable global prediction tools are currently available for photoinduced toxicity. Derek for Windows (DfW) is one such system containing structural alerts for photoinduced toxicity. Sub-endpoints covered include: phototoxicity, photoallergenicity, photomutagenicity, photogenotoxicity, photoinduced chromosome damage, and photocarcinogenicity. The current version (DfW ver. 11.0.0) contains 20 alerts, some of which have been evaluated. Pelletier and Greene [10] performed an evaluation with DfW ver. 8.0 (12 alerts). They concluded that the predictive performance of DfW was reasonably good but there was room for improvement as many of these alerts had been developed with Barratt photoallergens [11]. New data relating to sub-endpoints mentioned above would help in refining and enlarging existing alerts.

19.3.2
Local Models

Some structure–activity relationship (SAR) studies have been performed on specific classes of chemicals, including fluoroquinolones, quinine derivatives, pyrroles, thiophenes and polycyclic aromatic hydrocarbons (PAHs).

In this context, interesting exhaustive QSAR studies dealing with the assessment of phototoxic hazards of PAHs to aquatic organisms such as *Daphnia* were published some years ago [12–14]. Authors chose a descriptor based on the energy difference between the highest occupied molecular orbital (HOMO) and the lowest unoccupied molecular orbital (LUMO). They proposed that aromatic chemicals with a HOMO-LUMO gap energy in a window of $7.2\,eV \pm 0.4\,eV$ have a high phototoxic potential.

These statements were confirmed in a study dealing with the substituent effects on PAH phototoxicity. Compounds with a HOMO-LUMO gap in the range 6.7–7.5 eV were predicted phototoxic [15]. Interestingly, they showed that the effect of most substituents (e.g., alkyl or hydroxyl) was negligible and that phototoxicity in PAHs depended essentially on the parent aromatic structure. However, substituents that added to delocalization of electron density (e.g., nitrochloro, alkenyl) could shift the HOMO-LUMO gap into the domain of potential phototoxicity. It should also be noticed that this predictive model was extended to more complex molecules other than PAHs: α-terthienyls and some substituted derivatives. The same QSAR model was further studied by Ribeiro *et al.* [16] who solved the problem of the nonlinear relationship between the electronic descriptors and phototoxicity by using exponential transformations and proposed a new scale for toxic compounds, particularly for PAHs, through a new gap range ($7.2 \pm 0.7\,eV$). To our knowledge, this HOMO-LUMO model has not been tested yet for a large panel of compounds such as those used for the validation of the *in vitro* phototoxicity test 3T3 NRU shown in Table 19.1, and no other QSAR studies were recently published using this approach.

Table 19.1 Chemical structures of some phototoxic compounds used in the 3T3 NRU validation.

Compound	Structure
5-MOP	
8-MOP	
Angelicin	
Anthracene	
Bithionol	
Nalidixic acid	
Norfloxacin	

Table 19.1 (Continued)

Ofloxacin	
Tiaprofenic acid	
Ketoprofen	
Fenofibrate	
Amiodarone	
Chlorpromazine	

Table 19.1 (Continued)

Compound	Structure
Promethazine	(phenothiazine with N-CH(CH3)-CH2-N(CH3)2 side chain)
Neutral red	(phenazine derivative: H3C-N(CH3)– ...–NH+ ...–NH2, Cl−, with CH3 substituent)
Demeclocycline	(tetracycline structure with Cl, OH, N(CH3)2, NH2, and multiple OH groups)

19.4
Photoreactivity *In Tubo*: Prescreening of Compounds Producing ROS Upon Sunlight Exposure

19.4.1
Biochemical Detection of Photoinduced ROS

As mentioned in the introduction, the main process leading to phototoxicity is the production of ROS such as $^1O_2$ or $O_2^{\bullet-}$ by a photoactivated substance after energy or electron transfer to oxygen.

Assays to detect reactive oxygen species (ROS) can be based on the analysis of changes in absorption of specific chromophores after photo oxidation. For instance, $^1O_2$ can be assessed by measuring the bleaching of pnitrosodimethylanilinein the presence of imidazole [17], whereas $O_2^{\bullet-}$ reduces nitrobluetetrazolium, and increases its absorbance at 560 nm [18]. A multiwell plate-based ROS assay was recently proposed as an adaptable approach to high-throughput screening HTS using such chemical detections [19]. Experimental conditions such as light intensity, temperature and nature of the solvent can significantly influence generation and detection of ROS in such a screening. However, this method can be convenient for evaluation of a large number of synthetic compounds. A second step using cells is necessary to check non-ROS-dependent phototoxicity, that is, direct photoreactivity or generation of toxic photoproducts.

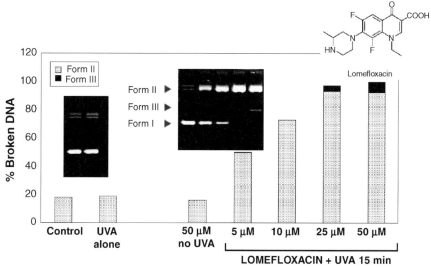

Figure 19.3 Use of supercoiled plasmid circular DNA for detection of ROS production by photo-activated lomefloxacin. Form I: supercoiled form (no DNA breaks); form II: relaxed form (few DNA single strand breaks); form III: linear form (high level of DNA single strand breaks leading to double strand breaks; see [38]).

19.4.2
Photo-Cleavage of Isolated Plasmid DNA

The high reactivity of ROS towards biomolecules (unsaturated lipids, DNA, proteins) can be used to evaluate in tubo the photoreactivity of substances absorbing in the sunlight range. For example, circular supercoiled DNA is a sensitive tool for detecting oxidative damage. In fact, just one single break in the DNA backbone (either induced directly by ROS or produced after excision of damaged bases or nucleotides by specific DNA repair enzymes) is sufficient to convert supercoiled plasmid into relaxed plasmid. Both forms may easily be separated and quantified by agarose gel electrophoresis.

This test does not require expensive equipment and permits screening of many compounds in a single day. It has been used for drugs such as fluoroquinolones as shown in Figure 19.3 [20–22], and even for insoluble pigments such as titanium dioxide [23, 24]. Poorly water-soluble chemicals can be tested as dispersions in organic solvents added to the buffer. However, solvents that may scavenge ROS (e.g., DMSO, ethanol) should be avoided, whereas acetone or acetonitrile are preferable.

19.4.3
Photo Red Blood Cells Test

The red blood cell phototoxicity test (photo-RBC test) is based on the ability of a light-activated substance to produce lysis of freshly isolated erythrocytes and to oxidize hemoglobin to oxyhemoglobin. Changes in optical density at 525 nm for photoinduced hemolysis (suggesting release of hemoglobin) and at 630 nm for methemoglobin formation are used to predict the phototoxic potential. In spite of a low specificity and low negative predictivity, a good overall *in vitro/in vivo* correlation was reported in prevalidation studies [25]. Given that erythrocytes may be considered as biomembranes containing hemoglobin, the photo-RBC test is an interesting system to obtain information on photooxidation/photoinduced changes of lipids and proteins during the photodynamic process. Erythrocytes may be exposed to more intense UV irradiation than other mammalian cells and are not susceptible to photogenotoxic effects since they do not contain a nucleus. The main limitation of this test is the supply of erythrocytes from animal blood and the difficulty to preserve them for a long time in the laboratory.

19.5
Microbiological Models for Photomutagenesis Assessment

19.5.1
Photo-Ames Test

Microbiological models (bacteria or yeast cells) are very convenient because they are cheap, easy to use and can tolerate chemicals with various physical/chemical properties. In order to assess photogenotoxicity, an extension of the Ames test, used already as a regulatory test for assessment of mutagenesis in the dark, is one possibility. However, the test encounters some difficulties, such as the high UV sensitivity of the DNA repair-deficient strains used and the inconvenient protocol for evaluating cytotoxicity. Moreover, the bacterial model cannot detect photoinduced recombination triggered by high levels of DNA damage such as double-strand breaks and inter-strand crosslinks. As a consequence, the use of the bacterial mutation assay under somewhat "realistic" UV exposure conditions (i.e., with a solar simulator providing attenuated UVB and total UVA radiation) is restricted to excision-proficient strains such as *Salmonella typhimurium* TA102 or *Escherichia coli* WP2 [26–28]. A recent paper described the use of *E. coli* Dh5α strain to assess the phototoxicity of drugs or cosmetic products in combination with an agar gel diffusion assay in order to test antibiotics [29]. A few publications described methods where test substances were irradiated prior to incubation with bacteria. This approach can be useful if stable genotoxic compounds are produced during exposure, but it fails to detect short-lived photoproducts.

19.5.2
The Yeast Model

The yeast *Saccharomyces cerevisiae* is a useful microbiological alternative to bacteria, especially in the field of photobiology [30–32]. Several endpoints such as colony-forming ability (lethal effects), nuclear and cytoplasmic mutations (reversion due to

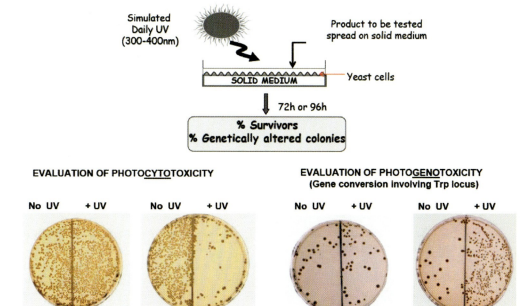

Figure 19.4 Experimental procedure for the assessment of phototoxicity of formulations using the yeast assay. Formulations are spread on agar previously seeded by yeast cells. Photocytotoxicity is assessed by colonies counting after growth on complete medium, whereas genetically altered colonies (here gene conversion involving the tryptophan locus) are detected using selective growth medium (here tryptophan-free), [39].

genomic mutations, or "petite" mutation due to damage to mitochondrial DNA) as well as genetic recombination can be studied in a single set of experiments. Very different kinds of products, including galenic formulations (ethanolic or oily solutions, cosmetic formulations), may be spread over solid media, which is useful for substances that are not easily dissolved in aqueous buffers or hardly mixed with top agar used in the Ames test. The *Saccharomyces* test is thus not restricted to pure ingredients. Similar approaches based on diffusion of test chemicals from a paper disc placed upon agar were previously described for fragrance materials or psoralen-containing products [33–35]. The yeast phototoxicity test is particularly convenient for detection of furocoumarins such as psoralens in perfumes or in any formulation containing fragrance ingredients [36].

As shown in Figure 19.4, the D7 strain of *S. cerevisiae* is a particularly useful tool because of its ability to assess various genotoxic events such as intergenic and intragenic mitotic recombination as well as point mutagenesis [37, 38]. In a recent paper, we showed that the D7 yeast strain could detect the phototoxicity of most of chemicals used in the validated phototoxicity test 3T3 NRU, except the antibiotics domeclocycline and lomefloxacin, that is, substances that are difficult to evaluate in the Ames test due to their anti-bacterial activity. Interestingly, the yeast assay was sensitive enough to detect traces of furocoumarins (a few ppm) in commercial fragrances as well as in a cosmetic formulation [39]. This approach could be used as a prescreening method in order to reduce the number of compounds to be tested on mammalian cells in culture and even to confirm or support chemical analysis of perfumed materials used in skin care products.

19.6
Photocytotoxicity and Photogenotoxicity in Mammalian Cells: Regulatory Tests and Beyond

19.6.1
The 3T3 NRU Assay: a Validated Test for the Assessment of a Photoirritation Potential

Much research has been invested to identify a common and validated test method that may be used in all industrial laboratories concerned by phototoxicology. Cultured mammalian cells constitute an essential model for the evaluation of phototoxicity. Such systems include all biological targets (lipids in membranes, proteins, nucleic acids) as well as active pathways likely to modulate the phototoxic impact (apoptotic pathways, cellular defenses, endogenous antioxidants, repair pathways, metabolism).

The phototoxicity test 3T3 NRU was proposed in 1994 and is so far the only *in vitro* method that has been validated by European regulatory authorities for predicting the photoirritant potential of substances [5, 40, 41]. In this test, the mouse fibroblasts cell line Balb/c 3T3 is exposed to simulated solar UV (or, more frequently, solar UVA) in the presence of the test compound after an incubation of 1 h in the dark. Evaluation of cytotoxicity is performed 24 h post-exposure using the neutral red uptake (NRU) method. NRU permits to distinguish live and dead cells, since intact cells retain this dye (detailed method in INVITOX protocol 78). The validation was performed with substances selected on the basis of their *in vivo* photoirritant or phototoxic properties. Some of these structures are shown in Table 19.1.

The classification of substances in the 3T3 NRU test is based on the photo irritation factor (PIF), defined as the ratio between cytotoxicity in the dark versus cytotoxicity in the presence of UV: $PIF = IC_{50} (dark)/IC_{50} (+UV)$. A substance is considered as photoirritant when its PIF exceeds a value of 5, and as a possible photoirritant when $2 < PIF < 5$. Interestingly, the 3T3NRU test is able to correctly predict phototoxicity of poorly water-soluble compounds: interactions between substances and biomembranes appear more important than their water solubility. However, some questions may be raised when comparing chemicals with different physicochemical properties. For example, UV screening effects may occur due to light absorption of the buffer containing water-soluble chemicals, or the density of the compound (e.g., oily solutions) may affect their availability to the test cells. Most likely, the 3T3 NRU test mainly measures the phototoxic impact of test substances on membranes, although damage to proteins or DNA may also lead to cell death. For this reason some researchers consider that the 3T3 NRU test is sufficiently reactive to also permit the evaluation of a photogenotoxic or photoallergic potential of substances.

The 3T3 NRU test may easily be performed under GLP conditions in contract research organizations (CROs); and a high-throughput screening (HTS) method was recently reported in the literature. The HTS method produced no false positives, although some false negatives were observed, suggesting that the standard 3T3 NRU test protocol remains necessary for the final selection of nonphototoxic compounds [42].

Although very convenient, the 3T3 NRU test has some limitations. First, Balb/c 3T3 fibroblasts are neither human nor normal cells. Therefore, the extrapolation of test results to responses of the human epidermis is sometimes problematic, especially for compounds displaying borderline phototoxicity ($2 < PIF < 5$). For example, it was shown that the susceptibility to the phototoxicity of low concentrations of lomefloxacin varies according to skin cell types: keratinocytes being the most sensitive, possibly due to their higher susceptibility to enter apoptosis in response to photogenotoxicity [43]. In contrast, keratinocytes were shown to be more resistant to bithionol-induced phototoxicity when compared with that predicted from the 3T3 NRU test. This discrepancy may be due to higher glutathione levels of keratinocytes when compared with those in Balb/C 3T3 fibroblasts, resulting in a higher capacity of keratinocytes to detoxify electrophilic substances [44]. A study comparing the phototoxicity of substances used in the validation study in 3T3 fibroblast and human keratinocytes concluded that both cell types yielded comparable results, except that keratinocytes were able to produce cytokines in response to phototoxic stress, which could yield additional and potentially more sensitive test endpoints than cytotoxicity and cell death alone [45]. Second, with PIF values between 2 and 5, it is difficult to determine whether the test substance is acceptable in terms of safety. Such results suggest that, although the substance may be photoactivated, it produces few toxic effects. In such cases, our laboratory investigates phototoxicity in normal human keratinocytes and normal human fibroblasts using two different methods for cytotoxicity assessment (MTT assay, NRU assay).

19.6.2
Photogenotoxicity: an Endpoint Without Corresponding *In Vivo* Equivalents

It is well established that solar radiation causes genotoxic effects as a consequence of DNA damage induced mainly by UVA and UVB. UVB absorption induces pyrimidine dimers which are mutagenic lesions, whereas UVA essentially produces oxidative damage such as strand breaks or oxidative base damage, such as 8-oxo-dG, which contribute to genomic instability. Exposure to high UV doses from sunlight or chronic exposures are an important risk factor for skin cancer development [46]. Numerous studies have reported that some photoreactive compounds could strongly enhance the DNA-damaging impact of low UV doses. Unfortunately, current knowledge does not provide genuine *in vivo* evidence on substance- or drug-induced photocarcinogenesis that would be necessary to establish a relevant validation for *in vitro* photogenotoxicity testing.

Clinical data from drugs used in phototherapy suggest that some may produce photocarcinogenic effects in humans, in particular psoralens such as 8-methoxypsoralene (8-MOP) used in PUVA therapy for treatment of vitiligo or psoriasis. However, little is known about adverse effects of other photogenotoxic compounds, especially those inducing oxidative damage. The analysis of photocarcinogenic effects is also limited by the fact that in current *in vivo* (hairless mice) models, the actual carcinogen is UV light, whereas the main endpoints are the time of appearance and number/severity of UV-induced skin tumors. Therefore, the test is unable to distinguish between genuine photocarcinogenicity (substance in combination with UV light producing skin tumors) and photo(co)carcinogenicity (substance promoting UV induced skin tumors). Among published data, the fluoroquinolone lomefloxacin was shown to be photocarcinogenic and/or photo(co)carcinogenic in mice [47], possibly due to its ability to photosensitize the formation of mutagenic pyrimidine dimers by UVA [43, 48]. Similarly, data were published on basal cell carcinoma induced by amiodarone, a phototoxic anti-arrhythmic drug [49, 50]. In this context, recommendations for the assessment of photogenotoxicity were issued by ECVAM and the European Medical Agency [41, 51]. However, the current paucity of experimental or epidemiological data defining thresholds (absorption, chemical structure, photochemical or photogenotoxic activity) was recently reviewed [52].

In addition to tests yielding information about the ability of a substance to damage DNA upon UV exposure (plasmid DNA) or to produce mutations in prokaryotic or eukaryotic systems (bacteria and/or yeast cells), methods in mammalian cells are necessary. Maybe one of the most appropriate tests using cultured cells is the comet assay that was first described more than 20 years ago [53]. In this assay, treated cells are embedded in an agarose microgel (generally on slides used for microscopy), lysed and subjected to alkaline electrophoresis. Damaged DNA generates fragments as the consequence of direct breakage by reactive species such as ROS (especially OH$^{\bullet}$) or as a result of incisions produced during the first step of endogenous DNA repair. After electrophoresis and staining with fluorescent dyes, the migration of DNA and DNA fragments produces a characteristic comet shape: the comet head is formed by the bulk of undamaged genomic DNA, whereas the comet tail contains fragments resulting from DNA breakage migrating away from the nucleus. Comets can be quantified using image analysis software measuring the distance of DNA migration and the fluorescence intensity of the comet tail (see Figures 19.5 and 19.6 for the impact of lomefloxacin on human keratinocytes).

The comet assay is increasingly used in genotoxicity testing and is being validated; a guideline for its conduct has been proposed [51, 53]. Furthermore, specific DNA repair enzymes may be used in this test, in order to investigate the presence of specific DNA damage such as 8-oxoguanine using the repair enzyme FPG [54]. The photocomet assay was predominantly used to study photogenotoxicity of fluoroquinolones, and the results published by different laboratories were in good agreement even for different cell types. It should be noted that furocoumarins such as 8-MOP and 5-MOP had negative results in the photocomet assay, probably due to their DNA

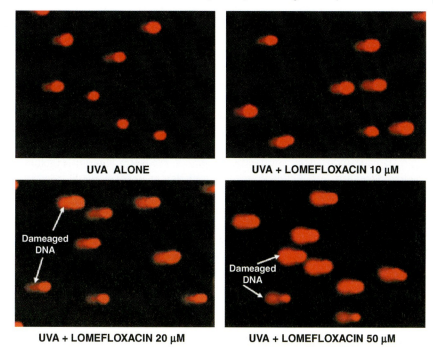

Figure 19.5 Visualization of DNA damage induction in cultured human keratinocytes by photo-activated lomefloxacin using the comet assay. The presence of DNA breaks (induced either by ROS or by excision of DNA lesions) leads to fragmentation and electrophoretic migration to produce the comet tails, whereas bulky genomic DNA remains in the comets heads.

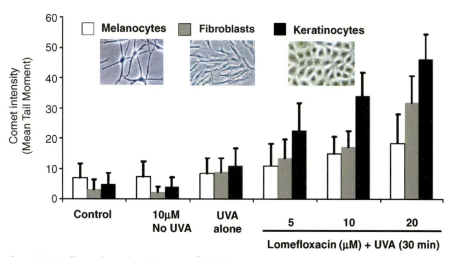

Figure 19.6 Cell type-dependent induction of DNA damage as revealed by the comet assay performed on melanocytes, fibroblasts and keratinocytes (see [43]).

cross-linking activity under UVA exposure, which would prevent the migration of fragments during single cell electrophoresis. Other compounds tested in this assay, (including the NSAID tiaprofenic acid [55], chlorpromazine, tetracyclines, titanium dioxide [23]) gave positive results, and recent papers proposed a protocol based on a 96-well plate HTS comet assay in which various chemicals were tested [56, 57]. Overall, the photocomet assay has the potential to become a rapid screening method for the detection of photogenotoxic potential of substances, especially for those with a borderline photocytotoxic potential in the 3T3 NRU test.

However, even when taking into account that the photocomet assay is able to detect DNA damage induced by substances under UV exposure, it is not a genuine photomutagenesis test. Although an increased risk of mutagenesis is associated with high induction of DNA lesions, the type of these lesions is of great importance: for example, DNA adducts tend to be more mutagenic than DNA single-strand breaks. Thus, there is the need for additional tests in regulatory test batteries clarifying these questions, such as *in vitro* photo-micronucleus or -chromosomal aberration tests, which may obtain more pertinent conclusions on the photogenotoxic potential of test substances. These tests assess the photoclastogenicity of a compound, that is, its ability to induce chromosomal damage upon UV exposure, at doses where irradiation itself displays no or only a very slight adverse effect.

A protocol for the *in vitro* micronucleus test in the dark has been established using Chinese hamster V79 cells and is currently being validated [58, 59]. An adaptation of this test including exposure to appropriate UV radiation was proposed as an *in vitro* approach for photogenotoxicity assessment [60, 61]. The photoclastogenic potential of different photosensitizers has been investigated. For example, some furocoumarins (5-MOP, angelicin), the NSAID tiaprofenic acid, the fluoroquinolone lomefloxacin and chlorpromazine were found to induce micronuclei when exposed to UV. Interestingly, photogenotoxic compounds consistently showed photocytotoxic activity, but not vice versa. For example, the NSAID ketoprofen which is strongly photocytotoxic was negative in the photo-micronucleus test [61].

The test for photoinduced chromosomal aberrations (CA) is another suitable alternative for photogenotoxicity assessment. The clastogenic effects of 8-MOP or 5-MOP under UV irradiation, but not in the dark, in these test systems have been known for many years [30, 62]. More recently, a large study on quinolones using this method has been published [63]. However, this method is relatively labor-intensive.

Finally, all photogenotoxic tests do not have a corresponding *in vivo* model, which raises the question how positive *in vitro* results could be clarified. There is an urgent need for development of suitable, short-term models that may validate positive *in vitro* data.

19.7
Reconstructed Skin: a Model for Mimicking Phototoxicity in the Target Organ

To overcome the limitations of cells in culture, the use of reconstructed skin models is an interesting alternative. Several studies have reported their capacity to predict photoirritancy [64–70]. In contrast to the 3T3-NRU test, reconstructed skin allows topical application of compounds with different physicochemical properties, such as water-insolubility or substances with extreme pH values, finished cosmetic products or complex formulations.

Moreover, by their three-dimensional (3-D) structure involving intercellular communication, the presence of an (albeit weakened) barrier function (stratum corneum) and an extracellular matrix, these models derived from human skin cells resemble the actual target organ. Indeed, previous studies on reconstructed skin models have shown their ability to confirm or rebut positive results of the 3T3 NRU phototoxicity test [42, 71]. Moreover, chemicals can be evaluated in conditions closed to their use in humans: they can be added to the culture medium when drugs are supposed to reach skin by the systemic route or applied to the surface of the reconstructed epidermis in order to mimic topical skin applications of substances. In the latter case, the influence of penetration on phototoxicity can be checked, even if the barrier function of reconstructed skin is generally weaker than that of human skin [72, 73]. Histology can be performed on exposed and control samples, which may generate additional data on the (photo)toxic impact on skin structures. In a prevalidation study, an appropriate test protocol has been proposed which may be suitable for assessment of the potency of topically applied phototoxic substances in reconstructed skin models [74]. Due to technical difficulties (in particular, the interaction between neutral red and collagen matrix that interferes with the colorimetric analysis), the MTT assay was chosen instead of neutral red uptake (NRU) for assessing phototoxicity on reconstructed epidermis. The MTT assay is based on the conversion of the MTT by the mitochondrial dehydrogenase activity of viable cells. However, some chemicals may either directly reduce MTT or stimulate mitochondrial activity leading to false negative results. In a recent paper, where 17 chemicals were tested, Lelièvre et al. [75] proposed to combine the MTT assay with the measurement of the pro-inflammatorycytokine IL-1α to overcome this limitation.

Reconstructed skin models may also be used to study photogenotoxicity. In fact, the comet assay was recently adapted to such models, using a specific technique, that is, dissociation and separation of keratinocytes after UV exposure of the reconstructed epidermis. Using a mixture of specific enzymes cocktail, it was possible to obtain suspension of cells without damaging them. For instance, the photocomet assay could be successfully performed for lomefloxacin after UVA exposure of reconstructed epidermis [76], as shown in Figure 19.7.

Finally, use of more complex models is in progress. For example, Lee et al. [77] studied the phototoxic impact of chemicals on reconstructed skin models that were prepared from cultured keratinocytes and melanocytes on de-epidermized dermis. The authors claimed that a pigmented epidermis showed a stronger resistance to UVA and possesses a photobiological response closer to *in vivo* human skin. Considering that pigmented reconstructed epidermis has become commercially available, one might envisage that such models will be more and more studied and used. Possibly, stimulation of melanogenesis in response to inflammation may become an interesting marker to evaluate chemical-induced phototoxic stress. Development of other models including Langerhans cells is in progress. These

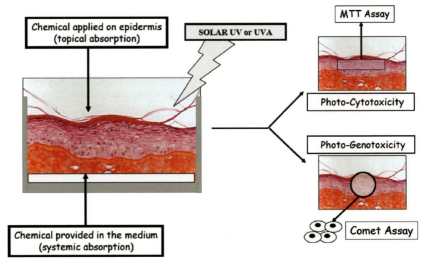

Figure 19.7 Experimental procedure for the assessment of photo-cytotoxicity (MTT assay) and photo-genotoxicity (comet assay) on reconstructed epidermis. Drugs or formulations can be applied on the skin surface (topical route) or provided in the culture medium (systemic route; see [76]).

innovative models could lead to future, highly sophisticated screening techniques for photosensitizers. Reconstructed skin models are not expected to totally replace the use of cultured cells given their substantial costs and the complex experimental design. However, they are becoming essential as a final step in phototoxicity screening (particularly for "borderline" phototoxicity and for formulations applied on skin surface), allowing the performance of experiments in more realistic conditions resembling those of human skin.

19.8
Conclusions

Light-mediated adverse effects reported by dermatologists stress the importance to evaluate the phototoxic potential of substances or drugs that come into contact with areas of the skin likely to be exposed to sunlight. In response, during recent years, methods for the assessment of phototoxic hazards have been developed. Today, it is possible to define screening strategies involving complementary *in vitro* models. This should prevent phototoxicity-related problems in the future, in particular in a context where *in vivo* experiments will be banned (European regulation for cosmetic industry, seventh amendment). Although it is possible that different strategies will be developed by different laboratories, we propose the *in vitro* strategy shown in Scheme 19.1.

The use of *in tubo* tests or microbiological models could be helpful when a large number of chemicals needs to be screened. The 3T3 NRU test remains central for

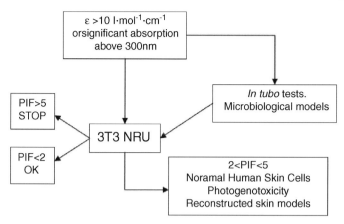

Scheme 19.1

phototoxicity testing. However, assessment of photogenotoxicity and use of reconstructed skin models will be necessary when results obtained in the 3T3NRU test are ambiguous.

In the future, more accurate *in silico* methods will hopefully become available in order to orientate chemical synthesis. Moreover, some new approaches should be developed or improved such as the detection of photoallergic potential and the production of more sophisticated industrial reconstructed skin models.

Acknowledgments

The authors deeply acknowledge: (i) R. Note and S. Ringensen (L'OREAL Safety Research Department, Aulnay, France) for their precious advice in writing the section about *in silico* models; (ii) F. Christiaens (L'OREAL Applied Research, Clichy, France) for his help about optical considerations; (iii) A. Labarussiat (L'OREAL Safety Research Department, Aulnay, France) for her important contribution in preparing the final manuscript; (iv) D. Averbeck (Institut Curie, Orsay, France) for critical reading of the manuscript.

References

1 Ferguson, J. (2002) Photosensitivity due to drugs photodermatol. *Photoimmunology & Photomedicine*, **18**, 262–269.
2 Moore, D.E. (2002) Drug-induced cutaneous photosensitivity: incidence, mechanism, prevention and management. *Drug Safety*, **25**, 345–372.
3 Kochevar, I.E. (1995) Photoimmunology: primary processes, in *Photobiology and Photosensitization*, Blackwell Sciences, Oxford, pp. 19–33.
4 Moore, D.E. (1998) Mechanisms of photosensitization by phototoxic drugs. *Mutation Research*, **422**, 165–173.

5 Spielmann, H., Balls, M., Dupuis, J., Pape, W.J., Pechovitch, G., De Silva, O., Holzhutter, H.G., Clothier, R. et al. (1998) The international EU/COLIPA in vitro phototoxicity validation study: results of phase II (blind trial). Part 1: the 3T3 NRU phototoxicity test. *Toxicology In Vitro: An International Journal Published in Association with BIBRA*, **12**, 305–327.

6 Commission directive 67/548/EEC: 3T3 NRU phototoxicity test Regulation: included into Annex V of Council Directive 67/548/EEC part B.41 on phototoxicity in April 2000; and OECD Test Guideline 432, adopted April 2004.

7 OECD (2004) *In Vitro* 3T3 NRU Phototoxicity. Guideline TG 432. Revised and approved by the National Co-ordinators in May 2002, approved by Council April 2004. Organization for Economic Coopération and Development, Paris.

8 Christiaens, F.J., Chardon, A., Fourtanier, A. and Frederick, J.E. (2005) Standard ultraviolet daylight for non extreme exposure conditions. *Photochemistry and Photobiology*, **81**, 874–878.

9 Commission directive 2000/33/EC of 25 april 2000 adapting to technical progress for the 27th time Council Directive 67/548 E on the classification, packaging and labeling of dangerous substance, 2000. Annex V method B41 phototoxicity – *in vitro* 3T3 NRU phototoxicity test. Official Journal of the European Communities L136, 90.

10 Pelletier, D. and Greene, N. (2007) Evaluation of phototoxicity alerts in DEREK and use of a fingerprint-based decision tree approach to identify potential novel alerts. *The Toxicologist*, **96**, 223.

11 Barratt, M.D. (2004) Structure-activity relationships and prediction of the phototoxicity and phototoxic potential of new drugs. *Alternatives to Laboratory Animals*, **32**, 511–524.

12 Newsted, J. and Giesy, J. (1987) Predictive models for photoinduced acute toxicity of polycyclic aromatic hydrocarbons to Daphnia Magna, strauss (Cladocera, crustacea). *Environmental Toxicology and Chemistry/SETAC*, **6**, 445–461.

13 Mekenyan, O.G., Ankley, G.T., Veith, G.D. and Call, D.J. (1994) QSARs for photoinduced toxicity: 1. Acute lethality of polycyclic aromatic hydrocarbons to Daphnia Magna. *Chemosphere*, **28**, 567–582.

14 Lampi, M.A., Gurska, J., Huang, X.D., Dixon, D.G. and Greenberg, B.M. (2007) A predictive quantitative structure-activity relationship model for the photoinduced toxicity of polycyclic aromatic hydrocarbons to Daphnia magna with the use of factors for photosensitization and photomodification. *Environmental Toxicology and Chemistry/SETAC*, **26**, 406–415.

15 Veith, G.D., Mekenyan, O.G., Ankley, G.T. and Call, D.J. (1995) A QSAR analysis of substituent effects on the photoinduced acute toxicity of PAHs. *Chemosphere*, **30**, 2129–2142.

16 Alves De Lima Ribeiros, F. and Castro Ferreira, M. (2005) QSAR model of the phototoxicity of polycyclic aromatic hydrocarbons. *Journal of Molecular Structure*, **719**, 191–200.

17 Kraljic, I. and El Mohsni, S. (1978) A new method for the detection of singlet oxygen in aqueous solutions. *Photochemistry and Photobiology*, **28**, 577–581.

18 Pathak, M.A. and Joshi, P.C. (1984) Production of active oxygen species ($1O_2$ and O_2-.) by psoralens and ultraviolet radiation (320–400 nm). *Biochimica et Biophysica Acta*, **798**, 115–126.

19 Onoue, S. and Tsuda, Y. (2006) Analytical studies on the prediction of photosensitive/phototoxic potential of pharmaceutical substances. *Pharmaceutical Research*, **23**, 156–164.

20 Martinez, L. and Chignell, C.F. (1998) Photocleavage of DNA by the fluoro-quinolone antibacterials. *Journal of Photochemistry and Photobiology. B, Biology*, **45**, 51–59.

21 Marrot, L. and Agapakis-Causse, C. (2000) Differences in the photogenotoxic potential of two fluoroquinolones as shown in diploid yeast strain (Saccharomyces cerevisae) and supercoiled plasmid DNA. *Mutation Research*, **468**, 1–9.

22 Viola, G., Facciolo, L., Dall'Acqua, S., Di Lisa, F., Canton, M., Vedaldi, D., Fravolini, A., Tabarrini, O. et al. (2004) 6-Aminoquinolones: photostability, cellular distribution and phototoxicity. *Toxicology In Vitro: An International Journal Published in Association with BIBRA*, **18**, 581–592.

23 Dunford, R., Salinaro, A., Cai, L., Serpone, N., Horikoshi, S., Hidaka, H. and Knowland, J. (1997) Chemical oxidation and DNA damage catalysed by inorganic sunscreen ingredients. *FEBS Letters*, **418**, 87–90.

24 Ashikaga, T., Wada, M., Kobayashi, H., Mori, M., Katsumura, Y., Fukui, H., Kato, S., Yamaguchi, M. et al. (2000) Effect of the photocatalytic activity of TiO2 on plasmid DNA. *Mutation Research*, **466**, 1–7.

25 Pape, W.J., Maurer, T., Pfannenbecker, U. and Steiling, W. (2001) The red blood cell phototoxicity test (photohaemolysis and haemoglobin oxidation): EU/COLIPA validation programme on phototoxicity (phase II). *Alternatives to Laboratory Animals*, **29**, 145–162.

26 Dean, S.W., Lane, M., Dunmore, R.H., Ruddock, S.P., Martin, C.N., Kirkland, D.J. and Loprieno, N. (1991) Development of assays for the detection of photomutagenicity of chemicals during exposure to UV light–I. *Assay development, Mutagenesis*, **6**, 335–341.

27 Henderson, L., Fedyk, J., Bourner, C., Windebank, S., Fletcher, S. and Lovell, W. (1994) Photomutagenicity assays in bacteria: factors affecting assay design and assessment of photomutagenic potential of para-aminobenzoic acid. *Mutagenesis*, **9**, 459–465.

28 Gocke, E. (2001) Photochemical mutagenesis: examples and toxicological relevance. *Journal of Environmental Pathology, Toxicology and Oncology*, **20**, 285–292.

29 Verma, K., Agrawal, N., Misra, R.B., Farooq, M. and Hans, R.K. (2008) Phototoxicity assessment of drugs and cosmetic products using E. coli. *Toxicology In Vitro: An International Journal Published in Association with BIBRA*, **22**, 249–253.

30 Chetelat, A., Albertini, S., Dresp, J.H., Strobel, R. and Gocke, E. (1993) Photomutagenesis test development: I. 8-Methoxypsoralen, chlorpromazine and sunscreen compounds in bacterial and yeast assays. *Mutation Research*, **292**, 241–250.

31 Moysan, A., Miranda, M.A., Morlière, P., Peno-Mazzarino, L., Averbeck, D., Averbeck, S., Clément-Lacroix, P. et al. (1994) *Utilisation of In Vitro Techniques in the Evaluation of Phototoxicity of New Compounds*, IOS Press, pp. 85–105.

32 Marrot, L., Belaidi, J.P., Chaubo, C., Meunier, J.R., Perez, P. and Agapakis-Causse, C. (1998) An *in vitro* strategy to evaluate the phototoxicity of solar UV at the molecular and cellular level: application to photoprotection assessment. *European Journal of Dermatology*, **8**, 403–412.

33 Weinberg, E.H. and Springer, S.T. (1981) A quantitative *in vitro* assay for the evaluation of phototoxic potential of topically applied materials. *Journal of Society of Cosmetic Chemists*, **32**, 303–315.

34 Tenenbaum, S., DiNardo, J., Morris, W.E., Wolf, B.A. and Schnetzinger, R.W. (1984) A quantitative *in vitro* assay for the evaluation of phototoxic potential of topically applied materials. *Cell Biology and Toxicology*, **1**, 1–9.

35 Sugiyama, M., Itagaki, H. and Kato, S. (1994) Photohemolysis test and yeast growth inhibition assay to assess phototoxic potential of chemicals, in *Alternative Methods in Toxicology* (eds A. Rougier, A.M. Goldberg and H.I. Maibach), Mary Ann Liebert, Inc., NY, **10**, pp. 213–221.

36 Averbeck, D., Averbeck, S., Dubertret, L., Young, A.R. and Morliere, P. (1990)

Genotoxicity of bergapten and bergamot oil in Saccharomyces cerevisiae. *Journal of Photochemistry and Photobiology. B, Biology*, **7**, 209–229.

37 Zimmermann, F.K., Kern, R. and Rasenberger, H.A. (1975) Yeast strain for simultaneous detection of induced mitotic crossing over, mitotic gene conversion and reverse mutation. *Mutation Research*, **28**, 381–388.

38 Marrot, L., Belaidi, J.P., Chaubo, C., Meunier, J.R., Perez, P. and Agapakis-Causse, C. (2001) Fluoroquinolones as chemical tools to define a strategy for photogenotoxicity *in vitro* assessment. *Toxicology In Vitro: An International Journal Published in Association with BIBRA*, **15**, 131–142.

39 Marrot, L., Labarussiat, A., Perez, P. and Meunier, J.R. (2006) Use of the yeast Saccharomyces cerevisiae as a pre-screening approach for assessment of chemical-induced phototoxicity. *Toxicology In Vitro: An International Journal Published in Association with BIBRA*, **20**, 1040–1050.

40 Spielmann, H., Lowell, W.W., Hölzle, E. et al. (1994) *In vitro* phototoxicity testing. The report and recommendations of ECVAM workshop 2. *Alternatives to Laboratory Animals*, **22**, 314–348.

41 Spielmann, H., Muller, L., Averbeck, D., Balls, M., Brendler-Schwaab, S., Castell, J.V., Curren, R., De Silva, O. et al. (2000) The second ECVAM workshop on phototoxicity testing. The report and recommendations of ECVAM workshop 42. *Alternatives to Laboratory Animals*, **28**, 777–814.

42 Jones, P.A. and King, A.V. (2003) High throughput screening (HTS) for phototoxicity hazard using the *in vitro* 3T3 neutral red uptake assay. *Toxicology In Vitro: An International Journal Published in Association with BIBRA*, **17**, 703–708.

43 Marrot, L., Belaidi, J.P., Jones, C., Perez, P., Riou, L., Sarasin, A. and Meunier, J.R. (2003) Molecular responses to photogenotoxic stress induced by the antibiotic lomefloxacin in human skin cells: from DNA damage to apoptosis. *The Journal of Investigative Dermatology*, **121**, 596–606.

44 Reid, L., Clothier, R.H. and Khammo, N. (2001) Hydrogen peroxide induced stress in human keratinocytes and its effect on bithionol toxicity. *Toxicology In Vitro: An International Journal Published in Association with BIBRA*, **15**, 441–445.

45 Clothier, R., Willshaw, A., Cox, H., Garle, M., Bowler, H. and Combes, R. (1999) The use of human keratinocytes in the EU/COLIPA international *in vitro* phototoxicity test validation study and the ECVAM/COLIPA study on UV filter chemicals. *Alternatives to Laboratory Animals*, **27**, 247–259.

46 IARC (1992) Solar and ultraviolet radiation. *IARC Monographs on the Evaluation of Carcinogenic Risks to Humans*, **55**, 1–316.

47 Klecak, G., Urbach, F. and Urwyler, H. (1997) Fluoroquinolone antibacterials enhance UVA-induced skin tumors. *Journal of Photochemistry and Photobiology B, Biology*, **37**, 174–181.

48 Traynor, N.J. and Gibbs, N.K. (1999) The phototumorigenic fluoroquinolone lomefloxacin photosensitizes pyrimidine dimer formation in human keratinocytes *in vitro*. *Photochemistry and Photobiology*, **70**, 957–959.

49 Monk, B.E. (1990) Amiodarone-induced photosensitivity and basal-cell carcinoma. *Clinical and Experimental Dermatology*, **15**, 319–320.

50 Monk, B.E. (1995) Basal cell carcinoma following amiodarone therapy. *The British Journal of Dermatology*, **133**, 148–149.

51 EMEA (2002) note for guidance on photo safety testing.

52 Brendler-Schwaab, S., Czich, A., Epe, B., Gocke, E., Kaina, B., Muller, L., Pollet, D. and Utesch, D. (2004) Photochemical genotoxicity: principles and test methods. Report of a GUM task force. *Mutation Research*, **566**, 65–91.

53 Tice, R.R., Agurell, E., Anderson, D., Burlinson, B., Hartmann, A., Kobayashi,

H., Miyamae, Y., Rojas, E. et al. (2000) Single cell gel/comet assay: guidelines for in vitro and in vivo genetic toxicology testing. *Environmental and Molecular Mutagenesis*, **35**, 206–221.
54 Marrot, L., Belaidi, J.P. and Meunier, J.R. (2005) Importance of UVA photoprotection as shown by genotoxic related endpoints: DNA damage and p53 status. *Mutation Research*, **571**, 175–184.
55 Agapakis-Causse, C., Bosca, F., Castell, J.V., Hernandez, D., Marin, M.L., Marrot, L. and Miranda, M.A. (2000) Tiaprofenic acid-photosensitized damage to nucleic acids: a mechanistic study using complementary in vitro approaches. *Photochemistry and Photobiology*, **71**, 499–505.
56 Kiskinis, E., Suter, W. and Hartmann, A. (2002) High throughput Comet assay using 96-well plates. *Mutagenesis*, **17**, 37–43.
57 Struwe, M., Greulich, K.O., Suter, W. and Plappert-Helbig, U. (2007) The photo comet assay–a fast screening assay for the determination of photogenotoxicity in vitro. *Mutation Research*, **632**, 44–57.
58 Kirsch-Volders, M., Sofuni, T., Aardema, M., Albertini, S., Eastmond, D., Fenech, M., Ishidate, M., Lorge, E. et al. (2000) Report from the in vitro micronucleus assay working group. *Environmental and Molecular Mutagenesis*, **35**, 167–172.
59 Von der Hude, W., Kalweit, S., Engelhardt, G., McKiernan, S., Kasper, P., Slacik-Erben, R., Miltenburger, H.G., Honarvar, N. et al. (2000) In vitro micronucleus assay with Chinese hamster V79 cells – results of a collaborative study with in situ exposure to 26 chemical substances. *Mutation Research*, **468**, 137–163.
60 Gocke, E., Muller, L., Guzzie, P.J., Brendler-Schwaab, S., Bulera, S., Chignell, C.F., Henderson, L.M. et al. (2000) Considerations on photochemical genotoxicity: report of the international workshop on genotoxicity test procedures working group. *Environmental and Molecular Mutagenesis*, **35**, 173–184.

61 Kersten, B., Kasper, P., Brendler-Schwaab, S.Y. and Muller, L. (2002) Use of the photomicronucleus assay in Chinese hamster V79 cells to study photochemical genotoxicity. *Mutation Research*, **519**, 49–66.
62 Natarajan, A.T., Verdegaal-Immerzeel, E.A.M., Ashwood-Smith, M.J. and Poulton, G.A. (1981) Chromosomal damage induced by furocoumarins and UVA in hamster and human cells including cells from patients with ataxia telangiectasia and xeroderma pigmentosum. *Mutation Research*, **84**, 113–124.
63 Itoh, S., Nakayama, S. and Shimada, H. (2002) In vitro photochemical clastogenicity of quinolone antibacterial agents studied by a chromosomal aberration test with light irradiation. *Mutation Research*, **517**, 113–121.
64 Cohen, C., Dossou, K.G., Rougier, A. and Roguet, R. (1994) Episkin: An in vitro model for the evaluation of phototoxicity and sunscreen photoprotective properties. *Toxicology In Vitro: An International Journal Published in Association with BIBRA*, **8**, 669–671.
65 Edwards, S.M., Donelly, T.A., Sayre, R.M., Rheins, L.A., Spielmann, H. and Liebsch, M. (1994) Quantitative in vitro assessment of phototoxicity using a human skin model, Skin2. *Photodermatology Photoimmunology & Photomedicine*, **10**, 111–117.
66 Liebsch, H.M. and Spielmann, H. (1995) Balb/c 3T3 cytotoxicity test. *Methods in Molecular Biology*, **43**, 177–187.
67 Jones, P.A., King, A.V., Earl, L.K. and Lawrence, R.S. (2003) An assessment of the phototoxic hazard of a personal product ingredient using in vitro assays. *Toxicology In Vitro: An International Journal Published in Association with BIBRA*, **17**, 471–480.
68 Bernard, F.X., Barrault, C., Deguercy, A., De Wever, B. and Rosdy, M. (2000) Development of a highly sensitive in vitro phototoxicity assay using the SkinEthic

reconstructed human epidermis. *Cell Biology and Toxicology*, **16**, 391–400.

69 Medina, J., Elsaesser, C., Picarles, V., Grenet, O., Kolopp, M., Chibout, S.D. and De Brugerolle de Fraissinette, A. (2001) Assessment of the phototoxic potential of compounds and finished topical products using a human reconstructed epidermis. *In Vitro & Molecular Toxicology – A Journal of Basic and Applied Research*, **14**, 157–168.

70 Portes, P., Pygmalion, M.J., Popovic, E., Cottin, M. and Mariani, M. (2002) Use of human reconstituted epidermis Episkin for assessment of weak phototoxic potential of chemical compounds. *Photodermatology Photoimmunology & Photomedicine*, **18**, 96–102.

71 Liebsch, M., Spielmann, H., Pape, W., Krul, C., Deguercy, A. and Eskes, C. (2005) UV-induced effects. *Alternatives to Laboratory Animals*, **33** (Suppl 1), 131–146.

72 Schafer-Korting, M., Bock, U., Gamer, A., Haberland, A., Haltner-Ukomadu, E., Kaca, M., Kamp, H., Kietzmann, M. et al. (2006) Reconstructed human epidermis for skin absorption testing: results of the German prevalidation study. *Alternatives to Laboratory Animals*, **34**, 283–294.

73 Netzlaff, F., Lehr, C.M., Wertz, P.W. and Schaefer, U.F. (2005) The human epidermis models EpiSkin, SkinEthic and EpiDerm: an evaluation of morphology and their suitability for testing phototoxicity, irritancy, corrosivity and substance transport. *European Journal of Pharmaceutics and Biopharmaceutics*, **60**, 167–178.

74 Liebsch, M., Traue, D., Barrabas, C., Spielmann, H., Gerberick, F., Cruse, L., Diembeck, W., Pfannenbecker, U. et al. (1999) Prevalidation of the EpiDerm phototoxicity test, in *Alternatives to Animal Testing II: Proceedings of the Second International Scientific Conference Organised by the European Cosmetic Industry* (eds D. Clark, S. Lisansky and R. Macmillan), CPL Press, Newbury, UK.

75 Lelievre, D., Justine, P., Christiaens, F., Bonaventure, N., Coutet, J., Marrot, L. and Cotovio, J. (2007) The EpiSkin phototoxicity assay (EPA): development of an in vitro tiered strategy using 17 reference chemicals to predict phototoxic potency. *Toxicology In Vitro: An International Journal Published in Association with BIBRA*, **21**, 977–995.

76 Flamand, N., Marrot, L., Belaidi, J.P., Bourouf, L., Dourille, E., Feltes, M. and Meunier, J.R. (2006) Development of genotoxicity test procedures with Episkin, a reconstructed human skin model: towards new tools for *in vitro* risk assessment of dermally applied compounds? *Mutation Research*, **606**, 39–51.

77 Lee, J.H., Kim, J.E., Kim, B.J. and Cho, K.H. (2007) *In vitro* phototoxicity test using artificial skin with melanocytes. *Photodermatology Photoimmunology & Photomedicine*, **23**, 73–80.

Index

a

abberration   256
- assay   256
absorption
- assay   49
- prediction of *in vivo* absorption   135
accessibility   119
accuracy   105
acetaminophen (APAP)   147, 373
acetanilide   147
active transport   51
active transporter   119
- cell model   123
acyl glucuronide (AG)   152
ADME (absorption, distribution, metabolism, and excretion)/Tox (ADMET)   3ff.
- assay   6ff.
- materials for screening   14f.
- methods   16ff.
ADMET Predictor   131
advanced compartmental absorption and transit (ACAT) model   121, 224
advanced drug absorption and metabolism (ADAM) model   121, 224
adverse drug reaction (ADR)   44, 58, 149, 315
- bone marrow toxicity (BMT)   433
- classification   150, 276
- *in silico* prediction   298
adverse immune effect   439ff.
- profiling   439ff.
adverse reaction enzyme   280
aggregation   83ff.
- partitioning   87
- solubility   83
aggregation number   88
alanine aminotransferase (ALT)   369ff.
ALIAS   22
alkaline phosphatase (ALP)   369ff.

allergy
- *in vitro* assay   452
- testing for induction   445
AlogP   307
ALOGPS method   96, 307
Ames test   251ff.
- photo-Ames test   480
- variant   255
aneugenesis   245
antibiotics   33
area under the first moment curve (AUMC)   208
area under the plasma concentration–time curve (AUC)   198, 291
aromatic hydrocarbon, halogenated   450
aromatic/aryl hydrocarbon receptor (AhR)   418, 450
artificial membrane   125, 134
aspartate aminotransferase (AST)   369ff.
assay robustness   48
assay validation   47
atabrine   148
attrition   326
- rate   308
autoimmunity, testing for induction   446
autoimmunity potential, evaluation of chemicals   447
azithromycin   33

b

barrier solubility diffusion theory   126
basic absorption assay   49
bile acid   365
bile acid salt   89
bile salt efflux protein (BSEP)   365
- *in vitro* and *in vivo* measurement of inhibition   365
- inhibition   368
binding assay   284

Hit and Lead Profiling. Edited by Bernard Faller and Laszlo Urban
Copyright © 2009 WILEY-VCH Verlag GmbH & Co. KGaA, Weinheim
ISBN: 978-3-527-32331-9

bioactivation   151, 349ff.
– bioactivation potential   347ff
– cytochrome P450-mediated   355
bioactivity spectra, data mining   314
BioEpisteme   252
biological dialysis   205
biomarker   369ff.
– discovery   372
– ex vivo   443
– hepatotoxicity   369ff
– immune suppression   443
– immunotoxicity   452ff.
– in vitro   373, 452
– in vivo   373, 443
– safety   329
– validation   374
Biopharmaceutics Classification Scheme (BCS)   49
BioPrint   60
– database   300
bis(tri-n-butyl)tinoxide (TBTO)   456
blood brain barrier (BBB)
– brain-penetration   45
– cell culture model   122
bone marrow toxicity (BMT)   433
Boudinot equation   204
broad safety   280

c

^{14}C cyanide trapping   157
C10-tetraethylammonium (C10-TEA)   398f.
CACO-2 cell   121
– assay   7, 29, 51
calcium channel, L-type   390ff.
candidate selection   351
capillary electrophoresis (CE)   104
cardiosafety   387ff.
– cardiosafety assessment   401ff.
– cardiotoxicity   326
– nonclinical assay   396
– non-hERG ion channel assay   395
cell biology   6
cell death, measurement   330
cell model
– active transporter   123
– in vivo brain penetration   124
– toxicity   331
cell mutation test, mammalian   256
cell-free competition binding assay   392
cellular dielectric spectroscopy (CDS)   292
chemical database, data mining   314
chemical profiling   305
chemical sensitization   454
– in vitro cell culture   454

chemogenomics database   309
ChemSpider   316
cholestasis, drug-induced   365ff.
cholestatic injury   370
chromatographic hydrophobicity index (CHI)   102
chromatographic method   100
chromosomal aberration (CA), photoinduced   485
chromosome damage   256
– assay   262
clastogenesis   245
clearance   213
clinical candidate (CC)   290
Cloe PK   224
clofilium   398
ClogP method   94
CNS (central nervous system)   45
coenzyme A (CoA), depletion   360
comet assay   258, 488
complete bioactivity data matrix   298
complete data matrix   298
compound
– management   5
– profile   42
– profiling   415ff.
– in silico tool   307
– in vitro and ex vivo   415ff.
– prediction   304ff.
– promiscuity   303ff.
computational approach   130
CoMSIA (conformational analysis and molecular alignment) approach   133
π-constant method   92
constant neutral loss (CNL)   156
constitutive androstane receptor (CAR)   177ff.
contact dermatitis (CD)   445
contract research organization (CRO)   280, 482
covalent binding   154
– determination   348
– detoxification   154
– liver microsome   157
– non-toxicological   154
– study   348
cutaneous reaction, immune-mediated   153
CYP enzyme, see cytochrome P450
– inhibition screen   170
– inhibitor   171ff.
cyclosporine   32
cytochrome P450 (CYP enzyme)   148, 168
– assay   7ff.
– recombinant human   181

cytokine 454
cytotoxicity 325ff.
– acute 331
– assay 335
– biomarker 335
– in vitro, see in vitro cytotoxicity
– marked 331
– sublethal 331
cytotoxicity assessment 329
cytotoxicity testing 340

d

danger hypothesis 153
data analysis 18, 305
data matrix 298
data mining 59
data reporting 59
database 311
– similarity search 313
– target prediction 312
– web-based 278
DDI, see drug–drug interaction
degree of flatness (DF) 120
delayed type hypersensitivity (DTH) 445
dendritic cell (DC) 454f.
DEREK 35, 251, 347, 451, 475
detection and analysis 17
detoxication 350
– covalent binding 154
development candidate (DC) 287
dexfenfluramine 274
diffusion coefficient 86
DILI (drug-induced liver injury) 57, 356ff.
dilution range 249
discovery cytotoxicology 329
discovery safety assessment 327
discovery screening 326
discovery toxicology screening 325ff.
dissolution 86
distribution 51
distribution coefficient 98f.
DMPK (drug metabolism and pharmacokinetics)
– testing strategy 8
– workflow 4
DNA adduct assessment 258
dofetilide 399
dose 248
drug candidate, hepatotoxic potential 348
drug delivery 43
drug design, volume of distribution 208
drug discovery
– candidate selection 351
– covalent binding study 348

– HCA cytotoxicity testing 339
– in vitro safety pharmacology profiling 287
– PAMPA (parallel artificial membrane assay) 127
– PBPK (physiologically based pharmacokinetic) model 226
– PK/PD model 227
– reactive metabolite trapping 348
drug discovery process
– challenge 221
– delivery 43
– drug-likeness 35
drug metabolism 145ff.
– prediction 149
drug–drug interaction (DDI) 53, 165ff., 179
– assessment of risk 165
– cocktail assay 173
– in silico modelling 167
– magnitude 184f.
– perpetrator 169ff., 183
– plasma protein binding 197ff.
– prediction 182
– screening for liability 165
– single point 172
drug-induced liver injury, see DILI
drug-likeness
– computational prediction 26
– filter 35
– natural product 32
– prediction 25ff.
DrugBank 316

e

E-state descriptor 95
effective parameter 334
efficacious free plasma concentration (EFPC) 403f.
efficacy 105
– screening 329
efflux 51
efflux ratio (ER) 53
electrochemical oxidation 158
electron transport system (ETS) 357
elimination 51
empirical rule 30
environment and management 19
enzyme induction 176
enzyme inhibition 169ff.
equilibrium dialysis 204
ex vivo compound profiling 415ff.
ex vivo covalent binding 157
experimental filtering 98

exposure
– assay   49
– plasma protein binding   197ff.

f
fatty acid β-oxidation   360
felbamate   349
fenfluramine   274
fexofenadine   62
fialuridine   275
flip-flop model   126
fluorescent inhibition screen   172
fluorescent polarization (FP)   284, 392f.
fluorescence resonance transfer (FRET)   284
fluorofelbamate   349
fold expansion (FE)   119
fraction absorbed data   124
2D fragmental approach   92ff.
free radical   152
functional assay   284
functional parameter   333

g
gastrointestinal transit absorption model (GITA)   121
GastroPlus   131, 224ff.
gene expression assay   259
– eukaryotic   259
– prokaryotic   259
gene mutation assay   254ff.
general safety profile   280
general side effect profile   280
general solubility equality (GSE)   30
genetic toxicity (genotoxicity)   57, 243ff., 264
genotoxicity assay, screening   253
genotoxicity assessment   250ff.
genotoxicity profiling   248, 263
genotoxicity testing   246
genotoxin   245
Gibbs–Donnan effect   204
glutathione (GSH)   151
– conjugate   151
– glutathione-S-transferase (GST)   151
– mass spectrometric detection   155
GPCR (G protein coupled receptor)   34, 307
growth arrest and DNA damage, see GADD

h
H bonding   30
HAART (highly active antiretroviral therapy) treatment   360ff.
hapten hypothesis   153
HCA cell model   337
HCA cytotoxicity assay   338

– drug discovery   339
HCS cytotoxicity assay   340f.
hematotoxicity   415ff.
– inducing compound   416
– potential   417
– testing   419ff., 431
hepatocellular injury   370
hepatotoxic potential
– covalent binding study   348
– reactive metabolite trapping   348
hepatotoxicity   57, 326
– idiosyncratic   337
– mitochondrial   275
– predicting drug-induced   345ff.
hERG (human ether-a-go-go related gene) channel   35, 56ff., 388ff.
– blocker   299, 399
– CoMFA model   400
– computational model   398
– CoMSiA model   401
– GRIND model   401
– homology model   399
– hypothesis   298
– inhibition   387ff.
– patch clamp assay   396
– pharmacophore model   398
– profiling assay   391
– QSAR model   400
hierarchical testing, concept   46
high content screening (HCS)   7
high throughput induction assay   179
high throughput screening (HTS)   25ff., 98, 284
– in vitro   104
Hildebrand parameter   77
hit
– collection   98
– profiling   265
hit and lead profiling   264
– in silico method   252
– in vitro approach   243ff.
hit rate parameter   305
hit-to-lead in silico profiling   135
hit-to-lead phase   287
hormesis   338
human equilibrative nucleoside transporter (hENT1, adenosine transporter)   275
human leukocyte antigen (HLA)- haplotype   448
human toxicity data   336
– validation   336
hydrophilic interaction liquid chromatography (HILIC)   103
hydrophobicity   103

i

ICH (International Conference on Harmonisation of Technical Requirements for Registration of Pharmaceuticals for Human Use) guideline 247ff., 440
idiosyncratic drug reaction (IDR) 150
idiosyncratic liver injury, see liver injury
idiosyncratic toxicity 153
immobilized artificial membrane (IAM) 102
immune system 439ff.
– toxicity study 443
immunostimulation 450
immunosuppression 453
– gene profiling 453
– in vitro assay 452
immunotoxicity/immunotoxicology 439ff.
– biomarker 452ff.
– chemicals 441
– detection 442ff.
– in silico approach 451
– in vitro approach 451
– structure 449
– target organ and cell 458
immunotoxicogenomics 456
in silico assessment 250
– genotoxicity assessment 250
in silico intestinal device (ISID) 131
in silico modeling 130ff.
– drug–drug interaction (DDI) 167
in silico prediction 92
– adverse reaction 298
– human VD 213
– phototoxicity 474
– plasma protein binding (PPB) 206
in silico safety profiling 303
in silico target fishing 313
in vitro assay 49, 59
– limitation 128
– species specificity 58
in vitro assessment 360
in vitro cellular membrane system 132
in vitro compound profiling 415ff.
in vitro cytotoxicity 325ff.
in vitro metabolism 146
– system 149
in vitro photogenotoxicity testing 483
in vitro phototoxicity testing 471ff.
in vitro reactive metabolite trapping study 347
in vitro safety pharmacology 273ff.
– computational approach 297ff.
– knowledge-based 297ff.
– profiling 273ff.
– safety profiling assay 280
in vitro–in vivo extrapolation 119
in vivo assessment 360
in vivo brain penetration 124
in vivo model 260
in vivo profiling 264
in vivo system 130
in vivo toleration (IVT) study 327
indicator variable 134
indirect acting agent 245
inhibition
– chemical 180
– competitive 169
– IC_{50} 172
– mechanism-based (MBI) 169ff.
intestinal cell culture model 121
intestinal membrane 118
intrinsic clearance 186
ion channel 389ff.
ionic species, prediction 97
iterative assay 54
IVIVC (in vitro/in vivo correlations) 53

l

LC/MS (liquid chromatography/mass spectrometry) 7
lead identification 227
lead optimization 231, 287
– profiling 266
lead profiling 7
lead selection 287
– clinical 235
LeadProfilingScreen 280
library, profiling 265
ligand 34
ligand binding assay 177
LIMS (laboratory information management system) 21
linear free energy relationship (LFER) 96
Lipinski's rule of five 30
lipophilicity 92, 106
– coefficient 92
– 3D lipophilicity prediction 107
– neutral substance 92
liquid handlers 17
liver injury, idiosyncratic 364ff.
liver microsome 157
– covalent binding 157
local lymph node assay (LLNA) 445
long QT (LQT) syndrome 387ff.

m

machine learning 26
– algorithm 29
mammalian cell mutation test 256
MAO (monoamine oxidase) inhibitor 275

mass spectrometric detection 155
materials for screening 14f.
MATLAB 225
MC4PC 252
MCASE 251
MDCK (Madin–Darby Canine Kidney) cell line 122
MDLmolfile standard 34
MDL-QSAR 252
mean residence time (MRT) 210
mechanism of action (MOA) 313
mechanism-based inhibition (MBI) 169ff.
membrane
– binding 129
– permeability 118
– permeation 117
– structure, physiology, and chemistry 117
membrane potential-sensitive fluorescent dye 394
mercapturic acid 155
meta analysis, safety pharmacology 304
metabolic intermediate complex (MIC) 169
metabolic stability assay 7
metabolism 51
– hepatic 62
metabolite
– electrophilic 151
– measurement of reactive metabolite 155
– reactive 153ff., 346
Metafer MSearch 257
MetaSite 347
method 16
– ADME/Tox screening 20
5-methoxypsoralene (5-MOP) 476, 485
8-methoxypsoralene (8-MOP) 476, 483
microfluidics 17
micronuclei 257
microsome 149ff.
mitochondrial DNA (mtDNA) 359ff.
– synthesis 359
mitochondrial dysfunction, drug-induced 360
mitochondrial permeability transition pore (MPT) 359
mitochondrial protein synthesis 359
mitochondrial respiration, uncoupler 358
mitochondrial target 334
mitochondrial toxicity 356
MLOGP method 95
molecular field interaction (MIF) 107
molecular group surface area approach (MGSA) model 78
molecular hologram 26
molecular lipophilicity potential (MLP) 95

molecular mechanics (MM) 134
morphological parameter 333
mouse lymphoma assay 254
MTT (3-(4,5-dimethylthiazol-2-yl)-2,5-diphenyltetrazolium bromide) assay 486ff.
multi-parameter optimization (MPO) 168
MULTICASE 35
mutagenesis 245

n
NCE, see new chemical entity
neomycine 33
new chemical entity (NCE) 98, 165
no observed adverse effect level (NOAEL) 375
non-aqueous solvent, solubility 78
non-hERG ion channel assay 395
non-steroidal anti-inflammatory drug (NSAID) 358, 418
nuclear magnetic resonance (NMR) technique 362
nucleophile
– hard 155
– soft 155
nucleotide reverse transcriptase inhibitor (NRTI) 359f.

o
OCT-PAMPA 99
octanol-water partition coefficient 30, 125
ochratoxin A (OTA) 199
off-target effect 291
organic anion transporter (OATP) 199
oxidative phosphorylation (OXPHOS) 356ff.
– inhibition 358
oxidative stress 152, 363
– measurement 363
– source 363

p
PAMPA (parallel artificial membrane permeability assay) 99, 126, 205
– measurement 10, 29
– variation 127
paracellular pathway 118ff.
paroxetine 350
partition 125
partition coefficient 92
– measurement technique 106
partitioning 87
passive transcellular pathway 117
passive transcellular permeability 119
PBPK, see physiologically based pharmacokinetics
peace pill 274

penetration, brain 45
peptide transporter PEPT1 130ff.
permeability 49
– UWL 128
permeability assay 7, 50
permeation 125
P-glycoprotein (P-gp) 51
pH partition theory 118
pharmacological promiscuity, clinical interpretation 288
phospholipid vesicle PAMPA 127
phospholipid–octanol PAMPA 127
photo irritation factor (PIF) 482
photo red blood cells test (photo-RBC test) 479
photo-Ames test 480
photo-cleavage, isolated plasmid DNA 479
photoallergy 471
photocytotoxicity 481
photogenotoxicity 471, 481ff.
photoirritation potential 481
– 3T3 NRU assay 481ff.
photomutagenesis assessment
– microbiological model 480
– yeast model 480
photoreactivity, in tubo 478
phototoxic compound 476f.
phototoxicity/photoinduced toxicity 57, 471ff.
– global model 475
– in silico method for prediction 474
– local method 475
– mimicking 485
– substance 474
phototoxicity screening, artificial sunlight source 472
physical integration
– complete 21
– federated 22
physicochemical determinant 206
physiologically based pharmaco–kinetics (PBPK) 131, 222ff.
– limitation 237
PipelinePilot 60, 307
PK/PD (pharmacokinetic pharmacodynamic) model 225ff., 375
– limitation 237
PK-Sim 224
plasma protein binding (PPB) 197ff., 213
– in silico prediction 206
– measurement 201
polar surface area (PSA) 30
polarity 103
polychlorinated biphenyl (PCB) 450

polychlorinated dibenzo-p-dioxin (PCDD) 450
polychlorinated dibenzofuran (PCDF) 450
polymorphism, CYP enzyme 44
polymyxin B1 33
popliteal lymph node assay (PLNA) 448
potassium channel 390
potency 290
potency screen, plasma protein binding 197ff.
prediction 96
– activity spectra for substances (PASS) 314
– compound promiscuity 304
– 3D molecular structure 95
– drug-likeness 25ff.
– drug metabolism 145ff.
– in silico 96
– in vivo absorption 135
– ionic species 97
– model 27, 96f.
– phototoxicity 474
– target 312
– toxicogenomics 457
– volume of distribution (VD) 210
Predictive Data Miner 252
predictive toxicology 337
pregnane X receptor (PXR) 177ff., 369
principal component analysis (PCA) 53
process logistics 3
profiling
– adverse immune effect 439ff.
– hit 265
– lead optimization 266
– library 265
– primary assay 49
– test 253
profiling assay quality 48
progression, criteria 160
promiscuity, see compound promiscuity
prontosilto 146
protein binding 454
PubChem 316
purity 249

q
quantitative structure–activity relationships (QSAR) 252, 451, 474f.
– 3D QSAR model 133

r
RAD54-GFP yeast assay 260
radiolabeled soft nucleophile trapping 158
radiolabeled covalent binding experiment 160

radioligand binding 393
radiometric assay 156
rapid equilibrium dialysis (RED) 204
RCA, see root cause analysis
reaction phenotyping 179
reactive metabolite 153ff., 346
– minimizing risk 159
– trapping 348
reactive nitrogen species (RNS) 357
reactive oxygen species (ROS) 357ff., 478f.
– photoinduced 478
reference compound 46
relative activity factor (RAF) 181
reporter gene assay 178, 263
reverse-phase liquid chromatography (RP-LC) 100
risk assessment 401
– integrated 387, 401
– integrative 61
RNA-based technique 10
root cause analysis (RCA) 13
Rowland–Matin equation 182ff.
rubidium efflux 393
rule of five 30

s

Σf method 93
Saccharomyces cerevisiae mutation assay 256
safety assay
– sensitivity 58
– specificity 58
safety assessment 260
safety attrition 326
safety margin 338, 403
– plasma protein binding 197ff.
safety pharmacology data 298
– meta data analysis 304
safety pharmacology profiling 273ff.
– *in vitro* 273
safety profiling assay 56
scintillation proximity assay (SPA) 177, 284, 392
screening
– ADME/Tox 17ff.
– genotoxicity assay 253
– hierarchical 9
– parallel 9
screening data 261
– positive 262
secondary pharmacology 274
sentinel 49
sensitization, chemical 454
sertindole 399
serum chemistry marker 370

Simcyp 224
simulated biological fluid, solubility 89
single-cell monitoring 333
skin, reconstructed 485
SMARTS 34
sodium taurocholate 89
software 18, 93
solid phase microextraction (SPME) 206
solubility 49, 71ff.
– aggregation 83
– calculation 77
– determination 74
– equilibrium 50
– function of pH 79
– influence 72
– kinetic 50
– low 129
– non-aqueous solvent 78
solubility assay 50
solubility product 85
solvatochromic equation 96
solvent accessible surface area (SASA) 95
SpotFire 60
stress response 330
structure–activity relationship (SAR) 354, 475
structure-based drug design (SBDD) 168
structure–toxicity relationship 353

t

3T3 NRU assay 481ff.
target annotation 276
target compound profile (TCP) 41
target family 34
target hit rate (THR) 58, 289, 305
target organ, reconstructed skin 485
target prediction, database 312
target selection 275
terfenadine 62
testing
– hierarchical 45
– tiered cascade 419ff.
thallium influx 393
therapeutic index (TI) 42, 290, 403
thiazolidinedione (TZD) 354
threshold of toxicological concern (TTC) 250
TLOGP method 95
TOPKAT 251, 451
topological descriptor 95
TOPS-MODE 451
toxicity
– genetic, see genetic toxicity
– idiosyncratic 153

– mitochondrial 356
toxicogenomics 456
– prediction 457
toxicology 56
– predictive 337
– screening 325ff.
toxicophore 352
transactivation assay 178
TRANSIL technology 206
translocation 245
transporter 51
trapping assay 155
trend analysis 60
tri-layer PAMPA 127
triangulation 396f.
troglitazone 354ff.

u

unstirred water layer (UWL) 117
– permeability 128
UV exposure 480ff.

v

validation 336
– biomarker 374
– human toxicity data 336

vancomycin 33
variability, interlaboratory 129
vascular leak syndrome (VLS) 450
vehicle 248
villi expansion (VE) 119
virtual filtering 92
VLOGP method 96
volume of distribution (VD) 208ff.
– prediction 210
– prediction of human VD from animal pharmacokinetic data 210
– prediction of human VD from *in silico* method 213
– prediction of human VD from *in vitro* data 212
– steady state (VD$_{ss}$) 208ff.

w

whole-process approach 20

x

xenobiotic metabolism 147

y

yeast model, photobiology 480
yeast mutation assay 256